AJN/MOSBY

Question
& Answer
Book

For the NCLEX-RN Examination

AJN/MOSBY

Question & Answer Book

For the NCLEX-RN Examination

FIFTH EDITION

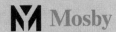 Mosby

St. Louis Baltimore Boston
Carlsbad Chicago Naples New York Philadelphia Portland
London Madrid Mexico City Singapore Sydney Tokyo Toronto Wiesbaden

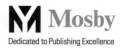

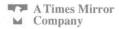

Vice President and Publisher: Nancy L. Coon
Senior Editor: Susan R. Epstein
Senior Developmental Editor: Beverly J. Copland
Associate Developmental Editor: Jerry Schwartz
Project Manager: Dana Peick
Senior Production Editor: Stavra Demetrulias
Designer: Amy Buxton
Manufacturing Supervisor: Linda Ierardi

FIFTH EDITION

Printed in the United States of America
Composition by Clarinda Company
Printing/binding by Courier Corporation

Mosby–Year Book, Inc.
11830 Westline Industrial Drive
St. Louis, Missouri 63146

International Standard Book Number 0-8151-0081-7

96 97 98 99 00 / 9 8 7 6 5 4 3 2 1

Contributors

COORDINATORS

Deborah Antai-Otong, RN, MS, CS
Psychiatric Clinical Specialist;
Program Director, EAP
Department of Veterans Affairs Medical Center
Dallas, Texas

Steven Jones, MS, RN, C, PNP
Averville Park, New York

Roberta Kordish, RN, MSN
Principal
Professional Nurse Associates, Inc.
Cleveland, Ohio

Paulette D. Rollant, RN, MSN, CCRN, PhD
President
Multi-Resources, Inc.
Grantville, Georgia

Marybeth Young, RNC, PhD
Associate Professor
Loyola University, Niehoff School of Nursing
Chicago, Illinois

Contributing Authors

Deborah Antai-Otong, RN, MS, CS
Psychiatric Clinical Specialist;
Program Director, EAP
Department of Veterans Affairs Medical Center
Dallas, Texas

Deborah A. Ennis, RN, BSN, MSN, CCRN
Professor of Nursing
Harrisburg Area Community College
Harrisburg, Pennsylvania

Peg Gray-Vickrey, RN(C), BSN, MS, DNS
Assistant Professor
Lycoming College
Williamsport, Pennsylvania

Debra Jeffs, MS, RN
Troy, New York

Katherine Jones, MS, RN
Averville Park, New York

Stephen Jones, MS, RN, C, PNP
Averville Park, New York

Roberta Kordish, RN, MSN
Principal
Professional Nurse Associates, Inc.
Cleveland, Ohio

Paulette Rollant, RN, MSN, CCRN, PhD
President
Multi-Resources, Inc.
Grantville, Georgia

Judith K. Sands, RN, BS, MS, EdD
Associate Professor, Director of
Undergraduate Students
University of Virginia
Charlottesville, Virginia

Marybeth Young, RNC, PhD
Associate Professor
Loyola University, Niehoff School of Nursing
Chicago, Illinois

Reviewers

Karen Bowers, BSN, Med
Lancaster, Ohio

Linda Fasciani, MSN
Assistant Professor
County College of Morris
Randolph, New Jersey

Lynette Jack, PhD, RN, CARN
Assistant Professor
University of Pittsburgh
Pittsburgh, Pennsylvania

Allison B. Jones, MSN, RN
Assistant Professor
Troy State University
Montgomery, Alabama

Mary Kunes-Connell, PhD, RN
Omaha, Nebraska

April Sieh, MSN
Delta College
Flushing, Michigan

Paula Smith, BSN, MNSc
Assistant Professor of Nursing
Arkansas State University
Jonesboro, Arkansas

Margaret Tufts, MS, RNC
Assistant Professor
Quinnipiac College
Hamden, Connecticut

Introduction

This volume completes a trio of offerings from the American Journal of Nursing Company and Mosby–Year Book. Here you will find a whole book of practice questions to use alone or in combination with the *AJN/Mosby Nursing Boards Review* text and the AJN/Mosby Nursing Boards Review course.

Section 1 explains in detail the NCLEX/RN testing format and scoring methods. Strategies on how to read questions more carefully and clues to help you select the correct answer are included to increase your test-taking skills. Techniques to help you reduce stress on the day of the examination are also presented. Read this section first, and refer to it as often as necessary for reinforcement.

Sections 2 through 5 include more than 1100 questions organized according to the broad clinical content areas of Psychosocial and Mental Health Nursing, Care of the Adult, Care of the Childbearing Family, and Care of the Child. Within each clinical area, questions are grouped by specific health problem.

Section 6 contains ten practice tests of 75 questions each. These integrated exams reflect the same kind of overview of content you can expect on the NCLEX-RN. When you feel ready, set aside time to practice taking the examination. The goal is to answer each section within about 75 minutes. Although the computerized NCLEX is not strictly a timed test, you will have an unlimited amount of time for the exam. Pacing yourself to answer each question in about one minute will ensure that you have ample time to complete the test. Following each section of questions are the correct answers and rationales that explain why the correct answers are right and the other options are incorrect. Rationales include the step of the nursing process and client needs category tested by the question. For questions in Section 6, a reference is provided to the appropriate section of the *AJN/Mosby Nursing Boards Review* text for those requiring additional content review.

Develop a system for review that meets your needs. Based on your answers and your understanding of the answer rationales, you may decide you need to review content in a specific area using your textbooks or the *AJN/Mosby Nursing Boards Review*.

Computer disks for both IBM and MAC can be found inside the back cover. These disks include a 120-question practice test that is not included in the book; this test can be used in both a study/review and test format. To reinforce learned information and build confidence, it is recommended that you practice answering questions on a computer to simulate the NCLEX-RN.

The test items in this book have been prepared by the national faculty who teach the AJN/Mosby Nursing Boards Review course. All are instructors, clinical specialists, or authors in the clinical specialty. They, along with all of us involved in the production of this book at the AJN Company and at Mosby–Year Book, wish you every success on the NCLEX-RN and in your career as a registered professional nurse.

Contents

1 **Preparing for the NCLEX-RN,** 1

Marybeth Young, PhD, MSN, RNC

Pretest, 2
Know the Test Format, 2
   Nursing Process, 2
   Categories of Human Needs, 2
How the Test is Scored, 3
Where Should You Begin?, 4
Cognitive and Affective Keys to Success, 4
   Cognitive Strategies to Promote Success, 4
   Affective Strategies for Success, 6
   Answer Key for Pretest Questions, 7
Acing Multiple-Choice Tests, 8

2 **Nursing Care of the Client with Psychosocial and Mental Health Problems,** 12

Deborah Antai-Otong, MS, RN, CS

Questions, 14
Correct Answers, 36
Correct Answers with Rationales, 39

3 **Nursing Care of the Adult,** 58

COORDINATOR   *Paullette D. Rollant, PhD, MSN, RN, CCRN*
Contributors   *Deborah A. Ennis, MSN, RN, CCRN*
     Peg Gray-Vickrey, MS, RNC
     Paullette D. Rollant, PhD, MSN, RN, CCRN
     Judith Sands, BS, MS, EdD

Questions, 60
Correct Answers, 98
Correct Answers with Rationales, 103

4 **Nursing Care of the Childbearing Family,** 128

COORDINATOR   *Roberta Kordish, MSN, RN*

Questions, 130
Correct Answers, 145
Correct Answers with Rationales, 147

5 **Nursing Care of the Child,** 156

COORDINATOR   *Stephen Jones, MS, RN, C, PNP*

Questions, 158
Correct Answers, 175
Correct Answers with Rationales, 178

6 **Practice Tests**

Instructions for Taking the Test, 189
Practice Test 1, 190
Practice Test 2, 196
Practice Test 3, 203
Practice Test 4, 209
Practice Test 5, 216
Practice Test 6, 222
Practice Test 7, 229
Practice Test 8, 236
Practice Test 9, 242
Practice Test 10, 248
Answers and Rationales, 255
Key to Abbreviations, 255
Answers and Rationales: Practice Test 1, 256
Answers and Rationales: Practice Test 2, 260
Answers and Rationales: Practice Test 3, 265
Answers and Rationales: Practice Test 4, 269
Answers and Rationales: Practice Test 5, 273
Answers and Rationales: Practice Test 6, 277
Answers and Rationales: Practice Test 7, 282
Answers and Rationales: Practice Test 8, 286
Answers and Rationales: Practice Test 9, 290
Answers and Rationales: Practice Test 10, 294

Contents

Pretest .... p. 2

Know the Test Format .... p. 2

How the Test Is Scored .... p. 3

Where Should You Begin? .... p. 4

Cognitive and Affective Keys
to Success .... p. 4

Acing Multiple-Choice Tests .... p. 8

Chapter *1*

Preparing for the NCLEX-RN

COORDINATOR
Marybeth Young, PhD, MSN, RNC

PRETEST

1. Test items on the NCLEX-RN
   a. describe actual or potential patient health problems.
   b. emphasize knowledge of physiology and safe care.
   c. focus on situations encountered by entry-level nurses.
   d. all of the above choices are correct.
2. The examination requires the graduate nurse to select
   a. one single, best resolution to a problem.
   b. several answers from multiple-choice options.
3. Computer Adaptive Testing (CAT)
   a. requires advanced computer skills.
   b. allows flexibility in changing responses.
   c. individualizes testing by ability level.
   d. penalizes the slow reader.
4. The integrated nursing examination *equally* tests the ability to apply knowledge of
   a. pediatrics, maternity, and medical-surgical nursing.
   b. all five phases of the nursing process.
   c. acute and chronic health problems.
   d. risk factors and measures to promote health.
5. Which of the following test-taking strategies does *not* apply to CAT?
   a. Try to narrow possible responses to two options.
   b. Focus on key words such as *initially* or *least effective.*
   c. Ignore difficult items and return to them later.
   d. Avoid "reading into" the item.

KNOW THE TEST FORMAT

Just as the novice driver needs to know what to expect on the state driving test, each graduate nurse needs a clear idea of the professional licensure exam format. Knowing that you have some questions about the test itself or are unsure of your responses on the pretest, the following brief summary will provide answers.

Success on the national examination is required for entry into professional practice. NCLEX-RN CAT has replaced the paper-and-pencil state boards. This new format reduces the environmental stressors of massive testing rooms by allowing for small-site testing and flexible scheduling.

The framework for the examination continues to follow published guidelines established by the National Council of State Boards of Nursing. Two types of questions are included. The first follows a case study format, in which a situation briefly describing a client's health problems is followed by a multiple-choice question. Each case and subsequent question is discrete; for example, you may need to shift focus from identifying care priorities of an acutely ill adult to teaching an adolescent parent. The second format asks a question that is unrelated to a client case study. Among many possibilities, this type of item may address delegation of care or the responsibilities of a professional nurse.

Graduates may complete the minimum 75 items quickly or continue to test for the maximum of 5 hours or 265 questions. The length of testing is not an indication of performance. The flexibility of CAT tailors each person's exam to a specific ability level.

The test continues to be organized around a broad framework comprised of "Nursing Process" and "Categories of Human Needs." Each part of this plan is summarized briefly; implications for review are suggested.

Nursing Process

The nursing process provides organization for the test as it does for care planning in every clinical setting. Each nursing process phase is equally important in resolving health problems. This consistency is immediately evident to test takers who perceive this equal emphasis. These same graduates are quick to point out that the numbers of items testing maternity and psychiatric nursing are not equal; medical-surgical nursing is heavily emphasized. Table 1-1 suggests a possible test item focus for each phase of the nursing process.

Categories of Human Needs

Concepts that contribute to understanding human needs are another exam focus. Among these are basic human

Table 1-1 Test item focus suggested by the nursing process

Phase	Possible item focus
Assessment	Identifying database
	Selecting appropriate means to gather data
	Gathering information from client/family
	Noting significant observations/data
	Considering environmental factors
	Communicating findings
Analysis	Formulating a nursing diagnosis
	Interpreting data and reporting results of analysis
Planning	Prioritizing nursing diagnoses
	Setting measurable long- and short-term goals
	Involving client/family in planning
	Determining outcome criteria
	Reviewing/modifying plan
Implementation	Carrying out nursing actions safely
	Understanding rationale for care
	Prioritizing care
	Promoting self-care
	Calculating/administering medications safely
	Suggesting diet modifications
	Ensuring safety/comfort
	Preventing infection/injury
	Promoting health
	Responding to emergencies
	Recording/sharing information
	Teaching to client's intellectual level
	Communicating appropriately with client/family/staff
	Supervising/delegating care
Evaluation	Comparing outcomes to goals
	Examining response to therapy
	Seeking more information
	Identifying learning outcomes
	Recognizing risks/problems of therapy
	Communicating evaluation findings
	Evaluating staff learning/caregiving

needs, the teaching-learning process, therapeutic communication, crisis intervention, and developmental theory. Knowledge of anatomy, physiology and pathophysiology, asepsis, nutrition, accountability, the group process, and mental health concepts is basic to the practice of nursing and also is incorporated into many test items. The organization of client needs based on these concepts is identified by the National Council of State Boards of Nursing as "Categories of Human Needs" and is part of the test format. These four categories flow from the ANA Nursing Social Policy Statement and current research on job analysis for entry-level practitioners. The greatest NCLEX-RN exam emphasis is on the categories of physiologic integrity, followed by a focus on health promotion and maintenance. The safe care environment and psychosocial integrity are important, but fewer test items focus on these categories (Tables 1-2 and 1-3). Some overlap is evident as you look at the nursing process framework and the categories of client needs. For example, the nursing process phase of planning addresses both physiologic and psychosocial needs. However, if an individual has a severe fluid volume deficit related to dehydration, emotional needs are attended to *after* setting a goal to resolve life-threatening physiologic problems. Setting priorities is critical to exam success, just as it is in clinical caregiving.

Use your knowledge of the test format to help you identify and review concepts learned throughout your nursing education and to prepare thoughtfully for the examination. However, during the actual NCLEX-RN, do not attempt to identify whether safe, effective care or physiologic integrity is tested in a particular item.

Applied knowledge, rather than mere recall of facts, is measured in most test questions. As you read each question, use the knowledge gained from clinical experience and classroom learning to identify and resolve client problems. Expect to find questions at the beginning of the test fairly easy, followed by increasingly difficult and challenging items. This feature of the CAT allows for individualization of *your* test, and a fit with your ability level. Remember that the NCLEX-RN CAT is a test of competence.

HOW THE TEST IS SCORED

One feature of the CAT is relatively rapid feedback on your PASS/FAIL score. But you must wait several weeks for this information to arrive in the mail. Do not try to keep your own score during the examination; just proceed thoughtfully from one item to the next. If the computer takes a few extra seconds to select an item, remember that it is matching the question difficulty with your ability. Be careful in reading the case study so that you focus on key words. Select the best option thoughtfully. A helpful feature of the CAT is that you are asked to confirm an answer before it registers as your choice. This allows a second opportunity to rethink an answer before moving to another item. Remember, the successful graduate need not be a "computer whiz." Only two keys function during the exam: a space bar and an "enter" key. A brief tutorial will acquaint you with their use. Keep in mind that you will not be able to return to earlier items and change answers as you could on paper-and-pencil tests.

Remember, the NCLEX-RN test plan has been developed to measure critical thinking and nursing competence. Knowing the framework of the exam should dispel some of your fears and help you anticipate and prepare for the test. As you take the test, do not think about the "test plan,"

Table 1-2 Categories of human needs

Categories	Nursing focus
Safe, effective care environment	Coordinating care
	Ensuring quality
	Setting goals
	Promoting safety
	Preparing client for treatments/procedures
	Implementing care
Physiologic integrity	Promoting adaptation
	Identifying/reducing risks
	Fostering mobility
	Ensuring comfort
	Providing basic care
Psychosocial integrity	Promoting adaptation
	Facilitating coping
Health promotion/ maintenance	Promoting growth and development
	Supporting self-care
	Fostering support systems
	Prevention/early treatment of disease

Table 1-3 Test item focus suggested by categories of human needs

Human needs category	Possible test item focus
Safe, effective care environment	Understanding basic principles
	Using management skills
	Implementing protective measures
	Promoting safety
	Ensuring client/family rights
	Preventing spread of infection
Physiologic integrity	Recognizing altered body function
	Using body mechanics
	Providing comfort measures
	Using equipment safely
	Understanding effects of immobility
	Recognizing untoward responses to therapy/medication/procedures
	Documenting emergency actions
Psychosocial integrity	Identifying mental health concepts
	Recognizing behavior changes
	Referring to resources
	Communicating appropriately
Health promotion/ maintenance	Understanding family systems
	Teaching nutrition
	Promoting wellness
	Strengthening immune responses
	Recognizing adaptive changes to health alterations
	Considering cultural/religious impact on childbearing
	Supporting the dying/family

but concentrate on the challenge of each question. Just as the driver attends the road test without wondering, "What is being tested now?" you need only address the problem-solving task.

WHERE SHOULD YOU BEGIN?

When you are familiar with this text and the test format, map out a personal plan for preparation and review. If independent study is planned, set realistic goals within the time available. Ideally, reviewing content over several months is preferable to "cramming" in a few weeks. Studying regularly, over time, helps reinforce knowledge and improves your ability to apply that knowledge.

Begin your review plan by focusing on content that is less familiar to you or about which you feel insecure. Your results on standardized national tests, such as the Assess Test, could serve as a guide, or you may select several case studies from Chapter 6 and answer the questions that follow after reviewing related content. After completing the test items, refer to the correct responses, rationale, and test format classification; then compare your problem-solving abilities to those of content experts. You may find it helpful to return to the review book outline, to a nursing specialty or fundamentals text, or to your class notes to resolve doubts or increase understanding. Look for patterns of test-taking difficulties as you review responses. Becoming aware of your strengths and weaknesses in test taking is an important phase of review and gives more meaningful feedback than counting correct and incorrect responses. By beginning with the greatest challenge and reinforcing understanding, your confidence is renewed as the date of the exam approaches.

COGNITIVE AND AFFECTIVE KEYS TO SUCCESS

Three factors are important in achieving success: *reading,* which affects both reviewing and test taking; being *testwise,* which is defined as the ability to use a test situation to demonstrate learning; and the ability to *control tension* in a major examination, freeing the mind to concentrate on the written questions. Although these factors are interrelated, they are discussed separately. Suggestions and strategies are offered for use during your licensure exam experience (Table 1-4).

Cognitive Strategies to Promote Success

In addition to using this book, other media may meet your needs for review. Audiotapes and videotapes may be helpful in clarifying content or suggesting approaches to test items. You may wish to prepare for the CAT by using one of the many software programs available in schools, libraries, and bookstores.

Reading with concentration is a learned skill that is critical for study, review, and successful examination performance. When preparing for the NCLEX-RN, select an environment that is well lighted and suits your learning style. Avoid reading on a bed—its comfort may induce sleep rather than reinforce knowledge. Gather all materials in advance for the planned study session, including this review book, other appropriate texts, notes, and marker pens to highlight content needing subsequent review.

Skim the review text material, then read for understanding. Look up any unfamiliar terms. Make a note of further questions that come to mind as you review information. Use your knowledge of anatomy, physiology, and pathophysiology to visualize the impact of a specific health alteration. Review the disease process, preventive measures, restoration, and rehabilitation. Refresh your memory of procedures specifically used in treatment. Think about ways in which health might be improved.

While reading test items as practice or in a real situation, be especially observant of *key words.* Notice cues such as *age, risk factors,* and *coping mechanisms.* Clearly identify the question focus (e.g., the concerned parent, the ill child, or the caregiver). Use your knowledge of nursing to think through the question and consider possible responses even before reading all possible options.

Although you must read carefully to understand the questions, avoid reading into the words more than is actually stated. Assume that the health care agency described is ideal and well staffed. If you think that the client's needs would be met by a midnight snack of milk and crackers, do not qualify this with ". . . but it may be impossible to provide this at night."

During the exam, you have no resource for defining vocabulary. Use the sentence context to deduce the meaning of unfamiliar words. Refer to the case study for insight and clarification, and remember to apply your understanding of pathophysiology throughout the exam.

The following examples give you an opportunity to apply several testing strategies to varied questions typical of the NCLEX-RN. Priority setting can be a challenge on an exam. One approach is to view each option as a true/false statement. This is especially helpful if several nursing implementations are correct but you are asked to select a *best* or *initial* action. Ask yourself, "Will the client's health or recovery be affected if one action is *not* carried out initially?"

Consider these test items:

1. Ms. Travis, a 44-year-old kindergarten teacher, was admitted last evening with a medical diagnosis of endocarditis. History includes a cholecystectomy 2 years ago and childhood rheumatic fever. Two days ago her dentist extracted an infected molar after an unsuccessful root canal procedure. Although she usually takes prophylactic penicillin before dental treatment, she forgot to do so. Present temperature is 103°F. IV ampicillin is ordered every 6 hours. She seems uncomfortable and anxious, asking repeatedly if her son has arrived from a distant state. During the initial assessment of Ms. Travis, the nurse notes that 600 ml of 5% dextrose

Table 1-4   Cognitive strategies for success

Prepare	for safe practice
Plan a review	to broaden knowledge
Read carefully	for understanding
Identify key words	to focus attention
Narrow options	by critical thinking
Use an educated guess	not random choice
Set priorities	based on health risk

in 0.225% normal saline has infused in 2 hours. The physician ordered 1000 ml in 10 hours; therefore the *initial action* should be to
① notify the attending physician.
② assess respirations and breath sounds.
③ recalculate the infusion rate.
④ report the problem to the supervisor.

As you would do in a clinical setting, review the assessment data and filter out the information that has less impact on the client's present condition. Identify the actual and potential problems; then read the question and consider each option thoughtfully. As fluid volume is altered, physiologic integrity clearly dictates priority assessments and *immediate* interventions.

In this example say to yourself, "The priority action is to notify the physician. True or false?" Then proceed to the other options. Although responses 1, 2, and 3 are appropriate, the *priority action* is to detect signs of fluid volume excess related to rapid infusion (option 2). Pulmonary edema could further complicate the client's condition. Option 4 is not an initial action, nor should the supervisor be notified until after consulting with the head nurse or unit manager.

2. A physician orders 1000 ml of IV fluids to be infused in 10 hours. The drop factor is 10/ml. The nurse should adjust the rate to
① 2 drops per minute.
② 6 drops per minute.
③ 16 drops per minute.
④ 21 drops per minute.

Calculate the fluid rate using the standard equation. Be sure to label all values such as minutes and milliliters. The correct response is option 3. During the actual exam, use the scrap paper provided to work out the mathematics; never calculate from memory!

3. Mr. Kent had a bronchoscopic examination several hours ago. A topical anesthetic spray was used during the procedure. Because the physician ordered diet as tolerated and the client tolerated sips of water, he was given a general diet for lunch. As he begins to eat, his color turns gray; he appears to have difficulty breathing and then grasps his throat. Select the correct priority action.
① Notify the anesthesiologist.
② Suction secretions from his oral pharynx.
③ Perform a thrust maneuver.
④ Assess for other problems.

The priority action is to ensure a patent airway, option 3. Further reflection may lead you to question if the client's swallowing and gag reflexes were assessed before the meal. In this example, as in many NCLEX-RN test items, one choice suggests the need for further information. Be careful in selecting this response. Although it may be helpful to have more assessment data, this question provides sufficient data to direct quick and safe action.

Communication test items present a special challenge. As in actual practice, nonverbal cues and the environment affect the communication process. When reading questions focusing on nurse/client/family interactions, consider all information carefully. Realize that a reference to an interaction or the presence of quotation marks does not automatically imply therapeutic use of self. Refer to Table 1-5 for suggested ways in which communication test items might vary with *nurse-client* interactions. Apply basic principles and be aware of possible communication blocks. Base choices on a sound rationale, rather than selecting a response that "sounds like" what you actually might say.

4. Ms. Fox, 57, visits the clinic for a Pap smear and describes occasional hot flashes and irregular menstrual periods. She plans to discuss estrogen replacement therapy with her gynecologist. In response to questions about lifestyle, she describes regular activity and rest patterns and a well-balanced diet. A review of her history reveals that two sisters had breast cancer. When asked if she performs breast self-examinations regularly, Ms. Fox appears upset. "I am so afraid of cancer! I'd rather not know if there is a problem! I could not cope with finding a mass." Select an appropriate reply to the client:
① "Fear is no reason to neglect your health."
② "Your risk is very high because of family history."
③ "Tell me more about what you are feeling."
④ "You should not feel afraid; early detection is critical."

This question suggests an initial need for therapeutic communication. Although correct information should be

Table 1-5   Focus of communications test items

Type of interaction	Approach
Interview	Asking purposeful questions
	Identifying risk factors
	Using appropriate vocabulary
	Listening to responses
	Maintaining confidentiality
Information giving	Describing tests/procedures
	Clarifying data
	Explaining treatment to client/family/staff
Teaching/learning (to client, family, health care providers)	Assessing health, learning needs
	Using developmentally appropriate terms
	Giving instructions to promote safety
	Supporting self-care
	Reinforcing group learning
	Observing a return demonstration
	Involving family in basic care
	Evaluating learning outcomes
Therapeutic use of self	Establishing trust
	Identifying own communication skills
	Developing goal direction
	Listening actively
	Clarifying, reflecting
	Sharing observations
	Anticipating needs
	Reinforcing positive coping styles
	Supporting in loss
	Referring for help

conveyed, risk factors identified, and teaching emphasized, this client needs to express her feelings and concerns. Response 3 indicates the nurse's availability as a listener.

5. A nursing assistant (NA) from the ambulatory care unit is assigned to your acute care setting at a time when several staff have called in sick. He is assigned to work with you. Which of the following tasks could you assign to him?
   ① Changing sterile dressings
   ② Assisting with morning care
   ③ Suctioning tracheostomy tubes
   ④ Monitoring IV fluids

Delegation of care to unlicensed personnel is increasingly the responsibility of professional nurses. Such delegation involves trust and a knowledge of the skills of the assistive worker. In this case, the abilities expected of the NA should include providing for client hygiene, response 2. The other tasks are beyond the ability of an aide without advanced training.

Some questions focusing on Human Needs Categories address potential problems within the environment. Consider the following:

6. During a busy day in the outpatient clinic, the nurse suspects that a young child may have rubella. Of the following clients who were in contact with the child, which individual is at greatest risk?
   ① John Norris, HIV-positive, recovering from tuberculosis
   ② Celia Moran, 8 months pregnant; rubella titer positive
   ③ Lori Ruiz, 1 month old; breast-feeding
   ④ Frances Long, chronic alcoholic with cirrhosis

Rubella exposure is particularly dangerous for any immunosuppressed client (option 1). Although insufficient information is given about the 1-month-old baby's nursing mother and there may be a risk to the client described in option 4, you are asked to identify the individual for whom exposure is *most dangerous*. That client is John Norris.

7. As a nurse makes rounds on a pediatric unit, each of the following is observed. Which situation must be corrected immediately to ensure client well-being?
   ① A school-aged amputee leaves his wheelchair at the bedside.
   ② Several toddlers spread their toys on the playroom floor.
   ③ The stereo volume in the adolescent lounge is too loud.
   ④ The newborn step-down ICU is 68° F.

The low nursery temperature (option 4) is a serious problem and may lead to cold stress. Examine the other options for potential safety problems. The child with a disability should have access to his wheelchair. Although toys should not be left in an area where they create a hazard, risk is minimal in the playroom. The loud music may subsequently affect hearing, but this is typical for adolescents. The question does not mention that other clients are disturbed; therefore there is no need for immediate action.

Some test items ask you to consider potential or actual problems identified in several clients and then decide on an appropriate action. Consider this item:

8. Each of the following assessments is documented by a night nurse on an adult surgical unit. Which observation should be reported *immediately* to the physician?
   ① Jenny Bocci has a temperature of 100° F the night after surgery for a ruptured appendix.
   ② Karen Rosen's knee is hot and swollen 2 days after cartilage repair.
   ③ William Clifford's dressing has purulent drainage shortly after the incision of an abscess.
   ④ George Henderson has blood-tinged urine 12 hours after a transurethral prostatectomy.

In reviewing the data, visualize the operative procedure and expected recovery. Identify problems that may delay healing. The physician should be notified immediately about the orthopedic client's postoperative condition. Option 2 indicates a serious problem that may lead to subsequent bone or systemic infection. All other observations are expected during convalescence for the surgical procedures described.

Affective Strategies for Success

It is difficult to separate cognitive and emotional factors in test performance. There are, however, distinctly separate ways to prepare for the mental and emotional challenges of the examination. Long-range goal setting must include realistic life plans. Anticipate the time that study and review demand; avoid a major life change that increases tension. Because of the increased flexibility of NCLEX-RN CAT, you can schedule your test date so that it does not conflict with a wedding or a 3-week hiking trip.

Realistically evaluate your personal responses to test challenges. Look at past successes and ways you maintain energy and confidence under stress. How have you reacted to past major examinations? What physiologic or psychologic responses to stress are common for you? Many graduates report that tension headaches or gastrointestinal distress occur during the 2 days of testing. Some suggest that lapses of concentration are frequent during a tiring day of problem solving. Expect that your thoughts may "drift" or that you may experience a "failure fantasy," as many other nurses have described. Expect some anger about a specific test item. You may feel that you could have written "better answers than those!"

To use your mind to its fullest and to demonstrate your competence as a nurse, you need to control the effects of anxiety. Several effective ways exist to reduce tension; try one or more of the following:
- Relaxing and contracting muscles progressively from head to toe
- Slow, deep breathing and deliberate calming
- Guided imagery with focus on a peaceful scene
- Meditation, prayer, positive thoughts
- Focusing on a confident self

Select the method of stress reduction that has worked for you in the past, learn new approaches, and practice them during times of tension while studying. For example, to use imagery, see yourself in the setting that is most peaceful for you. Close your eyes and imagine the quiet, the scents, the scenery around you. Feel the warmth and energy. Relax and feel calm. Change the setting as you need to until it is

Table 1-6   Keys to success on the NCLEX-RN

Know the test format
  An integrated exam
  Pass/fail score
  Single-response, multiple-choice items
  Based on measurement of safe nursing behaviors for common
    health problems
Review concepts
  Growth and development
  Pharmacology and pathophysiology
  Effects of culture and nutrition on health
  The nursing process
  Categories of human needs
Where should you begin?
  Consider your strengths and your learning style
How should you prepare?
  Review course notes and texts
  Consider a review program
  Use human resources and support services
Strategies to promote success
  Begin with self-evaluation
  Sharpen test-taking skills
  Learn methods to reduce stress
  Be self-confident
Just before the exam
  Get a good night's rest
  Avoid late cramming
  Eat breakfast
During the NCLEX-RN CAT
  Concentrate on your screen
  Read items carefully
  Draw on your knowledge
  Use relaxation methods

1982, 1988, 1995 Young M, Kopala B.

the perfect relaxing pause. Recall these images during difficult moments in the exam when you need a brief recharge. You will feel your spirits lift and will experience clearer thinking.

Close to the exam date, plan your travel to the testing center. If distance allows, visit the area in advance so that you know the best route and alternates. Consider seasonal problems that may affect travel time. It is critical to arrive at the testing site ahead of time, or you may be refused entry.

Anticipate that even a small test setting may be overwhelming. Plan ways that you can deal with environmental stressors, such as security measures. This is one time in your professional life when *your* needs are a priority. Do what you must to remain calm and confident.

On the exam day, consider your own comfort and nutritional needs. Dress in nonconstricting and attractive clothing that helps you feel good about yourself. It is wise to carry a jacket in anticipation of temperature changes within the testing room. Eat a high-protein breakfast, but avoid excessive caffeine and fluids so that an emergency trip to the restroom is not necessary. Pack fruit, a can of juice, and headache remedies or cough drops so that they are available at the required and optional breaks.

Expect to encounter at least one unfamiliar health problem in the NCLEX-RN CAT. Remain confident that you can use your knowledge of anatomy, physiology, pathophysiology, and nursing to solve the problem. Do not allow anger to destroy your concentration with thoughts such as "Why didn't we learn about that condition in school?" Rather, think to yourself, "I can try to answer these questions." Above all, do not be distracted by the individual who leaves after 1 hour of testing! That person may have a different ability level, or may even be taking a different professional exam.

The keys to success are within you (Table 1-6). Discover your strengths and potential by preparing thoroughly—mentally and emotionally. Study, review, practice test-taking strategies, and learn how to reduce personal tension. The rewards begin with your license to practice as a professional nurse. You are needed in the changing health care field, and you are welcomed as a caregiver and a colleague!

Answer Key for Pretest Questions, p. 2

1. d
2. c
3. d
4. b
5. c

REFERENCES

Changes incorporated into the NCLEX-RN Test Plan, *Issues* 15(4):1, 1994.
Chornick N, Yocom C, Jacobson J: *1992-1993 job analysis study of newly licensed entry-level registered nurses,* Chicago, 1993, National Council of State Boards of Nursing.
Questions and answers on the methodology of the computerized adaptive testing for the NCLEX, Chicago, 1995, National Council of State Boards of Nursing.
Test plan for the national council licensure examination for registered nurses, Chicago, 1995, National Council of State Boards of Nursing.

ACING MULTIPLE-CHOICE TESTS

Just remember confidence, control, content, *and* common sense—*it'll be easier to focus on the questions and answers.*

BY PAULETTE D. ROLLANT

D o multiple-choice exams make your heart race? Do exams on computers challenge your coping skills? Do you have trouble choosing the best answer?

All of the above?

Turn your stress into success! Use the stabilization approach, or what I call the four-point success system.

Houses, cars, chairs, tables, and other useful items are usually based on this system. Each has four points of reference. For example, a car has four tires; if one goes flat, one point of reference is removed. The car can still be driven but not for long. If two tires are damaged, you're out of luck.

Likewise, there are four points of reference to pass exams: the four Cs—*confidence, control, content, and common sense.* If you prepare for multiple-choice exams by using only one or two of these points of reference, you'll lessen your chances of passing. To see how this success system can work for you, let's take a look at each of the points of reference.

CONFIDENCE

You can gain confidence in test taking by learning to read and answer questions precisely. Practice the following easy steps.

Step 1: Be a Detective

Look for clues in the stem, the question, and the responses. Clues include:

Paulette D. Rollant, RN, CCRN, PhD, is president, Multi-Resources, Inc., Atlanta, a firm that develops, presents, and evaluates educational programs.
Modified from AJN: Nursing career guide, Jan. 1994.

Key words: *most, first, initially, immediately, late, toxicity, side effect, toxic effect, complication, usual problem*

Nursing process: assessment, analysis, plan, intervention, evaluation

Time parameters: day one versus day three, preop, postop, during, after

Age group of a patient: the decade determines the developmental need, normal physiologic changes, and will guide an approach for teaching or discharge planning

Absolutes: *always, never, every, none, all, all the time*

Words of essence: *acute, chronic, partial, total,* or diseases that indicate acute or chronic conditions

Locations: outpatient, clinic, hospital, home, postanesthesia unit

Distractors: mystery diseases, absurd situations, content that clashes with your personal beliefs; that is, questions that evoke an emotional response and obscure your thinking

Let's apply these clues to questions. **A patient begins to experience a severe gastrointestinal bleed. The plan of care to meet the patient's fluid needs should include, as a priority, which of the following?**

a. accommodating the patient's frequent need for the bedpan or emesis basin

b. monitoring vital signs on an hourly basis

c. maintaining the gastric pH

d. rapidly administering blood and fluid

When questions include key words such as *first* or *priority,* you don't need to look for an incorrect response: All the responses are correct. You must choose the *best response.* Think of us-

ing the ABCs or the nursing process. For the ABCs approach, airway, breathing, and circulation take precedence over any other factors. If the information in the stem defines a situation, try the nursing process. The most likely answer is to do further assessment before an intervention or evaluation. So look for the assessment response. If all the assessment data have been included in the stem, then an intervention response is the likely correct answer.

In the question above, essential words—*priority* and *severe bleed*—guide your selection of the answer. Think ABCs. The only answer that deals with circulation or fluid needs is d. If you are thinking that d is incorrect because at your hospital blood is rarely given, you're reading into the question, as well as letting personal experience influence your answer. Thus, you have answered *a* question rather than answering *the* question asked.

A nurse is caring for a patient with acute myocardial infarction whose recovery is uncomplicated. To prevent complications on the third day, the nurse would do which of the following?

a. Monitor the patient's ability to turn, cough, and deep breathe.

b. Have the patient walk a short distance.

c. Apply antiembolic hose to the patient's legs.

d. Give the patient sublingual nitroglycerin prior to all out-of-bed activity to prevent chest pain.

During a patient's seizure the nurse should

a. suction as needed.

b. ensure safety.

c. elevate head with a pillow.

d. observe the length and aftereffects of the seizure.

The answer to the first question is b. If you read it too quickly, you may have overlooked the time clue of *third day.* If you selected answer c, which is the answer for *a* question about an action on the *first day* post–myocardial infarction, you didn't answer *the* question. By the third day this patient should be walking short distances to prepare for discharge. Answer a might be a good choice for a patient with complications. Response d is incorrect because of the word *all,* an absolute. Not all activity needs preventive medication.

The answer to the second question is b. The key word is *during.* This makes answer d incorrect because it includes information after the seizure. *The* question is asking for general information; select a more general or global response. Response a is too specific, and suctioning is commonly not done during a seizure because the patient's jaws are usually clamped. Elevating the head with a pillow (c) flexes the neck and closes the patient's airway.

The initial content for discharge teaching of a patient, age 26, after the repair of a ruptured appendix with an open incision would be focused on concerns about

a. loss of functional ability.

b. the effects of surgery on intimacy.

c. alterations in body image.

d. fears of not being able to attain life's goals.

The correct answer is c; body image is a major concern of people aged 20 to 29. If the age was changed to 36, b would be correct; if 46, d would be correct; and if 76, a would be correct.

Patients over 60 years of age typically have difficulty with seeing small print, hearing, and manipulating equipment, whereas teenagers may have these abilities but lack the interest or motivation.

A family member of a post–myocardial infarction patient sat in on the discharge teaching session. Which of the following statements indicates the family member understands the steps to successful recovery?

a. "Before we do any activity around the house, a nitroglycerin needs to be taken to avoid chest pains."

b. "We will plan to take a one-hour nap every day."

c. "When we go fishing we'll need to alternate moderate activity with periods of rest."

d. "We have a calendar to mark down the blood pressure and weight in the morning and in the evening."

When a response contains absolutes, it's usually incorrect. Response a is incorrect because of the word *any.* Nitroglycerin should be taken before *strenuous* activity, not just *any activity.* There's no reason for the patient to take a nap every day, so b is incorrect. In response d the activities mentioned are usually done once a day in the morning. The correct response is c.

Ms. Murphy, age 80, who's had diabetes for more than 25 years, visits the clinic for education. She says, "I've cooked the same way for 20 years. I know what I like to eat and I don't plan to change now." At this time, patient teaching for Ms. Murphy should be based on the results of an evaluation of

a. the condition of her feet.

b. her activity level.

c. her serum glucose level.

d. the foods she's eaten.

The correct response is a. Ms. Murphy has a chronic condition and is at the clinic. Her statement indicates that diet education at this time would be ineffective. The clinic nurse would have the most influence on behaviors related to foot care. If the feet were in good condition the nurse could give positive reinforcement. If the feet were in bad condition, the clinic nurse could initiate physical care, then refer Ms. Murphy to a foot specialist. The patient may be more likely to follow up since bad feet are uncomfortable, and this physiologic need commonly supersedes other needs. (Don't forget Maslow's hierarchy of needs.) Response c is incorrect since it's too general—a more specific answer would refer to *when* the glucose was checked (that is, fasting or nonfasting levels). The patient's activity level (b) may be least likely to change due to her age and psychosocial limitations.

The patient with acute disease may be more anxious and have fewer effective coping mechanisms. A patient with a chronic condition, on the other hand, usually has greater coping skills, more available support systems, and a deeper knowledge of the condition to allow for adaptation. These factors will influence your nursing actions in different clinical settings.

Step 2: Read the Stem Systematically

Relax! A tense body results in a tense mind that misses important words and can't think or make decisions. Read the question first. Then read the information above the question. Note any clues in the stem and give all words equal attention. Read the question again. Think of what the answer would be. Then read the given responses.

As you go from question to question, read at an even pace. Avoid spending too much time on a question. Avoid "hangover," which is thinking about prior questions while you're now on a new question.

In the first few seconds of reading a question, avoid the "I know" or "I don't know the content" approach. Remember that your biases from life experiences or emotions may influence how you read the question. For example, if you dislike neuro and had an awful instructor for neuro, when you get to a neuro question this bias automatically kicks into gear. You tense up and can't think. To counter this reaction, for neuro questions tell yourself, "I'm familiar with some part of this situation. I can relate the information. I can make an educated decision." Besides, the question may be asking about something else other than neuro—if you're tense you may not even notice.

After you read the stem, try to act out the situation mentally. Close your eyes, visualize the scenario. Often the correct response will come to mind immediately. For questions about adduction, abduction, flexion, extension, and so forth, you can help yourself choose the right answer by moving your arm or leg in the described manner.

While reading the stem, determine if the background information is important or even related to the question asked. Decide if the question is asking about assessment, planning, intervention, evaluation, or communication content. Or is the question asking about *normal* or *abnormal?* Identifying the focus at this point will help you screen the four responses. Remember that "quotations" don't always indicate a communication or psych question. Be aware that teaching-type questions could be testing correct or incorrect information. For example, questions may be worded "needs additional teaching" or "needs no additional teaching." If you read too quickly or haven't controlled your anxiety, you may overlook small but crucial words like the "no."

Step 3: Read All the Responses, Then Select the Answer

Look for those clues mentioned above in step 1! Concentrate on each word in each response. If possible, narrow your choices to two responses. That will increase your chance of answering the question correctly by 50%. In some cases, you might try to cluster the responses to select the correct answer. That is, categorize the responses: general versus specific, internal/external, immediate/late, drugs/nondrugs, and assessment/intervention. If three of the responses can be grouped, the one outside the category is usually correct.

A patient is constipated and dehydrated. Which intervention would the patient most likely comply with?

a. drinking Ensure between meals
b. drinking extra fluids with meals
c. drinking 8 oz of water every hour between meals
d. drinking adequate amounts of fluid during the day

The correct answer is c. Note that a, b, and d can be clustered since they are general statements without specific fluid amounts. Or perhaps you found the correct response based on the teaching theory that specific goals more likely result in completion of tasks. (You may want to keep this theory in mind for yourself in preparation for passing those exams.)

With responses that have series of items, read "vertically." For example:

Which set of arterial blood gases should the nurse expect to find in a patient with metabolic acidosis?

a. pH 7.28, PCO_2 55, HCO_3 26
b. pH 7.50, PCO_2 30, HCO_3 31
c. pH 7.48, PCO_2 30, HCO_3 22
d. pH 7.30, PCO_2 36, HCO_3 18

First, read only the pHs down vertically and look for a lowered pH, acidosis. Using this technique, you can narrow the responses to either a or d. Now look at the HCO_3, since you can recall the rules: for metabolic imbal-

ances the pH and the bicarb move in the same direction and for respiratory imbalances the pH and the CO_2 move in the opposite directions. Note that *the* question is about a metabolic imbalance. Compare the bicarbs in responses a and d. You know the answer is d. By using the vertical technique, you have saved time, energy, and maintained a clearer mind.

If you're stumped by the question, sometimes simply matching similar words or ideas in the stem and response will result in a correct answer. Try these questions.

The patient had his blood pressure taken in lying and standing positions. The nurse explains to him that this is a test for

a. central nervous system depression.
b. malignant hypertension.
c. orthostatic hypotension.
d. vascular insufficiency.

A patient in acute renal failure develops pulmonary edema. Which of the following interventions would be inappropriate to include in this patient's care?

a. Administer oxygen.
b. Encourage coughing and deep breathing.
c. Place the patient in high Fowler's position.
d. Replace lost fluids.

In the first question, by matching the idea of *position* in the stem with the associated word *orthostatic,* you choose the correct response, c. In the second question, by matching the concept *edema* in the stem to the word *fluid,* you choose d. (A word of caution: Reserve this technique for when you have no idea what the answer may be.)

When you select an answer, your first hunch is usually correct! Don't change answers unless you're sure that you misread the question or missed some important clues the first time around.

Step 4: Review Practice Questions

When you're preparing for an exam, correct your practice questions. Read all the rationales of all questions if they're available. Rationales frequently include clinical pearls stated in a precise and easy-to-recall manner along with essential factors to consider for the correct response.

Look for patterns of missed questions. For example, you might find

clusters of missed questions at the beginning, middle, or end of the exam. This could reflect periods of fatigue or anxiety. On your next practice test, make a mental note to consciously relax at these times. Take a mental minivacation. Also, if you have the opportunity, review the questions at these patterned intervals to make sure you correctly read the questions before turning in the test. On computer exams you can't go back, so it's best to pause every 15 questions or so for minivacations, deep breathing, or the relaxation exercises that work best for you.

Note the questions for which you have changed answers. Did this help or hinder the number of questions that you got right? If it helped, you have a pattern of changing answers to better your score. Change answers. However, if it didn't help, don't change your answers—no matter what!

Some authorities say that if you have no idea what the answer is, choose "c." The rationale given is that more item writers use "c" as the correct answer. I think that if you would rather choose "a," then do so. In the end it doesn't matter because some research findings report that 25% of any number of multiple-choice questions will be correctly answered by random selection—on a 100-item exam you will get at least 25 questions correct by guessing. Add that to at least 50 questions you will get correct by having studied. You pass the exam.

Review your incorrect responses. For each correct answer you missed, ask yourself: Why did I miss this?

Did I know the content? Make a list of the unfamiliar content. Look it up. Then try to categorize unfamiliar content. Was it cardiac? Renal? If you have time, read parts of the chapter that you think would be most helpful to you.

Ask yourself: What step in the nursing process was more frequently missed? Assessment? Evaluation? The next time you do practice questions pick those types of questions to do. Or be sure when you are doing practice questions to identify these questions, read them more carefully, and try to relax before selecting your response.

Did I misread the questions or responses? Most people fall into this category. Did you overlook a key word in the stem or in one of the responses?

Did you answer *a* question instead of *the* question? When you get your exams back do you say, "I knew that! Why did I choose this"? If you do, you need to sharpen and to more frequently apply confidence skills. Or maybe you need to sharpen and more frequently apply your control skills to lessen your anxiety during exams. Or maybe you need to do both! Your analyses of why you're missing questions will guide you. When you're very nervous, your concentration and perception are below par. You then need to reduce your anxiety through techniques such as deep breathing.

If you practice these strategies for controlling errors in reading test questions, you will certainly boost your confidence in your ability to pass exams. And, as you work on confidence, you can also develop your skills of control.

CONTROL

Control is your ability to maintain a minimum stress level so that your perceptions and decisions are accurate. You're able to read the questions objectively, to think, and to problem-solve. The three most common categories of exam stressors are mental, physical, and psychosocial.

Mental stressors are those messages you play over and over in your mind. Frequently, these messages are negative, draining your confidence, energy, and thinking ability. First, you have to consciously work at becoming aware of these messages. Then you can counter them with positive ones. For example, if you go in to take a test playing the mental message of "I didn't study enough. I know I'll have trouble on this test," counter that thought immediately with something more positive, such as, "I studied as much as I could. I know that content and will use it to figure out related items on the test." Other positive messages might be: "I will slow down and read the questions more carefully." "I will ignore the distractions in the room."

Physical stressors include the environment and your body. The exam room may be too cold, hot, noisy, or crowded, the chairs uncomfortable, and the lighting poor. Plan on the worst. Dress in layers so clothing can be added or removed. You may want to use ear plugs if you find noises distracting. When you do test questions at home, select days when it's hot, cold, or noisy. Practice tuning out the distractions.

To diminish your body's stress, stay away from spicy, fatty, and high-sugar foods, which can make you feel sluggish and heavy, and give you indigestion. Caffeine can make you feel hyper, tense, and anxious, and cause you to make frequent trips to the bathroom. Alcohol depresses the central nervous system as well as dehydrating and depleting important minerals.

Psychosocial stressors result from the behaviors or comments of your colleagues either during study time or right before the exam. Suggest to your group that you have a rule to allow only positive comments during study times or before exams. You may want to distract yourself before testing by listening to music through a headset or by reading something fun or "nonnursing." Also, be aware that a family member's physical problems that are similar to your test material may cause you to answer the question based on your personal experience rather than general theory.

CONTENT

To help you remember content for later application, try this process. Before class on a given topic simply read the introduction and summaries of the chapter that covers the content. Go to class and listen as well as take notes. Every night read over your notes before bedtime. You're more likely to retain content in long-term memory if you study for no longer than an hour and then sleep for at least a few hours. On the following days do some practice questions in that content area, guided by the ones you missed. Refer to your text as much as needed. It's usually students' goal to read all the pages in the text; however, in reality, it's next to impossible. Remember that the content includes facts and the application of facts to clinical situations.

COMMON SENSE

Common sense—don't leave home without it. Pick it up each morning from the kitchen counter and put it in your pocket. Common sense says, "I'll figure this out. I know something. That something will get the answer." Let's practice:

How long does it take to dissolve fibrin?
a. 1-3 days
b. 7-10 days
c. 25-30 days
d. 60-90 days

If you have no idea what the correct answer is, use common sense plus a little content knowledge. You recall that fibrin has something to do with clotting. So you think of what might be a common situation when a clot forms in the body. You remember that this morning you bumped into the table and bruised your leg. Yes, a bruise is a clot. Then think. You remember that your bruises usually last about a week. Yes! The answer is certainly b.

Another commonsense approach for this question is to look at the numbers in the given responses. Throw out the extremes, the highest and the lowest, answers a and d. Use a conservative approach and select the numbers in b. Try another question.

In the elderly patient sympathetic responsiveness
a. increases with age.
b. remains equal to that of a young adult.
c. decreases with age.
d. no longer occurs.

As people get older they slow down. Similarly, the sympathetic system most likely does also. The correct answer is c.

The key to becoming a successful test taker? Practice, practice, and more practice in using the four reference points: confidence, control, content, and common sense. Pick up stamina, speed, and steam in thinking and decision making. Remember—that which has your attention determines your direction. Pay attention to these details. I'm sure you'll do well!

Contents

Questions *14*

Correct Answers *36*

Correct Answers with Rationales *39*

Chapter 2

Nursing Care of the Client with Psychosocial and Mental Health Problems

COORDINATOR
Deborah Antai-Otong, MS, RN, CS

Questions

1. During the first meeting for a group of elderly nursing home residents, Ms. Brooks, R.N., the facilitator, introduces herself and asks each member to do the same. What information might be useful to the nurse at this time?
   ① The reasons for each resident's admission
   ② A sociocultural history of each resident
   ③ The usual activity patterns of each resident
   ④ The interaction patterns in the group

2. Judy Mason, R.N., is leading a grief group for senior citizens. When she asks the group what kinds of things they would like to focus on, the only responses she receives are comments such as "You tell us; you're the leader," and "Why do we need to come to this group anyway?" This behavior is probably explained by which of the following statements?
   ① The purpose of the group was not clearly explained.
   ② The residents are anxious, a typical response.
   ③ The residents are expressing disinterest in the group.
   ④ Interpretation of these comments is not possible after one meeting.

3. During a group therapy meeting for elderly residents in a retirement home, one of the residents tells everyone of his apprehension about going to visit his daughter for a weekend. What would your best response be?
   ① "There is no reason to feel anxious about this visit."
   ② "Maybe others in the group have had similar feelings."
   ③ "Have you ever had those feelings before?"
   ④ "Why are you so anxious?"

4. Mr. Armie, a 63-year-old man admitted to the psychiatric unit for depression, has monopolized most of the conversation in group therapy. How might the group facilitator best handle this?
   ① Take him aside and kindly tell him that others deserve a chance to talk, too.
   ② Ignore Mr. Armie's comments, and they will occur less often.
   ③ Tactfully share your perception with the group and wonder aloud why they let it occur.
   ④ Point out the inappropriateness of his behavior in the group.

5. Melissa Kern is a 50-year-old woman who was admitted to the psychiatric unit over the weekend. She says she is quite angry and frustrated, even though she is smiling. Which of the following best describes Mrs. Kern's behavior?
   ① Suspicious
   ② Demanding
   ③ Incongruent
   ④ Reluctant

6. What is the best response when dealing with clients whose behavior does not parallel expressed feelings?
   ① "Your behavior does not match what you are saying."
   ② "Tell me what is really on your mind."
   ③ "Tell me more about your feelings."
   ④ "What were you thinking just now?"

7. The nurse notices Mrs. Dillard, a 62-year-old depressed woman, in the dayroom. The client looks upset but continues to sit and not notice the nurse's presence. The nurse says, "Mrs. Dillard, you look upset." The client reflects on what the nurse has said and begins to think, but does not say anything. What would be an appropriate nursing response?
   ① Remain silent to allow her time to formulate her thoughts.
   ② Ask her, "Did you understand my question?"
   ③ Tell her, "I'm concerned about your silence, Mrs. Dillard."
   ④ Tell her, "Just say the first thing that comes to mind, Mrs. Dillard."

8. The team talks about Mrs. Jeffers, a newly admitted woman who is angry but refuses to talk to the staff. Which of the following information would be most useful to discuss at today's treatment planning meeting?
   ① Psychiatric diagnosis
   ② Case history
   ③ Psychologic testing
   ④ Approaches for present behavior

9. When a client begins to become more isolative and refuses to leave the room, what is the best initial nursing response when making contact?
   ① "Come, let's go play some cards."
   ② "Have I done something to frighten you?"
   ③ "I'll stay with you for awhile."
   ④ "It is important for you to mingle with other clients."

10. 52-year-old Renee Sanders comes to the mental health clinic and relates that since the death of her husband she feels really miserable. She says in a loud voice, "How could he leave me? I can't deal with this!"

Which of the following stages of the grief reaction is Mrs. Sanders most likely displaying at this time?
① Denial
② Anger
③ Bargaining
④ Resolution

11. Which of the following statements made by a client whose husband has just died would be the most important in determining whether her response is normal or delayed or extended?
① "My husband died 1 week ago."
② "I feel sad and want to cry all the time."
③ "We were married for 40 years."
④ "We grew apart during the later years."

12. Lynn Colby's husband died 2 months ago. She was brought to the unit by her son, who said his mother is not eating, paces the floor at night, and tells her son about plans she and her husband are making to go to Hawaii. Which of the following is the most appropriate statement of the client's problem?
① Prolonged grief reaction related to death of husband
② Anger related to loss of husband
③ Denial of the loss
④ Powerlessness over the situation

13. What is the most therapeutic *initial* nursing intervention in helping a grieving client deal with feelings after the loss of a spouse?
① Help the client see the positive aspects of the relationship with the spouse.
② Describe the stages of the grieving process.
③ Support the client's expression of feelings.
④ Explain that in time the hurt feelings will lessen.

14. 39-year-old Mrs. Killman has a history of cancer of the breast and had a radical mastectomy 6 years ago. Recent examination and surgery have revealed inoperable cancer, and she has been admitted for palliative chemotherapy and radiation treatment. She is quiet and withdrawn, a thin, frail woman. She speaks only when spoken to and eats and drinks only when someone feeds her. What is the nurse's *highest priority* in caring for the client at this time?
① Help the client focus on managing personal affairs.
② Encourage verbal expression of the client's anger.
③ Ensure that the client receives adequate nutrition and hydration.
④ Allow the client to use any form of denial that she chooses.

15. When any client becomes depressed, loses weight, and refuses to move from bed or turn, this behavior may result in three of the following consequences. Which is *least* likely to occur?
① Formation of decubitus ulcers
② Decreased staff interaction with the client
③ Anger and hostility from the nursing staff toward the client
④ Contractures of the extremities

16. When a dying client refuses to see or talk with family members, such behavior may be understood as
① The family not being able to meet the client's emotional needs.
② The client moving through the grief process more quickly to resolution.
③ Emotional distancing resulting from the pain of separation and loss.
④ A lack of understanding by children, who are too young to know the difference.

17. One evening, the physician meets with Mrs. Tess, a 61-year-old woman who has uterine cancer and has been told she has 2 months to live. They discuss discharge and subsequent hospice care. The client is visibly troubled, and later that night she suffers an episode of respiratory arrest. Her medical condition is treated and stabilized, but she is obviously weakened and remains withdrawn. Which of the following nursing actions is the *least* therapeutic at this time?
① Turning and positioning the client as needed
② Having the nurse consider her own feelings and beliefs about dying
③ Sitting quietly with the client
④ Encouraging her to feed and bathe herself to regain autonomy

18. When working with the dying client and significant others, the nurse believes that three of the following are very likely to occur. Which one is *not*?
① The family will respond to the dying member much as they have handled other major crisis situations.
② The client will proceed through each of the stages of dying, regardless of outside help.
③ The family's greatest needs may be for competent physical care for the ill member and empathy for their situation.
④ Young children may see death as something experienced by others, but not themselves.

19. Mr. and Mrs. Jacobs have learned recently that their 3-year-old daughter Amy has an untreatable malignant tumor. The nurse can expect Amy to have which of the following views of death?
① Someone bad will carry her away.
② Death occurs, but is not permanent.
③ Death and absence are the same.
④ Everyone must die.

20. In the case of a 3-year-old with an untreatable malignant tumor, which of the following would probably be nontherapeutic in helping the child express her reactions and feelings about her situation?
① Provide dolls and puppets for symbolic play.
② Provide paper and crayons to draw with, and have her describe her drawings.
③ Set up a regular time each day to talk about her feelings and concerns.
④ Read stories and talk about how the children in the stories feel.

21. LeAnn Mellin is a 29-year-old woman admitted to the surgical unit after an accident in a small airplane. Her husband, the pilot, was killed. Mrs. Mellin has some minor abrasions and contusions, but she is physically

stable. She has a 2-year-old son. The day after admission, the nurse enters the client's room to find the shades drawn and her in bed sobbing quietly. The most therapeutic nursing response is
① "It's a beautiful day outside. Let's get some sunshine in here."
② "Obviously you are upset, let's talk about what you're feeling now."
③ "I'll come back when you are feeling better, you seem too upset."
④ "It's not good for you to sit in here in the dark."

22. Which of the following would most likely be considered an *abnormal* grief response?
① A period of preoccupation with the deceased
② Initially idealizing the deceased
③ Hoarding sleep medications
④ Expressing angry feelings

23. Which of the following would be most helpful in facilitating the grief process?
① Allow long periods of solitary activity.
② Schedule numerous activities to keep the client's mind occupied.
③ Arrange an unannounced visit from a relative.
④ Allow the client to work through the grief process at the client's own pace.

24. The nurse enters the room of a client who is overtly upset and crying. Which of the following would be the most effective nursing intervention?
① Tell the client you will return later when the client gains control.
② Tell the client you will stay around until the client is ready to talk.
③ Administer a sedative immediately.
④ Attempt to understand the meaning of the client's behavior.

25. Several days after learning of her pregnancy, a recently widowed client tells the nurse, "I'm going to have an abortion. I can't bear the thought of raising this child alone." What is the best response?
① "Well, it sounds as though you already have made a decision."
② "You may be acting too hastily."
③ "Let's talk about it."
④ "You might be sorry in a year or two."

26. Amber Garcia, a newlywed, comes to the mental health clinic because of "nervousness." She relates to the nurse that "my stomach is tense most of the time. I haven't missed any work, but it's getting harder because I can't concentrate very long on anything." What level of anxiety is Mrs. Garcia likely experiencing?
① Mild
② Moderate
③ Severe
④ Panic

27. Which of the following would be the best way to gather a psychosocial history from a client with moderate anxiety?
① "Identify any recent changes in your life."
② "What are you feeling now?"
③ "Have you ever felt this way before?"
④ "Does anyone else in your family ever get these feelings?"

28. Jennifer Dewey calls out to the nurse's station every 10 minutes asking for something. She is a 67-year-old client who underwent a hip pinning 2 days before. The nursing staff is planning behavior modification techniques to deal with her persistent requests. Which of the following is the *first action* for the nurse to take regarding Miss Dewey's behavior?
① Observe her behavior at regular intervals to obtain a baseline.
② Observe her ability to carry out her activities of daily living.
③ Assess her need for pain medicine or tranquilizers.
④ Assess her reaction to the anesthetic.

29. Which of the following is an effective plan of nursing care for a demanding client?
① Confront the client about the inappropriateness of numerous calls.
② Encourage the client to take a mild tranquilizer at regular periods.
③ Seek out the client at consistent intervals.
④ Explain that the nurse has other clients to care for.

30. The effectiveness of behavior modification in managing demanding behaviors lies in the nurse's ability to
① Allay the client's anxiety.
② Present reality to the client.
③ Respond to the client's need for safety.
④ Avoid reinforcing the behavior.

31. Which of the following explains the *major difference* between normal anxiety and anxiety disorders?
① Normal anxiety is constant; an anxiety disorder is intermittent and short-lived.
② Normal anxiety is experienced as a natural human response; in an anxiety disorder, there is an impending sense of doom.
③ An anxiety disorder is seldom controllable and usually must run its course.
④ Normal anxiety is a fact of life and rarely becomes an anxiety disorder.

32. A client says to the nurse, "Dr. Sims has surely botched my case. I can't believe they'd let her continue to practice." Which of the following is an appropriate response?
① "Dr. Sims is a fine doctor and one worthy of respect."
② "Dr. Sims has been sued before, and her practice is questionable."
③ "You seem to have some concerns about Dr. Sims."
④ "Dr. Sims usually provides good care."

33. Major signs and symptoms of anxiety disorders include which of the following?
① Complaints of apprehension, impaired cognitions, diaphoresis, stomach pains, and restlessness
② Inability to get to sleep, early morning awakening, 10-pound weight loss, and lack of energy
③ Ideas of reference, grandiose delusions, hallucinations, and delusions
④ Tangential speech, intrusiveness, spending or giving away large amounts of money

34. Merlin Landrin is experiencing anxiety. He is married, has three children, and just lost his job as a coal miner.

He comes into the hospital with severe indigestion and fears that he has a serious stomach disorder. If Mr. Landrin experiences a panic attack, the nurse would most likely note which of the following symptoms?

① Persecutory delusions, ideas of reference, and rhyming
② Greatly reduced perception, extreme discomfort, and extreme agitation
③ Fugue state, amnesia, and dissociation
④ Extreme agitation, mood depression, and immobilization

35. Nursing care during a panic attack would most likely include which of the following?
① Providing an unhurried approach while encouraging expression of thoughts and feelings
② Encouraging discussion of childhood events and their impact on the client's inability to cope
③ Talking with the client about the future and how the present situation is a temporary setback
④ Establishing rapport and helping the client express and deal with anger

36. Amelia Terr comes to the university's health clinic complaining of anxiety, insomnia, and trouble eating. Which of the following criteria should the nurse use to develop a plan for care?
① Coherence of thought processes, reality orientation, and anxiety level
② Reduction of behavioral signs of nervousness and effective use of coping mechanisms
③ Cycle of mood swings and their impact on self-care
④ Self-reports of experiencing less fear

37. Elmore Johnson, a 46-year-old married man, has demonstrated increased reluctance to leave his home over the past 3 months. He had been absent from his job frequently, and 1 month ago his employment was terminated. Since that time, he has not been outside his home. Mr. Johnson most likely displays symptoms of which of the following disorders?
① Acrophobia
② Agoraphobia
③ Astraphobia
④ Claustrophobia

38. The ego-defense mechanism thought to be used by clients with phobic disorders is which of the following?
① Sublimation
② Displacement
③ Substitution
④ Suppression

39. What is the most effective technique in treating a client with a phobia?
① Confrontation to determine if the fear is based on reality
② Immediate exposure to the feared situation
③ Distraction each time the client complains of a fearful situation
④ Gradual desensitization by controlled exposure to the feared situation

40. Which of the following would most likely be prescribed for a client with agoraphobia?
① The antipsychotic fluphenazine (Prolixin)
② The antipsychotic haloperidol (Haldol)

③ The anti–manic-drug carbamazepine (Tegretol)
④ The anxiolytic clonazepam (Klonopin)

41. Which of the following activities attended by a client with agoraphobia indicates an improvement in the client's condition?
① Milieu group in the dayroom
② Occupational therapy in the adjunctive-therapy room
③ Recreational therapy on the outside volleyball court
④ Friday lunch in the hospital cafeteria

42. Lucinda Lopez is a 16-year-old high school student brought to the psychiatric hospital by her mother. She has been preoccupied with excessive cleanliness, refusing to go in areas where she might soil her clothing, and bathing several times a day. She is diagnosed with obsessive-compulsive disorder. The primary reason for Lucinda's symptoms is represented by which of the following?
① A pattern of receiving attention
② A means of reducing anxiety
③ A learned childhood behavior of staying clean
④ A manipulative method of avoiding socialization

43. Which ego-defense mechanisms are most prominently used in obsessive-compulsive disorders?
① Introjection and projection
② Compensation and sublimation
③ Displacement and undoing
④ Rationalization and suppression

44. When formulating the nursing diagnosis for a client experiencing anxiety, which of the following is the *most* important?
① Take a detailed history of the client's panic responses.
② Gather information about what preceded the anxiety reactions.
③ Distinguish nursing interventions that reduce the anxiety by one level.
④ Evaluate the effectiveness of the nursing interventions used to reduce anxiety.

45. Which are the most important factors for the nurse to assess concerning a client with obsessive-compulsive disorder?
① Actions, current stressors, level of function, and activities of daily living
② Silly behavior, thought patterns, associations, and delusions
③ Nervousness, vital signs, body language, and level of anxiety
④ Involvement of involuntary muscles, fears, attention level, and sleeping disorders

46. When planning the initial nursing care plan of a client with obsessive-compulsive hand-washing behaviors, which of the following should receive the highest priority?
① Client will maintain a role in the family
② Client will discontinue the washing behavior
③ Client will verbalize major causes of the washing behavior
④ Client will reestablish skin integrity

47. During early stages of treatment the nurse will most likely consider which of the following in planning care for a client with obsessive-compulsive disorder?
    ① The client will require strict limit setting in order to conform to scheduled unit activities.
    ② The client will need extra time to perform rituals so that anxiety will be manageable.
    ③ The client will need to be isolated in order to feel less anxious about proximity to other clients.
    ④ The client will need to be confronted about the senselessness of the compulsive behavior.

48. Which of the following is most important in planning nursing care for a client with obsessive-compulsive disorder?
    ① Use continuous reality orientation.
    ② Set limits on compulsive behaviors.
    ③ Administer Lorazepam (Afivan), 2 mg as ordered.
    ④ Teach assertiveness training.

49. Maribeth, a 31-year-old with obsessive-compulsive disorder, relates that she likes to play chess but is fearful of sitting on the chairs in the dayroom. What would be the most therapeutic intervention?
    ① Sterilize one of the chairs in the dayroom and reserve it for her.
    ② Move the chess game into Maribeth's room.
    ③ Allow Maribeth to stand while playing chess.
    ④ Insist that she sit in the chair.

50. Three of the following interventions are useful in reducing ritualistic behaviors in clients with obsessive-compulsive disorder. Which one is *not*?
    ① Allow the client to complete the ritual once it has begun.
    ② Assist the client with self-care and activities of daily living.
    ③ Stop ritualistic behaviors immediately and encourage expression of feelings.
    ④ Provide protection from physical discomfort caused by the ritualistic behavior.

51. Which statement would be the most appropriate guideline when considering possible outcomes of care for a client with obsessive-compulsive disorder?
    ① The antipsychotic haloperidol will completely eliminate symptoms.
    ② Psychotherapy will deal with repressed feelings and completely eliminate symptoms.
    ③ Given sufficient opportunities to succeed in activities, self-esteem will improve, and all symptoms will be eliminated.
    ④ The tricyclic clomipramine (Anafranil) will reduce obsessions and ritualistic behaviors.

52. Which of the following criteria would be used to evaluate the client's progress during treatment of obsessive-compulsive checking behaviors?
    ① A reduction of ritualistic behaviors and resumption of daily activities
    ② Intact thought processes grounded in reality
    ③ Able to go to the shopping mall without fear of open spaces
    ④ Self-reports of decreased anxiety and ability to redirect obsessive thoughts

53. Nineteen-year-old Tamara washes her arms and legs constantly. She has been diagnosed with obsessive-compulsive disorder. Which statement best demonstrates Tamara's understanding of her problem?
    ① "I suppose washing all the time is a crazy thing to do."
    ② "I feel so clean when I get done washing, but it just doesn't last very long."
    ③ "I know I'm getting better, because I smell cleaner."
    ④ "I really don't think I have a problem. It's important to be clean if you want to have dates."

54. Three of the following conditions are frequently characteristic of the client with anorexia nervosa. Which one is *not*?
    ① Intense fear of gaining weight and becoming fat
    ② Absence of at least three consecutive menstrual cycles
    ③ Loss of appetite
    ④ Strenuous exercise

55. Which of the following behaviors could be considered *atypical* of anorexia nervosa?
    ① Hoarding food
    ② Eating only low-calorie foods
    ③ Napping frequently to conserve energy
    ④ Abusing laxatives and diuretics

56. Which of the following is the *most* critical treatment strategy of a client with anorexia nervosa?
    ① Negotiate a behavioral contract with the client.
    ② Teach the importance of maintaining proper nutrition.
    ③ Institute immediate measures to restore electrolyte and nutritional balance.
    ④ Observe closely for 2 hours after each meal.

57. In setting up a treatment plan for the treatment of clients with anorexia nervosa, three of the following would be appropriate. Which one would be *inappropriate*?
    ① Provide opportunities to make choices from an appropriate menu.
    ② Provide positive reinforcement for each pound gained.
    ③ Encourage more autonomy.
    ④ Provide solitary time in a room after each meal.

58. When monitoring the eating patterns of the client with anorexia nervosa, it is vital for the nurse to recognize that the client
    ① Has total control over sense of hunger and experiences a sense of independence.
    ② Is aware of a distorted self-image, which helps the client understand the need to eat properly.
    ③ Has alterations in the hypothalamus producing aphagia and decreased body weight.
    ④ Is never aware of the sensation of hunger.

59. Twenty-two-year-old Patrice Perney has been admitted to the hospital for anorexia nervosa. She is started on a behavior modification program. She is encouraged to eat three well-balanced meals each day and to attempt to gain at least one-half pound each day. Each time she accomplishes this, she is allowed an additional privilege on the unit. This is an example of

which of the following behavior modification techniques?
① Avoidance of punishment
② Positive reinforcement
③ Negative reinforcement
④ Desensitization

60. Clients with anorexia nervosa often deny problems and maintain distant relationships with the staff and peers on a unit. Which of the following nursing approaches would be the most effective?
① Point out that the client will be force-fed if there is no improvement in eating habits.
② Let the client eat when necessary because there will be no weight loss after an optimal weight is reached.
③ Involve the client in the preparation of a treatment plan, assisting in decisions concerning food, exercise, and hygiene,
④ Assign a roommate who has good eating habits so that there will be more interest in proper nutrition.

61. Which of the following is the most suitable nursing response when a female client with anorexia nervosa describes her hips as fat?
① "Actually you're too skinny; your appearance is not very attractive."
② "Look here in the mirror. Now, you can see your hips are not fat."
③ "I understand that your hips seem fat to you, but to others you appear very thin."
④ "It's difficult for me to understand how you can do this to yourself."

62. Larry Moorehead is seen in a primary health care setting complaining of a 6-year history of numerous medical admissions for severe, intermittent headaches. Despite medical reassurance and extensive diagnostic workups and tests that have revealed no physical basis for his symptoms, he continues to be preoccupied with the belief that he is seriously ill. He holds a responsible job as a pharmacist, is married, and is the father of two young children. Mr. Moorehead's symptoms are most characteristic of which of the following diagnostic categories?
① Hypochondriasis
② Dissociative disorder
③ Conversion disorder
④ Psychological factors affecting medical condition

63. Mr. Lidstrom has been admitted to the psychiatric unit for severe anxiety and headaches. The day after admission, he tells the nurse that he will be unable to participate in group therapy because his headaches have increased. What is the most therapeutic response from the nurse?
① "You sure do complain a lot, so let's discuss what is wrong."
② "Go to your room and lie down. I'll call your doctor."
③ "You must go to group therapy. It's part of your treatment."
④ "Let's sit down and talk a bit about what group therapy involves."

64. Lorazepam (Ativan) is primarily effective in treating which of the following?
① Hallucinations
② Delusions
③ Anxiety
④ Incoherent speech

65. When teaching clients how to take lorazepam (Ativan), the nurse would *exclude* which of the following instructions?
① "Do not combine medication with alcohol."
② "If you need to take any other medication while taking this drug, consult with your physician first."
③ "Ativan decreases muscular coordination and mental alertness, so use caution when driving."
④ "Drink at least eight glasses of water daily because Ativan will dehydrate you."

66. Marcie Merle, a 36-year-old widow and mother of four children, was visiting a neighbor when her house burned down. The two oldest children, age 12 and 10, died in the fire. The baby, Cedric (8 months old), and Carlin (6 years old) survived, but they were badly burned. Four months later, Marcie is still waking at night with nightmares about the incident. She keeps remembering the sight of the firemen carrying her children out of the burning home. She cannot turn on a stove and see flames without becoming extremely anxious and scared. She visits a local mental health clinic and receives a diagnosis of posttraumatic stress disorder. When describing the fire to the nurse at the clinic, Mrs. Merle clearly leaves out part of the story. The best nursing response at this time would be to
① Encourage her to answer questions to help her remember what happened.
② Allow her to tell as much of the story as she is comfortable relating.
③ Realize that she probably does not remember those parts of the story that are not painful.
④ Tell her that she must not hold back information if she wants to improve.

67. Mr. Coleman is a father of three children and is being seen at the mental health clinic because two of his children have recently died in a car accident during which he was the driver. He is complaining of feeling guilty about the children's deaths. He says, "I wish it had been me that died." Which of these responses is most appropriate for the nurse to make?
① "Your feelings are normal for this type of accident, and we can talk more about them."
② "Your feelings are different from most parents in this type of situation, let's explore the meaning of them."
③ "Then who would take care of your surviving child?"
④ "Do you have a plan to kill yourself?"

68. Which of the following interventions would be most effective in helping parents who have experienced the death of a child?
① Join a Parents Without Partners group.
② Take a 2-week trip out of town.

③ Plan to go on a weekly outing.

④ Join a group of parents whose children have died.

69. A number of mental health clinics have emergency crisis intervention teams to provide immediate care to reduce the incidence of posttraumatic stress disorder. According to the community health model, this is an example of which of the following?
    ① Primary prevention
    ② Secondary prevention
    ③ Tertiary prevention
    ④ Early diagnostic care

70. Lydia Lemmon, age 62, is admitted to the hospital with symptoms of increasing forgetfulness, irritability, decreasing concentration, and feelings that others are out to get her. Based on the medical (Axis III) diagnosis of Alzheimer's disease, which of the following data would be most useful to obtain for immediate nursing care?
    ① Family history concerning other members with similar disorders
    ② Her previous occupation, interests, and social activities
    ③ Her past medical history
    ④ Recent major stressors in her life

71. Three of the following statements are true about Alzheimer's disease. Which one is *inaccurate?*
    ① There is degeneration of the cortex and atrophy of the cerebrum.
    ② Death usually occurs 1 to 10 years after onset.
    ③ There is progressive deterioration of intellectual function and change in personality and behavior.
    ④ The etiology of this disease is well-known and documented in research findings.

72. Memory loss of recent events is the most common early symptom of Alzheimer's disease. Of the following actions, which one will probably *not* help?
    ① Answer questions repeatedly as needed using direct, short, simple sentences.
    ② Place a large calendar and boldface clock next to the client's bed.
    ③ Place the client's name in large letters outside the door to the client's room.
    ④ Remind the client of the forgetfulness.

73. Mrs. Lemmon, a 62-year-old with Alzheimer's disease, has difficulty remembering where her room is on the unit. Which of the following would best help her alleviate this problem?
    ① Paint the door to her room light pink.
    ② Assign her a peer who will help her when she gets lost.
    ③ Put her picture and her name in large letters on the door to her room.
    ④ Assign her a room next to the nurses' station so the staff can assist her as necessary.

74. Mr. Lesson is a 66-year-old man admitted to the geriatric unit. His food intake is only marginally adequate, in part because of his inability to sit at the table and concentrate for the length of time necessary to eat. Which approach would be most likely to ensure a nutritionally adequate intake?
    ① Order a pureed diet that will take him less time to eat.

    ② Feed Mr. Lesson while encouraging him to pay attention.
    ③ Order six small, nutritionally balanced meals.
    ④ Offer small amounts of food whenever he appears ready to eat.

75. Mrs. Kendall is a 74-year-old admitted to the geriatric unit because of Alzheimer's disease. During a visit, her husband asks to speak to the nurse. He tearfully tells her that his son and daughter are urging him to place Mrs. Kendall in a nursing home. Which of the following is the best response?
    ① "Your wife will eventually improve. Just be patient."
    ② "Our social service department has a list of the best nursing homes in the area that you may want to consider."
    ③ "When you are finished visiting your wife, come up to the nursing station. I'll find a quiet place where we can talk."
    ④ "I'm sure you will be able to take care of your wife at home without that much difficulty."

76. Mr. Hope, a 31-year-old client admitted to the psychiatric unit with a diagnosis of recurrent major depression with psychomotor retardation, seems less lethargic today and agrees to participate in the occupational therapy program. To help make the session most successful for Mr. Hope, the nurse would do which one of the following?
    ① Set up a large number of projects for Mr. Hope to choose from.
    ② Introduce Mr. Hope to the other clients in occupational therapy.
    ③ Structure his activities to facilitate successful completion of a small task in occupational therapy.
    ④ Stay away from the client while he is in occupational therapy so that he is free to express himself.

77. Of the following side effects, which one is *not* expected with nortriptyline (Aventyl) 100 mg daily?
    ① Blurred vision
    ② Dry mouth
    ③ Urinary retention or delayed urination
    ④ Restlessness

78. Which of the following manifestations is common in a client with major depression?
    ① Lack of cooperation with staff
    ② Flight of ideas
    ③ Increased motor activity
    ④ Pressured and tangential speech

79. Which nursing intervention is considered *inappropriate* when caring for clients with a major depressive episode?
    ① Discussing changes that are important to the client
    ② Taking responsibility for the client's physical safety
    ③ Refusing to acknowledge or discuss irrational demands
    ④ Evaluating the effect of the antidepressant medication on the client

80. When orienting Mr. Festal, a 63-year-old depressed and withdrawn widower, to the unit, which of

the following guidelines would be most appropriate?
① Ensure that he meets everyone on the unit as soon as possible.
② Accompany him to his room and stay with him, giving concise information as needed.
③ Accompany him to all activities so that he will be encouraged to participate.
④ Assign him to a room with a talkative roommate so that he will not become bored.

81. In severe, major depression, which of the following defense mechanisms is most prominent?
① Introjection
② Projection
③ Sublimation
④ Rationalization

82. Which of the following is *most often* associated with the symptoms of depression?
① Episodic substance misuse
② A problem with sexual identity
③ An unresolved parental conflict
④ A sense of real or imagined loss

83. In planning activities for the client who is depressed and withdrawn during the *initial stages* of treatment, which of the following is *most* applicable?
① Give only one activity a day to reduce social interactions.
② Prepare a schedule of activities for the client to follow each day.
③ Encourage the client to select what he wants to do each day.
④ Wait until the client indicates a willingness to participate before providing any activities.

84. During the first few days of her hospitalization, Mrs. Morgan, a 49-year-old woman experiencing a major depressive episode, comes to the dayroom when escorted, but she remains silent. Which of the following statements would be most therapeutic when approaching this client?
① "I will sit with you, Mrs. Morgan. You may wish to talk later."
② "I will sit with you, Mrs. Morgan, so that you won't hurt yourself."
③ "You won't get better if you don't talk to others, Mrs. Morgan."
④ "I will leave you alone. If you want to talk come and get me."

85. The most appropriate choice of chemotherapeutic agents for a depressed older client would be which of the following?
① The selective serotonin reuptake agent paroxetine (Paxil) 10 mg every morning
② The neuroleptic haloperidol (Haldol) 10 mg tid
③ The tricyclic amitriptyline (Elavil) 150 mg tid
④ The monoamine oxidase inhibitor phenelzine sulfate (Nardil) 50 mg tid PO

86. The possibility of suicide is a serious concern in the care of depressed clients. During which period is the client most likely to attempt suicide?
① When the client is mute and unlikely to tell anyone about it
② When the client is ready to go home

③ When the client's family goes on vacation
④ When the client's depressive symptoms begin to decrease

87. The greatest priority in caring for a client who is at risk for suicide is to do which of the following?
① Administer tranquilizers so that the client will be less suicidal.
② Monitor location and behavior constantly.
③ Avoid discussing suicide because this puts ideas into the client's head.
④ Isolate the client to prevent other clients from witnessing a possible suicide attempt.

88. Mr. Regan, a 69-year-old man who was admitted for depression, consents to a series of electroconvulsive therapy (ECT) treatments. Before the first treatment, he becomes anxious and states that he does not wish to go to the treatment room. Which of the following is the most appropriate response?
① "You'll be asleep, Mr. Regan, and won't remember anything."
② "I'll call your doctor if you want, Mr. Regan, and let him know you have suddenly changed your mind about the treatment."
③ "You don't have to go, Mr. Regan. You have the right to refuse any treatment. You seem anxious. Let's talk about it."
④ "I'll go with you, Mr. Regan, and I'll be there throughout the treatment."

89. The most common side effects of ECT include which of the following?
① Aphasia and gait difficulties
② Nausea and vomiting
③ Confusion and memory loss
④ Diarrhea and gastrointestinal distress

90. Which of the following medications is used in conjunction with ECT?
① Succinylcholine (Anectine) as a muscle relaxant
② Methohexital (Brevital) as an anesthetic
③ Atropine sulfate as an anticholinergic
④ All of the above

91. The most important advantage a depressed client gains from group therapy is
① Improved social interactions and focus on others' problems.
② Improved reality orientation.
③ Greater insight into problems through the concept of universality.
④ Greater insight and knowledge of self through feedback provided by group members.

92. One of the chief benefits of ECT is that it
① Shortens the hospitalization and follow-up periods.
② Often serves as an adjunct to psychotherapy and other treatment.
③ Decreases the need for medication and psychotherapy.
④ Enables the client to terminate psychiatric treatment.

93. Which of the following is *not* a nursing responsibility for ECT?
① Remove dentures, hairpins, and other objects.
② Administer medications, such as sedatives, as ordered.

③ Prep the client as if the client were going to the operating room.
④ Carry out the ECT treatment.

94. To deal effectively with the side effects that follow ECT, the initial nursing action would be to do which of the following?
① Reintegrate the client into the therapeutic milieu.
② Orient the client to place, time, and person.
③ Provide environmental stimulation when treatment is completed.
④ Initiate bed rest for the client for the remainder of the day.

95. Marian Helper has been admitted to a locked unit; her diagnosis is major depressive episode with history of agitation and suicidal ideation. She is a 50-year-old unemployed divorced woman. She expresses feelings of hopelessness, anger at hospitalization, and self-deprecation. She also reports persistent suicidal ideations and has a plan to "crash my car and die." After completing the initial assessment, the nurse most accurately determines that Mrs. Helper's suicidal risk is at which level?
① Low
② Medium
③ High
④ In remission

96. Which of the following is *not* a high-risk group for suicidal behavior?
① The elderly
② Adolescents
③ Clients who use alcohol and other drugs
④ Nonpsychiatric populations

97. Which of the following is *not* considered a suicide precaution?
① Searching personal effects for toxic agents (drugs or alcohol)
② Removing sharp instruments (razor blades, sewing equipment, glass bottles, and knives)
③ Removing clothes that could be made into straps (belts, stockings, and pantyhose)
④ Asking the client to remain in his or her room when feeling depressed

98. Severe depression is categorized and considered as which of the following?
① Amnestic disorder
② Mood disorder
③ Anxiety disorder
④ Personality disorder

99. All of the following are essential characteristics of a major depressive episode *except*
① Loss of interest or pleasure in activities.
② Increased sexual drive (libido).
③ Depressed, irritable mood.
④ Feelings of worthlessness.

100. Which of the following short-term goals is *not* appropriate for a client with insomnia who chooses to sleep during the day?
① Client will discuss feelings and concerns about sleep.
② Client will state an ability to sleep during the night.

③ Client will take several naps during the day.
④ Client will participate in exercise and activity in the daytime.

101. Nursing actions for insomnia should include which of the following?
① Ignore sleep patterns and complaints of insomnia because they are normal during stressful periods.
② Reassure the client that insomnia is not a serious problem.
③ Encourage short naps during the day.
④ Help the client establish a bedtime routine to promote rest and sleep.

102. Bupropion hydrochloride (Wellbutrin) is classified as which of the following?
① Selective serotonin reuptake inhibitor
② Nonserotonergic antidepressant
③ Monoamine oxidase inhibitor antidepressant
④ Anxiolytic agent

103. Which statement is correct about sertraline (Zoloft)?
① May take 2 weeks to produce an antidepressant effect
② May cause urinary frequency
③ May cause increased salivation
④ Should be taken intermittently when the client is severely depressed

104. Which of the following would *not* be an appropriate question for the nurse to ask when assessing the depressed client?
① "What do your friends think of you?"
② "How do you cope with anger?"
③ "What kinds of things are pleasurable for you?"
④ "Don't you know that it is a sin to kill yourself?"

105. Which of the following would be the most appropriate goal for a nursing diagnosis of "ineffective individual coping related to feelings of despair and anger"?
① The client will deny feelings of despair and anger.
② The client will demonstrate a happy disposition.
③ The client will voice no complaints.
④ The client will share feelings with nurse and others.

106. Which of the following actions would be *most* effective in helping a depressed client cope with painful feelings?
① Focus on the positive aspects of life.
② Discourage discussion of painful feelings.
③ Encourage social isolation so client can gather thoughts.
④ Challenge negative self-talk and overgeneralizations.

107. Mr. Ruth, a 49-year-old depressed man, is about to go home, but he refuses to discuss discharge plans. He states that he "can't go home alone, and no one wants to come live with me." Which of the following is the most appropriate action?
① Accept for now his appraisal of the situation.
② Continue working with the family and client on discharge planning.
③ Allow Mr. Ruth to discuss other topics of interest.
④ Insist that Mr. Ruth discuss discharge before he goes home.

108. Which of the following would be an *ineffective* intervention for rumination, a symptom often seen in depressed clients?
    ① Introduce communication that expands the client's limited frame of reference.
    ② Tell the client to stop ruminating about failure and to speak of positive goals.
    ③ Provide opportunities for activity and exercise.
    ④ Help the client reevaluate personal strengths and weaknesses.

109. When a depressed client becomes angry, three of the following nursing actions are appropriate. Which one is *not* appropriate?
    ① Encourage client to verbalize feelings and concerns.
    ② Use simple, direct explanations and open-ended questions.
    ③ Make plans with the client for physical activity and exercise.
    ④ Encourage the client to move to another room away from others.

110. Mr. Patterson, a 50-year-old man, is admitted to the intensive care unit. His wife tells the nurse that she recently asked the client for a divorce. She left the house yesterday to go on a 3-day business trip. Some of her meetings were canceled, and she returned home unexpectedly to find her husband unconscious. An empty bottle that had contained sleeping pills was on the bedside table. In assessing the seriousness of Mr. Patterson's suicide attempt, which of the following facts is the most important?
    ① He is unconscious.
    ② He used a potentially lethal method.
    ③ He planned the attempt for a time when he thought no rescue was possible.
    ④ He did not leave a suicide note.

111. Mr. Colledge, a 60-year-old client who tried to commit suicide with antidepressants, regains consciousness. He is in tears and tells the nurse, "I'm a failure at everything, as a man, as a husband; and I've even failed at killing myself." When interpreting this statement, which of the following is *least* likely to be correct?
    ① The client is depressed and feels guilty.
    ② The client is remorseful about the suicide attempt and is unlikely to make a second attempt.
    ③ The client is feeling hopeless, and the potential for another suicide attempt is likely.
    ④ The client is ambivalent about the suicide attempt.

112. Which of the following nursing interventions initially has the *highest* priority when caring for clients with a high suicide risk?
    ① Remove all potentially harmful items from the client's room.
    ② Allow the client to express feelings of hopelessness and helplessness.
    ③ Note the client's capabilities and strengths in order to increase self-esteem.
    ④ Assess the client closely for suicidal ideation or gestures.

113. After a week on a psychiatric unit, 32-year-old Les Miller, a man who was admitted after a suicide attempt, tells the nurse he is going to ask the physician

for a weekend pass. He is cheerful and well-groomed. What does the nurse need to know regarding this abrupt change in behavior and affect?
    ① Realize that the client is improving and discontinue suicide precautions.
    ② Realize that his first weekend at home will be difficult, and offer anticipatory guidance.
    ③ Realize that a decrease in depressive symptoms may indicate a renewed suicide potential, and monitor the client carefully.
    ④ Realize that depressed clients often have mood swings, and no intervention is probably necessary.

114. Which of the following is the most appropriate way of increasing self-esteem in depressed clients in the early stages of treatment?
    ① Suggest that the client make the bed and keep the room in order.
    ② Introduce the client to another client who is an excellent chess player and suggest that he teach the client to play.
    ③ Suggest that the client lead the evening monopoly game.
    ④ The client is an excellent seamstress; suggest that a sewing class for the other clients would be helpful.

115. Which of the following is the *least effective* way to increase independence in a depressed client?
    ① Frequently ask the client what he or she needs.
    ② Encourage the client to solve his or her own problems.
    ③ Assign the same staff to care for the client.
    ④ Encourage participation in program activities.

116. Dorothy Rush, a 53-year-old homemaker, was recently admitted to the psychiatric unit because of dramatic sleep, appetite, and concentration disturbances, subsequent weight loss of 10 pounds, and suicidal behavior over the past 2 weeks. She has also expressed feelings of hopelessness, social isolation, and somatic complaints before hospitalization. Mrs. Rush presents the typical symptoms of which of the following?
    ① Schizoid personality disorder
    ② Manic-depressive reaction, manic phase
    ③ Major depressive episode
    ④ Substance abuse

117. Which of the following is the most important nursing action for a severely depressed client?
    ① Encourage expression of feelings regarding cause of depression.
    ② Institute suicide precautions.
    ③ Encourage the client's interest in family.
    ④ Reassure the client that the physical complaints are imaginary.

118. A potential victim of suicide is most likely to commit suicide at which time?
    ① Immediately after admission
    ② At the point of deepest depression
    ③ When depressive symptoms decrease
    ④ Just before discharge

119. Of the following characteristics of monoamine oxidase inhibitors, which one should the nurse be most aware of?
    ① They are short acting.
    ② They produce profound drowsiness.

③ They cause an increase in appetite.
④ They produce potential serious drug interactions.

120. A client who is to begin electroconvulsive therapy (ECT) tells the nurse she is very afraid. The best response is which of the following?
① "Don't be afraid, your doctor has had 18 years of experience in giving ECT."
② "Do not worry, this is a very safe procedure."
③ "You do seem frightened; I will stay with you. Let's talk about it."
④ "Most people say the same thing, so you are not alone."

121. Fifty-seven-year-old Lydia Murray is admitted to the psychiatric unit with a diagnosis of major depressive disorder with agitation. Which of the following behaviors would the nurse expect to observe with this diagnosis?
① Pacing and easily angered
② Psychomotor retardation
③ Apathy and social withdrawal
④ Sleeping 10 to 12 hours a day

122. Which classification of psychotropic drugs includes sertraline (Zoloft)?
① Tricyclic antidepressants
② Monoamine oxidase inhibitors
③ Phenothiazines
④ Selective serotonin reuptake inhibitors

123. Dry mouth, constipation, and blurred vision are characteristic symptoms of the action of imipramine (Tofranil) on which of the following body systems?
① Cardiovascular system
② Endocrine system
③ Autonomic nervous system
④ Respiratory system

124. Three days after a client is started on a tricyclic antidepressant, the client still exhibits signs of agitation, anxiety, and restlessness. What is the most likely explanation for this?
① The client is not taking the medication.
② The client is not responding to the medication.
③ Therapeutic effects of these agents occur in 4 to 6 weeks.
④ The dosage is too small to be effective.

125. A client refuses to take the next scheduled dose of the antidepressant because the side effects are too annoying. Which of the following is the *most appropriate* nursing intervention?
① Tell the client that skipping one dose is not important.
② Explain that the side effects might diminish in a few days.
③ Ask the client to discuss the side effects with the physician.
④ Advise the client that electroconvulsive therapy is an alternative to noncompliance.

126. Lindy Perkins, age 32, is admitted to the hospital because of increasing feelings of extreme worthlessness. These problems began shortly after she learned that her husband was having an affair with her best friend. A diagnosis of major depression is made. During the initial interview, Mrs. Perkins states, "I really can't

blame him. He's such a fine person, and I'm such a terrible wife." How might the nurse best respond?
① "Everyone has good qualities, Mrs. Perkins. I'm sure you do too."
② "Tell me what makes you feel so terrible."
③ "Obviously you are not feeling well. Let's talk about it."
④ "You'll feel better about yourself after a few days in the hospital."

127. Mr. Irving was admitted to the hospital with a diagnosis of major depression with psychotic features. His symptoms appeared after his mother died. Mr. Irving's response to this situation most likely may be viewed as
① Normal, because of the severity of the precipitating stress.
② A reaction to what he perceives as a severe blow to his security.
③ The result of a maturational crisis.
④ Transitory and likely to be self-limiting.

128. Which approach would be most therapeutic in helping a depressed client develop effective decision-making skills?
① Firmly but kindly indicate that the client is expected to make decisions.
② Explain how important decision making is to the client's recovery.
③ Provide an opportunity for the client to make small decisions when ready to do so.
④ Avoid asking the client to make decisions.

129. Mr. Colby, an 80-year-old man with a diagnosis of major depression, stays in his room most of the time and is not interested in any activities or persons on the unit. Which *initial* action by the nurse would be most therapeutic?
① Allow him the time alone because it gives him some control.
② Require him to attend at least one activity per day.
③ Spend short, frequent periods of time with him.
④ Explain that becoming more active will help him feel better.

130. Which of the following explanations is the basis of preparing the client for electroconvulsive shock therapy (ECT)?
① The preparation for this is basically the same as for any procedure in which a general anesthetic is used.
② ECT is not effective in the treatment of severe depression, so clients should not get their hopes up.
③ ECT is highly controversial and is used only as a last resort.
④ ECT has no short-term side effects.

131. Most clients are anxious before they receive their first ECT treatment. Which action by the nurse would be most therapeutic?
① Administer oral lorazepam (Ativan).
② Encourage the client to sit quietly in the room and breathe deeply.
③ Take the client to the day room for a cup of coffee.
④ Remain with the client and respond to the client's concerns.

132. What nursing action would be *inappropriate* after ECT?
① Remain quietly with the client until the confusion subsides.
② Ask the client to remain in bed until the physician arrives.
③ Assess the client's orientation to time, place, and person frequently.
④ Call the client by name and reorient to the unit as soon as possible.

133. Jeremy Lord, a 14-year-old, was admitted to the day hospital with a diagnosis of conduct disorder. During the second week of treatment he says to his nurse, "I was thinking about what you said about hurting others. I think some of that is me getting nervous, but I want to talk to you about it." This statement best indicates which phase of the nurse-client relationship?
① Initiating
② Working
③ Terminating
④ Orienting

134. Gladys Moring, a 48-year-old homemaker, is admitted to the psychiatric unit with a diagnosis of major depression with psychotic features. The nurse's first priority is to
① Establish reality orientation.
② Ensure client safety.
③ Administer antidepressants.
④ Improve cognitive perceptions.

135. While interviewing Ms. Nelson, a woman with depression with psychotic features, the nurse asks what led her to consider hospitalization. Ms. Nelson says, "I'm wicked and it's God's wrath." The most appropriate therapeutic response by the nurse would be which of the following?
① "You are not wicked, Ms. Nelson."
② "What do you mean by that?"
③ "God does not punish people."
④ "We'll talk about this later."

136. A client scheduled for electroconvulsive therapy (ECT) asks the nurse what to expect. Which of the following is the most appropriate explanation to give her?
① "ECT is a relatively safe form of treatment that will reduce your depression over time."
② "Electrodes will be placed on your temples, and a light electrical shock will be delivered to your brain."
③ "The anesthesiologist will put you to sleep, and you will not feel a thing."
④ "You will be given something to help you relax, and you will not feel the actual shock."

137. After initially regaining consciousness, a client who has just had electroconvulsive therapy seems to go to sleep. What would the nurse do?
① Try to wake the client.
② Let the client sleep.
③ Summon the physician.
④ Administer a prescribed stimulant.

138. A depressed 28-year-old man is slow dressing and getting ready for breakfast. What should the nurse do?
① Permit him to take as much time as he wishes.
② Tell him that if he is late he will miss breakfast.
③ Serve breakfast in the client's room.
④ Assist him in dressing and preparing for breakfast.

139. A depressed 76-year-old man says to the nurse, "I'm really not worth all the time it takes for you to help me." What is the best response for the nurse to make?
① "Even though you feel that way, I am here to help you. I think it is worthwhile."
② "It is not healthy to think like this."
③ "Lets talk about this later since you are obviously upset."
④ "Soon you will be able to start doing more for yourself, so it won't take so much of my time."

140. After 2 weeks of treatment, Mrs. Reese, a 59-year-old homemaker who has been psychotically depressed, begins to take more responsibility for herself and expresses an interest in getting ready for discharge. What should the nurse do?
① Assess the client's current level of self-esteem.
② Institute suicide precautions.
③ Encourage her to become more involved with the activities on the ward.
④ Discuss with her denial of the long-term effects of her depression.

141. Mr. Lewis, a 68-year-old retiree who came into the hospital with a diagnosis of major depression with psychotic features, tells the nurse, "I feel guilty, now that my children are grown, because I didn't do more for them when they were little." Which is the most therapeutic response for the nurse to make?
① "What have your children done to make you feel that way?"
② "Parents often feel guilty when their children grow up."
③ "You probably did the best you could for them."
④ "What other feelings do you have toward your children besides guilt?"

142. The day before discharge, a client is late for the last interview with the nurse. When the nurse mentions the late arrival, the client blurts out, "You have no right to question me! I'm an adult." What is the best response for the nurse to make?
① "You seem angry; let's talk about anger and leaving the hospital."
② "Your behavior is inappropriate and unacceptable."
③ "Is it hard for you to think about leaving the hospital?"
④ "Being on time is part of being responsible for yourself."

143. The neurobiologic model of psychiatric illness is based on three of the following assumptions. Which assumption is *not* a tenet of this model?
① A client suffering from emotional disturbances has an illness or susceptibility.
② The illness has characteristic symptoms or syndromes.

③ Alterations in biologic processes and structures underlie most psychiatric disorders.

④ Psychiatric illness stems from social and environmental conditions.

144. Bipolar disorder, manic episode, is best explained by which of the following statements?
① High self-esteem is the core of this disorder.
② Manic behavior represents a serious treatable anxiety disorder.
③ Psychosocial factors are the basis of this disorder.
④ Complex biologic and psychosocial factors contribute to this disorder.

145. Marilyn Liston has been brought to the hospital by her husband, who states that she has become increasingly agitated and overactive during the past 2 weeks. She did not sleep last night. After admission, Mrs. Liston refuses to sit down and continues to move about rapidly, speaking in a loud, tense voice. Which of the following would be the best initial response to Mrs. Liston?
① "I'm glad to see you have so much energy today, Mrs. Liston."
② "I need you to help me pass the breakfast trays, Mrs. Liston."
③ "Let me introduce you to another new client, Mrs. Liston."
④ "I will go with you to your room, Mrs. Liston."

146. When managing manic behavior on the unit, which of the following actions would *not* be helpful?
① Suggest activities that require a long attention span.
② Attempt to minimize environmental stimuli.
③ Encourage the client to complete short projects in occupational therapy.
④ Use distraction techniques when necessary to channel attention appropriately.

147. The therapeutic blood level for lithium therapy is maintained between which of the following?
① 0.8 and 1.8 mEq/L
② 2.5 and 3.5 mEq/L
③ 5.0 and 7.5 mg/ml
④ 0.3 and 0.75 mg/ml

148. As part of a teaching plan on lithium carbonate, clients are instructed to have lithium levels determined every 1 to 3 months when they are outpatients. Which statement best describes the reason for this?
① Lithium carbonate can produce potassium and magnesium depletion.
② Triglyceride levels can increase as the lithium level increases.
③ Lithium carbonate in large quantities produces sedation resulting in safety risks.
④ A narrow margin of safety exists between therapeutic and toxic levels of lithium carbonate.

149. Mild lithium toxicity is manifested by which of the following?
① Urinary retention, increased appetite, and abdominal distention
② Dry mouth, decreased appetite, and constipation
③ Macular rash, fever, and hematuria
④ Diarrhea, muscle weakness, and polydipsia

150. Mr. Daniel is concerned about his wife, who has been hospitalized with bipolar disorder, manic episode. He asks the nurse what he can do to help his wife after discharge. Which of the following would be the most appropriate information to give Mr. Daniel?
① Get someone to stay with her, because she probably will not be stable enough to be left alone.
② While his wife receives lithium therapy, it is necessary to have her blood lithium levels monitored regularly.
③ Bipolar disorder is hereditary, so they should not have any children.
④ Ensure that she has a prescription for tranquilizers, so that she can start taking them if her symptoms of mania recur.

151. Mrs. Efiong, a client who has been newly diagnosed with bipolar disorder, manic episode, receives instructions about lithium before discharge. An understanding of these instruction is best reflected when she notifies the outpatient clinic registered nurse of which of the following?
① Vomiting and diarrhea for 48 hours
② Swollen lymph nodes
③ Dry mouth and urinary retention
④ Symptoms of a persistent dry cough

152. Johnnie Lyle, a 60-year-old investment analyst, was admitted to the psychiatric unit with a diagnosis of bipolar disorder, manic episode, and alcohol abuse. His wife left him a week ago. Two days ago, he was given a written reprimand by his work supervisor for telling several clients to sell all their stocks immediately and not to ask questions. In obtaining a family history, which of the following would the nurse most expect to find?
① Mr. Lyle had a high incidence of childhood illnesses.
② As a child he spent little time with his father.
③ His parents were divorced when he was a child.
④ He has a family history of a mood disorder.

153. Which of the following is *not* characteristic of bipolar disorder clients in a manic phase?
① Irritable and agitated mood
② Talkativeness
③ Decreased libido
④ Decreased need for sleep

154. Of the following, which is characteristic of a manic episode of bipolar disorder?
① Psychomotor retardation
② Relevant and logical thoughts
③ Social isolation and the need to be alone
④ Persecutory and grandiose delusions

155. Mr. Levy was admitted with a diagnosis of bipolar disorder. On Mr. Levy's admission, his daughter said to the nursing staff, "He's been really tough to handle. I hope you can calm him down, because I sure can't." Which of the following responses would be most helpful at this time?
① "You must really be fed up. I've never seen anyone this maniacal."
② "Sounds like this has been difficult for you. Hospitalization will be very helpful to both of you."

③ "I can appreciate your embarrassment. He is really high, isn't he?"

④ "You must wonder why your father is acting aggressively in order to gain attention."

156. Mr. Byrd, a 45-year-old man with a diagnosis of bipolar disorder, manic episode, tells the nurse, "Go get your money. The banks have failed. Only I know this." In assessing Mr. Byrd's behavior, what do his remarks most likely indicate?
① Short attention span
② Irritability and uncooperativeness
③ Impaired thought processes
④ Impaired social interaction

157. The client's current medication is lithium carbonate, 300 mg qid PO. The laboratory results indicate a serum lithium level of 1.5 mEq/L. The client does not exhibit or complain of any side effects. Which nursing action is most appropriate?
① Suggest that the psychiatrist repeat the lab test.
② Withhold the next dose of lithium and notify the psychiatrist.
③ Administer the next dose of lithium.
④ Observe the client's degree of pressured speech.

158. For clients taking lithium, it is critical that the nurse assess the client's nutritional status. Lithium toxicity is most likely to occur if the client has insufficient intake of which of the following?
① Fat and carbohydrates
② Potassium and iron
③ Sodium and fluids
④ Protein

159. Which of the following is most likely to contraindicate treatment of a client with lithium?
① Kidney damage
② High suicide risk
③ High level of physical activity
④ Hyperthyroidism

160. To provide clients with bipolar disorder, manic episode, with the most therapeutic environment during hospitalization, which of the following is the most important for the nurse to provide?
① Assign the client to a semiprivate room with another client who has a similar problem.
② Assign the client to a private room.
③ Realize that the presence or absence of a roommate is not particularly important.
④ Place the client in the seclusion-quiet room and in restraints as soon as possible after admission.

161. To intervene effectively during a manic episode, when the client is talking rapidly and indicating a flight of ideas, the nursing staff would consistently remind him to do which of the following?
① Verbalize how he feels about his work and his behavior.
② Tell himself that his behavior is indicative of depression.
③ Speak more slowly so that he can be understood better.
④ Describe as many details of his problems as possible.

162. To help reduce the overt aggression demonstrated by some clients during a manic episode, the nursing staff would use three of the following measures. Which measure would *not* be indicated?
① Participation in competitive games
② Physical exercise of large muscle groups
③ Reduction in environmental stimuli
④ Administer anti agents

163. With clients who exhibit manic behaviors, client education would best include which of the following aspects?
① Recognize conditions that increase the risk of anxiety and stress.
② Teach one family member to make most major decisions for the client.
③ Encourage the client to handle business matters quickly and aggressively.
④ Teach the client and family to call the nurse when a crisis arises.

164. Which of the following would *not* be indicative of readiness for discharge of a client with bipolar disorder, manic episode?
① Active participation in self-care activities
② Working effectively with staff and getting needs met
③ Frequent expressions of anger and hostility
④ A decrease in manipulative or acting-out behaviors

165. The psychiatric–mental health nurse assesses Mrs. Liden in the emergency department. The client was hospitalized 6 months ago for bipolar disorder. She is talkative, rude, hostile, and insulting to the emergency room staff. When conducting the initial nursing assessment, the most important question to ask early in the interview is which of the following?
① "What happened when you returned to work?"
② "Are you and your husband still separated?"
③ "Have you stopped taking your lithium?"
④ "What makes it difficult for you to talk about your problem?"

166. William Brown is a 40-year-old boat salesman. He has a history of mood swings. His wife reports that over the past 2 weeks he has slept only a few hours and is constantly on the go. His supervisor is concerned about his intrusiveness and irritability and has suggested that he take a few weeks off. When assessing Mr. Browns's behavior, the nurse will most likely note which one of the following behaviors?
① Sound judgment
② Overactivity
③ Delusions of persecution
④ Hallucinations

167. During the first few days on the unit, Mr. Taylor, a 69-year-old plumber who has a history of severe mood swings, comes up to the nurse several times and says, "You're a lousy cheap nurse." How would the nurse best deal with this inappropriate statement?
① Reflect that he seems to be upset about something.
② Interpret the defense to Mr. Taylor as projection.

③ Tell him that that kind of language is unacceptable.
④ Seclude him until his speech is less offensive.

168. Clients in the manic phase of bipolar disorder may fail to eat because they
① Feel that they do not deserve to eat.
② Feel that the food is poisoned.
③ Are too busy.
④ Do not like hospital food.

169. Typically, clients with manic behaviors lose weight. Which of the following will most likely decrease further weight loss?
① Increase the size of the client's portions at each meal.
② Remain with the client at meals to ensure that he eats everything.
③ Restrict between-meal snacks so that the client will be more hungry at mealtime.
④ Provide between-meal, nutritious foods that the client can eat in a short time.

170. A client with manic behavior refuses to eat, stating that he has too much to do. Which of the following is the best nursing response?
① "Come and eat at the table."
② "Here is a sandwich for you to eat."
③ "You will be able to work later."
④ "If you do not eat you will be medicated."

171. The *chief* aim of occupational therapy for clients with overactive behavior is to
① Teach social skills for group and home living.
② Stimulate interest and interaction with other clients.
③ Provide a constructive outlet for excessive energy.
④ Provide a safe setting for confrontation and improving treatment compliance.

172. Lisa McKay is a 17-year-old mother of an 8-month-old son. The nurse is discussing the baby's progress with Mrs. McKay during a regularly scheduled visit to the well-baby clinic. Mrs. McKay expresses her frustration over her baby's recent illness and reveals her fear of harming the baby and her feelings of wanting to throw the baby to the floor. When assessing the mother's potential for child abuse, which factor from the mother's history would be most important to know?
① Whether the mother has completed high school.
② The mother's age at menarche and last menstrual period.
③ Whether the mother, as a child, was physically abused by her parents.
④ The socioeconomic status of the mother's family of origin.

173. When assessing a mother's current potential for child abuse, which factor is the most important to determine?
① Is the mother currently pregnant?
② Has the mother actually harmed the baby?
③ Did the mother want the baby at the time of birth?
④ Does the mother currently live with her spouse?

174. Which of the following describes major qualities of teenage mothers?
① They often have unrealistic expectations about the love and caring they will receive from the baby.
② They often have realistic expectations of the baby's patterns of growth and development.
③ They often have adequate knowledge about the child care, nutrition, and health needs of the baby.
④ They usually have excellent role models for parenting from their own parents.

175. Which of the following clinic-sponsored programs would be the most appropriate referral for potential or actual child abusers?
① The birth control clinic
② The nutritional counseling program
③ Early childhood development and parenting classes
④ Marital or family therapy

176. Retha Lesser is a 45-year-old married mother of four children ages 24, 22, 19, and 11. Mrs. Lesser appears at the medical clinic this morning with a bandaged forehead and a black eye. As the nurse enters the examining room, Mrs. Lesser laughs, points to her face, and says, "Look at me! My husband did this. I was in the emergency room 5 hours the other night getting patched up. He really did a good job on me this time." With that comment, Mrs. Lesser becomes sad and stares at the wall. Which of the following approaches is most appropriate when responding to Mrs. Lesser's comment?
① Respect Mrs. Lesser's need to minimize the problem and do not probe further into the issue.
② Comment that if Mrs. Lesser is not going to put a stop to this situation there is not much the nurse can do to help.
③ Acknowledge Mrs. Lesser's sadness and ask directly about the circumstances surrounding this current battering incident.
④ Assess reasons for staying in an abusive relationship.

177. The nurse's attitude toward women who remain in relationships in which multiple battering incidents occur often interferes with an objective approach to these women. Which of the following feelings are most commonly experienced by the nurse?
① Apathy and rejection
② Frustration and disappointment
③ Guilt and shame
④ Denial and repression

178. Which of the following attitudes, if conveyed by health care professionals, is most likely to inhibit self-disclosure by the battered woman?
① Indifference to the seriousness of the situation.
② Concern over the detail of the situation.
③ Interest in previous medical records to determine the history of the battering incidences.
④ Feeling that the survivor must get something out of being battered.

179. When planning care, which of the following is most important for a battered woman?
① A list of local crisis hotlines and battered-women's shelters.
② Referral to a psychotherapist for an in-depth evaluation and treatment.
③ Referral to assertiveness training classes for women.

④ No referral will be needed unless the battering occurs again or is witnessed by an adult.

180. Terry Lindsay, a 14-year-old boy, is admitted to an inpatient psychiatric unit with the diagnosis of conduct disorder. He has been running away from home, taking illegal drugs, and skipping classes, and now he has been arrested for shoplifting. His family is very discouraged and does not feel he can be controlled at home. The nurse assigned to Terry can expect him to behave in which of the following ways the first few days on the unit?
① He will exhibit depressed behavior.
② He will express a desire to spend most of the time alone.
③ He will tease and bait the staff.
④ He will display good interpersonal skills.

181. The acting-out behavior of adolescents with conduct disorders is primarily a way to
① Avoid or express feelings of anger or depression.
② Attempt to be liked by peers.
③ Behave like a normal teenager.
④ Deny a lack of social and intellectual abilities.

182. The most appropriate initial goal of nursing care for the adolescent who acts out will be which of the following?
① Client will sit and talk with a primary nurse for 30 minutes daily.
② Client will verbalize understanding of the family's disappointment with him.
③ Client will decrease acting-out behavior.
④ Client will increase contact with other clients.

183. The most appropriate action for early treatment of a teenager with conduct disorder would be to
① Have the client's friends visit daily.
② Have the client discuss with the nurse why his family is upset with him.
③ Set firm and consistent limits on his acting-out behavior.
④ Allow the client to act out until he is able to regain some control.

184. Miss Limmer's alcohol history indicates that during her drinking bouts, she has periods of amnesia and blackouts; when she withdraws from drinking, she has delirium tremens. Given this history, the multidisciplinary health team assigned to this client would best conclude that her alcoholism is in which stage?
① Early
② Middle
③ Late or chronic
④ Recovered

185. When dealing with a possibly aggressive client, nursing staff would use three of the following alternatives to restraints and seclusion. Which one would be inappropriate?
① Identify the anxiety (e.g., say, "You look stressed out. Tell me what is going on.").
② Encourage the client to verbalize instead of act out (e.g., "What happened during your visit with your spouse that made you so upset?").
③ Sit close to client and provide reassurance (e.g., say "Things are really not as bad as you think.").

④ Tell the client she is getting out of control and will have to be restrained if she refuses to take the prescribed medication.

186. When there is ample time to prepare to restrain a client, staff should do all of the following. If it is vital to restrain the client quickly, which component can be done after the restraint procedure?
① Obtain a physician's order for restraints.
② Remove personal articles that the client can use to harm staff.
③ Continuously assess the client's level of dangerousness.
④ Have adequate staff available to prevent client and staff injury.

187. Mr. Deeley, a 40-year-old with alcoholism, has been on a rehabilitation unit for 2 weeks. He is given a pass but returns to the unit in an agitated state. He has dilated pupils, is diaphoretic, and is experiencing vivid hallucinations and persecutory delusions. He continues to be agitated and combative for several hours. Blood is drawn for drug screening. Which of the following is the most likely substance used by Mr. Deeley while on pass?
① Barbiturates
② Heroin
③ Diazepam (Valium)
④ Cocaine (crack)

188. Three of the following behaviors indicate that the goals regarding the use of physical restraints have been attained. Which one does not?
① The client tolerates physical restraints.
② The client expresses angry feelings and calms down considerably.
③ The client exhibits decreased aggression and abusive language.
④ The client agrees to cooperate and be quiet.

189. The initial treatment of a rape survivor can significantly affect the psychologic impact the assault will have on the survivor. The first information elicited from the client should be which of the following?
① Marital state of the survivor
② Survivor's perception of what occurred
③ Whether the rapist was known to her
④ How she feels about having an abortion if she becomes pregnant

190. Rape is generally considered to be an act of
① Violence.
② Pedophilia.
③ Exposure.
④ Sexual passion.

191. Which of the following statements is most often true about the reactions of significant others after rape has occurred?
① They are usually supportive and helpful to the survivor.
② They are usually apathetic because they do not empathize with the survivor.
③ They may require time and professional assistance for resolution of this crisis.
④ They may derive positive experiences by providing emotional support for the survivor.

192. Which of the following is most likely to decrease the severity of the trauma after a rape?
① Support from counseling
② Support from work colleagues
③ Support from friends
④ Support from spouse/significant others

193. Lucy Ortez, a 35-year-old electrician, is brought by the police to the emergency room. The officer tells the triage nurse that Miss Ortez called the police to report that a man had broken into her apartment and raped her. The nurse notes that Miss Ortez has several bruises and lacerations on her face and is very quiet; she gives only her name. What is the nurse's first action?
① Arrange for a gynecologic examination to assist in future legal matters.
② Suture lacerations and clean all wounds.
③ Call Miss Ortez's family.
④ Reassure Miss Ortez that she is safe and will not be harmed further.

194. In planning care for a rape survivor, the nurse's first actions should be oriented toward which of the following?
① Controlling symptoms
② Diagnosis
③ Client's response to the situation
④ Client's intellectual capacity

195. Which of the following would *not* be helpful during the early stages of crisis intervention with a rape survivor?
① Encourage the client to describe the frightening events.
② Help the client understand the response to the crisis.
③ Assess the client's thoughts of suicide.
④ Identify the client's resources and support systems.

196. The use of crisis intervention is based on several important assumptions. Which of the following is *not* characteristic of the crisis model?
① Interventions focus on here-and-now, concrete problems.
② Interventions are consistent with the client's culture and lifestyle.
③ Interventions include the client's significant others.
④ Interventions will be initiated by the nurse and not by the client.

197. Neal Collins is a 46-year-old married man who is chronically suspicious and distrusts people. In the past few months, he has become convinced that his brother is having an affair with his wife. Although he is still functioning in his position as an accountant, his family, marital, and social relationships have deteriorated. He is admitted to the hospital with a diagnosis of paranoid personality disorder. Mr. Collins demonstrates which of the following?
① Persecutory hallucinations
② Persecutory delusions
③ Persecutory illusions
④ Persecutory phobias

198. Which of the following ego-defense mechanisms are most pronounced in clients with paranoid disorders?
① Denial and projection
② Denial and repression
③ Displacement and projection
④ Displacement and repression

199. Mr. Sandburg is a 50-year-old man who is very mistrustful of others. Which nursing action would be most appropriate?
① Encourage him to participate in activities that increase interactions with clients and other personnel.
② Approach him with a smile so that he will sense positive feelings from the nursing staff.
③ Be consistent with personnel and schedules so that structure is provided for his daily activities.
④ Use touch, and sit next to him when appropriate to reinforce reality.

200. What is the *primary* reason for the use of psychotropic drugs with clients who are highly mistrustful and suspicious?
① To provide sedation and manage the client
② To reduce symptoms and increase the effectiveness of other therapies
③ To assist in developing insight into the presenting problems
④ To improve the self-esteem of clients

201. Twenty-four-year-old Ms. Leonard is taking chlorpromazine (Thorazine) 75 mg bid. The clients are going on a visit too the zoo. What information should Ms. Leonard be given regarding the side effects of her medication before she leaves?
① Wear a hat and a long-sleeved shirt.
② Report constipation and fatigue.
③ Report dry mouth and a stuffy nose.
④ Watch for signs of unusual sweating.

202. A client who has a history of suspiciousness and distrust tells the nurse, "I really have had problems trusting others all these years." Which response by the nurse is preferable during the working stage?
① "Why do you say that?"
② "With whom have you had problems trusting?"
③ "Tell me about it."
④ "What would you do differently now?"

203. What is the nurse's *first* priority in working with clients who are suspicious?
① Develop a trusting nurse-client relationship.
② Inform the client that stress can exacerbate suspiciousness.
③ Improve self-esteem.
④ Improve social functioning.

204. Mr. First, a 44-year-old man admitted because of suspiciousness, states that he consented to being admitted only to please his wife and that there is really nothing wrong with him. What is the best nursing response?
① "Surely she would not have referred you here if you didn't need help."
② "You have been creating some problems for her."
③ "The only way you will get help is if you admit you need it."
④ "What have your major stressors been lately?"

205. The nurse assigned to meet with Miss Fowler, who has a diagnosis of paranoid schizophrenia, is delayed 45 minutes by an emergency. Which of the following is the best action for the nurse to take?
① Acknowledge the lateness, but do not dwell on it.
② Explain the reason for the delay.
③ Make another appointment with the client.
④ Apologize for being late.

206. Mr. Leonard is a highly suspicious client. Two nurses are discussing his progress when the client unexpectedly walks around the corner and overhears his name. He says, "What were you saying about me?" Which is the best response for the nurse to make?
① "We were discussing your progress."
② "We often talk about clients."
③ "It would be better if we didn't talk about it."
④ "What makes you think that we are talking about you?"

207. Which indicates that a highly suspicious client is developing a trusting relationship with a nurse?
① He discusses his delusions with the nurse.
② The nurse can explain the reasons for his delusions.
③ He describes his feelings to the nurse.
④ The nurse feels more comfortable with him.

208. Lincoln Mays is 21 years old. He was found curled up in a corner under a bridge. When asked his name all he would say was "good boy." The police brought him to the psychiatric unit. According to the client's guardian, Mr. Mays has had similar episodes in the past. His condition has been managed with medication, and he has not had a psychotic episode in more than 2 years. The current episode began when he refused to continue taking prescribed medication. What should be the nurse's *initial* concern about this client?
① The client's perception of reality
② The client's physical condition
③ The client's perception of present stressors
④ The client's speech patterns

209. How can the nurse talk with a severely regressed client when the client responds with baby talk or gibberish?
① Correct the client's speech.
② Discontinue efforts to communicate with her.
③ Give simple, explicit directions.
④ Encourage the client to focus on the nurse's words.

210. Which of the following would the nurse do before administering 5 mg of IM haloperidol (Haldol)?
① Draw blood
② Do a neurologic check
③ Offer fluids
④ Take blood pressure

211. Haloperidol (Haldol), 5 mg IM every 30 minutes is prescribed for three doses. After the third dose of the medication, a severely regressed client is still agitated and hallucinating. What would the nurse do?
① Call the physician for further orders.
② Administer another dose of the medication.
③ Record the results of the medication.
④ Observe the client for an hour.

212. The best explanation for the nurse to give a client about the side effects of haloperidol (Haldol) is which of the following?
① "This medication may make you feel a little light-headed, especially in the morning, but it will help your symptoms."
② "You will probably experience considerable drowsiness with this drug, but it will help you think clearer."
③ "This medication has few side effects, and it will help you to tell what is real from what you may be imagining."
④ "You will be able to stop using this drug before very long, because it will get rid of your disordered thinking."

213. Miss Moriarity is a woman in her early thirties who has been regressed and withdrawn since entering the hospital. She appears to be listening and talking to someone. The nurse hears nothing. What is the most appropriate nursing response?
① Give her an additional dose of her antipsychotic medication.
② Ignore the behavior.
③ Contact her physician and request a seclusion order.
④ Talk with her about what she is experiencing.

214. Mrs. Vicar, a 65-year-old woman, admitted herself to the hospital after she began hearing the voices of her dead husband. She says to the nurse, "My Jerry says I shouldn't talk to you." Which of the following is the most appropriate response?
① "Your husband has been dead for over 10 years."
② "When did he say that?"
③ "The more you talk like this the more confused you will feel."
④ "I know that this is real to you. It would be helpful for us to talk about it."

215. Of the following, which is the most appropriate way to get a client who is psychotic and withdrawn to participate in recreational activity?
① Determine a list of competitive sports, and find ways for the client to join other clients in one of them.
② Assign a staff member to play checkers with the client.
③ Provide a list of available choices, and have the client select a preference.
④ Give the client time to develop an interest and initiate activity.

216. To what degree should the nurse encourage the involvement of adult clients' families in the treatment process?
① None; the client is an adult and is able to choose.
② Only as much as the client requests during the hospitalization.
③ As much as the family wants to participate.
④ Collaborate with client and family throughout the treatment process.

217. Lillie Banks was brought to the hospital by her husband. He reported that she had disrobed in the mall and had urinated on the floor. Mrs. Banks

called the nurse "Holy Mary" and said she finally was in a place where "there are lots of saints." She also whispered that God talks to her through the television. Which of the following nursing actions should be given the highest priority?
1. Concentrate on helping her relate to her husband.
2. Concentrate on helping her form a few trusting relationships.
3. Concentrate on having her improve her grooming and appearance.
4. Concentrate on getting her involved in social activities on the unit.

218. Mrs. Kravitz, a woman diagnosed with schizophrenia, says to an approaching nurse, "I don't want to talk." What is the best nursing response?
1. "That's your choice!"
2. "Why don't you want to talk to me?"
3. "There is no need to talk with me."
4. "I'll sit with you for awhile."

219. A nursing student and a 21-year-old woman with a diagnosis of schizophrenia passed a room where other nursing students and clients were involved in a grooming and makeup session. The nursing student explained to the client, "These sessions are on Tuesday and Thursday afternoons. Women learn how to apply makeup." What is the rationale for this nursing student's remark?
1. To impress the client and the instructor
2. To encourage the success of the nurse-client relationship
3. To orient the client to reality
4. To persuade the client to join the group

220. Mrs. Valle yells for the nurse. As the nurse arrives and enters her room, the client says, "Do you see? There! God is appearing." Which of the following is the best nursing response?
1. "No, I don't see him, but I understand he is real to you."
2. "He is not there. You must be imagining things."
3. "Show me where God appears to you."
4. "God is appearing?"

221. The nurse's response when a client is hallucinating is to
1. Question and challenge the content of the hallucination.
2. Tell the client to reexamine feelings.
3. Give an honest reply with the focus on what the client believes to be real.
4. Tell the client that he is imagining things.

222. Mrs. Laws, a 35-year-old diagnosed with schizophrenia, has become increasingly anxious since her admission several days ago. Which behavior is Mrs. Laws most likely to demonstrate?
1. Being receptive to psychotherapy
2. Showing insight about the causes of her illness and increased willingness to participate in treatment
3. Becoming less able to focus her attention on the reality of the situation
4. Becoming less inclined to talk with her husband

223. Vincent Stalletti is admitted to the hospital because of increasing withdrawal. He moves slowly and is largely quiet and isolative. His admitting diagnosis is schizophrenia, catatonic type. The best initial goal is which of the following?
1. Client will begin to establish a trusting relationship with the nurse.
2. Client will increase his social skills and ability to communicate with others.
3. Client will increase his level of communication.
4. Client will be oriented to reality and encouraged to seek out the staff.

224. The nurse begins to establish a relationship with a client whose diagnosis is schizophrenia, catatonic type. Which of the following would be most effective in establishing communication at this time?
1. Sit quietly with the client.
2. Talk about current world problems.
3. Ask about the problems the client is experiencing now.
4. Tell the client about all of the activities on the unit.

225. Which of the following activities would be most appropriate for a client diagnosed with schizophrenia in partial remission?
1. Square dancing in the gym
2. Learning to play chess
3. Picnicking on the hospital grounds
4. Playing video games

226. After a week of therapy with thioridazine (Mellaril), the nurse notices that a woman with a diagnosis of schizophrenia walks with a shuffling gait. What action should be taken by the nurse?
1. Take the woman's blood pressure before the next dose.
2. Withhold the drug until the symptom disappears.
3. Suggest a neurologic consultation.
4. Obtain an order for an antiparkinsonian drug.

227. After the nurse has discussed an upcoming 3-week vacation, Mr. Lepold, a man hospitalized with schizophrenia, stops coming to scheduled meetings and begins spending more time alone in his room. What best explains his response?
1. He feels threatened by the closeness of their relationship.
2. He is having a cyclical exacerbation of his illness.
3. He is responding to the impending loss.
4. He no longer feels that treatment is indicated.

228. Albert Page has been admitted to the substance-abuse unit. He is 54 years old and has a history of increasing alcohol consumption over the last 35 years. He currently drinks 1½ quarts of whiskey daily. He is married, but his wife has moved out of their home because of his drinking problem. Which of the following would most likely be included in Mr. Page's admission orders?
1. High-protein diet, vitamins C and B-complex, chlordiazepoxide (Librium)
2. High-fat diet, vitamins B-complex and E, chlorpromazine (Thorazine)
3. Liquid diet, vitamins A and E, meperidine (Demerol)
4. Liquid diet, vitamins C and B-complex, phenytoin (Dilantin)

229. Prolonged use of alcohol may result in neuronal damage to the central nervous system and subsequent cognitive impairment. This may result in Korsakoff's syndrome (severe memory loss and confabulation). What is the physiologic basis of this condition?
① Encephalomalacia
② Destruction of brain tissue and often a severe deficiency of vitamin B_1 (thiamin)
③ Convulsions during withdrawal in spite of decreased alcohol consumption
④ Dystonic reaction

230. The initial signs and symptoms of alcohol withdrawal are
① Hypotension, bradycardia, and decreased salivation.
② Fever, dehydration, and convulsions.
③ Tremors, nervousness, and diaphoresis.
④ Permanent cognitive impairment and ataxia.

231. If a client experiences hallucinations during alcohol withdrawal, which would be the *most appropriate* nursing intervention?
① A quiet room and prn benzodiazepine medication
② Bed rest, soft music, and fluids
③ Hot tea every 2 hours, blood pressure check every 30 minutes, and restraints
④ Ice cream every 2 hours, blood pressure check every 15 minutes, and restraints

232. A family member asks the nurse about Al-Anon. What is the most appropriate response?
① "Al-Anon is a support group for families of alcoholics. How do you feel about joining?"
② "Al-Anon is a support group for families of alcoholics. Do you feel you need this, since you haven't been living with your husband?"
③ "Al-Anon is a support group for families of alcoholics. I'm sure you'd get a lot of help from joining."
④ "Al-Anon is a support group for families of alcoholics. Everyone who has a spouse who abuses alcohol should join."

233. The chances of persons with alcoholism becoming continuously sober are variable. Which factor is most necessary for sobriety to be maintained?
① Willingness to make amends for past behavior
② Recognition of the problem and motivation to change
③ Support from family and employer
④ Membership in Alcoholics Anonymous

234. Which drugs should *not* be taken with disulfiram (Antabuse)?
① Aspirin and acetaminophen (Tylenol)
② Most antitussive and some liquid cold preparations
③ Heart and blood pressure medications
④ Antacids and antiemetics

235. Which of the following most accurately defines Alcoholics Anonymous?
① It is a therapy group in which membership is prescribed after discharge from a substance-abuse program.
② It is a self-help group in which members acknowledge their illness and share experiences concerning their abuse and control of alcohol intake.
③ It is a self-help group led by professionals who have achieved sobriety.
④ It is a therapy group that discourages relationships outside the organization.

236. Eight months after discharge, Mr. Hicks, a 54-year-old man with a previous hospitalization for alcoholism, returns to visit. He attends AA regularly, his wife has returned to him and attends Al-Anon regularly, and he remains on the disulfiram (Antabuse) regimen. Which is the best description of Mr. Hicks?
① A person cured of alcoholism
② A person who formerly suffered alcoholism
③ A person who is recovering from alcoholism
④ A person recovered of alcoholism

237. Mr. Jonsson is a 19-year-old who was admitted to the orthopedic unit from surgery after a motorcycle accident. When the nurse enters the room to hang the IV fluid to follow the unit of blood, Mr. Jonsson says, "How about a pint of rye instead?" Which of the following is the most therapeutic response?
① "Don't you think alcohol is the last thing you need right now?"
② "It's a little early in the day for that, isn't it?"
③ "It sounds as though you feel that you could use a drink."
④ "Sorry, but liquor is not allowed in the hospital."

238. Mr. Kossler, a 26-year-old who has just returned from surgery to repair a fractured femur incurred in an automobile accident, is trying to undo his traction. What is the most appropriate nursing response?
① "The traction must be left in place, or more damage will be done to your leg. What is bothering you about it?"
② "You're in an awfully big hurry to get up. What made you try to undo your traction?"
③ "If you aren't comfortable, maybe I can get you some sedation."
④ "The traction is necessary to immobilize your leg, so that it can heal. You must leave it alone."

239. Fifty-five-year-old Mr. Mars had surgery 12 hours ago for a compound fracture of the tibia, which he sustained in a fall in his bathroom. He seems anxious, has tremors, and is perspiring. When the nurse gives Mr. Mars an IM medication for nausea, he says, "Is that gonna put me out?" Which of the following is an appropriate nursing response?
① "Do you want to be put out?"
② "This is only for your nausea."
③ "Are you used to taking drugs?"
④ "You seem to be having a difficult time."

240. If a nurse suspects a postsurgical client is going through alcohol or drug withdrawal, what should the *initial* nursing response be?
① Call the physician and discuss the symptoms.
② Observe the client closely for worsening symptoms.
③ Arrange to transfer the client to the detoxification unit.
④ Administer the sedative prescribed and monitor.

241. Mr. Gendrich is brought to the hospital for alcohol detoxification. When the nurse enters the room, he is trying to get out of bed and is shouting, "They're all over the bed! Get me outta this bed!" Which of the following is the most *appropriate initial* nursing response?
① Gesture as if to brush off whatever Mr. Gendrich thinks he sees.
② Reassure the client that there is nothing in his bed. Talk calmly, stay with him, and orient him to his surroundings.
③ Speak in a calm voice until he has settled down; then get help to restrain him.
④ Administer a neuroleptic to deal with this psychiatric condition.

242. Mr. Markowitz is experiencing moderate alcohol withdrawal. He becomes increasingly agitated and confused. He says, "What's happening to me? Why are you keeping me here?" Which of the following is the best response?
① "We are trying to help you, but you must try to get control of yourself."
② "When was the last time you took drugs or had a drink? You seem to be going through substance withdrawal."
③ "You are having withdrawal symptoms. We are going to take care of you and help you through this."
④ "You must lower your voice and refrain from disturbing other clients. We are keeping you here because you are sick."

243. Which of the following supportive nursing measures is appropriate with clients who are acutely agitated and withdrawing from alcohol?
① Encourage exercise of large muscles.
② Assess hydration and offer fluids if dehydrated.
③ Provide distractions, such as television or radio.
④ Give mild, natural stimulants, such as coffee or tea.

244. Mr. Jackabee is suffering chronic alcoholism and had his first withdrawal experience 3 days ago. He says to the nurse, "I've been a heavy drinker since high school and I never went through withdrawal before. This is it! I'm giving the booze up for good!" Which of the following goals has *highest* priority for the client?
① Client will admit to a drinking problem.
② Client will give up the use of alcohol permanently.
③ Client will join Alcoholics Anonymous or similar self-help group and attend meetings.
④ Client will accept the support of others to give up drinking.

245. Mr. Petty has just completed a 4-week inpatient alcohol treatment program. The evening before discharge, the nurse enters his room and finds him drinking a can of beer. How should the nurse respond?
① "It really must be difficult for you to give up drinking when you've been doing it for a long time."

② "It is so disappointing to see that you are not willing to change your habits."
③ "After all the work you've done, how can you throw it away like this?"
④ "Are you testing me to see how I'll react?"

246. A person with a history of alcoholism who is admitted for relapse states, "Even though I slipped up, I know I'm gonna be able to quit for good." What is the most appropriate nursing reply?
① "No matter how much you want to quit, it's going to be tough. How do you feel about asking for help when you need it?"
② "I'm proud that you are getting back on track. We all slip sometimes."
③ "You haven't really committed yourself to giving up drinking. You're not going to get better until you do."
④ "Don't make promises you're not ready to keep. You're the only one you hurt when you act like you did last night."

247. Lysergic acid diethylamide (LSD) fits into which of the following classifications of drugs?
① Opiates
② Barbiturates
③ Hallucinogens
④ Stimulants

248. Which of the following is *most* characteristic of lysergic acid diethylamide (LSD)?
① Heightened sensory perceptions
② Severe depression
③ Psychomotor retardation
④ Physical addiction

249. Clients who misuse substances respond best to which of the following?
① Psychoanalysis
② Behavior modification
③ Family therapy
④ Self-help groups

250. Rory Trell, a 28-year-old man, is admitted to the hospital in an acute psychotic state. Friends revealed that the client took an unknown amount of lysergic acid diethylamide (LSD). Immediately after admission to the unit, Mr. Trell's psychotic symptoms intensify. He tears at his clothes and hair, attempts to smash the television set in the dayroom with a chair, and threatens to attack another client. The *best* immediate nursing action is to
① Turn off the TV to reduce stimulation.
② Place the client in seclusion.
③ Ask the physician for a stat order for sedation.
④ Restrain the client in a chair in the dayroom.

251. Of the following reasons for the use of seclusion, which one is *not* appropriate?
① To reduce environmental stimulation
② To prevent a client from hurting himself
③ To prevent a client from hurting others
④ To reduce the need for constant observation

252. Mr. Fong, a 25-year-old man admitted in an acute psychotic state caused by ingestion of lysergic acid diethylamide (LSD), sees red spiders crawling on his

bed. Which of the following is the appropriate nursing response?
1. "Come on, Mr. Fong, you're putting me on."
2. Swat at the red spiders as if to kill them in the client's presence.
3. "I understand you believe you see the red spiders, Mr. Fong. I am not seeing any."
4. Discuss details of the hallucination with him.

253. Mr. Lambert, an acutely psychotic man, states that he is the king of Siam, and as one of his subjects, the nurse should bow in his presence. Which of the following is the most appropriate nursing response?
1. Bow and pay respect to Mr. Lambert.
2. "Being a king might make a person feel very powerful."
3. "If you're the king of Siam, I am Queen Jezebel."
4. Place him in seclusion until he is able to control himself.

254. Select the medication that best helps control hallucinations and delusions.
1. Haloperidol (Haldol)
2. Isocarboxazid (Marplan)
3. Alprazolam (Xanax)
4. Paroxetine (Paxil)

REFERENCES

AJN/Mosby nursing boards review, ed 10, St Louis, 1996, Mosby.

American Psychiatric Association: *Diagnostic and statistical manual of mental disorders,* ed 4, revised, Washington, DC, 1994, American Psychiatric Association.

Antai-Otong D: *Psychiatric nursing: biological and behavioral concepts,* Philadelphia, 1995, Saunders.

Baumann A, Johnston NE, Antai-Otong D: *Decision-making in psychiatric and psychosocial nursing,* St Louis, 1990, Decker.

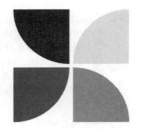

Correct Answers

1. no. 4
2. no. 2
3. no. 2
4. no. 3
5. no. 3
6. no. 1
7. no. 1
8. no. 4
9. no. 3
10. no. 2
11. no. 1
12. no. 3
13. no. 3
14. no. 3
15. no. 2
16. no. 3
17. no. 4
18. no. 2
19. no. 3
20. no. 3
21. no. 2
22. no. 3
23. no. 4
24. no. 4
25. no. 3
26. no. 2
27. no. 2
28. no. 1
29. no. 3
30. no. 4
31. no. 2
32. no. 3
33. no. 1
34. no. 2
35. no. 1
36. no. 2
37. no. 2
38. no. 2
39. no. 4
40. no. 4
41. no. 3
42. no. 2
43. no. 3
44. no. 2
45. no. 1
46. no. 4
47. no. 2
48. no. 2

49. no. 3
50. no. 3
51. no. 4
52. no. 1
53. no. 1
54. no. 3
55. no. 3
56. no. 3
57. no. 4
58. no. 3
59. no. 2
60. no. 3
61. no. 3
62. no. 1
63. no. 4
64. no. 3
65. no. 4
66. no. 2
67. no. 1
68. no. 4
69. no. 1
70. no. 2
71. no. 4
72. no. 4
73. no. 3
74. no. 3
75. no. 3
76. no. 3
77. no. 4
78. no. 1
79. no. 3
80. no. 2
81. no. 1
82. no. 4
83. no. 2
84. no. 1
85. no. 1
86. no. 4
87. no. 2
88. no. 3
89. no. 3
90. no. 4
91. no. 4
92. no. 2
93. no. 4
94. no. 2
95. no. 3
96. no. 4

97. no. 4			**158.** no. 3	
98. no. 2			**159.** no. 1	
99. no. 2			**160.** no. 2	
100. no. 3			**161.** no. 3	
101. no. 4			**162.** no. 1	
102. no. 2			**163.** no. 1	
103. no. 1			**164.** no. 3	
104. no. 4			**165.** no. 3	
105. no. 4			**166.** no. 2	
106. no. 4			**167.** no. 1	
107. no. 2			**168.** no. 3	
108. no. 2			**169.** no. 4	
109. no. 4			**170.** no. 2	
110. no. 3			**171.** no. 3	
111. no. 2			**172.** no. 3	
112. no. 1			**173.** no. 2	
113. no. 3			**174.** no. 1	
114. no. 1			**175.** no. 3	
115. no. 1			**176.** no. 3	
116. no. 3			**177.** no. 2	
117. no. 2			**178.** no. 4	
118. no. 3			**179.** no. 1	
119. no. 4			**180.** no. 3	
120. no. 3			**181.** no. 1	
121. no. 1			**182.** no. 3	
122. no. 4			**183.** no. 3	
123. no. 3			**184.** no. 3	
124. no. 3			**185.** no. 3	
125. no. 2			**186.** no. 1	
126. no. 3			**187.** no. 4	
127. no. 2			**188.** no. 4	
128. no. 3			**189.** no. 2	
129. no. 3			**190.** no. 1	
130. no. 1			**191.** no. 3	
131. no. 4			**192.** no. 4	
132. no. 2			**193.** no. 4	
133. no. 2			**194.** no. 3	
134. no. 2			**195.** no. 2	
135. no. 2			**196.** no. 4	
136. no. 4			**197.** no. 2	
137. no. 2			**198.** no. 1	
138. no. 4			**199.** no. 3	
139. no. 1			**200.** no. 2	
140. no. 1			**201.** no. 1	
141. no. 4			**202.** no. 4	
142. no. 1			**203.** no. 1	
143. no. 4			**204.** no. 4	
144. no. 4			**205.** no. 2	
145. no. 4			**206.** no. 1	
146. no. 1			**207.** no. 3	
147. no. 1			**208.** no. 2	
148. no. 4			**209.** no. 3	
149. no. 4			**210.** no. 4	
150. no. 2			**211.** no. 1	
151. no. 1			**212.** no. 1	
152. no. 4			**213.** no. 4	
153. no. 3			**214.** no. 4	
154. no. 4			**215.** no. 2	
155. no. 2			**216.** no. 4	
156. no. 3			**217.** no. 2	
157. no. 3			**218.** no. 4	

219. no. 3
220. no. 1
221. no. 3
222. no. 3
223. no. 1
224. no. 1
225. no. 3
226. no. 4
227. no. 3
228. no. 1
229. no. 2
230. no. 3
231. no. 1
232. no. 1
233. no. 2
234. no. 2
235. no. 2
236. no. 3

237. no. 3
238. no. 1
239. no. 4
240. no. 1
241. no. 2
242. no. 3
243. no. 2
244. no. 4
245. no. 1
246. no. 1
247. no. 3
248. no. 1
249. no. 4
250. no. 2
251. no. 4
252. no. 3
253. no. 2
254. no. 1

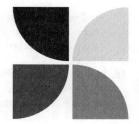

Correct Answers with Rationales

Editor's note: Three pieces of information are supplied at the end of each rationale. First, you will find a reference to a section in the *AJN/Mosby Nursing Boards Review* where a more complete discussion of the topic may be found, should you desire more information. A second reference indicates what part of the nursing process the question addresses. The third piece of information describes the appropriate client need category.

KEY TO ABBREVIATIONS

Section of the Review Book
P = Psychosocial and Mental Health Problems
T = Therapeutic Use of Self
L = Loss and Death and Dying
A = Anxious Behavior
D = Delirium, Dementia, and Amnestic and Other Cognitive Disorders
E = Elated-Depressive Behavior
PD = Personality Disorders and Other Maladaptive Behaviors
SC = Schizophrenia and Other Psychotic Behaviors
SU = Substance Use Disorders

Nursing Process Category
AS = Assessment
AN = Analysis
PL = Plan
IM = Implementation
EV = Evaluation

Client Need Category
E = Safe, Effective Care Environment
PS = Physiologic Integrity
PC = Psychosocial Integrity
H = Health Promotion and Maintenance

1. no. 4. The present interaction pattern allows the nurse to work in the here-and-now and not proceed based on preconceived ideas. Present interaction includes not only verbal aspects (who talks to whom), but also nonverbal ones (e.g., facial expressions, body movements, seating patterns). Options no. 1, no. 2, and no. 3 will be important later, once the group is established. P/T, IM, E

2. no. 2. The residents are anxious, and their response is not unusual. This is the establishing phase of the group. While the nurse may not have clearly explained the purpose of the group, a characteristic of this stage is anxiety related to uncertainty over what will actually occur in the group. The members may express anger; however, it is usually a manifestation of anxiety at the beginning of a new experience. P/T, AN, E

3. no. 2. The purpose of the group is member-to-member interaction. Option no. 2 will permit discussion and possible problem solving by the entire group. Option no. 4 singles out one resident, in effect closing the others out of the interaction. Option no. 1 is negation and false reassurance and cuts off further exploration. Option no. 3 keeps the focus on an individual rather than encouraging group interactions. Look for open-ended questions and statements. Option no. 4 challenges his feelings and might stimulate him into being defensive and guilty. P/T, IM, PC

4. no. 3. Commenting on your perceptions will allow the group members to discuss their feelings and has the potential for serving as a learning situation. Monopolizing the conversation is a group issue and should be addressed in the group, not on an individual basis. What are the dynamics occurring that allow only one person to talk? Ignoring the behavior does not help Mr. Armie learn how to be with other people appropriately. If transferred to another group, Mr. Armie might repeat the behavior, and it will give a message to other group members that exclusion can occur as a result of the decision of the facilitator alone. P/T, IM, E

5. no. 3. The client's verbal and nonverbal communications do not correspond. If she is angry and disgusted, she should not be smiling. Her words and behavior are incongruent. Mrs. Kern is not demonstrating suspicious (fear of harm from others), demanding (unnecessary and insistent requests), or resistive (unwilling to cooperate) behavior. P/T, AN, PC

6. no. 1. The best way to deal with incongruence is to point out in a nonhostile tone of voice the inconsistency observed between verbal and nonverbal communication to the client. Options no. 2, no. 3, and no. 4 do not address the incongruent behavior and are not as helpful to the client. P/T, IM, PC

7. no. 1. After the nurse has confronted her, the nurse should allow her some time to think about what was said before expecting her to respond. Rather than show concern, as in option no. 3, the nurse might do better to simply wonder why the client is silent. Option no. 2 reflects a lack of understanding about giving feedback and the need to provide the client time to reflect before responding. The suggestion of free

association (no. 4) would be more appropriate if the silence continued for a longer period of time. P/T, IM, PC

8. no. 4. The health care team can begin a plan of care based on initial assessment of the behavior. Part of the plan of care will include approaches or possible interventions for specific behaviors displayed by the client. It is most likely that options no. 2 and no. 3 have not been completed or even initiated yet. The diagnosis is provisional at this time and is based on the client's needs and behavior. P/T, PL, E

9. no. 3. Clients who become more withdrawn are frequently regarded as needing human contact. This can best be done through a one-to-one relationship, beginning at the client's level. The nurse offers physical presence, avoids probing questions, and does not demand options or premature participation. Option no. 1 attempts to engage the client in premature participation. Option no. 2 focuses on the nurse's rather than the client's feelings. Option no. 4 could make the client defensive by asking "why." Also, when people are in emotional turmoil, knowing why they are feeling the way they do is often difficult for them to understand or explain. P/L, AN, PC

10. no. 2. From the data presented, both affect and words indicate anger. "I'm sure he's really okay" would indicate denial. Bargaining would be suggested by "I would never argue with him again if he could come back." Depression would be demonstrated by crying, immobility, and inability to sleep and eat or sleeping and eating too much. Resolution would be shown by statements that acknowledge the death and view the deceased realistically. P/L, AN, PC

11. no. 1. This option provides information about the duration of the response. A commonly seen grief reaction generally resolves in 6 to 12 months and is usually resolved in 12 months. Options no. 2, no. 3, and no. 4 may be normal grief reaction statements, but they do not help to discern between normal and dysfunctional grief. P/L, AS, H

12. no. 3. The problem is denial of the loss (e.g., plans for Hawaii), which has also affected Mrs. Colby's somatic functioning (e.g., decreased sleep, loss of appetite). Because she is still grieving, this is not a prolonged reaction (no. 1). There is no evidence of anger at this stage (no. 2) or powerlessness (no. 4). P/L, AN, H

13. no. 3. The intensity and admixture of feelings during the initial grieving process may leave the client confused, sad, anxious, or guilty. Talking about feelings (ventilation) aids in recognition and resolution. Recounting the positive aspects of one's spouse occurs in the resolution stage. Educating the client to the normal grief process is important once the overwhelming feelings are explored. Option no. 4 is premature and might be experienced as negation and false reassurance, leaving the client feeling isolated and misunderstood. P/L, IM, H

14. no. 3. The client's basic physical needs must be met first. Helping the client deal with her feelings of loss and anger (no. 2) would be appropriate as her physical condition stabilizes. The staff can help the family deal with their feelings (no. 1), and the use of denial (no. 4) must be evaluated in terms of its constructiveness or destructiveness in the grieving process. P/L, PL, PC

15. no. 2. By "helpless" nonparticipation, the client has increased the chance of more staff interaction and assistance. Decubitus ulcers may result from immobility and associated stasis of blood flow. Nurses may feel anger toward client because this is not demonstrating "good client" behavior. Contractures in an already debilitated client are more likely with immobility. P/L, AN, PS

16. no. 3. The client's rejection is a defense (albeit unhealthy) against the pain and anxiety felt about the impending separation/loss. The client's behavior is not a reflection of the family's lack of empathy (no. 1) but rather a statement of the emotional pain experienced. There are no signs of moving through the grief process too quickly (no. 2), and children at very young ages are able to "sponge up" feelings. P/L, AN, H

17. no. 4. The client may be unable to achieve this physically or mentally. Nursing care measures in option no. 1 are necessary. The nurse who explores her own feelings usually gains greater awareness and self-control; thus she is able to focus more on the client's needs rather than her own needs. The presence of the nurse may be comforting and demonstrates acceptance of the client. P/L, IM, PS

18. no. 2. A client may or may not experience each of the stages of dying, in order or not. It is important for the nurse to remember the needs of the family (no. 3). A child's level of cognitive development will determine the response to death. (no. 4) P/L, AS, H

19. no. 3. To a 3-year-old, death is the same as going away for awhile. Children ages 6 to 9 personify death (someone bad carries them away). Children ages 5 to 6 believe death is reversible. Children ages 9 to 10 recognize that everyone must die. P/L, AS, H

20. no. 3. Children generally do not express their emotions or concerns in a verbal, direct manner as an adult does, especially to strangers such as the hospital staff. They are able to express their concerns better through stories, drawings, or other forms of play as indicated in options no. 1, no. 2, and no. 4. Through these media, children may state directly how they feel, or their emotions may be inferred through observation. P/L, IM, PC

21. no. 2. This approach is direct. It allows the client to talk about her feelings using broad statements. Options no. 1, no. 3, and no. 4 avoid dealing directly with Mrs. Mellin's sorrow and grief. This may foster the client's repressing her grief and developing a delayed grief reaction. P/L, IM, PC

22. no. 3. Thoughts of not wanting to live without the lost loved one are not uncommon in reactive depression, but hoarding sleep medications may indicate planning of a suicide attempt, which is an abnormal grief response. Options no. 1, no. 2, and no. 4 are common manifestations of a normal grief reaction. P/L, AS, H

23. no. 4. Although it is appropriate to offer support during the crisis period of a grief reaction, it is also im-

portant to allow clients to move through the process at their own pace. Depression is an expected stage of normal grief, and clients should be allowed to experience sorrow. Too little or too much introspection may be counterproductive. Additionally, involvement in numerous activities may delay the grief process. A "surprise" visit from a family member would not be part of a collaborative care plan. P/L, IM, PC

24. no. 4. This is the only option that initially affords the client broad openings for ventilation of affect. P/L, IM, PC

25. no. 3. This answer indicates the absence of a value judgment by the nurse, while encouraging the option of discussing the decision. Option no. 1 is a premature closure of the subject. Options no. 2 and no. 4 are judgmental statements and may elicit a defensive response to the decision rather than encouraging further consideration. All three (nos. 1, 2, and 4) discourage further discussion of her feelings. P/L, IM, H

26. no. 2. In moderate anxiety, the person's ability to perceive and concentrate is decreased. Physical discomforts increase, and overall level of functioning decreases. This client is still functioning and able to focus on work with effort, but her discomfort is increasing. At this point, the anxiety is moderate. Without intervention, it is likely to become severe, whereby the person's perceptual field is greatly reduced, sense of time is distorted, and all behavior is aimed at getting relief. During mild anxiety, the person is alert, and the perceptual field is increased. When in a panic, the person's emotional tone is associated with awe, dread, and terror. P/A, AN, PC

27. no. 2. This helps the client identify and express the feelings experienced at the time. It provides the nurse with more data to help the client recognize anxiety and begin to relate behavior to the feelings experienced. It is best in the beginning of assessment to focus on the here-and-now and start with a general perspective rather than being directive or asking about past experiences. P/A, IM, PC

28. no. 1. To establish an effective behavior-modification program, baseline data must first be collected about the behavior (e.g., frequency, amount, and time). Although options no. 2 and no. 3 are important because activities of daily living and pain contribute to the behavior, they themselves do not provide a complete picture of client behavior. Any reaction to the anesthetic already would have occurred. P/A, AS, PS

29. no. 3. Demanding clients often are afraid that they will not get the attention they need or that they will be left alone. Responding to the client at consistent intervals when the client is not demanding something will reduce the behavior and probably increase confidence that attention will be given. The underlying fears can be dealt with by checking on the client consistently and frequently. Option no. 1 reinforces the client's frequent requests. Option no. 2, offering medications to manage demanding behavior, is generally not the most effective approach, particularly when this behavior is not associated with a severe mental disorder, such as psychosis or agitation. Option no. 4 makes the client

feel guilty and does not address the underlying problem of fear of being alone or lacking attention. P/A, IM, E

30. no. 4. If demanding behavior is reinforced, it will be repeated. To change undesired behavior, reinforce more appropriate behavior. Options no. 1 through no. 3 address possible underlying dynamics for the behavior but are not considered essential for behavior change and are not as helpful for changing the behavior. P/A, PL, E

31. no. 2. During an anxiety reaction, the client thinks that something bad will happen; normal anxiety is experienced as a natural response. Both have physiologic and psychologic manifestations. Normal anxiety (no. 1) is not constant; there can be a wide range of levels, from mild to severe. An anxiety reaction can be controlled with proper interventions to reduce the level of distress (no. 3). Normal anxiety could become an anxiety reaction if stress renders normal coping mechanisms inadequate (no. 4). P/A, AS, PC

32. no. 3. The active listening techniques used in option no. 3 are reflection and restatement, which facilitate expression of feelings. Option no. 1 defends the doctor, no. 2 agrees with the client, and no. 4 is reassurance, all of which are nontherapeutic statements because they do not allow further exploration of the client's concerns and feelings. P/A, IM, PC

33. no. 1. These are the physiologic and psychologic manifestations of anxiety. Characteristics of depression are listed in option no. 2; no. 3 describes thought disorders related to psychosis; and no. 4 is also characteristic of mania and depression. P/A, AS, PC

34. no. 2. The person in panic is severely agitated, which shows in verbal and nonverbal behavior. Option no. 1 lists symptoms of psychotic behaviors; option no. 3 indicates a dissociative state. Option no. 4 is only partially correct; mood depression is not usually characteristic of a panic reaction. P/A, AS, PC

35. no. 1. Stay calm and help the client mobilize thoughts and feelings. Option no. 2, discussing early childhood issues, is inappropriate because of the immediate need to manage current symptoms. Option no. 3 is a cognitive skill that a person in panic may not be able to use. Clients in a panic state are usually experiencing fear, dread, and terror. Option no. 4, establishing rapport, is important during any nurse-client interaction, but expressing and dealing with feelings are not as significant during a panic attack as creating an immediate supportive and calm environment. P/A, IM, PC

36. no. 2. The nurse must assess the psychologic and physiologic indicators of anxiety and the client's effective use of coping mechanisms. Incoherent thought processes, mood swings, and lack of reality orientation have not been the problem. Although self-reporting is important, a more comprehensive evaluation is in order. P/A, EV, PC

37. no. 2. This is an increasingly recognized phobia. Literally "fear of the marketplace," agoraphobia is displayed by those who specifically fear being in a public place from which they feel they may not be able to escape. The "scope or territory" of what is consid-

ered the safety and security of home varies. Acrophobia is the fear of heights; astraphobia is the fear or dread of thunder and lightning; claustrophobia is the fear of closed places. P/A, AN, PC

38. no. 2. In a phobic disorder, the anxiety is displaced from the original source and then transferred, resulting in a phobia. Sublimation is a higher-order ego defense that involves the positive rechanneling of drives to a socially acceptable modality. Substitution involves replacing the original unacceptable wish, drive, emotion, or goal with one that is more acceptable. Suppression occurs when the client chooses not to think about something. P/A, AS, PC

39. no. 4. The most common behavior-modification technique used to treat phobic disorders is gradual desensitization. Under controlled conditions the client is slowly exposed to the object or situation feared. Confrontation is useful only when the client has the ability to hear the information and the readiness to work on the problem. Premature confrontation might result in panic or regression. Immediate exposure could create even greater anxiety. Distraction will not enable the client to overcome his fear and resume functioning. P/A, PL, PC

40. no. 4. Agoraphobia is classified as occurring with or without panic attacks. However, anxiety is experienced with exposure to the feared object or situation, and an anxiolytic may be prescribed at the beginning of desensitization. Fluphenazine and chlorpromazine are indicated for the treatment of psychosis. Lithium carbonate is used for bipolar disorders. P/A, IM, PS

41. no. 3. Because agoraphobia is fear of the outside, the client's presence on the volleyball court might be indicative of his increased ability to leave the hospital building. Milieu group, occupational therapy, and Sunday dinner are held on the unit in general and, although they are important elements of the treatment program, the client is still in a closed environment. P/A, EV, PC

42. no. 2. The ritualistic behavior demonstrated by the client with an obsessive-compulsive disorder is considered a symbolic attempt to control anxiety. Obsessive-compulsive behaviors may secondarily result in attention, but the behavior is an attempt to handle an anxiety-provoking situation. An obsessive-compulsive disorder reveals an uncontrollable thought and impulse pattern, and it may result in isolation. It may originate from a feeling of anxious dread and is persistently impelling, not manipulative. P/A, AN, PC

43. no. 3. Displacement of the ego-dystonic idea into an unrelated and senseless activity temporarily lowers the anxiety of the individual. By carrying out the act, the client attempts to undo the uncontrollable impulse. Counting compulsions and rituals are examples of undoing. Option no. 1: introjection is defined as a psychic representation of a loved or hated object taken into one's ego system; in projection, a person attributes to another ideas, thoughts, feelings, and impulses that are a part of his or her inner perceptions, but are unacceptable. Option no. 2: compensation is a conscious or unconscious defense mechanism by

which a person tries to make up for an imagined or real deficiency that is physical, psychologic, or both. Option no. 4: rationalization is an unconscious defense mechanism in which an irrational behavior, motive, or feeling is made to appear reasonable; suppression is a conscious defense mechanism by which a person deliberately forgets those ideas, impulses, and affects that are unacceptable. P/A, AN, PC

44. no. 2. When formulating the nursing diagnosis it is important to assess the events or circumstances that precipitate anxiety. This helps define a problem. Although the nurse would want to find out if there is a history of panic reactions (no. 1), a detailed history at this time is not appropriate. Nursing interventions should be identified (no. 3) after the nurse formulates the problem. The nurse would evaluate the nursing interventions only after defining the nursing diagnosis and actions (no. 4). P/A, AS, PC

45. no. 1. Obsessive-compulsive clients are assessed for the ritualistic behavior, possible sources of conflict in life situations, the degree to which the ritual or repetitive behavior interferes with activities of daily living, and potential unresolved conflicts. Assessment of thought patterns, associations, and delusions would be important if the nurse believed the client to be psychotic. Options no. 3 and no. 4 must always be assessed, but in determining whether or not the client has an obsessive-compulsive disorder, the nurse must first determine the client's specific daily actions. P/A, AS, PC

46. no. 4. It is necessary to reestablish and maintain physiologic integrity while working on the long-range goal of decreasing the washing behavior. If this is not focused on initially, infection could result. Option no. 1 is a higher level of functioning. Once the client has stabilized physically, it is helpful to begin working on the problem behavior. Expression of feeling is important, but understanding the causes may not be the equivalent of changing the behavior. Determining the "why" may or may not be a useful short-term goal. P/A, PL, E

47. no. 2. Plan sufficient time for the client to perform necessary rituals early in treatment; to prohibit or strictly limit this behavior would induce extreme anxiety, as would strict limit setting. Confrontation of irrationality and isolation may induce further defense of it. P/A, PL, E

48. no. 2. In dealing with ritualistic behavior, the nurse must help the client by setting limits on the destructive, repetitive behavior. Allow the client to carry out the behavior to some degree, but not to the point of injury. Options no. 1 and no. 3 are parts of the plan, but the key word that makes option no. 2 correct is *most*. The client also should be presented with reality in a matter-of-fact manner. The primary problem is not assertive behavior. Medication may be ordered to help the client with uncontrollable anxiety. P/A, PL, PC

49. no. 3. This allows some participation in a unit activity as tolerated by the client. Option no. 1 would be an overreaction by the nurse and is inappropriate. Moving the TV does not address the problem, encourages isolation, and elicits a reaction from others in the unit. Option no. 4 would likely result in the client becoming more anxious. P/A, IM, PC

50. no. 3. Abrupt cessation of ritualistic behaviors and expression of feelings are nontherapeutic because these clients are often resistent to focusing on feelings. Behavioral and cognitive therapy approaches are also useful in modifying ritualistic behaviors. Options no. 1, no. 2, and no. 4 are helpful in reducing ritualistic behaviors and promoting self-care and health maintenance. P/A, IM, PC

51. no. 4. Although medications to treat this disorder are being used, these behaviors are hard to extinguish altogether. Nursing care plans can aim at modifying or limiting ritualistic behaviors rather than attempting to eliminate them altogether. The obsessive-compulsive disorder is not a psychosis. Options no. 2 and no. 3 may be true, but initially the behavior must be controlled because of the threat to physical integrity. P/A, EV, PC

52. no. 1. To evaluate nursing care for the obsessive-compulsive client, look for a decrease in the ritualistic behavior and resumption of activities of daily living, such as personal care. Thought processes regarding obsessive beliefs and self-reports of reduced anxiety must also be evaluated. P/A, EV, PC

53. no. 1. Clients with obsessive-compulsive disorders usually recognize that the behavior is senseless and receive no pleasure from the activity. Anxiety and tension are only temporarily reduced. Option no. 2 indicates some beginning insight. Options no. 3 and no. 4 indicate no insight on the part of the client. P/A, AS, H

54. no. 3. Loss of appetite is rare in anorexia. Options no. 1, no. 2, and no. 4 are all DSM-IV criteria for anorexia nervosa. P/A, AS, PC

55. no. 3. These clients are not concerned with conserving energy; rather, they typically exercise frequently in order to expend the number of calories equal to the amount they estimate are consumed. Options no. 1, no. 2, and no. 4 are all commonly manifested behaviors in clients experiencing anorexia nervosa, who demonstrate an intense interest in food and the relentless pursuit of perceived thinness. P/A, AS, PC

56. no. 3. These clients are often in life-threatening electrolyte and nutritional imbalance. Death rates from 5% to 21% among diagnosed cases have been cited in the literature. Options no. 1, no. 2, and no. 4 are all important to implement after physiologic integrity is established. P/A, IM, PS

57. no. 4. It is important to keep the client with anorexia nervosa within view of the staff for at least 1 hour after meals to discourage induction of vomiting. Options no. 1 and no. 3 promote some positive control and independence, which the client needs instead of starving herself to gain control. Option no. 2, providing support and reinforcement, allays anxiety and increases compliance. P/A, IM, E

58. no. 3. Although much is still unknown about this disorder, studies suggest complex causes, including alterations in the hypothalamus that produce aphagia and decreased body weight. These clients have little control over their sense of hunger and lack a sense of independence. Additionally, cognitive disturbances contribute to their inappropriate perception of being fat. Despite not eating they are aware of the sensation of hunger. P/A, AN, PC

59. no. 2. A desired response is followed by a desired or positive consequence. Option no. 1 is the presentation of an aversive stimulus immediately after an undesired response. Option no. 3 occurs when the removal of a stimulus strengthens the tendency to behave in a certain way. Option no. 4 is the process of transferring learning from one situation to other, similar situations. P/A, IM, PC

60. no. 3. Involvement in preparation and management of the treatment plan will help the client gain control and mastery and practice responsibility for self. Threats create a power struggle that reenacts old, familiar, and pathologic family patterns. Option no. 2 can be life threatening because about 5% to 21% of clients with anorexia nervosa die from starvation. Option no. 4 is not helpful because the core issue is control and distorted self-image, not good eating habits. Indeed, the client may be extremely knowledgeable about nutrition. P/A, IM, PC

61. no. 3. Clients with anorexia nervosa see themselves as overweight regardless of how thin they are. Even when they look in the mirror, they see themselves as fat. The most appropriate nursing response is to tell them how the nurse sees their size in a factual way without judgments or statements that may decrease their self-esteem. Options no. 1, no. 2, and no. 4 are inappropriate because they are judgmental and reduce self-esteem. P/A, IM, PC

62. no. 1. Hypochondriasis is an exaggerated concern with one's physical health although no underlying medical condition or subjective loss of function (conversion disorder) exists. Other dissociative reactions are a mechanism for minimizing or avoiding anxiety by keeping parts of the individual's experience out of conscious awareness (e.g., amnesia, fugue state, dissociative identity disorder). The client does not have an underlying medical condition arising from psychologic factors. P/A, AN, PC

63. no. 4. These clients tend to react with increased anxiety and symptoms to new and different situations. Clear and concise explanations of treatments and procedures help allay the anxiety. The focus for intervention should not be the symptom (i.e., pain) but the precipitating event (i.e., group interaction). Option no. 2 fosters avoidance of the possible stressors and encourages reliance on others to relieve the symptom (pain). Option no. 3 avoids any interaction by exerting authoritative control and sets up a possible power struggle. P/A, IM, PC

64. no. 3. Lorazepam is a short-acting anxiolytic agent used in small doses to relieve anxiety. Hallucinations, delusions, and incoherent speech would be treated with antipsychotic medication, not lorazepam. P/A, IM, H

65. no. 4. Lorazepam does not produce dehydration, and increased fluid intake is not specifically indicated. Op-

tions no. 1, no. 2, and no. 3 are true for lorazepam (Ativan). Ativan and alcohol are both central nervous system (CNS) depressants; the combination could severely depress the CNS. Ativan can cause possible interactions or toxicity when taken with other medications. P/A, IM, PS

66. no. 2. As Mrs. Merle deals with her feelings of guilt, anger, and fear, she will begin to remember the rest of the painful event. Allow her time to remember without probing. Asking questions might help the client recall additional details of the story, but it might also increase her anxiety and contribute to a sense of being overwhelmed by the situation. It is common for clients experiencing posttraumatic stress disorder to have lapses in memory regarding details that are too painful to remember. Telling the client that she is withholding information may add to her sense of frustration, anxiety, and guilt. P/A, IM, PC

67. no. 1. For those with posttraumatic stress disorder, the pain of surviving and the accompanying guilt often lead to the wish that they too had died. For many survivors, the situation can compound their guilt if they feel they should have been at the scene of the trauma or were there but survived when others did not. The client's feelings are those normally expressed in this type of situation. Option no. 3 does not convey a sense of acceptance of the feelings and adds more guilt. It is always important for the nurse to assess risk of suicide; however, option no. 4 is not sensitive to the client's feelings of guilt at that moment. P/A, IM, PC

68. no. 4. Support groups of people who have suffered similarly can be helpful in teaching clients how to deal with the situation. They can also provide a forum where the client can express feelings shared by others in an accepting atmosphere. Although activities (options no. 2 and no. 3) may be helpful to get the parents involved in life again, the support group will help in the work of grieving. Parents Without Partners (no. 1) would be a good support group after the crisis period if the parent is single. P/A, IM, H

69. no. 1. Crisis intervention, a form of primary prevention, particularly in this situation, seeks to reduce the incidence by helping people cope adaptively with normal emotional reactions. Option no. 2, secondary prevention, refers to early case finding and treatment of symptoms. Tertiary prevention aims at reducing the long-term impact resulting from psychiatric disorders and includes health restoration and maintenance through reeducation and rehabilitation programs. P/A, PL, H

70. no. 2. Knowledge of past occupations and hobbies will help keep interactions based on reality. Present medical conditions and past methods of coping with stress are more immediately useful in planning nursing care than are prior medical history and stressors. Family history would be important later in assessing previous episodes of this disorder and how they are handled. P/D, AS, PC

71. no. 4. The etiology of Alzheimer's disease is currently unknown. Blood tests confirming the disorder are under investigation. Currently, it can only be truly diagnosed by an autopsy. Options no. 1, no. 2, and no. 3 are true of Alzheimer's disease because decreased immunity or a virus attacks the tissue of the cerebral cortex, causing progressive deterioration of intellectual functioning and behavior. P/D, AN, PC

72. no. 4. Realization that memory loss is occurring often causes anxiety and depression in these clients. The first three options will help the client remain oriented to time, person, and place and maintain self-esteem and dignity for as long as possible. P/D, IM, PC

73. no. 3. Her picture and name on the door draw on long-term memory, which is more likely to remain intact in the early stages. Mrs. Lemmon would have a difficult time remembering the light-pink door because of short-term memory loss. Assigning her a buddy or placing her close to the nurses' station is likely to reinforce her feelings of dependency and loss of control. P/D, IM, E

74. no. 3. Serving smaller amounts of food at more frequent intervals will increase the probability of an adequate intake, as well as preserve the dignity of the client. A full liquid diet would not be palatable and would decrease his appetite. Feeding Mr. Lesson would decrease his self-worth because of being forced to be in an unnecessarily dependent position. Serving food whenever Mr. Lesson is ready could lead to an unbalanced diet; it is difficult to monitor the type of food and amount eaten. P/D, IM, PS

75. no. 3. This response indicates a willingness to offer support and to allow Mr. Kendall to ventilate his feelings at a difficult time. Alzheimer's disease is a degenerating illness, and she will progressively worsen. Option no. 2 is poorly timed. Mr. Kendall has not come to terms with this alternative solution. Option no. 4 reflects denial on the nurse's part. Alzheimer's disease clients require demanding around-the-clock care, which may be too difficult for an elderly person. P/D, IM, H

76. no. 3. The client with major depression has low self-esteem, feelings of worthlessness, and little physical energy. A structured, positive experience will help increase self-esteem. Setting up too many tasks will overwhelm him. Introducing Mr. Hope to other people will make him feel more self-conscious. Staying away will reinforce the withdrawal and low self-esteem. Having him express himself freely is inappropriate in occupational therapy. P/E, IM, H

77. no. 4. Restlessness is a common side effect of the antipsychotic medications and the newer selective serotonin reuptake inhibitor antidepressants, not of tricyclic antidepressants. Options no. 1, no. 2, and no. 3 are all side effects of nortriptyline, a tricyclic antidepressant. P/E, AN, PS

78. no. 1. The depressed client is likely to demonstrate anger, withdrawal, or hostility at times. These behaviors will be perceived as a lack of cooperation. The other options are seen in mania and other psychotic disorders. P/E, AS, PC

79. no. 3. Refusal may be seen as rejection of the client. Focus on the client's needs. It is important to find out which changes the client wants to make. Depressed

clients are more likely to make suicidal attempts. The nurse monitors the blood levels of the antidepressant because they have a critical therapeutic window effect, meaning that at a certain range in the blood they are most effective. P/E, IM, E

80. no. 2. The severely depressed client can best understand simple information, given slowly and directly. The presence of the nurse will be comforting to him in new surroundings. Introducing him to everyone and asking him to perform too many activities will be overwhelming. Placing him next to a talkative client would be a mismatch that would exaggerate Mr. Festal's withdrawal. P/E, IM, E

81. no. 1. The depressed client may have hostile, angry, and primitive internal introjections. Projection is a defense mechanism used in personality disorders and by clients with paranoia. Sublimation and rationalization are mature adaptive defense mechanisms used in healthier individuals. P/E, AS, PC

82. no. 4. The perception that something or someone meaningful has been lost is frequently associated with depression. Option no. 1 (episodic substance misuse), option no. 2 (sexual identity problems may be related to either adolescent adjustment problems or homosexuality), and option no. 3 (personality disorders such as antisocial personality, resulting from unresolved parental conflict) can be associated with depression, but perhaps not as commonly as a sense of loss. P/E, AN, PC

83. no. 2. A regular schedule provides structure and removes the burden of making decisions from the depressed client. Limiting the client to one activity a day is likely to reinforce feelings of inadequacy and self-absorption, thereby worsening depression. A depressed client's thinking processes are slower, subsequently interfering with adept decision making (making choices) and taking initiative in participating. P/E, IM, E

84. no. 1. Nonverbal communication may be necessary with a severely depressed client. The presence of the nurse indicates to her that she is regarded as a worthwhile person. Option no. 2 assumes that Mrs. Morgan is self-destructive. At this point, the client lacks the energy to hurt herself. Option no. 3 is a judgmental response. The nurse must accept Mrs. Morgan's discomfort and not place demands on her when she does not feel comfortable around others. Option no. 4 conveys a lack of empathy and lack of sensitivity to the needs of depressed clients. Depressed clients often lack the initiative to seek out staff. Nurses must continuously assess the needs of depressed clients while providing emotional support. P/E, IM, PC

85. no. 1. A selective serotonin reuptake inhibitor (SSRI) antidepressant is used first because there are fewer restrictions with this class of drugs. The usual daily dosage of paroxetine (Paxil) is 20 mg. Amitriptyline has sedative side effects, and the dose stated is too high for initial administration. The monoamine oxidase inhibitors, isocarboxazid and phenelzine sulfate, are generally contraindicated in the elderly and would be used only if the tricyclic antidepressants and SSRIs

did not work. Haloperidol, a neuroleptic, is not indicated for treatment of nonpsychotic depression. P/E, IM, PS

86. no. 4. When depression is severe, the client has insufficient energy to plan and execute a suicide attempt. When depressive symptoms begin to decrease, the risk of suicide is the greatest. If the client is ready to go home, there is less suicide risk depending on how the client feels about home. When the client's family goes on vacation, the client might feel more depressed as a result of being left behind but would not necessarily become suicidal. P/E, AN, E

87. no. 2. Keeping the suicidal client under constant, close observation is mandatory protection from self-inflicted harm. Tranquilizers are contraindicated while taking antidepressants and will not eliminate the suicidal ideation. Suicidal feelings should be talked about and worked through until the internalized feelings of hostility are resolved. Encouraging clients to talk about suicide does *not* put ideas into their heads. Other clients could be helpful in monitoring a suicidal client's behavior by lending support and increasing concern regarding the client's whereabouts. P/E, PL, E

88. no. 3. The nurse is demonstrating a positive attitude toward the client, reality orientation, and respect for the client's participation in his treatment and is reinforcing his right to refuse treatment. The nurse offers self and an opportunity to clarify and ventilate concerns. Mr. Regan demonstrates anxiety about the unknown; option no. 1 does not address the unknown aspects of the electroconvulsive therapy (ECT) procedure and negates his anxiety. It is true that Mr. Regan does not have to go, but at his age, ECT might be safer than monoamine oxidase inhibitors in helping him overcome his depression. In option no. 4 the nurse offers emotional support by being with him throughout treatment but does not allow the client to participate in the informed consent process by giving him the option of refusing treatment. P/E, IM, E

89. no. 3. The most common ECT side effects are confusion and memory loss for recent events. It is reassuring to the client to know that this is a temporary condition. Aphasia and gait difficulties are symptoms of serious neurologic conditions, such as vascular dementia (stroke). Nausea and vomiting are common side effects of many drugs. Diarrhea and gastrointestinal distress are common side effects of lithium carbonate. P/E, AS, PS

90. no. 4. All of these drugs may be used for the safest and most effective administration of ECT. Electroconvulsive therapy causes seizures, so a muscle relaxant is given to prevent fractures. An anesthetic is used to reduce sensations of the seizure. Atropine sulfate is used to decrease secretions and to relax smooth muscles. P/E, IM, PS

91. no. 4. Group members provide feedback for each other through a variety of responses and reactions. This improves insight and self-knowledge. Group therapy's primary purpose is not to increase socialization skills; the focus is to work on one's own problems. Improved reality orientation is done through the use of calen-

dars, clocks, name tags, and reminiscence groups. Universality, or the feeling that other people have the same problem, provides comfort that one is not alone but does not provide insight (understanding) into what causes depression. P/E, EV, H

92. no. 2. Currently, the most frequent use of ECT is to treat severe depression and serve as an adjunct to psychotherapy and other treatment. After ECT, the client often becomes more accessible to psychotherapy. A shortened hospital stay is a benefit of ECT, but not the chief benefit. After the client has had some psychotherapy, the length of hospitalization may be shortened, but follow-up care is usually required. Electroconvulsive therapy does not necessarily lessen the need for medication. P/E, PL, PC

93. no. 4. Ordinarily, hospital policies and procedures require that the physician administer the shock to the client. Some of the nurse's responsibilities during ECT are cited in options no. 1 through no. 3. P/E, IM, E

94. no. 2. Immediately after ECT the client is given the same nursing care as that of any unconscious client. The client will experience drowsiness and confusion on awakening. Orienting the client will decrease anxiety or fears. There is no reason for the client to remain in bed after vital signs have stabilized. Resumption of normal activity on the unit by the client soon after treatment places ECT in its proper perspective as one of a number of therapeutic modalities. P/E, IM, PS

95. no. 3. Mrs. Helper exhibits behaviors or symptoms that are considered at high risk for suicide: severe depression, history of suicidal ideation, hopelessness, self-deprecation, anger at hospitalization, and a suicidal plan. Her age, sex, and divorced and unemployed status also place her at high risk. P/E, AN, PC

96. no. 4. The elderly, adolescents, and clients who misuse alcohol and other drugs are statistically high-risk groups for suicidal behavior; nonpsychiatric populations are not. P/E, AS, PC

97. no. 4. Suicidal clients often have problems talking about painful feelings; they need encouragement to express their feelings and concerns about suicide and hopelessness. Options no. 1, no. 2, and no. 3 are the responsibilities of a nurse when caring for a client with high risk of suicide. Also, suicidal clients generally must be observed, and if they remain in their room may be less likely to be observed. P/E, IM, E

98. no. 2. The DSM-IV classifies depression as a mood disorder. Amnestic disorders are conditions characterized by severe memory and cognitive impairment. Anxiety disorders are conditions characterized by feelings of fear and symptoms such as palpitations, tachycardia, and tremors. Personality disorders are conditions characterized by long-standing problems with relationships and maladaptive coping behaviors. P/E, AN, PC

99. no. 2. Persons experiencing depression often have decreased sexual drive. Options no. 1 and no. 3 are essential features of major depressive episode. Feelings of worthlessness (no. 4) are often associated with major depressive episode and may vary from inadequacy to negativism.

100. no. 3. Napping in the daytime encourages increased withdrawal from social activity and also prevents the client from being tired enough to sleep through the night. Encouraging discussion of feelings and concerns will reduce anxiety associated with lack of sleep. Option no. 2 will engage client in participating in self-care. Option no. 4 provides structure and normalization of routine for the client. P/E, PL, E

101. no. 4. Helping the client establish bedtime routines to promote rest and sleep will be a learning situation to practice in the hospital and to use at home; success builds hope and self-esteem. It would not be therapeutic to ignore sleep patterns and complaints because that discounts a client's concerns. Reassurance is rarely therapeutic. Option no. 3 would defeat the goal of normalization of sleep patterns. P/E, IM, PS

102. no. 2. Wellbutrin is a new-generation nonserotonergic antidepressant. It does not fall into the other categories listed in options no. 1, no. 3, and no. 4. P/E, IM, PS

103. no. 1. Zoloft may take 2 weeks or more to produce therapeutic antidepressant effects. The other side effects are not characteristic of those found in Zoloft. Zoloft cannot be taken on an as-needed basis because like other drugs, its effectiveness depends on a therapeutic blood concentration. P/E, IM, PS

104. no. 4. This option is a close-ended, judgmental question and is not appropriate, especially for depressed clients, who judge themselves harshly anyway. The remaining options all help the nurse to establish a useful data base. P/E, AS, PC

105. no. 4. Denying feelings and complaints would not be helpful. Sharing painful feelings is vital in learning to cope with them. P/E, PL, E

106. no. 4 is an effective cognitive therapy method that challenges negative or altered cognitive distortions. This process enables the client to gain a realistic perception of the situation, thereby reducing depressive symptoms. Option no 1, focusing on the positive aspects of life, has merit but is not effective in meeting the stated goal. Options no. 2 and no. 3 are nontherapeutic nursing interventions. P/E, IM, PC

107. no. 2. Current health care trends have reduced lengths of stays and encourage client and family involvement throughout treatment. Their input into discharge planning is critical to successful treatment outcomes. Option no. 1 does not consider the significance of collaboration with the family as part of treatment and the need to maximize hospital resources. Options no. 3 and 4 work against the nurse-client relationship and undermine the client's control over his life. P/E, IM, H

108. no. 2. Rumination can be mild to severe. It can be found in obsessive, depressive, and psychotic disorders. Telling a client to stop does little good. Introducing communication that expands a narrow frame of reference will enhance interaction and redirect thinking. Providing opportunities for activity and exercise will provide structure, encourage redirection, and broaden the use of energy for clients who ruminate. Option no. 4 enhances self-awareness and self-esteem. P/E, IM, PC

109. no. 4. <u>Nondestructive, verbal outbursts of anger are a positive behavior for depressed clients as they get better.</u> Options no. 1, no. 2, and no. 3 are all appropriate communication techniques and strategies for working with all clients. P/E, IM, H

110. no. 3. Most individuals who are intent on suicide still wish very much to be rescued. The fact that Mr. Patterson tried to eliminate the possibility of rescue indicates the seriousness of the attempt and should alert the staff to the possibility of another attempt. A client may be unconscious as a result of a suicide gesture that was not intended to be serious. Many clients who are not serious use a potentially lethal method and kill themselves accidentally. Not leaving a suicide note may indicate nonintent; however, it may also indicate impulsive and serious intent. P/E, AS, PC

111. no. 2. The client's response does not indicate remorsefulness about the suicide attempt but disappointment at his ineffectiveness in carrying it out successfully. He is depressed and feeling hopeless, so the potential for another suicide attempt is great. As with most suicidal people, he is probably ambivalent about whether he wants to live or die. P/E, AN, E

112. no. 1. Although all the options are appropriate, the first priority is to protect the client from suicidal gestures. Options no. 2 and no. 3 are correct actions; however, they are not the highest priority when dealing with a high-potential suicide risk. Option no. 4 is of a higher priority and would be implemented as soon as the safety needs addressed in option no. 1 were accomplished. P/E, IM, E

113. no. 3. Any change in behavior may mean that the client has worked out a suicide plan. The apparent lifting of his depression may mean that Mr. Miller now has the energy to carry out his plan. Any client's first weekend at home is stressful, but for this client and his history, a weekend pass at this time is contraindicated, premature, and potentially dangerous. Depressed clients may have mood swings; however, the abruptness of this client's change and his request for a weekend pass must be explored and considered cautiously. P/E, AN, PC

114. no. 1. In treating low self-esteem, it is important to begin by giving clients minimal tasks that they can accomplish without failure. All the other suggestions contain the possibility of failure, are too stressful when the client is feeling helpless, or both. P/E, IM, H

115. no. 1. Constantly asking clients what they need interferes with self-exploration, conveys a lack of confidence, and increases dependency on staff. Options no. 2 and 3 promote independence through various methods. Providing opportunities to problem solve and make decisions is critical to building confidence and a sense of accomplishment. Assigning one staff facilitates a sense of security and helps build a trusting relationship. Dependence on the staff can more appropriately be dealt with by firm limit setting and encouragement to be more independent. Option no. 4 is an early attempt to reduce dependent behavior. P/E, IM, PC

116. no. 3. Sleep, appetite, and concentration disturbances, hopelessness, somatic complaints, suicidal behavior, and a sense of loss are symptoms of a major depressive episode. Middle age, a life centered on family and home, and children leaving the "nest" are other clues. Paranoid schizophrenia is characterized by a concrete and pervasive delusional system that is generally persecutory. No data are presented to suggest a history of mood swings, manic behavior, or substance abuse. P/E, AN, PC

117. no. 2. Severely depressed clients are at a high risk for suicide. Encouraging expression of feelings regarding the cause of depression is important at some point during the treatment process but is not the most important action for the severely depressed client (no. 1). Encouraging interest in the family is inappropriate at this time because self-esteem has previously been attached to the caregiving role (no. 3), and physical complaints (no. 4) are real in people who are depressed. Saying they are imaginary devalues and minimizes the client's feelings.

118. no. 3. During times of deepest depression, the client lacks the energy to plan and carry out a suicide attempt. When depression lessens, the client has energy to act on self-destructive thoughts and impulses. P/E, AS, PC

119. no. 4. Serious drug interactions occur when monoamine oxidase (MAO) inhibitors are given in combination with tricyclic antidepressants, narcotics, alcohol, anticholinergics, antidiabetic agents, barbiturates, reserpine, sympathomimetics, and dibenzepin derivatives. Option no. 1 is incorrect because these drugs are slower to act than other antidepressants. Option no. 2 is also incorrect because MAO inhibitors do not produce profound drowsiness or (no. 3) increase appetite. P/E, AS, PS

120. no. 3. This comment by the nurse acknowledges the client's fear. Staying with the client also tends to allay anxiety. Telling the client who expresses fear to not be afraid discourages expression of the feelings. Options no. 2 and no. 4 are incorrect because they minimize the importance of these feelings. P/E, IM, E

121. no. 1. Depression with agitation causes the client to be hyperactive, restless, and easily angered. Agitated depression is characterized by psychomotor restlessness, pacing, and hand wringing. Characteristic symptoms of depression with psychomotor retardation include increased sleep, decreased energy and concentration, apathy, and social withdrawal. P/E, AS, PC

122. no. 4. Sertraline (Zoloft) is a selective serotonin reuptake inhibitor antidepressant. Although the monoamine oxidase inhibitors are also antidepressants, their mode of action is distinctly different from the tricyclic antidepressants. Phenothiazines are antipsychotic medications. P/E, AN, PS

123. no. 3. Dry mouth, constipation, and blurred vision are anticholinergic responses, indicative of side effects on the autonomic nervous system. Cardiovascular and en-

docrine system side effects such as dysrhythmias and impotence can occur with imipramine (Tofranil) but are not mentioned in this question. Respiratory system reactions are uncommon. P/E, AN, PS

124. no. 3. This is a major reason for noncompliance with tricyclic antidepressants. Therapeutic effects of tricyclic antidepressants do not usually occur until after 4 to 6 weeks of therapy, and clients often become noncompliant unless instructed about this time lag. Three days is an insufficient time to judge clinical effectiveness. P/E, AN, PS

125. no. 2. The side effects of tricyclic antidepressant medications are most apparent during initiation of treatment and diminish as therapy progresses. Drug therapy requires regularity of administration for effectiveness. Although the client may discuss the side effects with her physician, it also is appropriate for the nurse to provide health teaching. It is nontherapeutic and unprofessional to threaten clients with electroconvulsive therapy. P/E, IM, H

126. no. 3. This indicates to the client that her distress was heard and permits exploration of feelings she is experiencing now. The second option asks for an explanation that the client is probably unable to give. The first option may make the client feel that the nurse is minimizing or unaware of her feelings. The client with a major depression will not feel better about herself within a few days. P/E, IM, PC

127. no. 2. One theory regarding the etiology of major depressive episodes is that symptoms reflect the individual's response to a severe threat to security (a loss). The loss may be real or imagined and is perceived by an individual such as Mr. Irving as a threat to his very being. A psychotic depression is not a normal response regardless of the severity of the precipitating stress. The incident described is a situational, not maturational, crisis. Major depressions may last for a long time and require hospitalization. P/E, AN, PC

128. no. 3. Focusing on making small decisions such as "Do you want to wear the blue blouse or red blouse?" is a first step in building confidence in decision-making skills. The client may be unable to make decisions at this time and will need assistance. Explaining the importance of decision making is premature and likely to make her feel worse. Making all decisions will keep the client regressed and dependent. P/E, IM, H

129. no. 3. Short, frequent contacts, as tolerated, will assist in establishing the nurse-client relationship. Once this is accomplished, the client can be encouraged to participate in activities on the unit. Depressed clients need human contact. Aloneness will cause further alterations in the client's thought processes. However, he may be unable to attend activities yet. Explanations about the therapeutic value of activities are not a motivator for the depressed person. P/E, IM, PC

130. no. 1. The preparation is basically the same as for any procedure in which a general anesthetic is used, because electroconvulsive therapy (ECT) produces a loss of consciousness. Include all measures (e.g., NPO, removal of dentures) necessary to preserve the safety of the client. There is continuing controversy about the use of ECT, and many myths about it persist. Clients who have not responded to adequate trials of antidepressant medication may experience a reduction of symptoms after ECT. Short-term side effects of ECT are confusion, transient memory loss, and headache. P/E, AN, E

131. no. 4. The human contact provided by remaining with the client and conversing will help lighten the anxiety. Ativan and deep breathing lessen anxiety, but more important is the client's need to express fears and to be given proper reassurance by the nurse. A client receiving ECT must not eat or drink because an anesthetic will be administered. P/E, IM, E

132. no. 2. Option no. 2, remaining in bed until the physician arrives, is inappropriate in managing the care of a client after ECT. Options no. 1, no. 3, and no. 4 are effective interventions that facilitate prompt reorientation and lessen the anxiety generated by the confusion. Some degree of confusion may persist during the day; however, observations by staff can take place in the dayroom. The client will remain in bed or on a stretcher until the client is oriented and vital signs stabilize. The client can then safely join ward activities. P/E, IM, PS

133. no. 2. The working phase is characterized by the client's confronting problems and learning alternative methods of coping and problem solving. The relationship emerges during the orientation phase, where the purpose of the nurse-client interaction is given. In the terminating phase, the client and nurse summarize and evaluate the work of the relationship and express feelings and thoughts about termination. P/E, AN, E

134. no. 2. The first priority with any depressed client is to ensure safety because of a high risk of suicide. Promoting self-esteem, reducing cognitive distortion, presenting reality consistently, and administering antidepressants to the client are important, but safety is the highest priority. P/E, PL, E

135. no. 2. Encourage the client to express feelings in a realistic manner. It also allows the nurse to further assess the client so that the client can be understood and the appropriate interventions chosen. Do not accept irrational statements. Do not argue with the client, imply that personal beliefs are true, or end conversation. The client will become more determined in holding on to this delusion if the nurse tries to argue the client out of it (no. 1). Option no. 3 implies that the client's delusion is true. Option no. 4 evades the issue and dismisses the client's concern. P/E, IM, PC

136. no. 4. Before electroconvulsive therapy, give the client accurate information in a way that does not increase anxiety. Options no. 1, no. 2, and no. 3 are accurate but raise the client's anxiety by failing to provide any reassurance. P/E, IM, E

137. no. 2. It is normal for the client to fall asleep and therefore the client need not be disturbed. There is no reason to wake the client, give a stimulant, or call the physician. P/E, IM, E

138. no. 4. Assist the client in doing activities of daily living until he is able to do them on his own. Depressed

clients have psychomotor retardation and need help in mobilizing themselves. It may be beyond a depressed client's control to be punctual every day. P/E, IM, PS

139. no. 1. Acknowledge the client's feelings without implying that they are true or shared by the nurse. The depressed client cannot alter his/her way of thinking at this point in treatment. A client may feel devalued and unimportant by options no. 2, no. 3, and no. 4. P/E, IM, PC

140. no. 1. When a client shows a change in behavior, the nurse should assess the behavior to understand the nature of the change and how to respond. Such a change might imply suicidal intent, but this cannot be determined without further questioning. Data are insufficient to warrant suicide precautions, to warrant increased participation in ward activities, or to suggest denial of the client's depression. P/E, IM, PC

141. no. 4. Expressions of guilt often conceal unexpressed resentment and anger. The client must have the opportunity to identify and verbalize such feelings. Option no. 1 focuses on the children rather than the client. Options no. 2 and no. 3 make universal conclusions about parenting and give false reassurance. P/E, IM, PC

142. no. 1. Verbalizing the implied helps identify feelings and gives the client the opportunity to express them directly. Options no. 2 and no. 4 may be perceived by the client as punitive or as reprimands. Option no. 3 asks for a yes or no response, which tends to limit expression of feelings. P/E, IM, PC

143. no. 4. The first three options are all correct. A neurobiologic model does not address social and environmental conditions. However, some practitioners may consider that these conditions have some influence on the illness. The neurobiologic model assumes that alterations in biologic processes and structures and genetic predisposition underlie major psychiatric disorders. P/E, AN, PC

144. no. 4. Modern research suggests that the cause of this disorder is associated with an interplay between alterations in neurotransmitters and complex biologic structures, genetic transmission, and psychosocial factors. Option no. 1 is inaccurate because many of these clients have low self-esteem despite delusions of grandeur. Option no. 2. is incorrect because bipolar disorder, manic episode, is a mood disorder. Option no. 3 is also inaccurate because even though psychosocial factors contribute to exacerbation or worsening of symptoms, research suggests that alterations in complex biologic processes also play a major role in this psychiatric disorder. P/E, AN, PC

145. no. 4. The presence of the nurse may facilitate client adjustment to new surroundings and personnel. A decrease in environmental stimulation is necessary for its calming effect. The overactivity of Mrs. Liston should not be rewarded, because these clients are prone to self-injury and burnout. Involving the client in activities and introducing her to new people will increase her psychomotor activity. P/E, IM, PC

146. no. 1. A short attention span is characteristic of manic behavior, and a client with bipolar disorder, manic episode, would be unable to manage activities requiring extended concentration. Decreasing stimulation, channeling energy, and using distraction techniques are calming and therapeutic for manic clients. P/E, IM, PC

147. no. 1. The therapeutic blood-level range of lithium is 0.5 to 1.5 mEq/L. Lithium levels are not measured in mg/ml, but rather in mEq/L. P/E, AS, PS

148. no. 4. The therapeutic level and toxic level of lithium are so close that blood levels must be monitored carefully. The therapeutic level is 0.5 to 1.5 mEq/L. Above 1.5 mEq/L, significant side effects can occur. The toxicity level is 2.0 to 3.0 mEq/L. Options no. 1, no. 2, and no. 3 are not the accurate laboratory values for determining lithium levels. P/E, AN, PS

149. no. 4. These are symptoms of mild lithium toxicity. Options no. 1, no. 2, and no. 3 are not characteristic of lithium toxicity. P/E, AS, PS

150. no. 2. Once the therapeutic blood level is achieved, it should be monitored at least monthly for outpatients. The prognosis for bipolar disorder, manic episode, is good, so Mrs. Daniel probably does not need anyone to stay with her. Genetic research studies suggest there is a dominant X-linked factor present for the transmission of bipolar disorder. This factor is thought to occur in families in which one or more members have had both manic and depressive episodes of bipolar disorder. The decision to have children is a decision made by the couple and is not a discussion for discharge planning. Tranquilizers are not indicated. P/E, IM, H

151. no. 1. Vomiting and diarrhea may be signs of lithium toxicity or may be due to other causes. Loss of fluid will increase the concentration of medicine in the blood and may produce toxicity. Dryness of the mouth, although a side effect of lithium, is not serious. Swollen lymph nodes and a persistent dry cough would be associated with a health problem (e.g., infection) rather than with lithium toxicity. P/E, EV, H

152. no. 4. There is thought to be a genetic component to bipolar disorder. Bipolar disorder is a biochemical imbalance and is not related to childhood illnesses. Having parents divorce during one's childhood might contribute to an unresolved grief reaction leading to chronic depression. However, this past history is usually not the cause of manic excitement. P/E, AS, PC

153. no. 4. The mania seen in such clients is thought to be an attempt to ward off an underlying depression. These clients characteristically sleep very little during a manic episode. The other options describe manifestations of hyperactivity, confused thinking, aggressiveness, and poor judgment that are characteristic of manic behavior. P/E, AS, PC

154. no. 3. Decreased libido is not a characteristic symptom of bipolar disorder, manic episode. Options no. 1, no. 2, and no. 4 are all symptoms of a manic episode of bipolar disorder, according to the DSM-IV. P/E, AS, PC

155. no. 2. Providing empathy and indicating to the son that his actions will help his father are indicated. It would not be beneficial to the son to hear that his father is worse than anyone else the staff has dealt with or to have it implied that he is not capable of caring for his father. Interpreting the father's behavior will not help at this point. Option no. 3 assumes that the son is embarrassed by his father's illness. P/E, IM, H

156. no. 3. Although Mr. Byrd may be overly talkative and irritable, may have impaired social interactions, and may have a short attention span, his remark specifically typifies the delusion of grandeur that is a disorder of thought. P/E, AN, PC

157. no. 3. Administer the upcoming dose because the normal serum-level range is 0.5 to 1.5 mEq/L. The nurse would ask for the test to be repeated or withhold the next dose if the client showed signs of toxicity. If pressured speech were present, the nurse would record the observation and inform the physician. P/E, IM, PS

158. no. 3. With insufficient sodium, lithium is retained and toxicity occurs. The body needs sodium in order to excrete lithium. Insufficient fat and carbohydrates lead to weight reduction, and eventually the dosage may need to be readjusted; however, these foods are not critical to the proper absorption and elimination of lithium. Potassium is necessary when taking diuretics, and iron is important when anemia exists. Proteins are critical when damaged tissue is present. P/E, AN, PS

159. no. 1. Kidney damage occurs in association with lithium treatment in some clients. If the client already has a problem of this type, it is more appropriate to try other medication before using lithium. Lithium may be helpful in controlling suicidal urges when the client is coming out of the depression. Physically active clients should be advised to watch fluid and sodium intake. Lithium is known to decrease the amount of circulating thyroid hormones. P/E, AS, PS

160. no. 2. Clients with bipolar disorder, manic episode, tend to be disruptive, intrusive, irritable, and sometimes quarrelsome. Throughout a hospitalization, these clients need an atmosphere of decreased stimuli, which may be best achieved in a private room. In addition, client rights necessitate as unrestrictive an atmosphere as possible. Therefore seclusion and restraints are not used unless absolutely necessary. P/E, IM, E

161. no. 3. Having the client speak more slowly may help him to focus and identify some of his difficulties. Having him verbalize his feelings will only increase his anger and mania. Insight into the nature of his illness will not be absorbed because he is not able to hear too many details at this point. Therefore he needs to have support rather than insight. Encouraging the client to describe as many details as possible will also further increase incoherence or thought disorganization. P/E, IM, PC

162. no. 1. Competitive games are stimulating and escalate aggression; therefore physical exercise of a noncompetitive nature is the more constructive way to aid the client to discharge aggressive and angry feelings. Reduction of stimuli and ventilation of feelings are also therapeutic interventions for the client during the manic phase. P/E, IM, E

163. no. 1. Recognizing signs and symptoms of escalating, excited behavior will enable the client to seek early treatment of a recurrent episode of mania. By making most major decisions, a family member would increase the client's feelings of worthlessness. Option no. 2, teaching family members to make decisions, depends on the client's level of function and should not be done routinely. When the client's decision-making skills and judgment are impaired family members must take an active role in assisting in business matters. The client and family often feel reassured when they are taught crisis intervention skills, including knowing when to call the nurse. P/E, PL, H

164. no. 3. This kind of behavior is apt to be seen on admission, not discharge. For a client to be evaluated as ready for discharge, he must be able to perform activities of daily living. Options no. 2 and no. 4 indicate that the client has changed his behavioral pattern of aggressiveness to one of assertiveness, and that he believes in himself and feels worthy of asking for his needs directly. P/E, EV, PS

165. no. 3. Although at some point options no. 1, no. 2, and no. 4 must be assessed, the most important initial determination is the degree of compliance with the medication regimen, particularly because this is the most common reason for relapse. P/E, AS, PC

166. no. 2. Overactive motor behavior, speech, and thought patterns are characteristic symptoms of bipolar disorder, manic episode. Mr. Brown is not psychotic. He has distortions of reality but no associative looseness, delusions, hallucinations, or inappropriate affect. He also shows impaired judgment in his business practices. P/E, AS, PC

167. no. 1. Thought processes of the hypomanic client move rapidly. Focusing on inappropriate language only prolongs it. Mr. White is unable to grasp the meaning of his behavior at this time or to control it even when threatened or ordered to stop. Seclusion is a drastic measure for abusive language and not helpful in reducing its occurrence. P/E, IM, PC

168. no. 3. Hyperactivity is a behavior seen in the client with bipolar disorder, manic type. Option no. 1 indicates a psychotic depression with guilty delusions. Option no. 2 would be typical behavior of a paranoid schizophrenic, and no. 4 is a possibility but is unlikely. If he were not hyperactive, he would experience his hunger and request other food. P/E, AN, PS

169. no. 4. It is unrealistic to expect manic clients to sit and eat large quantities of food. Providing nutritious snack foods will increase the client's overall intake. Keeping the client company may intensify feelings of dependency, causing anger and more hyperactivity. P/E, IM, PS

170. no. 2. High-calorie finger foods and drinks can be consumed easily while standing or moving. Clients with bipolar disorder, manic episode, are not able to sit long enough to eat and will become irritated at the suggestion of putting off work. Option no. 1 sounds like a

demand and may be interpreted as such by the client and lead to increased agitation and irritability. Option no. 4 will put the client on the defensive and not facilitate eating. P/E, IM, E

171. no. 3. The aim of occupational therapy (OT) in the care of overactive clients is providing constructive outlets for excessive energy through large muscle motor skills such as painting, drawing, and rug making on a loom provide for appropriate discharge of energy and tension. Although options no. 1, no. 2, and no. 4 are offered by OT, they are not the chief aim for overactive clients. P/E, PL, H

172. no. 3. One important determinant of abuse by parents is whether they were abused as children. Child abuse can be a learned behavior. Education, age of menarche, and socioeconomic status are not of themselves indicators of potential or actual child abuse. P/PD, AS, E

173. no. 2. One important factor in assessing the current situation is to determine if the abuse has already occurred. If this has happened, more protective measures are necessary. This is the most important fact to determine when planning care. Being pregnant, not wanting a baby at the time of birth, and living without a spouse do not indicate potential or actual child abuse. P/PD, AS, E

174. no. 1. Most teenage pregnancies result because the teenager thinks her unmet needs for love and affection can be provided by a baby. These expectations are unrealistic and lead to anger, frustration, and possible abuse when the mother realizes that the child cannot fulfill her needs. Teenagers often have a lack of knowledge about patterns of growth and development, child care, nutrition, and health needs of a baby. The pregnant teenager may not have an excellent role model for parenting from her own parents. P/PD, PL, E

175. no. 3. The most helpful program to help child abusers is one that teaches about realistic growth and development of the child and appropriate child-care and parenting skills. Contraception, nutritional counseling, or family therapy are referral needs. P/PD, IM, H

176. no. 3. The most appropriate response is to acknowledge Mrs. Lesser's feelings and then explore the incident directly. By acknowledging the sadness, the nurse shows respect for her feelings and empathizes with Mrs. Lesser's pain. By exploring the issue directly, the nurse conveys concern and caring and reduces the client's embarrassment and shame over the incident. It is important that the nurse indicate that it is acceptable to talk about this problem. Talking directly about the problem conveys confidence and a sense of control. Mrs. Lesser has acknowledged, not denied, that she has a problem. Option no. 2 fails to address the client's feelings and will increase her shame and low self-esteem. Assessment about battering is an appropriate role and responsibility of nurses. A referral for psychotherapy can be made at a later point if the client wishes. P/PD, IM, PC

177. no. 2. The most common feelings experienced by the nurse are those of frustration and disappointment that the woman continues to remain in the destructive situation. These feelings influence the nurse's ability to remain nonjudgmental and objective. If the nurse is not aware of these feelings, it is easy to give up or avoid engaging the client in problem solving and exploration of alternative methods of dealing with the situation. It is unlikely that a nurse would experience apathy and rejection. Guilt, shame, denial, and repression are feelings that usually occur in battered women, rather than being a response of the nurse. P/PD, AN, E

178. no. 4. Blaming the victim is the most common response to victims of battering. When this attitude is conveyed the victim becomes reluctant to share the details of her experience, discuss her feelings, or engage in problem solving. This attitude often leaves the victim feeling helpless and powerless. Although indifference in the nurse is nontherapeutic, blaming the victim is a more powerful deterrant to self-disclosure by battered women. Some degree of concern over the detail of the situation may promote self-disclosure by the battered woman. Inquiring into the client's history should not affect self-disclosure. P/PD, AN, E

179. no. 1. The most important information to provide is the numbers of the crisis center and the battered-women's shelter, so the victim has resources available to her if the incident occurs again or if the battered woman needs support to help her come to a decision about the situation. Assertiveness training classes and psychotherapy are usually beneficial; however, the most important and highest priority referrals are no. 1. It is neither professional nor ethical to withhold information needed by the client. Battering recurs and needs no witnesses for proof. P/PD, IM, H

180. no. 3. Teasing is a way of testing the ability of staff to handle acting-out behavior. If staff members are consistent and can control his behavior, the client will learn trust. He will need to know, also, that staff members understand his underlying fears. If these two components are present, the adolescent will be in a climate conducive to helping him learn new behavior patterns. The client's pattern of behavior is acting out and will continue until firm limits are set. None of the information indicates that he is depressed or will want to be alone much of the time. Good interpersonal skills require more self-control than Terry's behavior demonstrates. P/PD, AS, PC

181. no. 1. The acting-out behavior can provide a diversion from the overwhelming fears the adolescent experiences. It can also be a way of channeling feelings or a way of asking adults for help. Conduct disorders, however, are not a normal part of adolescence. P/PD, AN, PC

182. no. 3. The adolescent will first need to decrease his acting-out behavior. He will then be ready to move on to other treatment goals. Acting out also pushes staff and peers away, so he will be unable to interact effectively with others until he can control his behavior. Acting-out behavior is an indication of anxiety. P/PD, PL, E

183. no. 3. Limit setting is the method staff can use to provide the necessary control over acting-out behavior.

Visits from friends could be disruptive. Such a visit could be used as a reward for showing self-control. The therapy should focus on the client at this time rather than his family because he may not understand or want to know why his family is upset with him. Limit setting should extend to control of abusive language. P/PD, IM, PC

184. no. 3. Delirium tremens is characteristic of the late stage of alcoholism. In the early stage, insomnia and tremors occur. In the middle stage, blackouts, amnesia, and physical changes such as chronic gastritis and fatty infiltration of the liver occur. A recovering alcoholic is not drinking and may be able to reduce some of the health problems that occurred as a consequence of alcohol ingestion. P/PD, PL, PS

185. no. 3. Options no. 1, no. 2, and no. 4 are appropriate interventions. Identifying feelings, encouraging expression, and setting limits are therapeutic. Sitting close to the client would be avoided because many potentially violent clients perceive closeness as an invasion of their territory and as a controlling maneuver on the part of staff. In response, the client is even more likely to assault the person who comes close. P/PD, IM, E

186. no. 1. Unless options no. 2 through no. 4 are carried out, the staff or the client may be at greater risk of injury. Rarely would a physician refuse to write this order after the fact. Such an order also can be included as part of an institution's protocol for care of the potentially violent client. P/PD, IM, E

187. no. 4. Clients who have ingested barbiturates, opiates, or diazepam (Valium) would have developed a general depressant-withdrawal syndrome. Crack cocaine intoxication is associated with intense agitation, diaphoresis, dilated pupils, hypervigilence, and persecutory delusions. P/PD, AN, PS

188. no. 4. The behaviors listed in options no. 1 through no. 3 indicate that the client may be regaining control. The behavior in no. 4 is more likely a way to manipulate staff. In short, the client may be promising to behave in an unlikely way. Because each client's potential for violence must be assessed individually, factors such as history of violence, substance misuse, cognitive impairment, and psychosis must be recognized as factors that decrease impulsivity and increase the likelihood of violence. P/PD, EV, E

189. no. 2. Determination of the survivor's perception of the rape is of value initially. Marital status and identity of rapist may be contributory, but they are not the most important information. To inquire about abortion is premature unless client indicates a wish to talk about this possibility. P/PD, AS, PC

190. no. 1. Rape is not considered a crime of passion, but rather one of violent aggression. The DSM-IV defines pedophilia as sexual arousal and fantasies involving sexual acts with a preadolescent child or children. Exposing one's sexual organs when socially inappropriate is called exhibitionism. Venting anger and hostility and exercising power and control motivate the rapist, rather than sexual passion. P/PD, AN, PC

191. no. 3. It is often a crisis for the significant other as well as for the survivor. It is difficult for the significant other to perceive the survivor as unchanged, and for this reason the significant other is supportive or empathic (options no. 1 and no. 2). Although option no. 4 is a possibility, no. 3 is more likely. P/PD, AN, H

192. no. 4. This will have the most significant effect in decreasing the trauma. Some survivors develop posttraumatic stress disorder after a severe trauma such as rape. Counseling and support from work colleagues and friends who are aware of the client's plight are also important. P/PD, IM, H

193. no. 4. The client who has been raped is extremely anxious and fears being harmed. Being touched is likely to be anxiety producing. First establish rapport, and then intervene to decrease the level of anxiety by providing reassurance about safety. Attention to lacerations, wounds, and obtaining a semen specimen can be done later in the visit. The decision to notify a family member can be made later in conjunction with the client. P/PD, IM, E

194. no. 3. Survivors of rape are in crisis and experience many changes. Nursing actions that focus on behavior deal with immediate needs. The symptoms will abate as the client's anxiety decreases. The client's diagnosis and intellectual capacity have implications for care, but actions that address presenting behaviors are most important initially. P/PD, PL, E

195. no. 2. During the early stages of crisis intervention, the client will be unable to clearly understand the crisis situation; the understanding will come later. If frightening events are identified, the client will be able to regain some feelings of control. Talking relieves anxiety for many people. A rape survivor feels much shame and repulsion for what has happened to his or her body. Sometimes, the survivor feel that the rape was his or her fault and suicidal thoughts may follow. Support systems and resource identification are necessary components of crisis intervention. P/PD, IM, PC

196. no. 4. Crisis theory is founded on the assumption that all plans will be developed in collaboration with the client. The underlying philosophy is that people have the resources to help themselves. The growth-and-development philosophy that is part of crisis theory is undermined when clients are not involved in their own decision making. The client's self-esteem will be lowered and she can feel devalued if decisions are made for her. Options no. 1, no. 2, and no. 3 describe important and necessary aspects of crisis intervention. P/PD, IM, PC

197. no. 2. He has symptoms of a persecutory delusional system. The idea that his brother is attempting to steal his property is almost certainly a false belief, a misunderstanding of reality. A hallucination is an imagined sensory perception that occurs without an external stimulus. An illusion is a misinterpretation of a sensory stimulus of a real experience. A phobia is a persistent, irrational, obsessive, intense fear of a situation or an object that results in increased tension and anxiety. P/SC, AN, PC

198. no. 1. Denial and projection are most common in paranoia. In denial, a person treats obvious reality factors as though they do not exist because these factors are intolerable to the conscious mind. In projection, a person attributes his or her own unacceptable emotions and qualities to others. Repression is the involuntary, unconscious forgetting of unacceptable or painful impulses, thoughts, feelings, or acts. Displacement refers to the transferring of unacceptable feelings aroused by an object or situation to a more acceptable substitute. P/SC, AN, PC

199. no. 3. As the client becomes more socially adapted, suspiciousness lessens. Structuring activities will help promote trust and safety. Ability for group participation comes slowly, if at all. Cheerful behavior on the part of others increases the suspiciousness of the paranoid client. These clients tend to misinterpret touch, experiencing it as control, anger, or invasion of their territory or person. P/SC, IM, PC

200. no. 2. Psychotropic drugs are used to lessen symptoms (e.g., paranoia, delusions, anxiety, and psychomotor excitement) so that clients can benefit more from milieu therapy and psychotherapy. Initially, psychotropic drugs may sedate a client. However, sedation is not the intention. Psychotropic medications do not of themselves assist clients in gaining insights. They contribute indirectly to improved self-esteem by enabling the client to benefit from therapy. P/SC, AN, PS

201. no. 1. Although the symptoms listed may all be side effects of chlorpromazine, protection from photosensitivity is most appropriate because the picnic is outdoors. Constipation, dry mouth, and stuffy nose occur because of the anticholinergic effect of chlorpromazine (Thorazine). Fatigue is usually transient and relieved as dosage is adjusted and individualized for each client. Unusual sweating is not a side effect of Thorazine. P/SC, IM, PS

202. no. 4. The client's statement demonstrates insight into past behavior. This response will help the client during the working stage of the relationship to work on patterns of more acceptable behavior. The nurse's response also gives the client an opportunity to tell the nurse about people and situations that the client thinks are tolerable. Generally speaking, it is better to avoid "why" questions because many clients feel as if they are being put on the spot or do not know why (option no. 1). It is more therapeutic to focus on ways to change behavior rather than a particular person (option no. 2). Although option no. 3 leaves a broad opening for further discussion it is less appropriate during the working stage. The client needs to learn effective ways to cope with people and situations. P/SC, IM, PC

203. no. 1. The first priority in working with suspicious clients is to establish a trusting relationship so that other goals can be accomplished. The reality of the situation cannot be dealt with and insight cannot be achieved until a trusting relationship is established. The client's self-esteem and social functioning should improve because there is improvement in functioning in a one-to-one relationship with staff. P/SC, PL, E

204. no. 4. Ask questions that encourage the client to explore his situation and gain a realistic perception of the situation. Option no. 1 would be too confronting and threatening to the client. If his anxiety is kept within reasonable control, he will be better able to explore his difficulties. In no. 2, the nurse sides with the wife, which the client may experience as accusatory. Option no. 3 is likely to cause the client to hold more firmly to his delusions. P/SC, IM, PC

205. no. 2. An explanation for the lateness is most important. Establishing trust requires giving accurate information about what is happening in the client's environment. This avoids the problem of the client's drawing conclusions that support a misinterpretation of events. If the nurse merely acknowledges lateness, the client's suspiciousness may lead her to conclude that the nurse does not want to see her. The nurse will not be viewed as a reliable person if the appointment is canceled after the delay. An apology rather than an explanation could be misinterpreted. P/SC, IM, PC

206. no. 1. Communications with clients should always be honest. This is even more important with suspicious clients; communications that are not honest will contribute to the suspicious delusions. Options no. 2, no. 3, and no. 4 may raise the client's anxiety needlessly, reinforce his delusional system, and increase his suspicions of others. P/SC, IM, PC

207. no. 3. When a suspicious client is willing to share feelings with a nurse, this is evidence that a trusting relationship is being formed. His delusions are an indication of anxiety and increase with greater anxiety. Trust with the nurse is not related to an explanation of the client's delusions by the nurse. Although desirable, the nurse's feeling at ease does not necessarily indicate that the client is developing a trusting relationship with the nurse. P/SC, EV, H

208. no. 2. The highest priority in assessment of a client experiencing psychosis is to evaluate physical well-being. Such a client may be suffering from an illness or fluid or electrolyte imbalances. He also may have physical injuries either self-inflicted or from an assault. His perception of reality is also important to assess potential safety risks and reality testing and to begin to set goals and plan the client's care. Observations at the bus station may or may not provide useful information. Speech patterns may provide useful information, but no. 2 has the highest priority. P/SC, AS, PS

209. no. 3. Establishing a therapeutic relationship with clients with psychosis requires communicating, even when they seem out of touch with reality. Make directions and expectations as clear and unambiguous as possible. The client is regressed, and baby talk or gibberish is part of the regression. It would not be therapeutic or effective to deal with the client's speech problem at this time. Therapeutic verbal and nonverbal communication by a professional person is a critical need of this client. Therapeutic communication and medication, not a speech therapist, will help the client. P/SC, IM, PC

210. no. 4. The most common side effect of antipsychotic or neuroleptic drugs is hypotension. Monitoring blood pressure is necessary to ensure that appropriate measures can be taken if blood pressure falls below safe levels. Lying and standing blood pressures should be taken for orthostatic hypotension before each dose. A blood specimen and neurologic check are not necessary before administering each dose of medication. Observation of parkinsonian side effects is important throughout hospitalization but is not necessary before each of these three doses. Fluids do not need to be offered. P/SC, AS, PS

211. no. 1. Control of psychotic symptoms may require as many as 10 doses of the medication within a matter of 5 to 6 hours. If the client is not experiencing any untoward side effects, further doses probably will be ordered by the physician. A nurse cannot administer any more haloperidol without a physician's order or a protocol. The nurse must always record the client's response to medication (both desired and adverse). The point of this question is the nurse's next action. It is not necessary to observe the client for an hour but rather to assess intermittently and to ensure that the client is safe. P/SC, IM, PS

212. no. 1. Mild hypotension may be present with haloperidol and may cause light-headedness when the client arises. This symptom usually disappears after 2 to 3 weeks. The drug controls psychotic symptoms. It is unlikely that the client will experience considerable drowsiness. Option no. 3 is inaccurate; the medication does have some major side effects, and the second part of the remark could be misunderstood by the client. Clients may need medication for an extended time period. P/SC, IM, E

213. no. 4. The nurse must make an assessment before assuming a client is hallucinating. A client should not be medicated before the nursing assessment and nursing diagnosis. The nurse must not jump to conclusions. It is not helpful to the client for the nurse to ignore the behavior; assessment is necessary. If hallucinating, the client may become worse if secluded, unless someone stays with her. P/SC, IM, PC

214. no. 4. Acknowledge that hallucinations are real to the client, but encourage the client to communicate with staff present in the unit. Although option no. 1 presents reality, it is not therapeutic to the client at this time. Option no. 2 does not address a relevant issue and does not provide the client with the direction (i.e., to talk with the nurse). In option no. 3, the nurse makes an assumption but has no data on which to base this conclusion. P/SC, IM, PC

215. no. 2. A client with psychosis may be unable to make choices or engage in activities with other clients without support. Assigning a staff member gives the client an opportunity to build a relationship. The client may not yet be able to describe what sports she enjoys, make choices, engage in activities with others, or develop an interest and initiate activity. P/SC, IM, E

216. no. 4. Involving the family enables the nurse to assess the family's ability to promote continued progress

for the client. Collaboration with the client and family throughout the treatment process is critical to developing positive treatment outcomes. Options no. 1 to 3 imply that family participation is passive or secondary to effecting positive treatment outcomes. P/SC, PL, H

217. no. 2. Building a one-to-one relationship with the client with schizophrenia is extremely important. A trusting one-to-one relationship with a staff member can serve as the basis of relationships with others. Sometimes it is difficult to assign the same staff, but the client should be assigned to as few staff members as possible. Options no. 1, no. 3, and no. 4 are important aspects of care but can be successful only after the client develops a trusting relationship with the nursing staff. P/SC, PL, E

218. no. 4. Perseverance and patience are essential when working with a schizophrenic client. The nurse must continue to demonstrate interest and sincerity until the client feels able to trust the nurse in increasing ways. The other options demand more verbalization and changes in behavior that are not appropriate at this time. P/SC, IM, PC

219. no. 3. The client with schizophrenia often mistrusts and is unable to interpret reality accurately. Here the nurse is orienting the client to the environment. Immediate involvement in unit activities may be too stimulating or demanding at this time and may cause the client's anxiety to escalate unnecessarily. P/SC, IM, PC

220. no. 1. The nurse should cast doubt on the client's perceptions, while at the same time not denying the validity of the perceptions to the client. Attempts to reason with the client or argue about, challenge, or reinforce the ideas serve only to entrench them more firmly. P/SC, IM, PC

221. no. 3. See the rationale for question 220. Options no. 1, no. 2, and no. 4 could precipitate an increase in the client's level of anxiety. P/SC, AN, PC

222. no. 3. Anxiety is one of the most crucial elements in the development of psychosis. As anxiety decreases, clients become more reality oriented and more approachable, and their behavior becomes more appropriate. Insight and receptivity to supportive psychotherapy are usually not seen when there is an increase in anxiety. Option no. 4 may be true; however, she probably would initially exhibit an attention or memory deficit. P/SC, AS, PC

223. no. 1. Establishing a trusting relationship will decrease the client's anxiety and make it possible for the nurse to work toward other goals, such as increasing communication and improving social skills. P/SC, PL, E

224. no. 1. Sitting quietly will promote interpersonal contact without pressuring the client to communicate beyond his level of readiness. Options no. 2, no. 3, and no. 4 will probably result in further retreat from socialization because the client is frightened about the level of interaction the nurse is attempting. P/SC, IM, PC

225. no. 3. A picnic on the hospital grounds provides the opportunity for interaction with other clients and staff

in a noncompetitive, nondemanding setting. Options no. 1, no. 2, and no. 4 are either physically demanding or require a high level of perceptual and cognitive awareness and may result in failure, further inhibiting socialization. P/SC, IM, E

226. no. 4. Parkinsonian side effects are common with phenothiazine drugs. Unless severe, their presence is not an indication to stop the drug. Option no. 1 would be an excellent intervention if the client were experiencing orthostatic hypotension, another side effect of thioridazine. Option no. 2 will not assist the client who is experiencing extrapyramidal effects of the antipsychotic agent. A neurologic consultation would be indicated only if there were additional focal symptoms and if an antiparkinson agent did not alleviate the extrapyramidal symptoms. P/SC, IM, PS

227. no. 3. People tend to respond to current or anticipated losses as they have responded to losses in the past. Clients with schizophrenia have difficulty dealing with closeness; however, a relationship has been established, and there is an impending absence of the client's primary nurse, which the client internalizes as loss and abandonment. Schizophrenia does not have a pattern of cyclic exacerbation as in bipolar disorders; this client is responding to a well-defined, precipitating event. The client apparently does feel a need for the relationship and is subsequently withdrawing from the nurse to get ready for the perceived loss of the relationship. P/SC, AN, PC

228. no. 1. A diet with extra protein and C and B vitamins is indicated to compensate for the poor nutritional state present in many clients who misuse alcohol and other psychoactive substances. Chlordiazepoxide (Librium) reduces the severity of withdrawal symptoms and incidence of seizures. Cirrhosis of the liver, a common side effect of chronic alcoholism, necessitates a low-fat diet. Vitamin E, a fat-soluble vitamin, is stored in the body and may not be depleted. Chlorpromazine (Thorazine) has not proven to be effective in alcohol detoxification, and this client is not psychotic. Although fluids are important to counteract dehydration, emphasis should be on high protein intake to build up the depleted nutritional state. Meperidine (Demerol) is an analgesic and is contraindicated with impaired hepatic function. Routine use of phenytoin (Dilantin) in the treatment of alcohol withdrawal is inappropriate. Benzodiazepines are more appropriate to treat withdrawal seizures. Short-acting benzodiazepines, such as lorazepam, may also be used to treat these symptoms in the elderly and in clients with compromised liver function. P/SU, IM, PS

229. no. 2. Poor dietary habits of clients who misuse psychoactive substances cause severe deficiency in thiamin. This results in symptoms of Korsakoff's syndrome. Encephalomalacia, convulsions, and dystonia are consequences of impaired central nervous system functioning, not the causative factors of Korsakoff's syndrome. P/SU, AN, PS

230. no. 3. These symptoms are accompanied by nausea and increased pulse rate and blood pressure. Alcohol withdrawal results in psychomotor agitation. The symptoms in option no. 1 are a result of autonomic nervous system depression. Option no. 2 lists manifestations of alcohol withdrawal, but they are not the first symptoms observed. The symptoms in option no. 4 would not be a direct result of alcohol withdrawal but may occur as a secondary consequence (e.g., from seizures). Permanent cognitive impairment and ataxia are associated with heavy and chronic alcohol consumption. P/SU, AS, PS

231. no. 1. Provide an environment with minimal stimulation. Remaining with the client provides reassurance and decreases anxiety. Soft music is an environmental stimulus and would therefore be contraindicated. Caffeine, a stimulant found in tea, and high fat content, found in ice cream, are contraindicated in alcohol withdrawal. Restraints are necessary only if client is a safety threat to himself or others. Use of restraints should be avoided because they tend to agitate and confuse the disoriented client. Vital signs should be monitored as necessary, but the nurse should minimize intrusions to maintain a quiet and calm environment. P/SU, IM, PS

232. no. 1. The nurse gives information but provides opportunity for the family member to ventilate feelings and decide. Option no. 2 implies that only the alcoholic is affected by the disease, whereas it is insidious to the family system. Although many find Al-Anon helpful, participation is not mandatory and should be an individual consideration. P/SU, IM, H

233. no. 2. The client must acknowledge the illness and be motivated to change his pattern of living. Atonement for past behavior is not nearly as important as motivation for change of future behavior. A strong support system is helpful in facilitating recovery; however, recovery is self-dependent. P/SU, EV, H

234. no. 2. Most cough and liquid cold medicines contain varying amounts of alcohol and would cause the client to become ill if she were to combine them with disulfiram. Aspirin, acetaminophen, antacids, and laxatives are over-the-counter drugs that do not contain alcohol and therefore would not cause adverse effects. Heart and blood pressure medications, which are also prescribed by the physician, may be medically indicated. Individuals taking disulfiram (Antabuse) must learn to read product labels to ascertain if alcohol is an ingredient. P/SU, IM, PS

235. no. 2. Alcoholics Anonymous is run entirely by persons with alcoholism who have achieved or are attempting to achieve sobriety. It is not group therapy, nor is it led by professionals. It does not discourage relationships, but instead recognizes the need for support. P/SU, AN, H

236. no. 3. A client who achieves sobriety after alcohol abuse is considered to be recovering from alcoholism. Alcoholism is not curable but can be controlled. Options no. 2 and no. 4 imply a resolved disease state, whereas the potential for active alcoholism remains throughout the client's life. P/SU, AN, PC

237. no. 3. Encourage the client to talk about feelings related to his drinking, using techniques such as reflection. Avoid judgmental responses, such as no. 2, that

close off communication. Options no. 1 and no. 4 do not allow exploration of Mr. Jonsson's feelings on drinking. P/SU, IM, PC

238. no. 1. Clear explanations about treatment are appropriate. The nurse would then assess the client's status. Option no. 2 sounds judgmental. Sedation may not be indicated. Although it is good to provide explanations to a client, option no. 4 does not allow the nurse to explore the reason why Mr. Kossler undid his traction. P/SU, IM, PS

239. no. 4. Reflection encourages the client to describe how he is feeling, so the nurse can assess, analyze, and plan care appropriately. Option no. 1 is a closed question and does not encourage exploration of the client's feelings. Option no. 2 does not allow the nurse to explore with the client what he is experiencing and therefore does not provide the nurse with the necessary information to make a complete assessment. In option no. 3, the nurse is making an assumption that could make the client feel judged and prevent further exploration. P/SU, IM, PC

240. no. 1. Collaborate with the physician in order to plan appropriately. Adequate assessment has been obtained by the nurse over the course of a shift. Option no. 3 is not a nursing decision. The physician will make this decision based on the diagnosis. If the client's condition has changed, the sedative may be medically contraindicated. The physician should be alerted to any dramatic changes in client status. P/SU, IM, PS

241. no. 2. Point out reality to persons who are having hallucinations from substance withdrawal. Reassure and orient them frequently. Option no. 1 serves to reinforce Mr. Gendrich's hallucinations. A physician's order is required to apply restraints, and reassurance may be all that is needed as an initial nursing action. Nursing measures to calm and orient Mr. Gendrich should be done first. If the behavior continues, the administration of a benzodiazepine, such as Librium, may be indicated. Neuroleptic or antipsychotic agents are not part of detoxification. P/SU, IM, E

242. no. 3. Persons in withdrawal need reassurance that they will be taken care of and will not be left alone. The client is unable to control himself at this time, and it is not an appropriate time to question him about his drinking habits. P/SU, IM, PC

243. no. 2. The highest priority of these measures is to prevent dehydration, but caffeine drinks would increase agitation. Exercise would overstimulate and may be injurious to a client in withdrawal. Keep the environment as quiet and distraction free as possible. P/SU, IM, PS

244. no. 4. The client has already admitted that he has a problem. The most realistic and highest priority goal for him is to accept the help of others. Options no. 2 and no. 3 are long-term goals, not the first or immediate concern. P/SU, PL, H

245. no. 1. Handle lapses nonjudgmentally and in a way that encourages the client to use the help of others to find new ways of coping. Option no. 2 is a judgment statement. The fact that the client is drinking does not imply that he is unwilling to change. The client needs

to be reassured that it is difficult, rather than chastised for his lapse. The focus should be on the client's needs and behaviors. He must assume responsibility and motivation for his recovery. P/SU, IM, PC

246. no. 1. Identify the difficulties associated with trying to stop alcohol intake so that the client does not continue to fall back on superficiality and denial. Continue to encourage the client to seek help from others. Option no. 2 supports the client's denial of the difficulty involved with abstaining from alcohol. Value judgments and threats are contraindicated and deny the client the necessary support needed. P/SU, IM, H

247. no. 3. Hallucinogens cause an individual to lose contact with reality and to hallucinate. Opiates are a class of drug that contain or are derived from opium. Barbiturates are a group of powerful sedative drugs that bring about relaxation and sleep. Stimulants are a class of drug whose major effect is to provide energy and alertness. P/SU, AN, PS

248. no. 1. There is no evidence that LSD is physically addicting. Heightened sensory perception can lead to an acute panic state. P/SU, AN, PC

249. no. 4. Successful treatment of persons using psychoactive substances continues to challenge health care professionals. Treatment by individuals who were once users of psychoactive substances continues to produce the most promising results. Examples of these groups are Alcoholics Anonymous (AA) and Narcotics Anonymous (NA). The aim of psychoanalysis is to restructure the personality. Behavior modification uses learning principles to improve behavior and has not proven to be effective in treating drug dependence. Family therapy does not focus on the drug abuser, but instead treats family roles and attitudes. P/SU, AN, PC

250. no. 2. One of the effects of LSD is heightened sensory perceptions, which can be frightening to the client and cause an acute panic state in which the client can hurt himself and others. Seclusion will reduce environmental stimulation and help protect both this client and others. Turning off the television and restraining the client are not sufficient. Client safety and dignity must be maintained. An order for sedation must be obtained as soon as possible. P/SU, IM, PS

251. no. 4. Clients should be observed constantly when in seclusion, and seclusion should be used only when it is the most effective therapy for the client at that time. The client needs a quiet and calm environment to counteract heightened sensory perception. The use of seclusion to protect the client from harming self or others is legitimate because safety is always a primary concern. P/SU, PL, PC

252. no. 3. The nurse must help the client sort out what is real and what is not by giving reality-based feedback. Option no. 1 belittles the client's feelings and is condescending. Option no. 2 does not help the client determine what is real and what is a hallucination. Discussing the hallucination, as suggested in option no. 4, will give it credence and increase the likelihood of recurrence. What the nurse discusses with a client reinforces it in the client's mind. P/SU, IM, PC

253. no. 2. Mr. Lambert is having a delusion. Delusions are created in the mind to make up for or meet an underlying need. Option no. 2 responds to the possible need underlying this client's delusion. Options no. 1 and no. 3 foster his grandiose and aberrant thinking and do not orient him to reality. The presence of delusions does not necessitate the use of seclusion. P/SU, IM, PC

254. no. 1. Haloperidol is a neuroleptic or antipsychotic agent, the purpose of which is to treat psychosis or thought disorders. Diazepam is an antianxiety drug. Imipramine (Tofranil) and isocarboxazid (Marplan) are antidepressants. P/SU, AN, PC

Contents

Questions 60
Correct Answers 98
Correct Answers with Rationales 103

Chapter 3

Nursing Care
of the Adult

COORDINATOR

Paulette D. Rollant, PhD, MSN, RN, CCRN

Contributors

Deborah A. Ennis, MSN, RN, CCRN

Peg Gray-Vickrey, MS, RNC

Paulette D. Rollant, PhD, MSN, RN, CCRN

Judith Sands, BS, MS, EdD

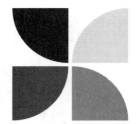

Questions

1. A nurse comes upon an auto accident and discovers a young man lying beside the road. He has a carotid pulse but does not seem to be breathing. Which action by the nurse indicates the need for a refresher course?
   ① Clear the mouth.
   ② Hyperextend the neck.
   ③ Perform a chin-lift maneuver.
   ④ Inhale deeply and smoothly deliver several rapid breaths.

2. If a victim had oral injuries, the nurse would deliver mouth-to-nose resuscitation. Which of the following techniques would be correct for mouth-to-nose resuscitation but incorrect for mouth-to-mask resuscitation?
   ① More force is required.
   ② The victim's mouth is closed during inspiration.
   ③ The victim's mouth is open during expiration.
   ④ The victim's neck is extended.

3. If during cardiopulmonary resuscitation (CPR) an Ambu-bag is used with one hand, how many milliliters of air can be delivered?
   ① 1000
   ② 800
   ③ 600
   ④ 400

4. A resuscitated client has a blood pressure of 60/0 mm Hg and a pulse of 140. After adequate ventilation, the nurse anticipates that the initial treatment priority is which of the following?
   ① Administration of sodium bicarbonate
   ② Insertion of a Foley catheter
   ③ Insertion of a nasogastric tube
   ④ Infusion of fluids

5. An 18-year-old client is admitted to the emergency room with chest injuries. Which piece of assessment data would be the most helpful in the assessment for blood loss and the decision for what action to take?
   ① Cause of the injury
   ② History of mentation since the accident
   ③ Time of injury
   ④ Sex of the victim

6. A thoracentesis is performed on a chest-injured client, and no fluid or air is found. Blood is administered intravenously (IV), but the client's vital signs do not improve. A central venous pressure line is inserted, and the initial reading is 20 cm H_2O. The most likely cause of these findings is which of the following?
   ① Spontaneous pneumothorax
   ② Ruptured diaphragm

③ Hemothorax
④ Pericardial tamponade

7. Below what systolic blood pressure level is perfusion to the vital organs sharply compromised in a usually normotensive client?
   ① 100 mm Hg
   ② 90 mm Hg
   ③ 80 mm Hg
   ④ 70 mm Hg

8. Blood levels of angiotensin and renin are increased during shock. What clinical findings would the nurse assess for as a result of these increased blood levels?
   ① Peripheral vasoconstriction
   ② Peripheral vasodilation
   ③ Increased respiratory rate
   ④ Decreased respiratory rate

9. A student nurse asked the experienced nurse to explain the use of dopamine to treat shock. Which of the following points should the experienced nurse include in the explanation?
   ① It is a powerful vasodilator.
   ② It has no unfavorable side effects.
   ③ Cardiac function is not affected.
   ④ Kidney perfusion is maintained.

10. What specific parameter would the nurse use to monitor for adequate fluid replacement in a client who is in shock?
    ① Systolic blood pressure above 100 mm Hg
    ② Systolic blood pressure above 90 mm Hg
    ③ Urine output of 30 ml/hr
    ④ Urine output of 20 ml/hr

11. A fluid bolus of 200 cc over 30 minutes is begun with a postoperative gastric surgery client. Which assessment methods will give the best indication of client response to this treatment?
    ① Central venous pressure (CVP) readings and hourly urine outputs
    ② Blood pressure and apical rate checks
    ③ Lung sounds and arterial blood gases
    ④ Electrolytes, blood urea nitrogen (BUN), and creatinine results

12. Which of the following points best describes why adrenergic agents are particularly useful in treating hypotension and controlling superficial bleeding?
    ① They cause dilation of peripheral vessels.
    ② They cause constriction of peripheral vessels.
    ③ They decrease cardiac output.
    ④ They block the effects of acetylcholine.

13. Epinephrine (adrenalin) is given in emergency situations for what primary reason?
    ① To increase cardiac output by increasing the rate and strength of myocardial contraction
    ② To increase tone and motility of the gastrointestinal tract
    ③ To prevent spasm and constriction of peripheral vessels
    ④ To prevent cardiac dysrhythmias

14. The most serious side effect of epinephrine that the nurse would monitor for is which of the following?
    ① Dilated pupils
    ② Headache
    ③ Cardiac dysrhythmias
    ④ Nervousness

15. A client in respiratory distress has the following arterial blood gas results: pH 7.30, Po_2 58, Pco_2 34, HCO_3 19. What primary acid-base imbalance would these results most likely indicate?
    ① Metabolic acidosis
    ② Metabolic alkalosis
    ③ Respiratory acidosis
    ④ Respiratory alkalosis

16. Why are acid-base imbalances life threatening?
    ① Enzyme activity is inhibited.
    ② Increased catecholamines cause cardiac stimulation.
    ③ Increased metabolites depress nerve activity.
    ④ Increased enzyme activity causes a hypermetabolic state.

17. A client's first line of defense when the body is attempting to compensate for an acid-base problem would be which of the following?
    ① Hormonal activity
    ② Changes in alveolar CO_2 diffusion
    ③ Retention of bicarbonate by the kidneys
    ④ Blood-buffering systems

18. A 64-year-old client has done well in surgery and returns to the unit after a cholecystectomy. During the night, the nurse assesses that the incisional area has become hard and elevated, the blood pressure is 80/60, and the pulse is 124. The nursing history reveals that this client took prednisone for a year before admission. Information is obtained from clients regarding previous use of corticosteroids to help identify
    ① Secondary adrenocortical insufficiency.
    ② Addison's disease.
    ③ Primary adrenocortical insufficiency.
    ④ Azotemia.

19. A client who sustained massive trauma begins to ooze blood at the IV site. Blood studies show that the hematocrit and hemoglobin are both low, the platelet count is 100,000/mm³, and the prothrombin time is prolonged. This client is most likely exhibiting signs of
    ① Acute tubular necrosis.
    ② Azotemia.
    ③ Disseminated intravascular coagulation (DIC).
    ④ Waterhouse-Friderichsen syndrome.

20. Drug therapy for a client diagnosed with addisonian crisis will probably include
    ① Tranquilizers and antispasmodics.
    ② Vitamins and pressor agents.
    ③ Adrenocorticosteroids and vitamins.
    ④ Adrenocorticosteroids and pressor agents.

21. A client diagnosed with diffuse microclotting will most likely need which of the following treatments?
    ① Heparin and packed red blood cells
    ② Whole blood and heparin
    ③ Peritoneal dialysis and fluids
    ④ Antibiotics and fluids

22. If a client who has hypercoagulation is not successfully treated, which of the following conditions would the nurse monitor for?
    ① Addisonian crisis
    ② Renal failure
    ③ Hemophilia
    ④ Neutropenia

23. A surgical client's fever climbs to 104.6°F (40.3°C). The physician orders hypothermia equipment and writes guidelines to maintain the client's body temperature at 99.6°F (37.5°C). At what body temperature would the nurse discontinue the hypothermia treatment?
    ① 97.6°F (36.4°C)
    ② 98.6°F (37°C)
    ③ 99.6°F (37.5°C)
    ④ 100.6°F (38.1°C)

24. A 55-year-old man arrives in the emergency room, complaining of crushing substernal chest pain, nausea, and sweating. He is quickly assessed by the nurse and the physician. The best initial nursing action is to
    ① Start an IV.
    ② Prepare and administer the pain medication as ordered by the physician.
    ③ Prepare him for immediate transfer to the coronary care unit.
    ④ Get a complete history from his wife.

25. The severe inner left arm and radiating neck pain experienced by a client is probably a result of
    ① Vasoconstriction because of arterial spasms.
    ② Myocardial ischemia.
    ③ Fear of death.
    ④ Irritation of nerve endings in the cardiac plexus.

26. The client's family asks the nurse to explain which area of the heart most frequently suffers the most damage in a myocardial infarction. What is the best response?
    ① The conduction system
    ② The heart valves
    ③ The left ventricle
    ④ The right ventricle

27. Because a client has a suspected myocardial infarction, which of the following would be included in the admission process?
    ① Contact the client's place of employment.
    ② Ensure that someone stays with the significant others.

③ Keep the family and significant others informed of the client's progress and status.
④ Secure information about client's medical insurance status.

28. During a conversation with a client's wife, the nurse learns that he had experienced some angina for months before admission but had not sought medical attention. What is the probable reason for the neglect of the pain?
① He has a high threshold for pain.
② He lacks knowledge about health maintenance.
③ He denied the significance of the pain.
④ He was afraid it would be interpreted as psychosomatic.

29. A client experiences a cardiac arrest. What would be the first nursing action in this situation?
① Call the physician on duty.
② Establish an airway.
③ Start closed-chest massage.
④ Give a bolus of sodium bicarbonate.

30. Which initial nursing assessment finding would best indicate that a client has been successfully resuscitated?
① Skin warm and dry
② Pupils equal and react to light
③ Palpable carotid pulse
④ Positive Babinski's reflex

31. Which of the following documentation items is nonsupportive of the characteristic pain with an acute myocardial infarction?
① Intense and crushing pain
② Pain relieved by nitroglycerin
③ Radiates to one or both arms, neck, or jaw
④ Pain of long duration and not relieved by rest

32. What is the narcotic of choice for a client with myocardial infarction?
① Morphine sulfate
② Meperidine (Demerol)
③ Codeine sulfate
④ Hydromorphone chloride (Dilaudid)

33. On admission to the coronary care unit, oxygen was ordered for a client with an acute myocardial infarction. The primary purpose of oxygen administration in this situation is to
① Relieve dyspnea.
② Relieve cyanosis.
③ Increase oxygen concentration in the myocardium.
④ Supersaturate the red blood cells.

34. The most dangerous period for a client after a myocardial infarction is
① The first 24 to 48 hours.
② The first 72 to 96 hours.
③ 4 to 10 days after myocardial infarction.
④ From onset of symptoms until treatment begins.

35. What is the most lethal complication associated with a myocardial infarction?
① Cardiogenic shock
② Ventricular dysrhythmias
③ Atrial dysrhythmias
④ Cardiac tamponade

36. Which fact is accurate about cardiogenic shock?
① It is easily treated with drugs.
② It can be prevented with close monitoring.
③ The mortality rate is very high.
④ It is difficult to identify high-risk clients.

37. Cardiac-enzyme studies are helpful in diagnosing a myocardial infarction. In these studies enzyme elevations are most indicative of which of the following?
① Cardiac ischemia
② Location of the myocardial infarction
③ Cardiac necrosis
④ Size of the infarct

38. A client with a 30% ejection fraction and cardiomyopathy has frequent premature ventricular contractions. Which drug would the nurse anticipate administering IV push and then hang a continuous infusion?
① Procainamide (Pronestyl)
② Diltiazem (Cardizem)
③ Lidocaine (Xylocaine)
④ Morphine

39. A client has had a lidocaine (Xylocaine) drip running at 3 mg/min over the past 8 hours. The nurse monitors for which most common initial sign of toxicity of the lidocaine (Xylocaine)?
① Bradycardia
② Suppressed respirations
③ Seizures
④ Confusion

40. Valsalva's maneuver can result in bradycardia, which can be dangerous for the client with cardiac muscle dysfunction. Which nursing action will prevent Valsalva's maneuver?
① Administer oral laxatives prn.
② Teach the client to hold his breath when changing position.
③ Serve liquids at room temperature.
④ Encourage the client to deep breathe frequently.

41. The client's wife tells the nurse that she is afraid her husband is going to die. Anticipatory grieving is important for her to experience at this time. Which of the following nursing actions would probably *hinder* her from the experience of anticipatory grieving?
① Have her participate in her husband's care when possible.
② Let her express her fears about the possibility of his dying.
③ Give her frequent reports about her husband's condition.
④ Tell her that the nurses are very competent.

42. A post–myocardial infarction client, now considerably improved, wants to talk about plans for his sexual activity at home. What would be the nurse's best approach?
① Give him some written materials and then answer questions.
② Plan a teaching session with the client and his significant other.
③ Answer his questions accurately and directly.
④ Provide enough time and privacy so that he can express his concerns fully.

43. Which of the following foods is appropriately selected as having the lowest amount of cholesterol by a client on a low-cholesterol diet?
① Liver
② Tuna fish
③ Shellfish
④ Rice

44. Which of the following items, if selected by a client, indicates knowledge of the lowest risk factor for the development of another myocardial infarction?
① Having a brother who had a myocardial infarction 2 years ago
② Having moderate control of the diabetes
③ Smoking a pack of cigarettes daily
④ Taking four baby aspirins daily

45. A client who had a myocardial infarction lives in a two-story house that has bathrooms upstairs and downstairs. Which of the following is the most appropriate to teach with regard to activity at home after discharge?
① "Do what you feel like."
② "Do not do any walking except to the bathroom from bed. Take your meals in the bedroom."
③ "Walk around in the house; do not walk up or down steps until you have discussed it with the doctor."
④ "Do all the walking you wish inside and outside. You can climb stairs inside the house."

46. The student nurse discusses with the experienced nurse that dyspnea is a characteristic, initial sign of congestive heart failure. The experienced nurse would explain that this is primarily the result of which factor?
① Accumulation of serous fluid in alveolar spaces
② Obstruction of bronchi by mucoid secretions
③ Compression of lung tissue by a dilated heart
④ Restriction of respiratory movement by ascites

47. In congestive heart failure, edema develops primarily because of which factor?
① Diffusion is inhibited.
② The capillary bed dilates.
③ Venous pressure increases.
④ Osmotic pressure increases.

48. How would the nurse most accurately document edema caused by cardiac failure?
① Painful
② Dependent
③ Periorbital
④ Nonpitting

49. To assess for left-sided heart failure, the nurse most often observes for which finding?
① Dyspnea
② Distended neck veins
③ Hepatomegaly
④ Pedal edema

50. The nurse notes that the client has a decreased cardiac output possibly caused by a decreased contractility. Which laboratory value might be checked for elevated serum levels?
① Calcium
② Chloride

③ Potassium
④ Sodium

51. The nurse would most likely document the respirations of the client with congestive heart failure as
① Rapid and shallow.
② Deep and slow.
③ Rapid with stridor.
④ Cheyne-Stokes.

52. The client with heart failure is assisted to bed and positioned by the care technician. Which bed position would indicate that the care technician needed no further instruction?
① Position of comfort, to relax the client
② Semirecumbent, to ease dyspnea and metabolic demands on the heart
③ Upright, to decrease danger of pulmonary edema
④ Flat, to decrease edema formation in the extremities

53. The student questions the use of IV drugs over IM or oral administration of drugs for a client with myocardial pump failure. The nurse's response would be based on which point?
① Altered circulation slows the action of IM and ingested drugs.
② Altered circulation speeds the action of IM and ingested drugs.
③ An enlarged heart needs stronger doses of medication.
④ No difference exists between IV, IM, and PO drug absorption in clients with heart failure.

54. The nurse's main concern when caring for the client receiving both digitalis and furosemide (Lasix) is to evaluate for
① Changes in the central venous pressure readings.
② Decreased edema.
③ Findings of hypokalemia and hypomagnesemia.
④ Findings of hyperkalemia and hypermagnesemia.

55. Chemical agents relieve the symptoms of acute pulmonary edema by
① Causing arterial vasoconstriction.
② Causing venous vasodilation.
③ Decreasing the preload and increasing the afterload.
④ Increasing the preload and decreasing the afterload.

56. A client receives nicardipine (Cardene) and metoprolol (Lopressor) concurrently to stabilize diastolic pressures. An essential nursing action before each time these medications are given is to take the client's
① Apical pulse while the client is lying flat and then in a high Fowler's position.
② Blood pressure while the client is lying flat and then in a high Fowler's position.
③ Blood pressure while the client is lying flat and then dangling on the side of the bed.
④ Blood pressure while the client is lying flat and then standing at the side of the bed.

57. A client with chronic heart failure has been placed on a diet restricted to 2000 mg of sodium per day. The client demonstrates adequate knowledge if behaviors

are evident such as not salting food and avoidance of which food?
1. Whole milk
2. Canned tuna
3. Plain nuts
4. Eggs

58. A client receiving digitalis and furosemide (Lasix) is counseled regarding potassium intake. Which of the following foods would be least important for the client to eat with regard to prevention of side effects of the medication?
1. Meats and milk
2. Citrus fruits
3. Potatoes
4. Cereals and breads

59. A client is being admitted with a diagnosis of thrombophlebitis. Which finding would the nurse be most likely to find at the initial assessment?
1. A negative Homans' sign
2. Pallor of the legs
3. Shiny, atrophic skin on the legs
4. Unilateral leg swelling

60. A student nurse is assigned to a client who has a diagnosis of thrombophlebitis. Which action by this team member is most appropriate?
1. Apply warm, dry packs to the involved site.
2. Elevate the client's legs 45 degrees.
3. Instruct the client about the need for bed rest for 10 to 14 days.
4. Provide active range-of-motion exercises to both legs at least twice every shift.

61. A client receiving heparin sodium asks the nurse how it works. Which of the following points would the nurse include in the explanation to the client?
1. It dissolves existing thrombi.
2. It prevents conversion of factors that are needed the formation of clots.
3. It inactivates thrombin that forms and dissolves existing thrombi.
4. It interferes with vitamin K absorption.

62. At 9:00 AM the first-semester student nurse asks the charge nurse what laboratory test needs to be checked today on the client with a heparin drip. The nurse's best response is which of the following?
1. Bleeding time
2. Activated partial thromboplastin time (APTT)
3. Prothrombin consumption test (PCT)
4. Prothrombin time (PT)

63. Which finding is inappropriately reported to the charge nurse as a manifestation of heparin overdosage?
1. Rectal bleeding
2. Positive Homans' sign
3. Smoky, dark urine
4. Epistaxis

64. An APTT >80 is called to the unit. Which drug would the nurse have available while waiting for the physician to return a call about the lab result?
1. AquaMEPHYTON
2. Atropine sulfate

3. Protamine sulfate
4. Vitamin B_{12}

65. A client will take iron supplements and warfarin sodium (Coumadin) for the next 2 years at home. Which point would the nurse include in the discharge instruction?
1. Keep a vial of vitamin K available.
2. Monitor for blood in the stool and notify the physician.
3. Take aspirin or Tylenol for headaches.
4. Use a firm toothbrush.

66. A client was admitted with complaints of sudden onset of chest pain and severe shortness of breath. Arterial blood gases on admission were pH 7.52, Pco_2 27, HCO_3 22, base excess 0, Po_2 53, O_2 saturation 91%. These arterial blood gas values suggest which acid-base disturbance?
1. Respiratory alkalosis
2. Respiratory acidosis
3. Metabolic alkalosis
4. Metabolic acidosis

67. The arterial blood gases of the client reflect respiratory alkalosis. The assessment of this client would most probably exhibit which findings?
1. Respiratory rate of 10 and shallow breathing
2. Respiratory rate of 26 and deep breathing
3. Central neurogenic hyperventilation syndrome
4. Cluster respiratory pattern

68. Which finding reported by the team member indicates that the client is at imminent risk for developing hypoxia?
1. Resonance over the chest on percussion
2. Expirations up to 2 times longer than inspirations
3. Central cyanosis
4. Increased tactile fremitus over the lung bases

69. The student nurse, reviewing for an exam, asks the nurse what the normal ratio is of Pco_2 to HCO_3. The nurse's best response is which of the following?
1. 1:10
2. 1:20
3. 10:1
4. 20:1

70. A 94-year-old with a history of chronic obstructive pulmonary disease has edema of the legs and feet, distended neck veins at 80-degree head-of-bed elevation, and a large, palpable liver. Considering these findings the nurse most likely suspects that the client is suffering from which condition?
1. Atelectasis
2. Pulmonary embolus
3. Cor pulmonale
4. Pleurisy

71. The nurse enters the room of a client with chronic obstructive pulmonary disease. The client's nasal cannula oxygen is running at a rate of 6 L per minute, the skin color is pink, and the respirations are 9 per minute and shallow. What is the best initial action?
1. Take heart rate and blood pressure.
2. Call the physician.
3. Lower the oxygen rate.
4. Position the client in a Fowler's position.

72. The reason to use pursed-lip breathing, included in the instruction for a client with pulmonary fibrosis, is that the prolonged exhalation
    ① Helps prevent air trapping.
    ② Trains the diaphragm to aid inspiration.
    ③ Improves the delivery of oral and nasal inhaler medications.
    ④ Facilitates the movement of thick mucus.

73. Chest percussion is ordered to facilitate the movement of thick mucus out of the lungs. In which situation would percussion be *contraindicated?*
    ① Hemoptysis
    ② Pneumonia
    ③ Cystic fibrosis
    ④ Atelectasis

74. A client with asthma develops respiratory acidosis. Based on this diagnosis, what would the nurse expect the client's serum potassium level to be?
    ① Normal
    ② Elevated
    ③ Low
    ④ Unrelated to the pH

75. A 45-year-old client is admitted through the emergency room with complaints of stabbing chest pain that becomes worse with coughing, diaphoresis, and productive sputum. The client states that it came on suddenly. Which condition would be inappropriate for the nurse to ask about during the initial assessment?
    ① Angina
    ② Congestive heart failure
    ③ Pneumonia
    ④ Pulmonary edema

76. A client complains of chills, fever, chest pain, and productive rust-colored sputum. Based on these symptoms, the nurse should suspect that the causative factor is related to which condition?
    ① A chemical irritant
    ② Coronary artery disease
    ③ Fluid overload
    ④ A pneumococcal infection

77. A client is diagnosed with pneumonia of the right middle lobe. What would the nurse expect to find on physical assessment?
    ① Egophony present at the right fourth intercostal space at the anterior axillary line
    ② Diminished breath sounds on the right posterior base
    ③ Diminished breath sounds on the right posterior base
    ④ Pericardial rub

78. A chest x-ray confirms consolidation in the right lower lobe. When percussing this area, what sound would the nurse most expect to hear?
    ① Tympany
    ② Resonance
    ③ Dullness
    ④ Hyperresonance

79. While inspecting a client's thorax, the nurse observes that the client is splinting. This means that the client
    ① Exhales with pursed lips.
    ② Holds his chest rigid.

③ Uses neck and shoulder muscles to exhale.
④ Flares the nares on inspiration.

80. Which finding would be included in a clinical pathway for a client diagnosed with pneumonia?
    ① Have client cough and deep breathe three times daily to minimize chest discomfort.
    ② Encourage incentive spirometer every hour without percussion to minimize chest discomfort.
    ③ Encourage client to drink 3 to 4 L of fluid a day.
    ④ Avoid analgesics to prevent the suppression of respirations.

81. The order reads to change a nasal cannula to a Venturi mask. The student nurse asks what the major advantage is of a Venturi mask over other types of oxygen masks. The nurse's response should include that the Venturi mask
    ① Can be used while the client eats.
    ② Delivers precise percentages of oxygen.
    ③ Requires no humidification of oxygen.
    ④ Allows for the administration of oxygen in concentrations of 95% to 100%.

82. Gentamicin (Garamycin), 60 mg PO q8h, is ordered for a client with a respiratory infection. Which laboratory values would the nurse monitor most closely for this drug therapy?
    ① BUN and serum creatinine
    ② Hemoglobin and hematocrit
    ③ SGOT and SGPT
    ④ PT and APTT.

83. Atelectasis develops in a client's right lower lobe. How would the nurse describe atelectasis to the client?
    ① Fluid in the air sacs
    ② Leftover secretions
    ③ Collapsed, mucus-filled air sacs
    ④ Collapsed, airless air sacs

84. When suctioning mucus from a client's lungs, which nursing action would be least appropriate?
    ① Lubricate the catheter tip with sterile saline before insertion.
    ② Use sterile technique with a two-gloved approach.
    ③ Suction until the client indicates to stop or no longer than 20 seconds.
    ④ Hyperoxygenate the client before and after suctioning.

85. During a skin test for tuberculosis with purified protein derivative, a client asks what causes tuberculosis. The nurse should answer that the cause is a
    ① Bacterium.
    ② Fungus.
    ③ Virus.
    ④ Spore.

86. Which indicates a positive tuberculin test?
    ① Induration is 0 to 4 mm in the general population.
    ② Erythema is 5 to 9 mm for the immunocompromised.
    ③ Erythema is 10 mm or larger for the health care givers.
    ④ Wheal is 10 mm or larger for the health care givers.

87. A positive reaction to purified protein derivative indicates that the client
    ① Has active tuberculosis.
    ② Has been exposed to *Mycobacterium tuberculosis*.
    ③ Will never have tuberculosis.
    ④ Has never been infected with *Mycobacterium tuberculosis*.

88. A physician prescribes oral rifampin (Rimactane) and isoniazid (INH) for a client with a positive purified protein derivative skin test. When informing the client of this decision, the nurse knows that the purpose of this choice of treatment is to
    ① Cause less irritation to the gastrointestinal tract.
    ② Destroy resistant organisms and promote proper blood levels of the drugs.
    ③ Gain a more rapid systemic effect.
    ④ Delay resistance and increase the tuberculostatic effect.

89. Which of these occurrences would probably be indicative of an untoward effect of isoniazid (INH)?
    ① Purpura
    ② Jaundice
    ③ Hyperuricemia
    ④ Optic neuritis

90. To prevent peripheral neuritis from isoniazid (INH), a second drug is added to a client's chemotherapy. Which drug is this likely to be?
    ① Vitamin B_{12}
    ② Vitamin B_1 (thiamin)
    ③ Vitamin C (ascorbic acid)
    ④ Vitamin B_6 (pyridoxine)

91. The nurse would teach a client that a fairly common side effect of the drug rifampin (Rimactane) is
    ① Reddish-orange color of urine, sputum, and saliva.
    ② Ectopic dermatitis.
    ③ Eighth cranial nerve damage.
    ④ Vestibular dysfunction.

92. A female client is skin-tested for tuberculosis and has a negative result. However, because of her husband's newly diagnosed tuberculosis, the physician recommends chemotherapy for her. What drug would the nurse anticipate teaching about for prevention therapy of tuberculosis?
    ① Streptomycin
    ② Paraaminosalicylic acid (PAS)
    ③ Isoniazid (INH)
    ④ Ethambutol (Myambutol)

93. Before starting on medication for tuberculosis, a client will probably need which of the following tests completed for a baseline test?
    ① Serum creatinine and BUN
    ② ALT and AST
    ③ Dexamethasone suppression test
    ④ Serum cortisol level

94. A client received a skin test for histoplasmosis. Histoplasmosis is often mistaken for
    ① Lung cancer.
    ② Pneumonia.
    ③ Tuberculosis.
    ④ Bronchitis.

95. The drug of choice in the treatment of histoplasmosis is
    ① Isoniazid (INH).
    ② Amphotericin B.
    ③ Paraaminosalicylic acid (PAS).
    ④ Streptomycin.

96. Steven Nelson undergoes a left thoracotomy and a partial pneumonectomy. Chest tubes are inserted, and one-bottle water-seal drainage is instituted in the operating room. In the postanesthesia care unit Mr. Nelson is placed in Fowler's position on either his right side or on his back to
    ① Reduce incisional pain.
    ② Facilitate ventilation of the left lung.
    ③ Equalize pressure in the pleural space.
    ④ Promote drainage by gravity.

97. Which finding would be considered most normal in the water-seal chamber within the first 24 hours postoperatively with a three-chambered water-seal drainage system?
    ① No fluctuation in the water-seal tube.
    ② Occasional intermittent, slight bubbling from the water-seal tube.
    ③ Bright-red bloody drainage.
    ④ Suction maintained at 20 cm H_2O.

98. A client has bilateral chest tubes. In discussing the drainage system to the client and family the nurse would explain that the water-seal chest drainage involves attaching the chest tube to a
    ① Bottle at a level above the bed.
    ② Tube that is submerged under water.
    ③ Tube that is open to the air.
    ④ Drainage bottle.

99. The student reports to the charge nurse that the fluid is oscillating in the water-seal chamber of a chest drainage system for a client who is 32 hours post–chest tube insertion for a pneumothorax. The nurse would identify that this situation indicates that
    ① The equipment is working well.
    ② The chest tube is clogged.
    ③ The chamber does not have enough water.
    ④ Air has leaked into the chest cavity.

100. The nurse is conducting an education session for a group of smokers in a stop smoking class. Which finding would the nurse state as a common symptom of bronchogenic carcinoma?
    ① Dyspnea on exertion
    ② Foamy, blood-tinged sputum
    ③ Wheezing sound on inspiration
    ④ Cough or change in a chronic cough

101. A client is scheduled for a bronchoscopy. When teaching the client what to expect afterward, what would be the nurse's highest priority of information?
    ① Food and fluids will be withheld for at least 2 hours.
    ② Warm saline gargles will be done q2h.
    ③ Coughing and deep-breathing exercises will be done q2h.
    ④ Only ice chips and cold liquids will be allowed initially.

102. A client has a left upper lobectomy. Which action by the nurse would best facilitate effective coughing and deep breathing postoperatively?
    ① Encourage the client to take a day at a time and to keep attempting to cough and deep breathe.
    ② Give the client a back rub to relax the muscles before coughing and deep breathing.
    ③ Administer pain medication 20 minutes before coughing and deep-breathing exercises.
    ④ Position the client for postural drainage with cupping and vibration 10 minutes before coughing and deep breathing.

103. What is the purpose of the long glass tube that is immersed 3 cm below the water level in a water-seal bottle?
    ① To humidify the air leaving the pleural space
    ② To allow the drainage to mix with sterile water
    ③ To monitor the respirations by visualization of the fluctuations
    ④ To prevent atmospheric air from entering the pleural space

104. Continuous bubbling in the water-seal chamber is observed during morning rounds. Which factor best accounts for this phenomenon?
    ① The system is functioning adequately.
    ② There is an air leak in the system.
    ③ The lung has reexpanded.
    ④ The suction pressure is too low.

105. A physician orders arterial blood gases for a client who is experiencing episodes of confusion. The respiratory therapist draws the blood and asks the nurse to apply pressure to the area so that the therapist can take the specimen to the lab. How long does the nurse apply pressure to the puncture site?
    ① 2 minutes
    ② 5 minutes
    ③ 8 minutes
    ④ 10 minutes

106. The arterial blood gas values drawn on a client who has asthma and increasing periods of confusion are pH 7.5, Pco_2 33.5, Po_2 45.7, HCO_3 22, and oxygen saturation 86.7%. Which value is within normal limits?
    ① Oxygen saturation
    ② Po_2
    ③ Pco_2
    ④ HCO_3

107. At the end of an hour of oxygen administration, a client's arterial blood gases are pH 7.45, Pco_2 34.7, Po_2 71.8, oxygen saturation 95.6%. The nurse will most likely expect this client to be
    ① Combative.
    ② Less confused.
    ③ More confused.
    ④ About the same.

108. John Baker, age 50, has experienced bouts of retrosternal burning and pain for 6 months. His condition has recently been diagnosed as esophagitis related to reflux of gastric contents into the esophagus with resultant mucosal injury. When documenting Mr. Baker's health history, the nurse would most likely expect him to report that his symptoms are worse
    ① When he is active and busy.
    ② While lying down.
    ③ While sitting.
    ④ When he is upset and under stress.

109. In assessing the nutritional status of a client with gastroesophageal reflux, the nurse finds that he has increased symptoms with foods that are associated with lowered esophageal-sphincter pressure. These foods include
    ① Poultry and yogurt.
    ② Fruits and vegetables.
    ③ Fried foods and chocolate.
    ④ High-fiber foods and vanilla.

110. Esophageal problems associated with reflux may necessitate a change in lifestyle. Which of the following would be appropriate to teach?
    ① Increase the amount of exercise.
    ② Discontinue smoking and alcohol.
    ③ Increase body weight.
    ④ Raise the foot of the bed to sleep.

111. Cancer of the esophagus occurs more commonly in men over age 50 and is associated with esophageal obstructions. Which statement guides the nurse's approach to client education?
    ① Histologically, the cells are very malignant.
    ② Symptoms develop late, and lymphatic spread occurs early.
    ③ Ulceration and hemorrhage occur.
    ④ Malnutrition and aspiration are present.

112. How can gastric regurgitation best be reduced?
    ① Eat small, frequent meals; avoid overeating.
    ② Have a small evening meal, followed by a bedtime snack.
    ③ Belch frequently.
    ④ Swallow air.

113. A client undergoes gastric endoscopy. When may food and fluids be given after this examination?
    ① At the client's request.
    ② When the gag reflex returns.
    ③ Within 30 minutes after the test.
    ④ As soon as the client returns to the ward.

114. A 47-year-old client is admitted with a diagnosis of possible gastric ulcer. The physician orders guaiac tests of all stools to determine the presence of
    ① Hydrochloric acid.
    ② Undigested food.
    ③ Occult blood.
    ④ Bile.

115. A client with a duodenal ulcer is most likely to complain of pain
    ① During a meal.
    ② 15 minutes after eating.
    ③ 1 to 4 hours after meals.
    ④ About 30 minutes after eating.

116. When a client with a gastric ulcer requests a cigarette during a follow-up visit, the best response of the nurse would be which of the following?
    ① One cigarette a day is all that is permitted.
    ② Nicotine increases gastric acid and stomach activity.
    ③ Nicotine decreases gastric acid and lessens stomach activity.
    ④ Cigars are less harmful than cigarettes.

117. A client with a gastric ulcer is advised by his physician not to drink coffee. The nurse explains that coffee
    ① Increases mental stress.
    ② Stimulates gastric secretions.
    ③ Increases smooth muscle tone.
    ④ Elevates systolic blood pressure.

118. A client with peptic ulcer disease does not respond to medical treatment. He is advised to have a subtotal gastrectomy. In preparing for client teaching, the nurse knows that this procedure involves removal of the
    ① Cardiac sphincter and upper half of the stomach.
    ② Pyloric region of the stomach and duodenum.
    ③ Entire stomach and associated lymph nodes.
    ④ Lower one half to two thirds of the stomach.

119. A client is scheduled for a subtotal gastrectomy. In anticipation of clarifying information for client education, the nurse knows that vagotomy is done as part of the surgical treatment for peptic ulcers in order to
    ① Decrease secretion of hydrochloric acid.
    ② Improve the tone of the gastrointestinal muscles.
    ③ Increase blood supply to the jejunum.
    ④ Prevent the transmission of pain impulses.

120. Which fact best explains why the duodenum is not removed during a subtotal gastrectomy?
    ① The head of the pancreas is adherent to the duodenal wall.
    ② The common bile duct empties into the duodenal lumen.
    ③ The wall of the jejunum contains no intestinal villi.
    ④ The jejunum receives its blood supply through the duodenum.

121. During the immediate postoperative period after gastric surgery, why must the nurse be particularly conscientious about encouraging a client to cough and deep breathe at regular intervals?
    ① Marked changes in intrathoracic pressure will stimulate gastric drainage.
    ② The high abdominal incision will lead to shallow breathing to avoid pain.
    ③ The phrenic nerve will have been permanently damaged during the surgical procedure.
    ④ Deep breathing will prevent postoperative vomiting and intestinal distention.

122. During gastric surgery a client has a nasogastric tube inserted. It will be removed when there is
    ① Inflammation of the pharyngeal mucosa.
    ② Absence of bile in gastric drainage.
    ③ Return of bowel sounds to normal.
    ④ Passage of numerous liquid stools.

123. Before having a subtotal gastrectomy, a client is told about the dumping syndrome. The nurse explains that it is
    ① The body's absorption of toxins produced by liquefaction of dead tissue.
    ② Formation of an ulcer at the margin of the gastrojejunal anastomosis.
    ③ Obstruction of venous flow from the stomach into the portal system.
    ④ Rapid emptying of food and fluid from the stomach into the jejunum.

124. When administering medication to a client with peptic ulcer disease, the nurse knows that aluminum hydroxide gel (Amphogel) is preferred to sodium bicarbonate in treating hyperacidity because, unlike sodium bicarbonate, aluminum hydroxide gel
    ① Is not absorbed from the bowel.
    ② Does not predispose to constipation.
    ③ Dissolves rapidly in all body fluids.
    ④ Has no effect on phosphorus excretion.

125. Which statement by a client recovering from a subtotal gastrectomy would indicate a need for additional teaching about the protocol for minimizing dumping syndrome?
    ① "I plan to eat a diet low in carbohydrates and moderate in protein and fat."
    ② "I plan to eat a diet high in carbohydrates and low in protein and fat."
    ③ "I will eat slowly and avoid drinking fluids during meals."
    ④ "I will try to assume a recumbent position after meals for 30 minutes to 1 hour to enhance digestion and relieve symptoms."

126. A client asks the nurse how he would know if he has dumping syndrome. The nurse would include which of the following clinical symptoms when discussing dumping syndrome?
    ① Nausea and vomiting
    ② Diarrhea and borborygmi
    ③ Ruddy skin color and hypertension
    ④ Headache and constipation

127. A client is started on propantheline bromide (Pro-Banthine). The nurse should monitor for the primary dose-limiting side effect of
    ① Dry mouth.
    ② Hiccoughs.
    ③ Visual blurring.
    ④ Urinary retention.

128. The most common precipitating cause of acute appendicitis is
    ① Chemical irritation by digestive juices.
    ② Mechanical obstruction of the lumen of the appendix.
    ③ Mechanical irritation of overlying pelvic viscera.
    ④ Ischemic damage from mesenteric thrombosis.

129. Peritonitis resulting from rupture of an inflamed appendix is primarily the result of
    ① Chemical irritation by digestive juices.
    ② Bacterial contamination by intestinal organisms.

③ Mechanical pressure exerted by the distended bowel.

④ Ischemic damage from mesenteric thrombosis.

130. To promote capillary proliferation and formation of scar tissue after an appendectomy, a client may be given a supplementary dose of which vitamin?
① E
② B₁
③ C
④ D

131. A 40-year-old female client has arrived in the postanesthesia room after a cholecystectomy and a common bile duct exploration. She is semiconscious. Her vital signs are within normal limits. Which action by the student nurse would need to be corrected?
① Apply a warm blanket to her body.
② Place her in a supine position.
③ Attach her T-tube to gravity drainage.
④ Set up low, intermittent suction for her nasogastric tube.

132. After a cholecystectomy, a client complains of abdominal pain. Her physician has ordered meperidine (Demerol), 50 to 100 mg q3h, prn for pain. Which criterion would be wrong to use when deciding how much analgesic to administer?
① Vital signs
② Anesthetics and drugs used during surgery
③ Nonverbal responses
④ The time and amount of any previous doses of Demerol

133. When planning care during the immediate postoperative period for a client who had a cholecystectomy, the nurse should select which of the following as the primary goal?
① Client will be free from respiratory complications.
② Client will maintain adequate nutrition.
③ Client will maintain full range of joint motion.
④ Client will return to normal bowel function.

134. Which finding would be most indicative of complications during the first 24 hours after a cholecystectomy?
① Serous drainage on the surgical dressing.
② Golden-colored fluid draining from the T-tube.
③ Urinary output of 20 ml/hr.
④ Body temperature of 99.8°F (37.6°C).

135. A client scheduled for a cholecystectomy is 50 pounds overweight. Because of her obesity, she would be most closely observed for which complication?
① Clay-colored, fatty stools
② Inadequate blood clotting
③ Cardiac irregularities
④ Delayed wound healing

136. The nurse knows that a client recovering from a cholecystectomy needs further discharge teaching if the client makes which statement?
① "I will not climb stairs for a month."
② "I will make a follow-up appointment with my surgeon."
③ "Eating fatty foods may cause me some discomfort for awhile."

④ "Redness or swelling in the incision must be reported to my surgeon immediately."

137. Which of the following signs and symptoms are most likely to be included in the initial assessment of a client with a diagnosis of possible cholecystitis?
① Abdominal pain, usually in the left upper quadrant
② Dyspepsia after carbohydrate ingestion
③ Fullness and eructation after protein ingestion
④ Nausea and vomiting

138. A client with acute cholecystitis is having severe pain. The physician has ordered morphine sulfate, 10 mg IM every 3 to 4 hours prn for severe pain or 6 mg IM every 3 to 4 hours prn for moderate pain. What would the nurse do?
① Ask her if she is allergic to morphine.
② Give 6 mg of morphine sulfate IM.
③ Give 10 mg of morphine sulfate IM.
④ Verify the order with the physician who wrote it.

139. A client is scheduled for a cholecystogram. The nurse should ask the client which question?
① "Are you on a low-sodium diet?"
② "Have you ever had a barium study?"
③ "Have you ever had a nasogastric tube inserted?"
④ "Are you allergic to any drugs?"

140. A client has an open cholecystectomy and is now ready to return to her room from the recovery room. An IV of 5% dextrose in 0.45% normal saline is infusing at 100 ml/hr, a T-tube is connected to gravity drainage, and a nasogastric tube is connected to low intermittent suction. What does the T-tube indicate?
① Stones were removed from the cystic bile duct.
② Stones were removed from the gallbladder.
③ The common bile duct was explored.
④ The cystic duct was removed.

141. During the first 2 hours after an open cholecystectomy, a client's nasogastric tube drains greenish liquid; then the drainage suddenly stops. What is the first action to take?
① Irrigate it as ordered with distilled water.
② Irrigate it as ordered with normal saline.
③ Notify the physician.
④ Reposition it.

142. After a cholecystectomy, a client asks the nurse how long it will be before she can have something to eat. The nurse replies
① "Are you hungry already?"
② "Since you are slightly overweight, now would be a good time for you to begin reducing."
③ "The doctor makes that decision."
④ "Usually clients start clear liquids after active bowel sounds return and the stomach tube is removed."

143. On the second postoperative day after an open cholecystectomy, the client's T-tube drains 30 ml during the day shift. What action should the nurse take?
① Irrigate the T-tube with 50 ml normal saline.
② Irrigate the T-tube with 50 ml distilled water.
③ Nothing; this is normal.
④ Notify the physician.

144. A postoperative cholecystectomy client asks when the T-tube will be removed. What would be best to tell her?
    1. Usually 3 to 4 days after surgery.
    2. Usually 5 to 6 days after surgery, after an x-ray of the cystic duct.
    3. Usually 7 to 10 days after surgery, after a T-tube cholangiogram.
    4. When the drainage exceeds 500 ml per day.

145. In assessing a client, the nurse knows that common causes of pancreatitis are
    1. Alcohol abuse and congestive heart failure.
    2. Alcohol abuse and biliary tract disease.
    3. Epileptic seizures and pancreatic fibrosis.
    4. Pancreatic fibrosis and chronic obstructive pulmonary disease.

146. Which description is an exocrine function of the pancreas?
    1. Secrete insulin and glucagon
    2. Secrete digestive enzymes
    3. Promote glucose uptake by the liver
    4. Facilitate glucose transport into the cells

147. What is the initial treatment plan for acute pancreatitis?
    1. Keep the gastrointestinal tract at rest to prevent pancreatic stimulation.
    2. Provide adequate nutrition to enhance healing.
    3. Prevent secondary complications such as peritonitis.
    4. Maintain adequate fluid and electrolyte balance.

148. Which drug is most commonly used in conjunction with analgesics to decrease the pain of pancreatitis?
    1. Magnesium hydroxide (Maalox)
    2. Prochlorperazine (Compazine)
    3. Propantheline bromide (Pro-Banthine)
    4. Pancreatin (Viokase)

149. Which diagnostic test best measures the response to treatment in the client with pancreatitis?
    1. Serum amylase
    2. Abdominal computed tomography (CT) scan
    3. Serum aspartate amniotransferase (AST)
    4. Erythrocyte sedimentation rate (ESR)

150. Initially, what laboratory test shows elevated values in viral hepatitis?
    1. Serum ammonia
    2. Serum bilirubin
    3. Prothrombin time
    4. Serum transaminase

151. A client is admitted to the hospital with a diagnosis of infectious hepatitis. Which goal would be given the highest priority during the initial hospitalization?
    1. Prevent decubitus ulcers.
    2. Limit physical activity.
    3. Eliminate emotional stress.
    4. Promote activity and diversion.

152. Which diet will be prescribed most often for a client with liver dysfunction?
    1. High fat
    2. Low sodium
    3. High calorie
    4. Low carbohydrate

153. Which statement by a student nurse indicates a need for further discussion?
    1. Cirrhosis is a chronic disease resulting in inflammation, destruction, and fibrotic regeneration of the liver.
    2. Cirrhosis causes obstruction of the venous and sinusoidal channels of the liver.
    3. Cirrhosis is frequently caused by alcohol abuse.
    4. Cirrhosis causes decreased resistance to blood flow through the liver.

154. A 48-year-old transient, unskilled laborer who has a 33-year history of alcohol abuse and a 12-year history of cirrhosis is admitted with the complaint of hematemesis and rectal bleeding. While in the emergency room, he has a bright-red emesis of approximately 400 ml, which is positive for blood. His admission diagnosis is bleeding esophageal varices with ascites. His blood pressure is 100/50 mm Hg, pulse 112, respirations 24, temperature 99°F (37.2°C) rectally. His breath smells of alcohol and he reports having drunk whiskey within the past 3 hours. He has an IV of 5% dextrose and water running at 125 ml/hr. The client's initial care plan would include which action?
    1. Elicit an alcohol consumption history.
    2. Obtain a social service referral.
    3. Secure information about nearest relative.
    4. Measure the abdomen for the degree of ascites.

155. Which action would the nurse be prepared to institute for the client who is experiencing delirium tremens?
    1. Provide a dark, quiet room; restraints; and side rails.
    2. Arrange a room away from the nurse's station and keep the TV on continuously.
    3. Keep the client's room door closed and a bright light on in the room.
    4. Provide a room with lighting that decreases shadows, and have someone in constant attendance.

156. Which findings would most likely be observed during an assessment of a client with cirrhosis?
    1. Cyanosis, headache, and lower abdominal pain.
    2. Peripheral edema, right upper quadrant pain, hemorrhoids, and decreased urine output.
    3. Hepatomegaly, decreased peripheral pulses, cool extremities, and intermittent claudication.
    4. Dyspnea, inspiratory stridor, and constipation.

157. Which laboratory result indicates a problem other than cirrhosis?
    1. Decreased serum folic acid and albumin
    2. Decreased platelets and increased bilirubin
    3. Decreased prothrombin time and leukocytes
    4. Elevated ALT, AST, and LDH

158. The most important pathologic factor contributing to the formation of esophageal varices that the nurse needs to consider when planning care for a client is
    1. Increased platelet count.
    2. Portal hypertension.
    3. Increased pulmonary artery pressure.
    4. Chronic renal failure.

159. The nurse knows that portal hypertension usually has little association with
    ① Esophageal varices.
    ② Pulmonary edema.
    ③ Ascites.
    ④ Hemorrhoids.

160. Before the insertion of a Sengstaken-Blakemore tube, what will the nurse need to do?
    ① Check each balloon for leaks, and label all tube ports.
    ② Clamp the lumen of the nasogastric tube.
    ③ Insert ice water into the gastric balloon.
    ④ Insert mercury into the esophageal balloon.

161. The nurse needs to make additional preparations before inserting the Sengstaken-Blakemore tube. Which action would be wrong to do before insertion?
    ① Place the client in a high Fowler's position.
    ② Administer a neomycin enema.
    ③ Instruct the client about the procedure.
    ④ Lubricate the tube with water-soluble lubricant.

162. A Sengstaken-Blakemore tube has been inserted and the balloons have been inflated. An *incorrect* action would be to
    ① Connect the gastric aspirating tube portal to intermittent suction.
    ② Tape the tube to provide some traction and decrease movement.
    ③ Place the client in a supine position.
    ④ Tape a scissors to the bedside to be used to cut the tube in the event of severe respiratory distress.

163. Complications resulting from the use of a Sengstaken-Blakemore tube can occur. The priority complication to monitor for would be
    ① Ulceration of the esophagus and gastric mucosa.
    ② Esophageal perforation.
    ③ Upward dislodgment of the esophageal balloon.
    ④ Downward dislodgment of the esophageal balloon.

164. If a client's esophageal bleeding is not controlled by mechanical means, the nurse would be prepared to administer which medication?
    ① Hydralazine (Apresoline)
    ② Vasopressin (Pitressin)
    ③ Meprobamate (Miltown)
    ④ Diazepam (Valium)

165. Which action would be least likely to be included in the clinical pathway of a client with esophageal bleeds from chronic liver dysfunction?
    ① Monitor intake and output carefully.
    ② Give frequent oral hygiene.
    ③ Maintain bed rest.
    ④ Sedate client.

166. When teaching about prevention of esophageal bleeding, what would the client be instructed to do?
    ① Eat a well-balanced, high-calorie, moderately high-protein, low-fat, low-sodium diet.
    ② Eat a low-protein, high-carbohydrate diet.
    ③ It is okay to maintain alcohol intake if diet is balanced.
    ④ Eat a general diet with no restrictions.

167. Knowing a client has a history of cirrhosis, what condition would the nurse most likely suspect when the client is admitted in a comatose state?
    ① Metastasis from hepatic tumors
    ② Hepatic encephalopathy
    ③ Acute cerebral bleeding
    ④ Acute hepatic insufficiency

168. The nurse must consider that the most important pathophysiologic factor contributing to a comatose state of a client with liver dysfunction is
    ① Increased prothrombin time.
    ② Portal hypertension.
    ③ Increased serum ammonia levels.
    ④ Increased serum bilirubin.

169. A central venous pressure (CVP) line is placed in a client's subclavian vein. What initial nursing intervention would be done after calibrating and zeroing the line?
    ① Check vital signs.
    ② Check CVP reading.
    ③ Check client's intake for the last 12 hours.
    ④ Measure output for 1 more hour.

170. Which finding is an unlikely assessment for clients with a diagnosis of hepatic encephalopathy?
    ① Asterixis
    ② Decreased level of consciousness
    ③ Muscle twitching
    ④ Exophthalmos

171. Which of the following would the nurse be prepared to administer to a client with hepatic encephalopathy?
    ① Neomycin and lactulose (Cephulac) enema
    ② Protein tube feeding
    ③ Phenobarbital (Luminal)
    ④ Phenytoin sodium (Dilantin)

172. What is the therapeutic effect of the treatment with neomycin in a client in liver failure?
    ① To decrease muscular twitching
    ② To induce sedation
    ③ To provide nutrition that promotes healing
    ④ To prevent formation of ammonia

173. In planning care for a client with liver failure, which of the following best describes the necessary dietary alterations?
    ① High carbohydrate, protein, and fat
    ② Low protein and low sodium
    ③ Low carbohydrate and low fat
    ④ High fiber

174. In planning discharge health teaching for a client recovered from liver failure, which of the following is *inappropriate* for the nurse to include?
    ① The need for a balance between activity and rest
    ② How to prevent bruising and bleeding
    ③ What kinds of foods to avoid
    ④ The need to drink 3 to 4 L of water each day

175. On the admission of a client with a chronic liver condition, which clinical manifestation is least likely to be observed by the nurse?
    ① Ascites
    ② Mild jaundice
    ③ Purpuric spots on client's arms and legs
    ④ Esophageal varices

176. Listed below are the most probable causes of cirrhosis. Which has the most important implications for long-term patient care?
① Obstruction of major bile ducts
② Chronic ingestion of alcoholic beverages
③ Long-term nutritional inadequacy
④ Viral inflammation of liver cells

177. Immediately after an intoxicated client's admission to the hospital, which action would be provided to make the client more comfortable?
① Vigorous back rub
② Scrupulous mouth care
③ Complete tub bath
④ Shave and haircut

178. The nurse anticipates that the client with alcoholism may experience nausea and vomiting. Which antiemetic would be the best to administer for the nausea and vomiting?
① Prochlorperazine maleate (Compazine)
② Hydroxyzine pamoate (Vistaril)
③ Hydroxyzine hydrochloride (Atarax)
④ Dimenhydrinate (Dramamine)

179. Accurate observation of a client's jaundice should be recorded because which of the following might likely be expected to develop?
① Hiccoughs
② Pruritus
③ Anuria
④ Diarrhea

180. A client with cirrhosis may be weighed daily to
① Allow correction of a nutritional deficiency.
② Monitor accumulation of edema and ascites.
③ Assess breakdown of tissue protein.
④ Monitor enlargement of the liver and spleen.

181. Because of a client's chronically poor physiologic state from cirrhosis, assessments and nursing actions would have the least amount of time spent to prevent
① Pneumonia.
② Decubitus ulcers.
③ Cystitis.
④ Gynecomastia.

182. A male client, 38 years old, is admitted with complaints of headache, hyperhydrosis (excessive sweating), and lethargy. After extensive diagnostic tests, acromegaly is diagnosed. In anticipating care of the client after his transsphenoid microsurgery for a small tumor, the priority nursing assessment postoperatively is to check for cerebrospinal fluid drainage from
① The dressing anterior to the right ear.
② The incision in the mouth between the upper gum and lip.
③ The nasal packing in the right nostril.
④ The occipital dressing.

183. Overproduction of which pituitary hormone can cause galactorrhea?
① Follicle-stimulating hormone (FSH)
② Estrogen
③ Progesterone
④ Prolactin

184. Which diagnostic test would provide the *least* helpful information in diagnosing a pituitary tumor?
① Hormonal assays
② CT scan
③ Visual fields
④ Serum calcium

185. A hypophysectomy is planned for a client. What would be the most important nursing action in the immediate postoperative period?
① Instruct client to cough and deep breathe.
② Assess urinary output hourly.
③ Keep client in a supine position.
④ Perform nasotracheal suctioning frequently.

186. What long-term problem may result from having had a hypophysectomy?
① Hypopituitarism
② Acromegaly
③ Cushing's disease
④ Diabetes mellitus

187. Before a 35-year-old client who has had a hypophysectomy leaves the hospital, she confides to you that she is worried that she will never be able to have children. What information relative to her case is most correct?
① The surgery has had no effect on her reproductive hormones.
② Her sexual libido may be decreased, but not her ability to conceive.
③ A decrease in gonadal hormones is common, but replacements can be given.
④ The ovaries can function independently without the pituitary hormones.

188. A client had a subtotal thyroidectomy today for removal of a nodule and is to return from the recovery room soon. Which question is the most important to ask the client postoperatively?
① "Do you feel uncomfortable?"
② "Do you have any tingling of your toes, fingers, or around your mouth?"
③ "Do your arms or legs seem heavier than usual?"
④ "Please tell me your name and where you are."

189. Which position would a client be placed in when the client returns from the recovery room after a thyroidectomy?
① Trendelenberg's position
② Left lateral recumbent with the upper part of the back supported
③ Semi-Fowler's with the neck supported
④ Supine with sandbags at the head

190. The nurse plans to assess for signs and symptoms of hypocalcemia. Which findings are most indicative of impending tetany?
① Poor coordination
② Dyspnea and cyanosis
③ Positive Chvostek's and Trousseau's signs
④ Muscular flaccidity and hypotension

191. Which piece of equipment would be kept on hand for a client who has just had a subtotal thyroidectomy?
① An arterial line
② A nerve stimulator

③ A tracheostomy set

④ An oral airway

192. Which drug would need to be readily available for a postparathyroidectomy client?
① Calcitonin
② Calcium gluconate
③ Calcium chloride
④ Saturated solution of potassium iodine

193. Which nursing action is inappropriate for the postoperative thyroidectomy client?
① Encourage minimal vocalization after surgery.
② Support the head with at least two or three pillows.
③ Check the back of the neck for drainage.
④ Encourage the client to cough and deep breathe.

194. The nurse is preparing to teach a 28-year-old, newly diagnosed diabetic. What nursing action is vital before implementing the teaching plan for this client?
① Determine if the client is a ketosis-prone or a ketosis-resistant diabetic.
② Assess the client's knowledge of the disease process.
③ Ask if there is a family history of diabetes.
④ Instruct the client that the client's lifestyle will never be the same.

195. Which statement is true regarding diabetes?
① Diabetes is an acute disorder that responds only to insulin treatment.
② Diabetes is a curable illness.
③ Diabetes is characterized by an abnormality of carbohydrate metabolism.
④ Diabetes is not a significant cause of mortality in the United States.

196. The nurse understands that a diagnosis of diabetes suggests that a client's symptom of polyuria is most likely caused by what physiologic change?
① Glucose, acting as a hypertonic agent, draws water from the extracellular fluid into the renal tubules.
② Increased insulin levels promote a diuretic effect.
③ Electrolyte changes lead to the retention of sodium and potassium.
④ Microvascular changes alter the effectiveness of the kidneys.

197. The client care plan includes teaching a client to prepare and give insulin injections. What is the most important reason for the nurse to instruct the client to rotate injection sites?
① Lipodystrophy can result and is extremely painful and unsightly.
② Poor rotation technique can cause superficial hemorrhaging.
③ Lipodystrophic areas can result, causing erratic insulin absorption rates from these areas.
④ Injection sites can never be reused.

198. Regular human insulin (Humulin-R) is ordered for a client. The first dose is administered at 7:30 AM. The nurse would monitor for a hypoglycemic reaction at what time?
① After breakfast
② After lunch

③ After dinner

④ After bedtime

199. Which symptom(s) of hypoglycemia would the nurse teach a client before discharge?
① Polydipsia and polyuria
② Elevated urine glucose
③ Rapid, deep respirations
④ Sweating, nervousness

200. A new diabetic client is now prepared for discharge. The client is concerned about continuing her aerobics program. What would the nurse suggest?
① Aerobic exercise is too strenuous for diabetics.
② An exercise program is an important part of diabetic management, when balanced with insulin and diet.
③ The client should limit exercise activities to walking.
④ Exercise increases the risk of diabetic complications (e.g., peripheral neuropathy).

201. Which finding is least characteristic of diabetes?
① Polyuria caused by the excessive amounts of glucose in the urine
② Polyphagia caused by starvation at the cellular level
③ Polydipsia caused by polyuria
④ Weight gain caused by excessive appetite

202. Which terms would best describe the most likely condition of the skin of a ketoacidotic client on admission?
① Warm, flushed, and dry
② Cool and clammy
③ Cool and dry
④ Warm, pale, and clammy

203. A 65-year-old woman is admitted with the diagnosis of hyperglycemic, hyperosmolar, nonketotic coma. Her blood glucose level is 1000 mg/dl. The highest priority of care when the client is admitted is to
① Force fluids orally to 4 L or more per 24 hours as ordered.
② Administer large doses of regular insulin SC as ordered.
③ Administer 2 to 3 L IV fluids in first 1 to 2 hours as ordered.
④ Administer large doses of NPH or Lente insulin as ordered.

204. A female client, age 30, is told she has diabetes. She replies, "I might as well be dead. I'll never be able to lead a normal life again." The best response to this is
① "After I teach you everything you need to know, you'll find out you're wrong."
② "Don't worry. Everything will be fine."
③ "The doctor gave you some medicine that will take care of everything."
④ "You will have to do some things differently to control this disease, but you can still lead a normal life."

205. The classic sign/symptom of arterial insufficiency of the lower extremities is
① Intermittent claudication.
② Peripheral paresthesias.

③ Shiny, atrophic skin over the tibia.

④ Pain on dorsiflexion of the foot.

206. Maintaining arterial blood flow to a client's feet is a nursing goal. Which nursing action would best achieve this?

① Encourage client to dorsiflex toes frequently.

② Keep client's feet covered with socks at all times.

③ Apply external heat to the feet.

④ Massage the feet briskly three times daily.

207. A client is scheduled for a left femoral-popliteal by-pass graft. The day before surgery, the client says to you, "I know this is only the beginning; soon they'll take my leg." Which response is most appropriate now?

① "Many persons who have had this surgery have not needed an amputation."

② "That may be a possibility some day, but don't worry about it now."

③ "I see this is worrying you. What would losing your leg mean to you?"

④ "There have been vast improvements in vascular surgery."

208. A client with non–insulin-dependent diabetes mellitus was scheduled for abdominal surgery. During the first few postoperative days, the client's diabetes can be best controlled by

① Restarting the oral agent as soon as possible.

② Administering an intermediate insulin daily.

③ Ensuring the client eats all the food on the trays.

④ Administering short-acting insulin on a sliding scale based on q4h blood glucose.

209. When the nurse goes into a diabetic client's room to give her morning care, the client is very irritable and tells the nurse to get out of her room. What is the best initial action?

① Assess her for other signs of hypoglycemia.

② Ask her if she would like you to come back later.

③ Allow her to express her anger and stay with her.

④ Recognize that she may be confused and orient her to her surroundings.

210. The nurse reviews a diabetic diet with the client in hospital. Which statement is most accurate?

① Recent research indicates that fats should be eliminated.

② Dietetic fruits may be eaten as free foods.

③ A regular meal pattern need not be followed because the client is not taking insulin.

④ Complex carbohydrates such as breads and cereals should be included in the diet.

211. Which action would be *inappropriate* to include in a diabetic teaching plan?

① Change position hourly to increase circulation.

② Inspect feet and legs daily for any changes.

③ Keep legs elevated on two pillows while sleeping.

④ Keep the insulin not in use in the refrigerator.

212. While completing the nursing history, the nurse anticipates that a client with Addison's disease would most likely complain of

① Weakness, decreased skin pigmentation, and weight gain.

② Weakness, increased skin pigmentation, and weight loss.

③ Weakness, pallor, and weight loss.

④ Insomnia, weight loss, and moist skin.

213. Which action would be most appropriate when administering care to a client with Addison's disease?

① Encourage exercise.

② Protect client from exertion.

③ Provide a variety of diversional activities.

④ Permit as much activity as client desires.

214. Which nursing action for the client with Addison's disease would be *inappropriate?*

① Observe for fluid and electrolyte imbalances.

② Administer varying amounts of cortisol as ordered.

③ Administer aldosterone as ordered.

④ Watch for symptoms of hypertension.

215. Which symptoms would alert the nurse to an addisonian crisis?

① Increased blood pressure, polyuria, and pulmonary edema

② Increased blood pressure and oliguria

③ Decreased blood pressure and urine output of 45 ml/hr

④ Decreased blood pressure and urine output of 10 ml/hr

216. A client with Addison's disease will be treated with replacement glucocorticoid, cortisone, and fludrocortisone acetate (Florinef). In developing the teaching plan, the nurse identifies which content as *inappropriate* to include?

① The different types and actions of medications.

② The need to wear or carry medical alert identification of condition and medications.

③ The use of hydrocortisone IM in an emergency.

④ The need for a lifestyle change, even with the use of replacement medications.

217. A 56-year-old personnel director is admitted for a cystoscopy. While admitting him, you learn that he has a urinary tract infection, smokes half a pack of cigarettes a day, and had a hernia repaired 20 years ago. He takes chlorothiazide (Diuril) for high blood pressure and follows a mild sodium-restricted diet. Which factor most increases the risk of the client's developing septic shock postoperatively?

① Cystoscopy in the presence of a urinary tract infection

② High blood pressure

③ Sodium-restricted diet

④ Smoking

218. While the nurse is preparing a client for a procedure, the client says, "I think I'm going to die." What is an appropriate nursing response?

① "Don't worry, your doctor is one of the best."

② "This procedure has a very low mortality rate."

③ "What ever gave you that idea?"

④ "You think you're going to die?"

219. A client returns from the recovery room at 9 AM alert and oriented, with an IV infusing. His pulse is 80, blood pressure is 120/80, respirations are 20, and all are within normal range. At 10 AM and at 11 AM, his vital signs are stable. At noon, however, his pulse rate

is 94, blood pressure is 116/74, and respirations are 24. What nursing action is most appropriate?
  ① Increase the IV rate.
  ② Notify his physician.
  ③ Take his vital signs again in 15 minutes.
  ④ Take his vital signs again in an hour.

220. Which finding is an *early* sign of septic shock?
  ① Cool, clammy skin
  ② Hypotension
  ③ Increased urinary output
  ④ Restlessness

221. The nurse shows a client with hypertension a list of foods and asks him to select any items included in his diet. His selection of which item probably indicates that he understands his dietary restrictions?
  ① Beef broth
  ② Cheese
  ③ Dried apricots
  ④ Peanut butter

222. Which statement best indicates that a client understands hypertension and the treatment?
  ① "I only add a little salt while preparing my food, and I salt my food lightly at the table."
  ② "I have blurred vision once in a while, but high blood pressure doesn't cause that."
  ③ "I know smoking increases my blood pressure and that I should stop, but it's very hard to do."
  ④ "I take my blood pressure pill whenever I get a severe headache."

223. During her hospitalization, Martha Cook acquires a urinary tract infection. Besides instructing Mrs. Cook on how, when, and why she should take her antibiotics, the nurse knows that the most important thing Mrs. Cook needs to learn to clear the infection is
  ① To drink up to 3 L of fluid each day.
  ② How to cleanse her perineum after voiding.
  ③ To limit fluids to increase the bacteriostatic activity of the urine.
  ④ To acidify the urine by drinking cranberry juice.

224. If a client experiences any of the following reactions after injection of the contrast material for an intravenous pyelogram, which one would have to be reported immediately?
  ① Feeling of warmth
  ② Flushing of the face
  ③ Salty taste in the mouth
  ④ Urticaria

225. An intravenous pyelogram reveals that a male client, age 35, has a renal calculus. He is believed to have a small stone that will pass spontaneously. To increase the chance of the stone passing, the nurse would instruct the client to force fluids and to
  ① Strain all urine.
  ② Ambulate.
  ③ Remain on bed rest.
  ④ Ask for medications to relax him.

226. Which factor predisposes the development of renal calculi?
  ① Bed rest for a client with multiple myeloma
  ② Use of a tilt table for a client who has a spinal cord injury

  ③ Forcing fluids in a client on bed rest
  ④ Decreasing calcium in the diet of a client with Paget's disease

227. Which of the following is a risk factor for bladder carcinoma?
  ① Cigarette smoking
  ② Family history
  ③ Low-bulk diet
  ④ Stress

228. What is the most common clinical finding in carcinoma of the bladder?
  ① Abdominal pain
  ② Gross, painless hematuria
  ③ Palpable tumor
  ④ Melena

229. Mr. Parker, diagnosed with bladder cancer, is scheduled for a cystectomy with the creation of an ileal conduit in the morning. He is wringing his hands and pacing the floor when the nurse enters his room. What is the best approach?
  ① "Good evening, Mr. Parker. Wasn't it a pleasant day, today?"
  ② "Mr. Parker, you must be so worried, I'll leave you alone with your thoughts."
  ③ "Mr. Parker, you'll wear out the hospital floors and yourself at this rate."
  ④ "Mr. Parker, you appear anxious to me. How are you feeling about tomorrow's surgery?"

230. In addition to emotional support, range-of-motion exercise is another nursing action that would be included in the nursing care plan for a client with a cystectomy. Why?
  ① Ambulation will be restricted for 1 week postoperatively.
  ② There is an increased risk of thrombophlebitis after pelvic surgery.
  ③ Cystectomies are extremely painful and limit the client's ability to move.
  ④ Range-of-motion exercise helps make the client feel that he is involved in his care.

231. After surgery, a client with a nasogastric tube in place continues to complain of nausea. Which action would the nurse take?
  ① Call the physician immediately.
  ② Administer the prescribed antiemetic.
  ③ Irrigate the tube to check for patency.
  ④ Reposition the client.

232. A nasogastric tube is present postoperatively for a client with a post-ileal conduit to
  ① Administer tube feedings.
  ② Test gastric secretions for bacteria.
  ③ Reduce the risk of paralytic ileus.
  ④ Increase the abdominal girth.

233. What color should a postoperative urinary stoma be?
  ① Brown
  ② Dark red
  ③ Light brown
  ④ Pink to red

234. A client's postoperative vital signs are a blood pressure of 80/40 mm Hg, a pulse of 140, and respira-

tions of 32. Suspecting shock, which of the following orders would the nurse question?
① Put the client in modified Trendelenberg's position.
② Administer oxygen at 100%.
③ Monitor urine output qh.
④ Administer morphine 10 mg IM q3-4h.

235. A female client is admitted with a diagnosis of acute renal failure. She is awake, alert, oriented, and complaining of severe back pain and abdominal cramps. Her vital signs are blood pressure 170/100 mm Hg, pulse 110, respirations 30, and oral temperature 100.4° F (38°C). Her electrolytes are sodium 120 mEq/L, potassium 7 mEq/L; her urinary output for the first 8 hours is 50 ml. The client is displaying signs of which electrolyte imbalance?
① Hyponatremia
② Hyperkalemia
③ Hyperphosphatemia
④ Hypercalcemia

236. The expected medical management for a client with a low sodium level would be which of the following?
① Fluid restriction
② Fluid replacement
③ Whole blood replacement
④ Sodium replacement

237. When taking a client's blood pressure, the nurse observes the presence of Trousseau's sign. This is an indication of which of the following?
① Hyponatremia
② Hyperkalemia
③ Hypocalcemia
④ Anemia

238. Which items are the most appropriate nursing actions for a client in acute renal failure?
① Intake and output, daily weight, and routine cardiopulmonary assessment.
② Intake and output, up ad lib, and restrict fluids.
③ Daily weight, force fluids, and daily measurement of dependent edema.
④ Daily weight, up ad lib, and restrict fluids.

239. A client suffering from acute renal failure has an unexpected increase in urinary output to 150 ml/hr. The nurse assesses that the client has entered the second phase of acute renal failure. Nursing actions throughout this phase include observation for signs and symptoms of
① Hypervolemia, hypokalemia, and hypernatremia.
② Hypervolemia, hyperkalemia, and hypernatremia.
③ Hypovolemia, wide fluctuations in serum sodium and potassium levels.
④ Hypovolemia, no fluctuation in serum sodium and potassium levels.

240. Which of the following best explains the elevation of the BUN in a client with acute renal failure?
① Increased protein metabolism
② Hemolysis of red blood cells
③ Inability of damaged nephrons to remove waste from the blood
④ Decreased protein metabolism

241. A low-protein diet is ordered for a client with chronic renal failure. The best explanation the nurse can give this client is that the diet will
① Minimize protein breakdown.
② Reduce the metabolic rate.
③ Decrease sodium intoxication.
④ Minimize the development of edema.

242. The nurse's aide assists with care of a client with chronic renal failure. It would be a priority for the nurse to check which of the aide's findings?
① Vital signs
② Intake and output
③ Amount of food consumed
④ Bowel movements

243. Assessing the laboratory findings, which result would the nurse most likely expect to find in a client with chronic renal failure?
① BUN 10 to 30 mg/dl, potassium 4.0 mEq/L, creatinine 0.5 to 1.5 mg/dl
② Decreased serum calcium, blood pH 7.2, potassium 6.5 mEq/L
③ BUN 15 mg/dl, increased serum calcium, creatinine 1.0 mg/dl
④ BUN 35 to 40 mg/dl, potassium 3.5 mEq/L, pH 7.35, decreased serum calcium

244. A likely cause of decreased serum calcium for a client with renal failure is
① Poor nutritional intake of calcium.
② Poor vitamin D intake.
③ Elevated serum phosphorus.
④ Elevated serum potassium.

245. A client with renal failure starts having Kussmaul's respirations. Which statement best describes the rationale for this occurrence?
① The kidneys cannot excrete the hydrogen ion or reabsorb bicarbonate.
② The kidneys cannot excrete the bicarbonate ion or reabsorb the hydrogen ion.
③ The kidneys are unable to excrete the potassium ion, resulting in acidosis.
④ The kidneys are unable to excrete sodium and phosphorus, resulting in alkalosis.

246. Laboratory studies on a client reveal hyperkalemia, the most serious electrolyte problem associated with renal failure. Hyperkalemia occurs for all but one of the following reasons. Which explanation is *not* accurate?
① Hyperkalemia results from failure of the excretory ability of the kidneys.
② Hyperkalemia results from the breakdown of the cellular protein that releases potassium.
③ Hyperkalemia results from acidosis, which causes the shift of potassium from the intracellular to the extracellular space.
④ Hyperkalemia results from decreased serum calcium because these electrolytes are inversely related.

247. Which drug would be *least effective* in lowering a client's serum potassium level?
① Glucose and insulin
② Polystyrene sulfonate (Kayexalate)

③ Calcium gluconate
④ Aluminum hydroxide

248. Peritoneal dialysis is considered as a possible means of treatment for a client. Which fact is the main *disadvantage* of peritoneal dialysis?
① Vascular access is required.
② The possibility of contracting hepatitis is great.
③ It is a slow method of treatment.
④ Fluid and electrolyte exchange is gradual.

249. A severe complication that requires frequent assessment during peritoneal dialysis is
① Respiratory distress.
② Peritonitis.
③ Hemorrhage.
④ Abdominal pain.

250. Treatment with hemodialysis is ordered for a client, and an external shunt is created. Which nursing action would be of highest priority with regard to the external shunt?
① Heparinize it daily.
② Avoid taking blood pressure measurements or blood samples from the affected arm.
③ Change the Silastic tube daily.
④ Instruct the client not to use the affected arm.

251. During the hemodialysis procedure, a client complains of nausea, vomits, and is disoriented. Which action would be the first nursing action?
① Slow the rate of dialysis.
② Administer protamine zinc.
③ Reassure the client; anxiety frequently accompanies the procedure.
④ Place the client in Trendelenburg's position.

252. Fredrick Rasmussen is a 69-year-old retired salesman. He is admitted with a diagnosis of urinary retention. His physician immediately inserts a Foley catheter. While being admitted, Mr. Rasmussen tells the nurse that he is going to have his prostate "shaved," because it is enlarged. Which parameter would be monitored throughout Mr. Rasmussen's preoperative period?
① Fluid intake
② Intake and output
③ Urinary output
④ Urinary pH

253. A client is scheduled for a transurethral resection of the prostate tomorrow. During outpatient preoperative teaching, he asks where his incision will be. What is the most appropriate response?
① "The incision is made in the abdomen."
② "The incision is made in the lower abdomen."
③ "The incision is made in the perineum between the scrotum and the rectum."
④ "There is no incision. The doctor inserts an instrument through the urethra, the opening in the penis."

254. A client returns from the recovery room after a prostatectomy. He has an IV infusing at 100 ml/hr, a three-way Foley catheter in place, and constant bladder irrigation. What would the nurse do first when increased blood in the urine is detected?
① Increase the speed of the irrigation.
② Release the traction on the Foley.

③ Irrigate the catheter manually.
④ Notify the physician.

255. A client who had a transurethral resection of the prostate complains of pain and bladder spasms. Which nursing action is most appropriate after determining that the drainage system is patent?
① Administer narcotics plus anticholinergic drugs, as ordered.
② Help him to a sitz bath.
③ Decrease the speed of the irrigation.
④ Decrease the traction on the Foley.

256. Nursing strategies can help prevent which complication associated with a transurethral resection of the prostate?
① Epididymitis
② Incontinence
③ Osteitis pubis
④ Thrombophlebitis

257. Which information would be included in the discharge teaching for a prostatectomy client?
① "Avoid straining at stools."
② "Avoid heavy lifting for approximately 2 weeks after surgery."
③ "Drive your car whenever you are ready to do so."
④ "Refrain from sexual intercourse for 12 weeks."

258. Which statement indicates that a prostatectomy client understands his discharge instruction?
① "I know my urine may be slightly pink tinged."
② "I know my urine should be clear all the time."
③ "I know my urine should be clear most of the time."
④ "I'll let my doctor know if I have any urinary dribbling."

259. Which finding is a common early symptom of prostate hypertrophy?
① Difficulty urinating
② Impotence
③ Urinary infection
④ Hematuria

260. The physician wants to examine a client's prostate gland. What equipment will be necessary for the exam?
① A Foley catheter
② Lubricant and gloves
③ Urethral dilators
④ A rectal tube

261. A client is scheduled to have an intravenous pyelogram (IVP) and cystoscopy. What nursing measure is essential to prepare the client for the IVP?
① Force fluids before the exam.
② Insert a Foley catheter.
③ Administer cleansing enemas.
④ Administer iopanoic acid (Telepaque) tablets the evening before.

262. A client undergoes a transurethral resection of the prostate under spinal anesthesia. He returns to his room with continuous bladder irrigation (CBI). Which of the following best explains the reason for the CBI?
① To decrease bladder atony
② To remove blood clots from the bladder

③ To maintain patency of the urethral catheter
④ To dilute the concentrated urine

263. The nursing assistant reports to the nurse that a client is confused. "He keeps saying he has to urinate, but he has a catheter in place." Which of the following responses would be most appropriate for the nurse to make?
① "His catheter is probably plugged. I'll irrigate it shortly."
② "He may be confused. What else did he say or do?"
③ "That may be a sign of internal bleeding."
④ "The urge to urinate is usually caused by the catheter. He may also have bladder spasms."

264. Which symptom can be expected temporarily when a client's urinary catheter is removed?
① Urgency
② Dribbling
③ Urinary retention
④ Decreased urinary output

265. Which assessment data is least important to consider when evaluating a client's ability to withstand surgery?
① Age
② Nutritional status
③ Race
④ Function of the involved area

266. Rennie Lacona, age 78, is admitted to the hospital with the diagnosis of benign prostatic hypertrophy (BPH). He is scheduled for a transurethral resection of the prostate (TURP). It would be *inappropriate* to include which of the following points in preoperative teaching?
① TURP is the most common operation for BPH.
② Explain the purpose and function of a two-way irrigation system.
③ Expect bloody urine, which will clear as healing takes place.
④ He will be pain free.

267. If a client has had a perineal prostatectomy, which item is the most appropriate during the postoperative period?
① Take rectal temperatures, not only to determine body temperature, but also to note the adequacy of perineal circulation.
② A Foley catheter with a 30 ml inflation bag is used to promote hemostasis.
③ For comfort, have the client sit in a semiinflated air ring.
④ Have the client sit on a hard surface to support the perineal incision.

268. Which item is least appropriate to include in the clinical pathway in the immediate postoperative period for clients with prostatectomies?
① Monitor for signs and symptoms of shock (e.g., vital signs, level of consciousness).
② Monitor for hemorrhage.
③ Observe patency of the catheter and color of the drainage.
④ Assess sexual potency.

269. Which daily nursing action would be *inappropriate* to include for a client with a urinary catheter in the early postoperative period after major surgery?
① Position the catheter to drain freely.
② Encourage adequate amount of fluids unless contraindicated by preexisting problems.
③ Ambulate the client.
④ Measure intake and output.

270. Which finding is the most common complication after a prostatectomy that has implications for nursing assessment and intervention?
① Urinary tract infection
② Cardiac arrest
③ Pneumonia
④ Thrombophlebitis

271. When beginning discharge planning for a client after a prostatectomy, what would be the highest priority?
① Diet
② Fluid restriction
③ Perineal exercises
④ Resumption of sexual relations

272. Which action is the most appropriate when preparing a client for a proctosigmoidoscopy?
① On the morning of the examination administer enemas until the returns are clear.
② Maintain the client NPO for 24 hours preceding the examination.
③ Give a strong cathartic on both the evening before and the morning of the examination.
④ Give sitz baths three times daily for 3 days preceding the examination.

273. What position is best for a client during a proctoscopic examination?
① Prone
② Right Sims'
③ Lithotomy
④ Knee-chest

274. Which nursing response is the most appropriate when preparing a client for a proctosigmoidoscopy?
① "You should not be anxious about this procedure. You will experience no pain or discomfort."
② "You will experience a feeling of pressure and the desire to move your bowels during the brief time that the scope is in place."
③ "You can reduce your discomfort during the procedure to a minimum by bearing down as the proctoscope is introduced."
④ "You will experience no discomfort during the procedure, because a topical anesthetic will be applied to the anus."

275. The physician wants a stool sample to check for amoebae. What is the correct procedure for obtaining a stool specimen for examination for amoebae?
① Deliver the specimen immediately to the laboratory while still warm and fresh.
② Mix the specimen with chlorinated lime solution before taking it to the laboratory.
③ Refrigerate the specimen until it is picked up by a laboratory technician.
④ Store the specimen in a warm-water bath until time for delivery to the laboratory.

276. Which findings are most characteristic of the stools of a client with ulcerative colitis?
① Diarrhea with blood and mucus
② Clay colored with blood and mucus
③ Gray and foamy
④ Semisolid, green with blood and mucus

277. The prothrombin time for a client with ulcerative colitis is considerably lowered. This most likely indicates
① Decreased absorption of vitamin K.
② Decreased absorption of vitamin C.
③ Decreased absorption of protein and potassium.
④ Decreased absorption of sodium, potassium, chloride, and fats.

278. Heidi Papps is a 25-year-old woman who has been experiencing intermittent bouts of diarrhea for the past 2 years. This condition has become increasingly worse for the past 2 months. She is seeking medical attention because her self-medication program is no longer working. Miss Papps is admitted to the hospital for diagnostic testing. Opiates and anticholinergic drugs are ordered for Miss Papps during her initial hospitalization, primarily to decrease
① Acute intestinal hypermotility and spasms.
② Gastric secretions.
③ Irritability and nervousness.
④ Pain.

279. A colectomy and ileostomy are proposed for a client. This surgery involves
① Removal of the rectum with a portion of the colon brought through the abdominal wall.
② Removal of the colon with a portion of the ileum brought through the abdominal wall.
③ Removal of the ileum with a portion of the colon brought through the abdominal wall.
④ A pull-through procedure.

280. Which finding is least anticipated after an ileostomy?
① Weight gain
② Liquid stool
③ Reestablishment of a regular bowel pattern
④ Irritation of the skin around the stoma

281. A 47-year-old computer programmer is admitted with a suspected small-bowel obstruction. He is 5 feet 7 inches tall and weighs 210 pounds. An IV of 5% dextrose in 0.45% saline with 20 mEq KCl is to infuse at 150 ml/hr. A nasogastric tube is inserted and connected to continuous low suction; it immediately begins to drain large amounts of gastric fluid. While taking a nursing history from the client the nurse would pay particular attention to any predisposition to bowel malignancy. Which disease of the bowel is least indicative of such a predisposition?
① Hemorrhoids
② Colitis
③ Amebiasis
④ Polyps

282. When examining a client's abdomen, which technique is performed last?
① Auscultation
② Inspection
③ Palpation
④ Percussion

283. Which factor is most consistent with a small-bowel obstruction?
① Diarrhea with blood and mucus
② Increased flatus
③ Malnutrition
④ Projectile vomiting

284. The priority nursing diagnosis for a client with a large bowel obstruction, without blood supply compromise, is
① Alteration in body image.
② Decreased tissue perfusion.
③ Fluid and electrolyte imbalance.
④ Pain.

285. A client has an intestinal tube, a Miller-Abbott tube, inserted in an effort to relieve a bowel obstruction. Which of the following is contraindicated?
① Position the client on his right side until the tube passes the pyloric sphincter.
② Tape the client's tube securely to the nose.
③ Connect the tube to suction.
④ Give mouth and nose care after any manipulation.

286. If a client needed emergency surgery, thus precluding thorough preoperative teaching, which content would be the most important for the nurse to review with the client?
① Deep-breathing exercises
② Painless movement from side to side
③ Relaxation techniques
④ Use of a splinting pillow

287. The physician constructed a transverse colostomy during a client's surgery. Based on the location of the colostomy, the nurse would most likely expect that the client's normal stool consistency 3 days after surgery would be
① Liquid.
② Semiformed.
③ Well formed.
④ Hard and solid.

288. When teaching a client how to irrigate his colostomy, which point would be incorrect to include?
① Use a catheter with a shield or cone.
② Hang the irrigation reservoir about 18 to 24 inches above the stoma.
③ Irrigate twice a day until regulated, then decrease to once a day.
④ Clear all air from the tubing before irrigation.

289. Skin care around a stoma is critical. In performing colostomy skin care, which action is contraindicated?
① Observe for any excoriated areas.
② Use karaya paste and rings around the stoma.
③ Apply mineral oil to the area for moisture.
④ Clean the area daily with soap and water before applying the bag.

290. Regulation of a colostomy will be most enhanced if the client
① Eats balanced meals at regular intervals.
② Irrigates after lunch each day.
③ Restricts exercise to walking only.
④ Eats fruit at all three meals.

291. When helping a client to accept his colostomy, which action is *inappropriate?*
① Encourage him to look at the stoma.
② Emphasize his positive attributes.
③ Involve the family in his care.
④ Have him do his own irrigations right from the start.

292. A gastric suction tube was inserted before a client was sent to surgery in order to
① Facilitate administration of high-calorie, nutritious liquids immediately after completion of the procedure.
② Prevent accumulation of gas and fluid in the stomach both during and after surgery.
③ Provide a reliable means of detecting gastrointestinal hemorrhage during the operative procedure.
④ Serve as a stimulus to restore normal peristaltic movement after recovery from anesthesia.

293. What is the primary purpose of inserting an indwelling Foley catheter before taking a client to the operating room for sigmoid colon removal?
① To facilitate distention of the bladder with saline during surgery
② To provide a ready check for renal function throughout surgery
③ To reduce the possibility of bladder injury during the procedure
④ To prevent contamination of the operative field from incontinence

294. Sections of colon both above and below the site of a tumor are removed to prevent
① Direct extension and metastatic spread of the tumor.
② Postoperative paralysis and distention of the bowel.
③ Accidental loosening of bowel sutures postoperatively.
④ Pressure injury to the perineal suture line.

295. The surgeon informs a client that he has cancer of the rectum and advises surgery for the removal of the rectum and formation of a permanent colostomy. When considering whether the client will receive tube feedings postoperatively, the nurse remembers that tube feedings are designed to provide adequate nutrition. Clients least likely to receive tube feedings are those who
① Have difficulty in swallowing.
② Are comatose.
③ Do not have a functioning gastrointestinal tract.
④ Are anorexic.

296. What preparational teaching would the nurse offer the client before the first irrigation of his colostomy?
① Explain that the procedure will be short and painless.
② Give him a pamphlet to read that outlines the procedure.
③ Talk with his spouse.
④ Show him pictures, and have him talk to a person with a well-regulated colostomy.

297. Which solution would be best suited for irrigation of a colostomy?
① 10% saline solution.
② Mild soap solution.
③ Warm tap water.
④ Dilute hydrogen peroxide.

298. Which factor is most likely to promote success when a client is irrigating his colostomy?
① Stoma size
② Excitement
③ Hunger
④ Relaxation

299. The symptoms of colon cancer vary depending on where in the colon the lesion is located. Which is *not* a classic symptom of colon cancer?
① Change in bowel habits
② Excessive flatus
③ Pain on the right side
④ Anorexia and nausea

300. Which diagnostic test will confirm the diagnosis of colon cancer most conclusively?
① Carcinoembryonic antigen
② Barium enema
③ Biopsy of the lesion
④ Stool examination

301. A male client, age 56, is found to have a lesion of the distal sigmoid colon and rectum. An abdominoperineal resection is planned. A bowel preparation is begun. After he has received three doses of neomycin, he complains of frequent stools. What would the nursing action be?
① See if there is an order for antidiarrheal medication.
② Explain to the client that this is the desired result.
③ Ask the client to record his stools.
④ Withhold the laxative that was ordered as part of the prep.

302. A client and his wife have been taught about the nature of a colostomy and removal of rectum. The nurse asks the client to repeat what he has learned. Which statement is most indicative of the need for follow-up by the nurse?
① "Maybe my colostomy won't have to be permanent."
② "My perineal wound may not be healed when I go home."
③ "I will be able to have normal bowel movements from my colostomy."
④ "I will have three incisions."

303. A postsurgical client with cancer is scheduled to return to the hospital in a month for a course of chemotherapy. Before leaving, he says to the nurse, "I'm not sure I want to come back. Maybe I'll just take my chances." What would be the best response?
① "It is your decision, and you should do what you feel is right."
② "What concerns you the most about coming back?"
③ "Have you discussed this with your wife and doctor?"

④ "The survival rate with adjuvant chemotherapy is quite high."

304. A client is to be started on a regimen of 5-fluorouracil (5-FU). During the time that he is receiving this drug, it is most important to
① Force fluids to maintain a good output.
② Practice good asepsis to prevent him from getting an infection.
③ Give frequent mouth care with lemon swabs.
④ Monitor his blood pressure during drug administration.

305. A 65-year-old retired teacher is admitted for tests. Her major complaints include crampy, lower left abdominal pain and frequent, bloody stools with mucus. Which diagnosis is likely to manifest these signs and symptoms?
① Appendicitis
② Cholecystitis
③ Diverticulitis
④ Pancreatitis

306. When assessing for a perforated bowel, the nurse would observe for
① Jaundice and clay-colored stools
② Rigid, tender abdomen and absence of bowel sounds
③ Nausea, vomiting, and pruritus
④ Dyspnea and chest pain

307. Which one of the following groups of diagnostic examinations is most likely to be ordered for a client with diverticulosis?
① Lower gastrointestinal series, barium enema, and colonoscopy
② Upper gastrointestinal series and gastric analysis
③ Cholecystogram and abdominal CT scan
④ Schilling test and sigmoidoscopy

308. A client is told that she has diverticulitis. Before her discharge, which of the following would be *inappropriate* to include in a teaching session?
① Practice stress-management techniques.
② Eat a high-residue diet.
③ Take psyllium hydrophilic mucilloid (Metamucil).
④ Eat foods that are highly refined.

309. A 52-year-old woman is admitted to the emergency room in an unconscious state. The client passed out while shopping with a friend. Her vital signs are stable, she has no apparent cuts or bruises, and her pupils react sluggishly to light. The friend reports that the client has a history of hypertension and complained of a headache while they were shopping. If admission orders include all of the following, which intervention should be performed first?
① Prepare for a lumbar puncture.
② Insert a nasogastric tube.
③ Check blood glucose level.
④ Insert a large-gauge intravenous line.

310. You are attending a high school baseball game. A wild throw veers into the spectators and strikes a woman near you in the head. She is conscious as you reach her side. You begin a quick neurologic assessment, re-

alizing that a person who has suffered a concussion is likely to exhibit which of the following?
① Nystagmus
② Unequal pupil responses
③ A dazed appearance and slowed response
④ Expressive dysphasia

311. Unequal pupillary light reflexes in the unconscious client are least likely to be a symptom of
① Ketoacidosis.
② Elevated intracranial pressure.
③ Epidural hematoma.
④ Brain tumor.

312. Cheyne-Stokes respirations can be best described as
① Shallow, then increasingly deep respirations that progress to a period of apnea.
② Extremely slow and fairly regular.
③ Several short breaths followed by irregular periods of apnea.
④ Rapid and deep.

313. A client with a severe head injury is reported to occasionally display decerebrate posture in response to stimulation. The nurse would recognize that decerebrate posture is present if the client exhibited
① Rigid extension of lower and upper extremities.
② Rigid extension of lower and flexion of upper extremities.
③ Flexion of lower and upper extremities into a fetal position.
④ Alternating flexion and extension of the upper and lower extremities.

314. A young man who was severely head injured in an automobile accident has extremely unstable intracranial pressure. To minimize changes in intracranial pressure it would be appropriate for the nurse to position the client
① With the head of the bed completely flat.
② With the head of the bed elevated 15 to 30 degrees.
③ On his left or right side and the head of the bed flat.
④ On his left or right side with the head of the bed elevated about 45 degrees.

315. A client is scheduled for craniotomy surgery. Which measure would be the most important aspect of the preoperative care?
① Teach the client about postoperative deep-breathing routines.
② Perform a thorough baseline neurologic assessment.
③ Determine the client's knowledge base about the planned surgery.
④ Teach the client about postoperative pain management.

316. Which interventions have the highest priority in the postoperative management of a client with a craniotomy?
① Deep-breathing exercises and positioning to support adequate respiratory function
② Frequent pupil and neurologic checks

③ Frequent position changes
④ Vital signs q4h

317. A client has an order for neurologic checks every 4 hours. When the nurse begins to assess the client's pupillary responses an important action is to
① Open the shades to ensure adequate room light.
② Shine the penlight into both eyes at the same time to record size and response.
③ Darken the room before beginning the pupil examination.
④ Instruct the client to close or cover one eye at a time.

318. Which statement is correct about cuffed tracheostomy tubes?
① The cuff should be deflated before suctioning.
② The pharynx needs to be suctioned before the cuff is deflated.
③ A hissing sound should be heard on each expiration.
④ Sterile normal saline should be used to inflate the cuff.

319. Level of consciousness is the most important aspect of neurologic monitoring. To make level of consciousness evaluation as accurate as possible it will be important for the nurse to
① Assess level of consciousness every shift.
② Consistently use the same tool and language used by other caregivers in the institution.
③ Use the Glasgow Coma scale for performing the assessment.
④ Use the Rancho Los Amigos scale for cognitive functioning to perform the assessment.

320. If an intubated client "fights" the ventilator, which actions by the student nurse would require correction?
① Remove the respirator, ventilate with an Ambubag, and then reinstate the respirator.
② Recheck the respiratory rate, air flow, and pressure settings.
③ Attempt to calm the client and assist him to relax.
④ Restrain the client.

321. During the first 8 hours after a head injury, a male client, age 25, excretes 3000 ml urine; his IV fluid intake has been 800 ml, and no diuretics have been given. These clinical signs probably indicate
① Cerebral edema.
② Diabetes insipidus.
③ Syndrome of inappropriate antidiuretic hormone.
④ Rising intracranial pressure.

322. The nurse is working with an unconscious client and has orders to assess the client's response to pain. The nurse realizes that pain assessment can result in tissue trauma to the client. Which actions are recommended for completing pain assessment?
① Shaking the client or application of pinprick
② Nailbed or supraorbital pressure
③ Sternal rubbing or nailbed pressure
④ Orbital pressure or application of pinprick

323. The client develops diabetes insipidus after a cran-

iotomy. Although not immediately life threatening, the syndrome can result in serious
① Increased intracranial pressure.
② Hypovolemia and electrolyte imbalance.
③ Cerebral infection.
④ Retrograde amnesia.

324. A young woman has come to the emergency department with complaints of high fever, photophobia, headache, and stiff neck of increasing severity. The physician proceeds to assess for signs of meningeal irritation. Brudzinski's sign would be said to be present if the client experienced
① Reflex flexion of the hip and knee when the head is flexed toward the chest.
② Severe pain when the neck is hyperextended.
③ Nystagmus when the head is turned from side to side.
④ Decerebrate posturing when the head is flexed and extended.

325. A 65-year-old woman is admitted for a workup after a series of transient ischemic attacks. Which finding is *not* commonly found in clients who have suffered a transient ischemic attack?
① Paresthesias
② Vertigo
③ Tachycardia
④ Disorientation

326. An 88-year-old female is admitted to the hospital with the diagnosis of a head injury. She fell and hit her head after suffering a transient ischemic attack (TIA). Which of the following tests would be a safe, noninvasive way of determining if the TIAs can be treated with endarterectomy?
① Electroencephalogram (EEG)
② CT scan
③ Doppler carotid studies
④ Arteriogram

327. Which action would be the best nursing intervention for a confused, head-injured client?
① Devise a reorientation program.
② Keep the client in bed with the side rails up.
③ Decrease the environmental stimuli.
④ Assign someone to stay with the client, and implement safety precautions.

328. A stroke client is experiencing mood swings and "crying jags," which are very distressing to his wife. She asks the nurse how she should respond when he behaves like this. Which advice would be most appropriate?
① "Be understanding and encourage him to express his grief."
② "Let him know that you understand that he cannot control his emotions and try to divert his attention to something else."
③ "Just ignore the behavior and go on with whatever you were doing."
④ "Explain to him that his behavior is unacceptable and he must get control of his behavior."

329. While caring for a client who has had a stroke, during the acute stage, the nurse performs frequent as-

sessments of the client's status. Which item is the most important assessment?

① Patency of airway and adequacy of respirations

② Pupillary reflexes

③ Level of awareness

④ Response to sensory stimulation, such as a pinprick on a lower extremity

330. To help prevent mouth odors and infections, stroke clients should be assisted to or taught to

① Avoid eating highly spiced foods.

② Brush their teeth before every meal.

③ Use antiseptic mouth washes at least twice daily.

④ Cleanse the affected side of the mouth with gauze wipes after eating.

331. A stroke client is experiencing expressive aphasia, and his family is very upset about his difficulties with oral communication. They want to know how to help. The nurse should instruct them that the most important thing that they can do is to

① Anticipate his needs as much as possible so he does not have to attempt to speak often.

② Encourage him to stop and rest whenever he shows signs of frustration.

③ Encourage him to practice verbal communication frequently despite its inherent frustrations.

④ Develop a set of gestures or signs that will allow him to successfully communicate without the need for speaking.

332. When preparing the room for a new stroke client, it would be most important to include which of the following?

① A footboard

② Suction

③ An egg crate mattress

④ Sandbags and trochanter rolls

333. Why should an unconscious client receive frequent mouth care?

① The client will experience severe thirst during the time that he is unable to take liquids orally.

② The oral mucosa will become dried and cracked because of mouth breathing during coma.

③ A dry mouth is more vulnerable to infections such as herpes simplex and *Candida.*

④ Tactile stimulation of the tongue and buccal mucosa will be needed to maintain minimal peristalsis.

334. The nurse knows that the most important action to prevent a decubitus ulcer in a client with a stroke is to

① Keep the skin clean, dry, and free from urine, feces, and perspiration.

② Place an alternating air pressure or water mattress on the bed.

③ Massage the reddened area with lotion or oil to stimulate circulation.

④ Turn and reposition the client at least q2h; avoid positioning the client on the affected side if possible.

335. Which is the most correct statement about positioning the stroke client?

① Flexor muscles are generally stronger than extensors.

② Extensor muscles are generally stronger than flexors.

③ The fingers should be positioned in moderate flexion.

④ The footboard should be flush with the mattress.

336. Which would be the most appropriate rehabilitation goal for a client who has experienced a major stroke?

① Achieve complete return of function in the affected limbs

② Prevent deterioration of current function and the development of complications

③ Achieve self-care capabilities in major activities of daily living

④ Successfully adapt all needed care activities to the remaining good limbs

337. A nurse is assigned to Mr. Perez, who experienced a recent right-sided cerebrovascular accident. His care protocol includes the notation to approach him from the right and reinforce the importance of visual scanning. What is the rationale for this instruction in this situation?

① Denial of the affected side is a common problem with stroke clients.

② Hemianopia, or partial blindness, is a common problem after stroke. The client loses a portion of the visual field and must be addressed from the side of intact sight.

③ Rehabilitation principles for stroke include encouraging the client to use the damaged side in self-care to the extent possible.

④ Mr. Perez is right dominant, and this approach builds on his strengths.

338. A client with suspected meningitis undergoes a lumbar puncture. After reviewing the lab results, the nurse recognizes that one of the following cerebrospinal fluid lab results is abnormal. Which result is abnormal?

① Appearance clear and colorless

② Glucose 60 mg/dl

③ Red blood cell count 40/mm^3

④ White blood cell count 2/mm^3

339. An elderly woman is in the rehabilitation phase after a stroke. As her condition improves her behavior becomes erratic. She frequently swears at the primary-care nurse and cries without apparent cause. The husband is upset about his wife's unpredictable and often unpleasant behavior. How would the nurse explain the client's behavior?

① She is probably suffering from emotional lability characteristic of clients after stroke.

② She is reacting to medications used to control blood pressure and cerebral edema, which frequently cause behavior changes.

③ She is reacting with anger and hostility to the consequences of her stroke.

④ She has experienced damage to her frontal lobe, which makes it impossible for her to control her behavior.

340. A young man is suspected of having suffered a spinal cord injury in an automobile accident. Which of the following would be the correct method of moving him while in the emergency room?
① Support the lower extremities because they are likely to be weak or paralyzed.
② Turn and immobilize the client on his side to protect the airway and prevent aspiration.
③ Support the back with additional pillows to prevent further spinal trauma.
④ Immobilize the head, neck, and back to prevent further spinal trauma.

341. Which finding would occur if a client has spinal shock?
① Spastic paralysis
② Hypertension
③ Diaphoresis below the level of the injury
④ Urinary retention

342. A client has experienced a complete cord injury at the level of C3-4. Which action would be the most important for a nurse caring for this kind of client in the acute stage after injury?
① Turn and position at least q2h.
② Immobilize the head and neck.
③ Monitor the patency of the airway and the adequacy of the tidal volume.
④ Monitor renal output.

343. Immediately after a spinal cord injury, the client's bladder will be
① Spastic.
② Atonic.
③ Likely to empty with the slightest stimulus.
④ Normal.

344. A client experiences a nondisplaced fracture of C7 and is placed on dexamethasone (Decadron) as part of his initial management. Stabilization surgery is planned for later in the week. Which intervention must be included in his care because of the use of Decadron?
① Vital signs and neurologic checks every 2 hours
② Guaiac all stools and emesis for blood
③ Maintain a nasogastric tube to low suction
④ Change positions every 2 hours

345. A client with a spinal cord injury to the cervical spine is admitted to the emergency department for initial management. The orders call for frequent assessment of tidal volume. If the client begins to experience difficulty breathing it will probably be the result of
① Edema in the cord above the level of the injury.
② Displacement of the parts of a fractured vertebra.
③ Severe anxiety as the reality of the severity of the injury becomes apparent.
④ Damage to the nerves that innervate the diaphragm.

346. A client who experienced a spinal cord injury 2 weeks ago has undergone surgery for spinal fusion and the application of a halo traction vest. The nurse has orders to begin the process of getting him out of bed. The first step will be raising the head of his bed to 15 degrees. The protocol calls for applying thigh-high elastic stockings and an abdominal binder. These actions are designed to prevent
① Spinal shock.
② Autonomic dysreflexia.
③ Pulmonary emboli.
④ Severe hypotension with position changes.

347. Two months after a serious spinal cord injury a young client begins to experience muscle spasms in his legs at regular intervals. His girlfriend becomes very excited when she notices these, saying "I just knew that you would walk again!" Which statement contains the most accurate information about the spasms?
① Two months is not enough time to evaluate the extent of the injury or its permanent effects.
② The beginning of muscle spasms are an excellent sign that recovery is proceeding well.
③ The muscle spasms are reflex movements that cannot be brought under conscious control.
④ The muscle spasms are a clear indication that the damage was not as severe as originally thought and some residual function remains.

348. The nurse is making a home health visit to a young man with a spinal cord injury that occurred over 6 months ago. While performing a routine skin assessment, the nurse notices that his face is red and he is becoming diaphoretic. Which should be the next action?
① Take his blood pressure immediately.
② Administer a muscle relaxant.
③ Catheterize him immediately.
④ Place him in Trendelenberg's position.

349. A 26-year-old male client with a spinal cord injury is progressing well with rehabilitation. He says that the dietitian has cautioned him about the amount of milk he drinks and told him that this could contribute to his problems with kidney stones. He says he is drinking no more than he did before the accident and wonders why it would be a problem now. The nurse's response would include which fact?
① The physiologic stress of the spinal cord injury decreases the excretion of calcium from his body.
② He has better absorption of calcium now than before the accident.
③ His kidneys are not clearing calcium as well as before surgery.
④ Demineralization of his long bones increases the amount of calcium to be cleared by the kidneys.

350. A client with C4 spinal cord injury asks how the injury is going to affect his sexual function. The nurse's response would include which of the following?
① His fertility will not be affected.
② His sexual functioning should not be impaired at all.
③ He will probably be able to have erections.
④ Ejaculation will occur, but he will not experience orgasm.

351. The nurse is caring for a woman who has just undergone a lumbar myelogram. The nurse realizes

that the most appropriate nursing diagnosis in her situation is

① Risk of infection related to disruption of the meningeal barrier of the spinal cord.

② Risk of acute pain, headache related to changes in cerebral spinal fluid pressure and volume.

③ Activity intolerance related to fatigue and weakness in the extremities.

④ Risk of injury related to dizziness and extremity weakness.

352. Jamal Reeves, a 22-year-old college student, was in an automobile accident and injured his cervical spine. The least likely finding during the period of spinal shock is

① Bradycardia.

② Hypotension.

③ Urinary retention.

④ Cool, clammy skin.

353. A 30-year-old homemaker fell asleep while smoking a cigarette. She sustained severe burns of the face, neck, anterior chest, and both arms and hands. Using the rule of nines, which is the best estimate of total body-surface area burned?

① 18%

② 22%

③ 31%

④ 40%

354. Which finding would be characteristic of a fresh, second-degree burn?

① Absence of pain and pressure sense

② White or dark, dry, leathery appearance

③ Large, thick blisters

④ Visible, thrombosed small vessels

355. If a client has severe burns on the upper torso, which item would be a primary concern?

① Debriding and covering the wounds

② Administering antibiotics

③ Frequently observing for hoarseness, stridor, and dyspnea

④ Establishing a patent IV line for fluid replacement

356. An IV narcotic was ordered to control the pain of a client with burns. Why was the IV route selected?

① Burns cause excruciating pain, requiring immediate relief.

② Peripheral circulation is constricted, delaying drug absorption from subcutaneous and muscle tissue.

③ Cardiac function is enhanced by adequate pain control.

④ Metabolism of the drug would be delayed because of decreased insulin production during extreme stress.

357. A major goal for the client during the first 48 hours after a severe burn is to prevent hypovolemic shock. The best indicator of adequate fluid balance during this period is

① Elevated hematocrit levels.

② Urine output of 30 to 50 ml/hr.

③ Change in level of consciousness.

④ Estimate of fluid loss through the burn eschar.

358. Mafenide acetate (Sulfamylon) is applied to a burned client's wounds every 12 hours. The nurse's assessment would include observation for which side effect of this drug?

① Metabolic acidosis

② Discoloration of the skin

③ Maceration of the skin

④ Dehydration and electrolyte loss

359. Autografts are applied to a full-thickness burn. Which action may be contraindicated during care of the donor site?

① Changing the dressing every shift

② Reporting any odor to the physician

③ Using a heat lamp to dry the wound

④ Exposing the mesh-covered wound to the air

360. Contractures are among the most serious long-term complications of severe burns. If a burn is located on the upper torso, which nursing measure would be least effective to help prevent contractures?

① Changing the location of the bed or the TV set, or both, daily

② Encouraging the client to chew gum and blow up balloons

③ Avoiding the use of a pillow for sleep, or placing the head in a position of hyperextension

④ Helping the client to rest in the position of maximal comfort

361. Diet and drug interactions are important with the use of antiparkinsonian drugs. Clients may be able to support maximum drug effectiveness if they follow a diet

① High in protein.

② With at least 10 glasses of water daily.

③ Low in fat.

④ With restricted quantities of meats and cheeses.

362. The symptoms of Parkinson's disease are believed to be primarily the result of

① Depletion of an essential neurotransmitter.

② An absence of histamine in the motor ganglia.

③ Blockage of the action of acetylcholine.

④ Failure of nerve impulses to bridge the myoneural junction.

363. Classic symptoms of Parkinson's disease include

① Ptosis of both eyelids.

② Visual impairment.

③ Involuntary resting tremor.

④ Vertigo.

364. A client's motor function can be best assessed by

① Checking Babinski's reflex.

② Assessing the strength of hand grips.

③ Having the client walk the length of the room.

④ Testing the knee-jerk reflex.

365. A shuffling propulsive gait is characteristic of Parkinson's disease. Which information describes that gait most accurately?

① A slumped-forward posture while walking

② Walking with increasingly quicker small steps

③ Staggering while walking

④ A stiff marching type of gait

366. A male client, age 62, has recently been placed on levodopa (Levopa), 250 mg bid. Which finding would

indicate that a therapeutic response had been achieved?
① Decrease in bradykinesia and rigidity
② Decrease in tremors
③ Presence of orthostatic hypotension
④ Increased strength and quality of the voice

367. Mrs. Patterson has had Parkinson's disease for over 5 years and has been admitted for readjustment of her medication. An atypical symptom of Parkinson's disease would be
① A stiff, blank facial expression.
② Severe, intentional hand tremors.
③ Soft monotone voice and drooling.
④ Bradykinesia and muscle rigidity.

368. A male client with multiple sclerosis, age 20, is started on a prednisone regimen. He states that he has never been treated with this drug before and asks for general information. Which piece of information would be incorrect to give?
① The drug should relieve or improve his symptoms.
② He will be taking it the rest of his life.
③ One theory is that the drug might be working by decreasing edema around involved areas of the nervous system.
④ The way in which it improves symptoms in multiple sclerosis is unknown.

369. A nurse in a department store notices a group of people gathered around a person lying on the floor having a seizure. The best immediate response would be for the nurse to
① Cradle the person's head in the nurse's lap.
② Place something in the person's mouth.
③ Hold the person's arms down.
④ Move the person to a place of safety.

370. A client with multiple sclerosis has been experiencing painful muscle spasms, which have responded only partially to muscle relaxant medication. She inquires about other self-care strategies that she could try to help relieve her spasms. Which strategy would be best to suggest?
① Use a prone position for sleep.
② Use assistive devices such as a cane to avoid falls and injury.
③ Take hot baths to relax the muscles when spasms are severe.
④ Use massage and stretching exercises to relax the muscles.

371. For a client with an exacerbation of multiple sclerosis, what would be the primary concern related to nutrition?
① Modifying the diet to make it easier to chew and swallow
② Maintaining a balanced body weight and optimal nutrition
③ Restricting the amount of protein in the diet
④ Supplementing the levels of vitamins B_6 and C

372. Multiple sclerosis causes a wide variety of symptoms. They are believed to be primarily the result of
① Patchy destruction of the nerve's myelin sheaths.
② Disturbances in the synapses at the myoneural junction.

③ Destruction of nerve cells in the basal ganglia.
④ Breakdown in the peripheral nerve fibers.

373. Which type of seizure is frequently preceded by an aura?
① Jacksonian (focal motor)
② Petit mal (absence)
③ Grand mal (tonic-clonic)
④ Myoclonic

374. Tom is a young man who is being placed on long-term seizure treatment with phenytoin (Dilantin). The importance of regular medical follow-up is emphasized. Which instruction is critical to include in the teaching for this client?
① The drug should always be taken on an empty stomach.
② Constipation is a common side effect, so he should increase his intake of fiber and fluids.
③ Good oral hygiene and gum massage should be incorporated into his daily routine.
④ Hyperactivity and insomnia are common early effects, but these should gradually decrease with time.

375. Which test would most likely be completed for diagnostic information on a client with seizures?
① Pneumoencephalogram
② Electroencephalogram
③ Cerebral angiogram
④ Cerebral tomography

376. What is the most common reason why clients suffer from sudden seizure recurrence?
① Extreme physical or emotional stress
② The use of alcoholic beverages in excess
③ Premenstrual fluid retention and hormone imbalances
④ Failure to consistently adhere to medication schedules

377. If one seizure occurs after another without the client's regaining consciousness between seizures, the nurse would recognize the development of which serious complication?
① Temporal lobe epilepsy
② Generalized repetitive seizures
③ Status epilepticus
④ Petit mal seizures

378. The nurse is working with a client with newly diagnosed generalized seizures who is overwhelmed by the diagnosis and expresses grave concerns about his future in regard to driving, employment, and having a family. The nurse acknowledges the reality of his concerns and reinforces to the client that most individuals with seizures should anticipate
① A restricted lifestyle with a slowly worsening prognosis.
② An unpredictable course to their condition necessitating frequent adjustments in medication, diet, and lifestyle.
③ A normal life with the seizures controlled effectively with medication.
④ A condition that gradually improves with time as seizure activity decreases.

379. Padded tongue blades are traditionally placed at the bedside of clients who are at risk for seizures. What is the appropriate use of the tongue blade in this situation?
① It should be inserted into the client's mouth at any time during the seizure.
② It is used during the postictal period when the major muscle movements have ended.
③ It is inserted only before the tonic-clonic movements begin.
④ It is inserted at the end of the tonic phase before the rhythmic clonic contractions begin.

380. In caring for a young woman who has been admitted for a workup for possible petit mal seizure activity, the nurse would be aware that the client's seizure activity will probably manifest itself as
① A vacant facial expression and lack of response.
② Sudden headache and dizziness.
③ Tonic-clonic muscle movements.
④ Antisocial behaviors such as beginning to disrobe in public.

381. The client just experienced a generalized grand mal seizure. During the postictal period, which actions would be appropriate nursing interventions?
① Perform a complete neurologic assessment and compare vital signs to evaluate for residual damage.
② Gently reorient and reassure the client about what has happened.
③ Encourage the client to get up and move around to regain strength and coordination in his extremities.
④ Take vital signs every 15 minutes and do not leave the client's bedside.

382. A client is placed on Mestinon for treatment of myasthenia gravis. In timing the administration of Mestinon, it would be most important to give it:
① One hour before meals.
② On an empty stomach.
③ With liquids, but not with milk.
④ Immediately before all planned activities.

383. A client is being admitted to the unit in probable myasthenic crisis. Which measure should the nurse implement?
① Place suction equipment at the bedside.
② Prepare for the transfusion of packed red blood cells.
③ Implement seizure precautions.
④ Prepare for a lumbar puncture.

384. Clients in myasthenic and cholinergic crises have many of the same symptoms, and an accurate diagnosis is often difficult. The two crises can be readily distinguished, however, by
① An EMG.
② An EEG.
③ Blood Mestinon levels.
④ Tensilon administration.

385. Routine nursing assessment of clients with exacerbations of myasthenia gravis might not include which measurement?
① Vital capacity
② Muscle strength of the extremities

③ Severity of ptosis
④ Swallowing ability

386. The drugs used in the treatment of myasthenia gravis exert cholinergic effects on multiple organ systems. Which findings are unexpected outcomes of cholinergic drug administration?
① Increased motility and tone of smooth muscles in the gastrointestinal tract
② Increased mucus secretion, sweating, and salivation
③ Increased heart rate and constriction of blood vessels
④ Miosis and a reduction in intraocular pressure

387. The nurse is assisting a student nurse to care for a client in a coma. While providing back care the student begins to express her feelings about the unfairness of the situation. The nurse reminds the student that hearing is thought to be the last sense to be lost and therefore the student should
① Speak more quietly to ensure that the client cannot hear her.
② Speak only to the other nurse and not speak about the client or the situation.
③ Remain respectfully quiet during all care.
④ Speak purposefully to the client, explaining all care provided and attempting to provide the client with meaningful stimulation.

388. Normal visual acuity as measured with a Snellen's chart is 20/20. A visual acuity of 20/30 indicates that
① At 20 feet, an individual can only read letters large enough to be read at 30 feet.
② At 30 feet, an individual can read letters small enough to be read at 20 feet.
③ An individual can read 20 out of 30 total letters on the chart.
④ An individual can read 30 out of 50 total letters on the chart at 20 feet.

389. Damage to the visual area of the occipital lobe of the cerebrum, on the *left* side, would produce what type of visual loss?
① Left eye only
② Right eye only
③ Nasal half of the right eye and temporal half of the left eye
④ Nasal half of the left eye and temporal half of the right eye

390. The anterior chamber of the eye refers to all the space in what area?
① Anterior to the retina
② Between the iris and the cornea
③ Between the lens and the cornea
④ Between the lens and the iris

391. As a person grows older, the lens loses its elasticity, causing which kind of farsightedness?
① Emmetropia
② Presbyopia
③ Diplopia
④ Myopia

392. If a person has a foreign object of unknown material

that is not readily seen in one eye, what would the first action be?
① Irrigate the eye with a boric acid solution.
② Examine the lower eyelid and then the upper eyelid.
③ Irrigate the eye with copious amounts of water.
④ Shield the eye from pressure, and seek medical help.

393. A client is admitted with a probable retinal detachment. The nurse recognizes that the client is most likely to report which symptom?
① Sudden loss of vision, as if a curtain were being drawn across the eye
② Sudden sharp throbbing eye pain
③ Loss of color perception leaving only gray vision
④ Development of acute tunnel vision

394. Postoperative care for the client after a stapedectomy would *not* include which client action?
① Out of bed as desired.
② No moisture in the affected ear.
③ Avoid sneezing.
④ No bending over or lifting of heavy objects.

395. Dimenhydrinate (Dramamine) is given after a stapedectomy to
① Accelerate the auditory process.
② Dull the pain exacerbated when the semicircular canal is disturbed.
③ Minimize equilibrium disturbances and imbalance.
④ Prevent nausea.

396. A client with chronic otitis is scheduled for a myringotomy. He asks the nurse why this procedure does not result in hearing loss. The response providing the most accurate data is that the procedure involves
① Just washing out the ear.
② Removing fluid from the outer ear.
③ Cutting the tympanic membrane, but it heals quickly.
④ Removing the tympanic membrane and putting a new membrane in.

397. If a client has Meniere's syndrome the client is most likely to complain of which of the following problems?
① Severe earache
② Many perceptual difficulties
③ Vertigo and resultant nausea
④ Facial paralysis

398. Treating a cataract primarily involves which action?
① Instillation of miotics
② Instillation of mydriatics
③ Removal of the lens
④ Enucleation

399. Preoperative instruction for cataract extraction would *not* include
① Type of surgery.
② How to use the call bell.
③ How to prevent paralytic ileus.
④ How to prevent respiratory infections.

400. A client is admitted for cataract extraction. In preparing to teach the client about adjustment to cataract lenses, the nurse needs to know that the lenses will
① Magnify objects in central vision by one third.
② Magnify objects in the peripheral vision by one third.
③ Reduce objects by one third with central vision.
④ Reduce objects by one third with peripheral vision.

401. When a client undergoes eye surgery, which standard postoperative intervention would be contraindicated?
① Coughing
② Turning on the unoperative side
③ Measures to control nausea and vomiting
④ Eating after nausea passes

402. Immediate nursing care after cataract extraction is directed primarily toward preventing which of the following?
① Severe pain
② Infection of the cornea
③ Bleeding
④ Prolapse of the iris

403. A client is confused during her first night after eye surgery. What would the nurse do?
① Tell her to stay in bed.
② Apply restraints to keep her in bed.
③ Explain why she cannot get out of bed, keep side rails up, and check her frequently.
④ Sedate her.

404. Discharge teaching for a postoperative eye surgery client would probably *not* include
① Staying in a darkened room as much as possible.
② Avoiding alcoholic drinks; limiting the use of tea and coffee.
③ Using no eye washes or drops unless they were prescribed by the physician.
④ Avoiding being too sedentary.

405. Which activity would be contraindicated after cataract surgery?
① Sewing
② Watching TV
③ Walking
④ Weeding the garden

406. A client visits her ophthalmologist and receives a mydriatic drug to facilitate the examination. After returning home, she experiences severe eye pain, nausea and vomiting, and blurred vision. During a visit to the emergency room, a diagnosis of acute glaucoma is made. The client's glaucoma may have been caused by
① Blockage of the outflow of aqueous humor by the dilation of the pupil.
② Blockage of the outflow of aqueous humor by the constriction of the pupil.
③ Increased intraocular pressure resulting from the increased production of aqueous humor.
④ Decreased intraocular pressure resulting from decreased production of aqueous humor.

407. Intraocular pressure is measured clinically by a

tonometer. What tonometer reading would be indicative of glaucoma?

① Decreased pressure bilaterally always
② Decreased pressure unilaterally or bilaterally
③ Increased pressure bilaterally always
④ Increased pressure unilaterally or bilaterally

408. What cranial nerve transmits visual impulses?
① I
② II
③ III
④ IV

409. Untreated or uncontrolled glaucoma damages the optic nerve. Which finding is least indicative of optic nerve atrophy?
① Colored halos around lights
② Severe pain in the eye
③ Dilated and fixed pupils
④ Opacity of the lens

410. Glaucoma is conservatively managed with miotic eye drops. Mydriatic eye drops are contraindicated for glaucoma. Which drug is a mydriatic?
① Neostigmine
② Pilocarpine
③ Timolol
④ Atropine

411. Glaucoma may require surgical treatment. Preoperative teaching would include
① Coughing and deep breathing every hour.
② Turning only to the unaffected side.
③ Medication for severe eye pain.
④ Restriction of fluids for the first 24 hours.

412. Clients with progressive undiagnosed wide-angle glaucoma are most likely to experience which symptom?
① Decreasing peripheral vision.
② Extreme pain in the eye.
③ Redness and tearing of the eye.
④ Seeing colored flashes of light.

413. If a client is placed on miotic eye drops for treatment of wide-angle glaucoma, it would be important to teach the client to
① Reduce fluid intake.
② Add extra home lighting to facilitate adjustment to dark rooms.
③ Wear dark glasses during the day.
④ Avoid exercise.

414. Miotics are used in the treatment of glaucoma. What is an example of a commonly used miotic?
① Atropine
② Pilocarpine
③ Acetazolamide (Diamox)
④ Scopolamine

415. What is the rationale for using miotics in the treatment of glaucoma?
① They decrease the rate of aqueous humor production.
② Pupil constriction increases the outflow of aqueous humor.
③ Increased pupil size relaxes the ciliary muscles.
④ The blood flow to the conjunctiva is increased.

416. When instilling eye drops for a client with glaucoma, what procedure would the nurse follow?
① Place the medication in the middle of the lower lid, and put pressure on the lacrimal duct after instillation.
② Instill the drug at the outer angle of the eye; have client tilt head back.
③ Instill the drug at the innermost angle; wipe with cotton away from inner aspect.
④ Instill medication in middle of eye; have client blink for better absorption.

417. Carbonic anhydrase inhibitors are sometimes used in the treatment of glaucoma because they
① Suppress production of aqueous humor.
② Dilate the pupil.
③ Paralyze the power of accommodation.
④ Reduce the production of vitreous humor.

418. When teaching a client with glaucoma, the nurse would omit what information?
① Vision in the affected eye will be restored once the drug regimen has been correctly established.
② Avoid excessive intake of stimulants (e.g., caffeine).
③ Adhere to the medication regimen.
④ Prevent constipation, and avoid heavy lifting and emotional excitement.

419. Glaucoma is a progressive disease that can lead to blindness. It can be managed if diagnosed early. Preventive health teaching would best include which point?
① Early surgical action may be necessary.
② All clients over 40 years of age should have an annual tonometry exam.
③ The use of contact lenses in older clients is not advisable.
④ Clients should seek early treatment for eye infections.

420. A client with progressive glaucoma may be experiencing sensory deprivation. Which action would best minimize this problem?
① Speak in a louder voice.
② Ensure that a sedative is ordered.
③ Orient the client to time, place, and person.
④ Use touch frequently when providing care.

421. Nursing management after rhinoplasty would omit which action?
① Elevate the head of the bed.
② Check the gag reflex.
③ Observe for frequent swallowing.
④ Apply warm compresses to the eyes and nose for comfort.

422. A 20-year-old college student is self-conscious about the appearance of her nose. She is admitted to the hospital for an elective rhinoplasty. After surgery the client reports that her bowel movement had a black appearance. What is the most appropriate nursing action?
① Call the physician immediately.
② Administer analgesics.
③ Observe for signs of fresh bleeding.
④ Check her gag reflex.

423. Before discharge, a postoperative client with rhinoplasty must be given which instruction?
① "Avoid blowing your nose for 3 to 4 days."
② "Resume your prior activities immediately."
③ "Limit your fluid intake for 1 week."
④ "Take aspirin if you observe increased pain and swelling."

424. Which medication would be used to promote vasoconstriction and control epistaxis?
① Epinephrine
② Lidocaine (Xylocaine)
③ Dopamine (Intropin)
④ Norepinephrine (Levophed)

425. Which position would be most desirable for a client with epistaxis?
① Trendelenberg's, to control shock
② Sitting, leaning forward, unless hypotensive
③ Side lying, to prevent aspiration
④ Prone, to prevent aspiration

426. If a physician decides to insert nasal packing in a client, which action would have the highest priority?
① Encourage the client to breathe through his mouth because he may feel panicky after the insertion.
② Advise the client to gently expectorate the blood in the nasopharynx and not to swallow it.
③ Periodically check the position of the nasal packing because airway obstruction can occur if the packing accidentally slips out of place.
④ Take rectal temperatures because the client must rely on mouth breathing and would be unable to keep his mouth closed on the thermometer.

427. The nurse instructs a client on the use of vasoconstrictive nose drops and cautions him to avoid too frequent and excessive use of these drugs. Which information provides the best rationale for this caution?
① A rebound effect occurs in which stuffiness worsens after each successive dose.
② Cocaine, a frequent ingredient in nose drops, may lead to psychologic addiction.
③ These medications may be absorbed systemically, causing severe hypotension.
④ Persistent vasoconstriction of the nasal mucosa can lead to alterations in the olfactory nerve.

428. A nasogastric tube is used to provide a client with fluids and nutrients for approximately 10 days after head and neck surgery. What is the rationale for this treatment?
① To prevent pain while swallowing
② To prevent stress on or contamination of the suture line
③ To decrease the need for swallowing
④ To prevent bleeding in the postoperative period

429. A client with laryngeal cancer has children who are concerned about their own risk of cancer. All but one of the following are facts that describe malignant neoplasia and must be considered by the nurse in her responses. Which fact needs to be omitted?
① Familial factors may influence an individual's susceptibility to neoplasia.
② Long-term use of corticosteroids enhances the body's defense against the development of cancer.
③ Sexual differences influence an individual's susceptibility to specific neoplasms.
④ Living in industrialized areas increases an individual's susceptibility to a malignant neoplasm.

430. A client is admitted with progressive Guillain-Barré syndrome. Which clinical manifestation would be unexpected in this syndrome?
① Muscle flaccidity of the arms and legs
② Loss of bladder tone
③ Decreased level of consciousness
④ Numbness and tingling in the extremities

431. Most clients who develop Guillain-Barré syndrome report a fairly recent history of which of the following?
① Autoimmune disease in the family
② Seizures
③ A viral illness
④ Recent trauma

432. Which goal would have the highest priority during the acute phase of Guillain-Barré syndrome management?
① To maintain an intact skin and full joint range of motion
② To reduce client anxiety over loss of function
③ To support normal growth and development and family relationships
④ To maintain adequate respiratory function

433. A 24-year-old client sustains a compound fracture of the shaft of the right femur in a motorcycle accident. Paramedics reach the scene and administer emergency treatment, which includes the application of a splint. How should any splint be applied?
① Apply it while the limb is in good alignment.
② Apply it to the limb in the position in which it is found.
③ Apply it extending from the fracture site downward.
④ Apply it extending from the fracture site upward.

434. A client is brought to the emergency room with a compound femur fracture. What is the first thing the emergency room nurse should do?
① Cover the open wounds.
② Take the client's blood pressure.
③ Clean the fracture site.
④ Assess the client's respiratory status.

435. After an open reduction of a femur fracture, a client displayed the following signs postoperatively: an increase in blood pressure, signs of confusion, and increased restlessness. Which pathology would the nurse most likely suspect?
① Concussion
② Impending shock
③ Fat emboli
④ Anxiety

436. A dry cast has which of the following characteristics?
① Gray, dull, and a musty odor
② Gray, shiny, and a musty odor
③ White, shiny, and odorless
④ White, dull, and tends to flake off when scratched

437. Which action is the recommended method of drying a cast?
① Place a radiation heat lamp about 1 foot from the cast.

② Cover the extremity with an electric heat cradle.
③ Place an electric fan at the foot of the bed.
④ Leave the cast uncovered in a well-ventilated room.

438. Which action is contraindicated during the first 24 to 48 hours after cast application?
① Handle the cast with the palms of the hand.
② Place the casted extremity in normal alignment.
③ Place rubber-covered pillows under the cast.
④ Elevate the entire extremity.

439. When a client returns from surgery, there are two small bloodstains on the cast. Four hours later, the stains double in size. What should the nurse do?
① Call the physician.
② Outline the spots with a pencil; note the time and date on the cast.
③ Cut a window in the cast to observe the site.
④ Record the amount of bleeding in the nurse's notes only.

440. On the first postoperative day, a client complains of a burning pain in one spot under the cast. The nurse should suspect which cause as the source of the discomfort?
① Skin irritation from a pressure spot
② A burn from the cast
③ An infection in the operative site
④ Hemorrhage from the incision

441. The first indication of an infection in a casted leg would most likely be
① An elevated temperature.
② An unpleasant odor from under the cast.
③ Redness and heat above and below the cast.
④ Purulent drainage on the cast.

442. Which finding is least characteristic of peroneal nerve palsy?
① Inability to dorsiflex foot and extend toes
② Numbness in the webbed space between the first and second toe
③ Inability to touch the heel to the floor when standing
④ Cyanotic toes

443. In response to a client's question regarding the cleaning of his cast, the nurse would reply
① "Cover the soiled area with shoe polish."
② "Spray the cast with shellac."
③ "Wipe the soiled area with a cloth moistened with alcohol."
④ "Clean soiled areas with a small amount of Bon Ami and a damp cloth."

444. A client slips on some grease on her kitchen floor and fractures the proximal end of the ulna. There is extensive soft-tissue damage in the fracture area. A cast is applied in the emergency department. Because of the location and type of fracture, the client is most at risk for the complication of compartment syndrome. Which finding would be the earliest indication of this phenomenon?
① Absence of the pulse distal to the fracture
② Pallor of the extremity
③ Paralysis of the hand
④ Progressive pain unrelieved by analgesics

445. If a client experiences the symptoms of compartment syndrome, which action is the recommended course of action?
① Bivalve the cast, and wrap it loosely with an elastic bandage.
② Apply hot packs to improve venous circulation.
③ Administer diuretics to reduce edema.
④ Encourage flexion and extension of the fingers on the affected arm.

446. If compartment syndrome is not recognized and treated early, what is the probable outcome?
① Gangrene will develop.
② A paralyzed and deformed arm with a clawlike hand results (Volkmann's contracture).
③ Healing of the fracture is delayed.
④ Cast syndrome will result.

447. What assessment is characteristic of a fat embolus after a fracture?
① Severe, stabbing chest pain 10 days after the fracture
② Frothy sputum
③ Petechiae across the chest and shoulders 24 hours after the fracture
④ Hypertension with coma

448. What is the most common reason why elderly women sustain hip fractures?
① Decreased intake of calcium
② Lack of muscles
③ Decreased production of bone marrow
④ Osteoporosis

449. Buck's extension is applied to a client's fractured leg. Which of the following is an *inappropriate* reason for using Buck's traction?
① It reduces muscle spasms and pain.
② It prevents further soft-tissue damage.
③ It reduces the fracture.
④ It immobilizes the leg while the dehydration is being treated.

450. Buck's traction would be contraindicated if a client experiences which of the following?
① Arthritis
② Bilateral lower leg ulcers
③ Pelvic pain
④ Deformity of the affected leg

451. A plan of care for a client in Buck's traction would include
① Removing the traction every shift to observe for pressure areas and provide skin care.
② Turning the client to the unaffected side for back care.
③ Elevating the head of the bed to apply counter-traction.
④ Raising the knee gatch to prevent the client from sliding down in bed.

452. When a client is immobilized, what is the most appropriate plan to prevent constipation?
① Encourage daily laxative use.
② Limit fluid intake.
③ Encourage frequent periods of sitting on the bedpan.
④ Increase the fiber in the client's diet.

453. Which statement is inappropriate concerning avascular necrosis of the femoral head?
    ① It is often a complication of total hip replacement.
    ② It results from impaired circulation.
    ③ Pain in the groin may be the first symptom in adults.
    ④ Restriction of abduction and internal rotation can occur.

454. When planning postoperative care for a client who has had a hip nailing, the nurse includes which of the following actions?
    ① Prevent internal rotation of the affected extremity.
    ② Prevent external rotation of the affected extremity.
    ③ Prevent hip flexion of greater than 10 degrees.
    ④ Prevent hip flexion of greater than 30 degrees.

455. Where would the nurse place the trochanter rolls on the affected extremity to prevent external rotation?
    ① From the hip to the ankle
    ② From the hip to the knee
    ③ From the knee to the ankle
    ④ From the knee to the midcalf

456. A client complains of severe burning in the right leg on the second postoperative day after a hip nailing. The nurse assesses the pulses, sensation, and movement of both legs, as well as vital signs. What is the next best action?
    ① Give the prn medication.
    ② Notify the physician.
    ③ Continue to monitor the assessments every 5 minutes.
    ④ Reassure the client that this is a normal response after this type of surgery.

457. Which of the following best describes the correct use of a walker?
    ① Always walk into the walker when all four of its legs are on the floor.
    ② Always walk into the walker when two of its legs are on the floor and the other two are off the floor.
    ③ Always have the walker legs at least 2 inches off the floor.
    ④ Always lift the walker up and down with each step.

458. An elderly man falls and breaks his hip. He is taken to surgery and receives a hip prosthesis. Positioning this client the first day postoperatively is best described by which of the following?
    ① Prevent external rotation and abduction of the affected extremity.
    ② Prevent external rotation and adduction of the affected extremity.
    ③ Prevent internal rotation and adduction of the affected extremity.
    ④ Prevent internal rotation and abduction of the affected extremity.

459. The second day after receiving a hip prosthesis, the client complains of the sudden onset of severe pain in the operative site. Assessment reveals that the affected extremity has a pulse, the color is pink, and the skin is warm. What is the next best action?
    ① Notify the physician.
    ② Give morphine as ordered.

③ Reposition the extremity.
④ Provide diversional activity.

460. After hip prosthesis surgery, a client asks to use the bedpan. Which approach would be the best for the nurse to use?
    ① Have the client lift up by using the overhead trapeze.
    ② Have the client use the bedside commode.
    ③ Have the client flex his legs and lift up his buttocks to slide the bedpan under him.
    ④ Get another nurse to help turn the client to his unaffected side. Place the bedpan under him and roll him back onto the pan.

461. A client has a standard above-the-knee amputation with an immediate prosthesis fitting. The surgeon's final decision on the level of the client's amputation is based on
    ① Saving all possible length and tissue of the extremity.
    ② Results of diagnostic tests such as an arteriography.
    ③ Observation of vascularity of tissue during surgery.
    ④ The best level to facilitate fitting with a prosthesis.

462. On the fifth postoperative day after above-the-knee amputation with immediate prosthesis fitting, the client's rigid dressing falls off. What would be an appropriate course of action for the nurse to take?
    ① Call the physician.
    ② Apply an elastic bandage firmly.
    ③ Apply a sterile saline dressing.
    ④ Elevate the limb on a pillow.

463. The nurse includes the important measures for stump care in the teaching plan for a client with an amputation. Which measure would be excluded from the teaching plan?
    ① Wash, dry, and inspect the stump daily.
    ② Treat superficial abrasions and blisters promptly.
    ③ Apply a "shrinker" bandage with tighter arms around the proximal end of the affected limb.
    ④ Toughen the stump by pushing it against a progressively harder substance (e.g., pillow on a footstool).

464. A young man's left arm is badly injured in a boating accident and is amputated just below the shoulder. While the nurse is checking the client's dressing, he says he is anxious and asks to have both his hands held. Which statement is the nurse's best response?
    ① "Mr. Gillman, I'm holding your hand."
    ② "Your left hand and arm were amputated the day of the boating accident."
    ③ "Your dressing is dry and clean where the doctors removed your arm."
    ④ "Many persons think their missing extremity is still present immediately after surgery."

465. How can the nurse best help a client adapt to an amputation?
    ① Have him think of how he would like to look.
    ② Talk about his change in body image.
    ③ Have him write about his feelings.
    ④ Have him touch and reorient himself to his body.

466. Which of the following is *least* characteristic of osteoarthritis?
   ① It most commonly affects the weight-bearing joints.
   ② Stiffness lasts about 15 minutes after a period of inactivity.
   ③ Joint effusion and crepitus are often present.
   ④ Inflammation and systemic symptoms are apparent.

467. A 65-year-old female comes to the clinic for a routine checkup. She is 5 feet 4 inches tall and weighs 180 pounds. Her major complaint is pain in her joints. She is retired and has had to give up her volunteer work because of her discomfort. She was told her diagnosis was osteoarthritis about 5 years ago. Which would be excluded from the clinical pathway for this client?
   ① Decrease the calorie count of her daily diet.
   ② Take warm baths when arising.
   ③ Slide items across the floor rather than lift them.
   ④ Place items so that it is necessary to bend or stretch to reach them.

468. The drug of choice for the treatment of arthritis is aspirin. A client's knowledge concerning aspirin is correct if she states which of the following?
   ① Avoid enteric-coated aspirin if gastrointestinal discomfort occurs.
   ② Take as many as 12 to 16 tablets every day on a regularly scheduled basis.
   ③ Increase the amount taken if there is ringing in the ears.
   ④ Absence of sensitivity to aspirin over time ensures continued safety with no risk of reactions.

469. Which statement is most characteristic of gout?
   ① It may be a familial metabolic disorder of purine metabolism.
   ② Ninety-five percent of the clients with gout are men between ages 18 and 30.
   ③ Urate crystal deposits cause a foreign body reaction in the plasma.
   ④ It usually occurs in previously traumatized joints.

470. A client is admitted from the emergency department with severe pain and edema in the right foot. His diagnosis is gouty arthritis. When developing a plan of care, which action would have the highest priority?
   ① Apply hot compresses to the affected joints.
   ② Stress the importance of maintaining good posture to prevent deformities.
   ③ Administer salicylates to minimize the inflammatory reaction.
   ④ Ensure an intake of at least 3000 ml of fluid per day.

471. Which dietary practice would be most appropriate for a client with gouty arthritis?
   ① Permanently eliminate foods high in purine.
   ② Eliminate foods high in purine only during the acute phase.
   ③ Permanently eliminate ingestion of alcohol and all rich foods.
   ④ Ingest foods that will keep the urine acidic.

472. What information is appropriate to include in discharge planning for a client taking allopurinol (Zyloprim)?
   ① He should drink at least 1000 ml of fluids per day.
   ② He should eliminate all foods with purine for the rest of his life.
   ③ He should take the medication before meals.
   ④ He should take the medication immediately after eating.

473. When teaching about the side effects of allopurinol (Zyloprim), the nurse should be sure to include monitoring for the first sign of a severe hypersensitivity reaction, which is
   ① Dizziness.
   ② A skin rash.
   ③ Aplastic anemia.
   ④ Agranulocytosis.

474. A client had a laminectomy and spinal fusion yesterday. Which statement is to be excluded from the plan of care?
   ① Before log rolling, place a pillow under the client's head and a pillow between the client's legs.
   ② Before log rolling, remove the pillow from under the client's head and use no pillows between the client's legs.
   ③ Keep the knees slightly flexed while the client is lying in a semi-Fowler's position in bed.
   ④ Keep a pillow under the client's head as needed for comfort.

475. The nurse in a cancer prevention and screening clinic is responsible for teaching clients about early detection of cancer. Which finding is *not* one of the seven warning signs of cancer cited by the American Cancer Society?
   ① Indigestion or difficulty swallowing
   ② Nagging cough
   ③ Unusual bleeding or discharge
   ④ Unusual tenderness in breast tissue

476. In a health education class, the American Cancer Society Guidelines for cancer-related checkups are discussed. Which response from a group member indicates correct understanding of these guidelines?
   ① "I should have a cancer-related checkup every 5 years after I reach age 50."
   ② "Women should have a baseline mammogram taken between the ages of 45 and 50."
   ③ "Adults over the age of 50 should have a stool guaiac slide test done on a yearly basis."
   ④ "A Pap smear needs to be done only on sexually active women."

477. A 40-year-old woman in a class asks what part of her body the cell sample is taken from for a yearly Pap smear. The nurse replies that the cells are scraped from the
   ① Cervix.
   ② Uterus.
   ③ Cul-de-sac.
   ④ Fallopian tubes.

478. If a client receives a Pap smear report that is class 1, what should the nurse advise?
   ① Call the physician to discuss treatment options.
   ② Prepare to go to the hospital for surgery.
   ③ Refrain from sexual activity.

④ Return for another Pap smear in 1 to 3 years, as directed by physician.

479. A female, 52 years old, is diagnosed with ovarian cancer. She is likely to have which manifestation?
① Changes in bowel elimination
② Postcoital bleeding
③ Dyspnea
④ Night sweats

480. A 67-year-old man is admitted to the hospital with a tentative diagnosis of bronchogenic carcinoma. His chief complaint is dyspnea and a chronic cough. The physician orders a sputum sample for cytologic testing. Important nursing implications involved with obtaining a sputum sample for cytology should include which of the following?
① Obtain the specimen in the evening hours.
② Collect the specimen in the morning before the client eats and drinks.
③ Have the client brush his teeth before collection of the specimen.
④ Keep the client NPO for 24 hours before collection of the specimen.

481. Which statement is incorrect regarding lung cancer?
① The 5-year survival rate depends on tumor histology and disease stage at the time treatment is initiated.
② Small-cell lung cancer has an excellent prognosis.
③ The 5-year survival rate for lung cancer is less than 15%.
④ Lung cancer is usually widespread by the time it is detected on chest x-ray.

482. A client is scheduled for external radiation treatment for laryngeal cancer. Of the following, which is *not* a common systemic side effect of this treatment?
① Nausea
② Fatigue
③ Malaise
④ Dry desquamation of the skin

483. When teaching the client about upcoming external radiation treatments, the nurse should stress the importance of
① Massaging the area daily.
② Exposing the area to sunlight for 30 minutes each day.
③ Not using soap on the treatment area and ink markings.
④ Applying cosmetic creams over the area to conceal reddened areas.

484. Which medication would be used to decrease a chemotherapy client's nausea and vomiting?
① Dexamethasone (Decadron)
② Methylcellulose (Citrucel)
③ Phentolamine mesylate (Regitine)
④ Metoclopramide (Reglan)

485. A 54-year-old man is admitted to the hospital for a colostomy related to a recent diagnosis of colon cancer. During the preoperative period, what is the most important aspect of this client's nursing care?
① Assure the client that he will be cured of cancer.
② Assess understanding of the procedure and expectation of bodily appearance after surgery.

③ Maintain a cheerful and optimistic environment.
④ Keep visitors to a minimum, so that he can have time to think things through.

486. Which instruction should be given in a health education class regarding testicular cancer?
① All males should perform a testicular exam after the age of 30.
② Testicular exams should be performed on a daily basis.
③ Reddening or darkening of the scrotum is a normal finding.
④ Testicular exams should be performed after a warm bath or shower.

487. During surgery, it is found that a client with adenocarcinoma of the rectum has positive peritoneal lymph nodes. What is the next most likely site of metastasis?
① Brain
② Bone
③ Liver
④ Mediastinum

488. The chemotherapeutic agent 5-fluorouracil (5-FU) is ordered for a client as an adjunct measure to surgery. Which statement about chemotherapy is true?
① It is a local treatment affecting only tumor cells.
② It is a systemic treatment affecting both tumor and normal cells.
③ It has not yet been proved an effective treatment for cancer.
④ It is often the drug of choice because it causes few if any side effects.

489. A client develops stomatitis during the course of methotrexate (MTX). Nursing care for this problem should include
① A soft, bland diet.
② Restricting fluids to decrease salivation.
③ Rinsing the mouth every 2 hours with a dilute mouthwash.
④ Encouraging the client to drink hot liquids.

490. A client who is getting chemotherapy asks the nurse why these sores developed in the client's mouth. What is the most appropriate response?
① "Don't worry; it always happens with chemotherapy."
② "Your oral hygiene needs improvement."
③ "It is a sign that the medication is effective."
④ "The sores result because the cells in the mouth are sensitive to the chemotherapy."

491. A 24-year-old woman who has been told about her diagnosis of acute granulocytic leukemia has an acute upper respiratory infection and bleeding gums. When her husband is told that she has leukemia, he insists that other family members not be told of her diagnosis. Which approach is best?
① Tell the husband that it is the family's right to be told.
② Suggest that he talk with the hospital chaplain.
③ Allow him to express his feelings and explain how they and their family can benefit from being told.
④ Be patient with him, hoping he will feel differently when his anger subsides.

492. A client begins a regimen of chemotherapy. Her platelet counts falls to 98,000. Which action is least necessary at this time?
   ① Test all excreta for occult blood.
   ② Use a soft toothbrush or foam cleaner for oral hygiene.
   ③ Implement reverse isolation.
   ④ Avoid IM injections.

493. High uric acid levels may develop in clients who are receiving chemotherapy. This is caused by
   ① The inability of the kidneys to excrete the drug metabolites.
   ② Rapid cell catabolism.
   ③ Toxic effects of the prophylactic antibiotics that are given concurrently.
   ④ The altered blood pH from the acid medium of the drugs.

494. The drug of choice to decrease uric acid levels is
   ① Prednisone (Colisone).
   ② Allopurinol (Zyloprim).
   ③ Indomethacin (Indocin).
   ④ Hydrochlorothiazide (HydroDiuril).

495. Nursing care for the client undergoing chemotherapy includes assessment for signs of bone marrow depression. Which finding accounts for some of the symptoms related to bone marrow depression?
   ① Erythrocytosis
   ② Leukocytosis
   ③ Polycythemia
   ④ Thrombocytopenia

496. Which finding is *not* a predisposing factor for cervical cancer?
   ① Early sexual experience with multiple partners.
   ② History of genital herpes, chronic cervicitis, or venereal disease.
   ③ Menarche before the age of 11.
   ④ Multiple pregnancies at an early age.

497. Medical treatment for a client with cervical cancer will include a hysterectomy followed by internal radiation. Although she is 32 years old and has three children, the client tells the nurse that she is anxious regarding the impending treatment and loss of her femininity. Which interaction is most appropriate?
   ① Tell the client that now she does not have to worry about pregnancy.
   ② Provide the client with adequate information about the effects of treatment on sexual functioning.
   ③ Refer her to the physician.
   ④ Avoid the question. Nurses are not specialists in providing sexual counseling.

498. A client receives a cervical intracavity radium implant as part of her therapy. A common side effect of a cervical implant is
   ① Creamy, pink-tinged vaginal drainage.
   ② Stomatitis.
   ③ Constipation.
   ④ Xerostomia.

499. A client's care plan during the time that she has a cervical implant in place would include which intervention?
   ① Frequent ambulation
   ② Unlimited visitors
   ③ Low-residue diet
   ④ Vaginal irrigations every shift

500. Which finding is a long-term side effect of a cervical radium implant?
   ① Shortening and narrowing of the vagina
   ② Nausea
   ③ Uterine cramping
   ④ Diarrhea

501. A 34-year-old client has recently had a mastectomy. Before discharge from the hospital, the nurse encourages the client to look at the incision. She turns her head and cries, "It is horrible." How should the nurse respond?
   ① "I know, I'd feel the same way, too."
   ② "I think we should talk about something less upsetting to you."
   ③ "Your feelings are normal; it's all right to cry."
   ④ "Look on the bright side, your physician was able to remove the cancer."

502. An important part of a postoperative mastectomy client's rehabilitation is teaching her the techniques of breast self-examination. Why is this important?
   ① Breast cancer can be bilateral.
   ② It will help the client confront the deformity.
   ③ It helps the client become more involved in care.
   ④ Teaching breast self-examination really is not important as long as the client has her physician do a thorough breast exam every 6 months.

503. A client who found a lump in her breast is admitted for a biopsy of the right breast with possible mastectomy and node dissection. While the nurse is doing preoperative teaching, the client says, "I'm sure this surgery will make me look like half a woman." What is the most appropriate nursing response?
   ① "I'm sure no one will know you've had a mastectomy."
   ② "Today's prosthetic devices are very realistic."
   ③ "You're concerned about how you'll look after surgery?"
   ④ "Everything will be all right. Your husband will still love you."

504. The nurse is preparing a client for a modified radical mastectomy. What does the nurse do after premedicating a client for surgery?
   ① Teach the client coughing and deep-breathing exercises to prevent postoperative complications.
   ② Have the client sign the operative permit.
   ③ Have the client void.
   ④ Put the side rails up.

505. A client's postoperative diagnosis is breast cancer, treated with a right, modified mastectomy. She returns from the recovery room in supine position, with an IV infusing, an elastic bandage wrapped around her chest, and a continuous portable suction device in place. The nurse monitors the client's vital signs and her dressing. Which part of the dressing does the nurse particularly observe for drainage?
   ① Back
   ② Front
   ③ Left side
   ④ Right side

506. Which discharge instruction is essential for the nurse to give a postoperative right mastectomy client?
① "Don't shave your right axilla."
② "Don't wear your bra until after the first visit to your doctor's office."
③ "Increase your sodium and fluid intake."
④ "Wash the incision every day with a soft cloth and an antiseptic solution."

507. A 40-year-old client recently visited her gynecologist for her annual examination. During the visit, the nurse practitioner palpated a lump in her right breast. She has now been admitted to the hospital for a breast biopsy. Which data would be excluded in the admission assessment?
① Prior sexual relationships
② Quality of present sexual relationship
③ Body image
④ Occupational role

508. During her admission interview for a breast biopsy, a client states, "This is really nothing to worry about. After all, I had a normal checkup last year. I expect to be back home tomorrow night." The client is most likely experiencing which of the following?
① Anger
② Denial
③ Depression
④ Bargaining

509. Depression may follow a mastectomy. Which observation would most alert the nurse to depression in this client?
① Disorientation during afternoon hours
② Increased agitation or restlessness
③ Verbalization of hopelessness or helplessness
④ Increased suspiciousness

510. A 49-year-old client is scheduled for a lumpectomy for breast cancer. Which nursing diagnosis is this client most likely to have after her lumpectomy?
① Disturbance in self-concept
② Self-care deficit
③ Impaired verbal communication
④ Alteration in cardiac output

511. Lymphedema is the most common postoperative complication after axillary lymph node dissection. Which action would minimize this problem?
① Avoid blood pressure measurements and constrictive clothing on the affected arm.
② Allow a liberal fluid and sodium intake.
③ Discourage feeding, washing, or hair combing with the affected arm.
④ Support the affected arm on pillows below the level of the heart.

512. It has been decided that a client will have antineoplastic chemotherapy after a mastectomy. Which purpose of this chemotherapy will also help best explain to the client the possible side effects of the therapy?
① It offers the only hope of cure.
② It attacks the fastest-growing cells of the body.
③ It is always indicated after a mastectomy.
④ It is a new treatment with few side effects.

513. When is the most appropriate time for a premenopausal client to perform a breast self-examination?
① Just before the time of menstruation
② The day menstruation begins
③ One week after the start of each menstrual period
④ Varying times throughout the month

514. A 40-year-old client has had a mammogram and biopsy for bleeding from the nipple of her left breast. The physician diagnosed intraductal breast cancer and explained that a modified radical mastectomy is necessary. The client has agreed to the surgery, which is scheduled for the following morning. What would be the most important aspect of the nurse's preoperative teaching?
① Discuss with the client how her sexual relations will be altered.
② Discuss the skin graft that will be necessary.
③ Explore the client's feelings and expectations about the surgery, and correct any misconceptions.
④ Explain that most breast masses are benign, and hers will most likely be nonmalignant.

515. A continuous portable suction device is in place at a surgical site postoperatively. Which nursing action would be *incorrect* when working with this equipment?
① Report bright-red, bloody drainage to the physician immediately.
② Maintain aseptic technique.
③ Curl the tubing, and tape firmly against the skin.
④ Check the drum frequently, and empty it when one-third to one-half full.

516. In the early postoperative period after a mastectomy, the surgeon encourages a client to begin using her left arm. She tells the nurse it hurts too much to move. What would be the best nursing action to reinforce the physician's instructions?
① Put the left arm in a sling to provide support.
② Initiate slow, passive range-of-motion exercises.
③ Teach the client full, active range of motion.
④ Tell the client she can postpone her exercises until after discharge when she is feeling better.

517. Which nursing action is *least* appropriate in planning for a postoperative mastectomy client's discharge from the hospital?
① Provide information on a local Reach to Recovery group.
② Discuss the availability of permanent prosthesis.
③ Discuss the possibility of a breast reconstruction in the future.
④ Discuss activities the client will have to discontinue.

518. Which statement is correct concerning Hodgkin's disease?
① It is a malignancy of the lymphoid system.
② It is a malignant neoplasm of the plasma cells.
③ It is a syndrome characterized by a defect in cell-mediated immunity.
④ It is a malignant disease that is associated with diffuse abnormal growth of leukocyte precursors in the bone marrow.

519. A 21-year-old female is admitted to the hospital for

suspected Hodgkin's disease. During the nursing history, the client's chief complaints are night sweats, not feeling hungry, not eating well, frequent abdominal cramps, diarrhea, and enlarged lymph nodes in her neck. Which of the following is *not* considered a sign or symptom of Hodgkin's disease?
① Night sweats
② Anorexia
③ Diarrhea
④ Enlarged lymph nodes

520. A client is scheduled for a lymphangiography. To prepare her for the procedure the nurse would tell her that
① She will be NPO after midnight.
② She will be allowed to move about freely during the examination.
③ She will need to keep her leg in a dependent position after the procedure.
④ Her stools and urine will be blue tinged for several days.

521. Which statement is correct regarding acquired immunodeficiency syndrome (AIDS)?
① It is caused by a retrovirus that destroys CD4 lymphocytes.
② It is a malignancy of the lymphoid tissue.
③ It is caused by a bacterial infection that produces fatal endotoxins.
④ It is a malignancy of the skin.

522. The initial screening test for AIDS is
① Lymphangiography.
② Enzyme-linked immunosorbent assay (ELISA).
③ Western blot assay.
④ Schilling's test.

523. Which finding is an opportunistic disease frequently seen in AIDS clients?
① Pancreatitis
② Prostatic cancer
③ Hodgkin's disease
④ *Pneumocystis carinii* pneumonia (PCP)

524. A 24-year-old man makes an appointment at the health clinic for his complaints of fatigue, diarrhea, and weight loss. He is concerned that he might have acquired immunodeficiency syndrome (AIDS). Mr. Evans is diagnosed as being HIV positive. When preparing for discharge, an important nursing goal is that he be knowledgeable about methods to prevent HIV transmission to others. Which response from the client indicates that he has a correct understanding of this?
① "I can donate blood 1 year after my therapy with zidovudine (Retrovir) is started."
② "I should avoid casual contact with all males."
③ "I need to wear gloves and a mask at all times."
④ "I should not donate my plasma, sperm, or organs."

REFERENCES

Beare PG, Myers JL: *Principles and practice of adult health nursing,* ed 2, St Louis, 1994, Mosby.

Mosby's medical, nursing, and allied health dictionary, ed 4, St Louis, 1994, Mosby.

Pagana KD, Pagana TJ: *Mosby's diagnostic and laboratory test reference,* ed 2, St Louis, 1994, Mosby.

Pagana KD, Pagana TJ: *Diagnostic testing and nursing implications: a case study approach,* ed 4, St Louis 1994, Mosby.

Rollant PD: Success on the NCLEX-RN exam: try this tripod approach, *Nursing* 22(10):6, 1992.

Rollant PD: Acing multiple-choice tests, *AJN career guide for 1994,* 1994, American Journal of Nursing.

Skidmore-Roth L: *Mosby's nursing drug reference,* St Louis, 1996, Mosby.

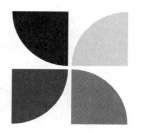

Correct Answers

1. no. 2.
2. no. 2.
3. no. 4.
4. no. 4.
5. no. 1.
6. no. 4.
7. no. 3.
8. no. 1.
9. no. 4.
10. no. 3.
11. no. 1.
12. no. 2.
13. no. 1.
14. no. 3.
15. no. 1.
16. no. 1.
17. no. 4.
18. no. 1.
19. no. 3.
20. no. 4.
21. no. 1.
22. no. 2.
23. no. 4.
24. no. 2.
25. no. 2.
26. no. 3.
27. no. 3.
28. no. 3.
29. no. 2.
30. no. 3.
31. no. 2.
32. no. 1.
33. no. 3.
34. no. 1.
35. no. 2.
36. no. 3.
37. no. 3.
38. no. 3.
39. no. 4.
40. no. 1.
41. no. 4.
42. no. 4.
43. no. 4.
44. no. 4.
45. no. 3.
46. no. 1.
47. no. 3.
48. no. 2.

49. no. 1.
50. no. 3.
51. no. 1.
52. no. 2.
53. no. 1.
54. no. 3.
55. no. 3.
56. no. 4.
57. no. 2.
58. no. 4.
59. no. 4.
60. no. 2.
61. no. 2.
62. no. 2.
63. no. 2.
64. no. 3.
65. no. 2.
66. no. 1.
67. no. 1.
68. no. 3.
69. no. 2.
70. no. 3.
71. no. 3.
72. no. 1.
73. no. 1.
74. no. 2.
75. no. 3.
76. no. 4.
77. no. 1.
78. no. 3.
79. no. 2.
80. no. 3.
81. no. 2.
82. no. 1.
83. no. 4.
84. no. 3.
85. no. 1.
86. no. 4.
87. no. 2.
88. no. 4.
89. no. 2.
90. no. 4.
91. no. 1.
92. no. 3.
93. no. 2.
94. no. 3.
95. no. 2.
96. no. 2.

97. no. 2.		**158.** no. 2.	
98. no. 2.		**159.** no. 2.	
99. no. 1.		**160.** no. 1.	
100. no. 4.		**161.** no. 2.	
101. no. 1.		**162.** no. 3.	
102. no. 3.		**163.** no. 3.	
103. no. 4.		**164.** no. 2.	
104. no. 2.		**165.** no. 4.	
105. no. 2.		**166.** no. 1.	
106. no. 4.		**167.** no. 2.	
107. no. 2.		**168.** no. 3.	
108. no. 2.		**169.** no. 2.	
109. no. 3.		**170.** no. 4.	
110. no. 2.		**171.** no. 1.	
111. no. 2.		**172.** no. 4.	
112. no. 1.		**173.** no. 2.	
113. no. 2.		**174.** no. 4.	
114. no. 3.		**175.** no. 4.	
115. no. 3.		**176.** no. 3.	
116. no. 2.		**177.** no. 2.	
117. no. 2.		**178.** no. 4.	
118. no. 4.		**179.** no. 2.	
119. no. 1.		**180.** no. 2.	
120. no. 2.		**181.** no. 4.	
121. no. 2.		**182.** no. 2.	
122. no. 3.		**183.** no. 4.	
123. no. 4.		**184.** no. 4.	
124. no. 1.		**185.** no. 2.	
125. no. 2.		**186.** no. 1.	
126. no. 2.		**187.** no. 3.	
127. no. 4.		**188.** no. 2.	
128. no. 2.		**189.** no. 3.	
129. no. 2.		**190.** no. 3.	
130. no. 3.		**191.** no. 3.	
131. no. 2.		**192.** no. 2.	
132. no. 3.		**193.** no. 2.	
133. no. 1.		**194.** no. 2.	
134. no. 3.		**195.** no. 3.	
135. no. 4.		**196.** no. 1.	
136. no. 1.		**197.** no. 3.	
137. no. 4.		**198.** no. 1.	
138. no. 4.		**199.** no. 4.	
139. no. 4.		**200.** no. 2.	
140. no. 3.		**201.** no. 4.	
141. no. 2.		**202.** no. 1.	
142. no. 4.		**203.** no. 3.	
143. no. 4.		**204.** no. 4.	
144. no. 3.		**205.** no. 1.	
145. no. 2.		**206.** no. 2.	
146. no. 2.		**207.** no. 3.	
147. no. 1.		**208.** no. 4.	
148. no. 3.		**209.** no. 1.	
149. no. 1.		**210.** no. 4.	
150. no. 4.		**211.** no. 3.	
151. no. 2.		**212.** no. 2.	
152. no. 3.		**213.** no. 2.	
153. no. 4.		**214.** no. 4.	
154. no. 1.		**215.** no. 4.	
155. no. 4.		**216.** no. 4.	
156. no. 2.		**217.** no. 1.	
157. no. 3.		**218.** no. 4.	

219. no. 3.
220. no. 4.
221. no. 3.
222. no. 3.
223. no. 1.
224. no. 4.
225. no. 2.
226. no. 1.
227. no. 1.
228. no. 2.
229. no. 4.
230. no. 2.
231. no. 3.
232. no. 3.
233. no. 4.
234. no. 4.
235. no. 2.
236. no. 1.
237. no. 3.
238. no. 1.
239. no. 3.
240. no. 3.
241. no. 1.
242. no. 1.
243. no. 2.
244. no. 3.
245. no. 1.
246. no. 4.
247. no. 4.
248. no. 3.
249. no. 1.
250. no. 2.
251. no. 1.
252. no. 2.
253. no. 4.
254. no. 1.
255. no. 1.
256. no. 4.
257. no. 1.
258. no. 2.
259. no. 1.
260. no. 2.
261. no. 3.
262. no. 2.
263. no. 4.
264. no. 2.
265. no. 3.
266. no. 4.
267. no. 2.
268. no. 4.
269. no. 3.
270. no. 1.
271. no. 3.
272. no. 1.
273. no. 4.
274. no. 2.
275. no. 1.
276. no. 1.
277. no. 1.
278. no. 1.
279. no. 2.

280. no. 3.
281. no. 1.
282. no. 3.
283. no. 4.
284. no. 3.
285. no. 2.
286. no. 1.
287. no. 2.
288. no. 3.
289. no. 3.
290. no. 1.
291. no. 4.
292. no. 2.
293. no. 3.
294. no. 1.
295. no. 3.
296. no. 4.
297. no. 3.
298. no. 4.
299. no. 2.
300. no. 3.
301. no. 2.
302. no. 1.
303. no. 2.
304. no. 2.
305. no. 3.
306. no. 2.
307. no. 1.
308. no. 4.
309. no. 3.
310. no. 3.
311. no. 1.
312. no. 1.
313. no. 1.
314. no. 2.
315. no. 2.
316. no. 1.
317. no. 3.
318. no. 2.
319. no. 2.
320. no. 4.
321. no. 2.
322. no. 2.
323. no. 2.
324. no. 1.
325. no. 3.
326. no. 3.
327. no. 4.
328. no. 2.
329. no. 1.
330. no. 4.
331. no. 3.
332. no. 2.
333. no. 2.
334. no. 4.
335. no. 1.
336. no. 3.
337. no. 2.
338. no. 3.
339. no. 1.
340. no. 4.

341. no. 4.
342. no. 3.
343. no. 2.
344. no. 2.
345. no. 1.
346. no. 4.
347. no. 3.
348. no. 1.
349. no. 4.
350. no. 3.
351. no. 2.
352. no. 4.
353. no. 4.
354. no. 3.
355. no. 3.
356. no. 2.
357. no. 2.
358. no. 1.
359. no. 1.
360. no. 4.
361. no. 4.
362. no. 1.
363. no. 1.
364. no. 3.
365. no. 2.
366. no. 1.
367. no. 2.
368. no. 2.
369. no. 1.
370. no. 4.
371. no. 2.
372. no. 1.
373. no. 3.
374. no. 3.
375. no. 2.
376. no. 4.
377. no. 3.
378. no. 3.
379. no. 3.
380. no. 1.
381. no. 2.
382. no. 1.
383. no. 1.
384. no. 4.
385. no. 2.
386. no. 2.
387. no. 4.
388. no. 1.
389. no. 4.
390. no. 3.
391. no. 2.
392. no. 4.
393. no. 1.
394. no. 1.
395. no. 3.
396. no. 3.
397. no. 3.
398. no. 3.
399. no. 3.
400. no. 1.
401. no. 1.

402. no. 4.
403. no. 3.
404. no. 1.
405. no. 4.
406. no. 1.
407. no. 4.
408. no. 2.
409. no. 4.
410. no. 4.
411. no. 2.
412. no. 1.
413. no. 2.
414. no. 2.
415. no. 2.
416. no. 1.
417. no. 1.
418. no. 1.
419. no. 2.
420. no. 4.
421. no. 4.
422. no. 3.
423. no. 1.
424. no. 1.
425. no. 2.
426. no. 3.
427. no. 1.
428. no. 2.
429. no. 2.
430. no. 3.
431. no. 3.
432. no. 4.
433. no. 2.
434. no. 4.
435. no. 3.
436. no. 3.
437. no. 4.
438. no. 3.
439. no. 2.
440. no. 1.
441. no. 2.
442. no. 4.
443. no. 4.
444. no. 4.
445. no. 1.
446. no. 2.
447. no. 3.
448. no. 4.
449. no. 3.
450. no. 2.
451. no. 1.
452. no. 4.
453. no. 1.
454. no. 2.
455. no. 2.
456. no. 2.
457. no. 1.
458. no. 3.
459. no. 1.
460. no. 4.
461. no. 3.
462. no. 2.

463. no. 3.
464. no. 2.
465. no. 4.
466. no. 4.
467. no. 4.
468. no. 2.
469. no. 1.
470. no. 4.
471. no. 1.
472. no. 4.
473. no. 2.
474. no. 2.
475. no. 4.
476. no. 3.
477. no. 1.
478. no. 4.
479. no. 1.
480. no. 2.
481. no. 2.
482. no. 4.
483. no. 3.
484. no. 4.
485. no. 2.
486. no. 4.
487. no. 3.
488. no. 2.
489. no. 1.
490. no. 4.
491. no. 3.
492. no. 3.
493. no. 2.

494. no. 2.
495. no. 4.
496. no. 3.
497. no. 2.
498. no. 1.
499. no. 3.
500. no. 1.
501. no. 3.
502. no. 1.
503. no. 3.
504. no. 4.
505. no. 1.
506. no. 1.
507. no. 1.
508. no. 2.
509. no. 3.
510. no. 1.
511. no. 1.
512. no. 2.
513. no. 3.
514. no. 3.
515. no. 3.
516. no. 2.
517. no. 4.
518. no. 1.
519. no. 3.
520. no. 4.
521. no. 1.
522. no. 2.
523. no. 4.
524. no. 4.

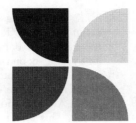

Correct Answers with Rationales

Editor's note: Three pieces of information are supplied at the end of each rationale. First, you will find a reference to a section in the *AJN/Mosby Nursing Boards Review* where a more complete discussion of the topic may be found, should you desire more information (e.g., A/E). A second reference indicates what part of the nursing process the question addresses (e.g., PL). The third piece of information describes the appropriate client need category (e.g., PS).

KEY TO ABBREVIATIONS
Section of the Review Book

A = Adult
H = Healthy Adult
S = Surgery
O = Oxygenation
NM = Nutrition and Metabolism
E = Elimination
SP = Sensation and Perception
M = Mobility
CA = Cellular Aberration

Nursing Process Category

AS = Assessment
AN = Analysis
PL = Plan
IM = Implementation
EV = Evaluation

Client Need Category

E = Safe, Effective Care Environment
PS = Physiologic Integrity
PC = Psychosocial Integrity
H = Health Promotion and Maintenance

1. no. 2. Hyperextending the neck can cause a spinal injury if the vertebrae have been fractured. The other options are correct, based on CPR standards. A/O, IM, PS

2. no. 2. The mouth is kept closed during inspiration. No more force than normal is required. The victim's neck is extended, not hyperextended. In both approaches, the mouth is open during expiration. A/O, IM, PS

3. no. 4. Using one hand, only approximately 400 ml of air can be delivered. Almost 1000 ml can be delivered if both hands are used. A/O, AN, PS

4. no. 4. Fluid volume is the first priority after adequate ventilation. The blood pressure and pulse indicate that the client is in a volume-depleted state. Sodium bi-carbonate may be given only after arterial blood gas results, usually when the pH is 7.1 or less and bicarbonate levels are low. Options no. 2 and no. 3 are not considerations of therapy in postarrest situations. A/O, PL, PS

5. no. 1. The type of instrument involved (blunt vs. sharp) and where it hit is the most valuable information because it will help define the type of injury. A sharp injury tends to bleed more quickly; a blunt injury tends to leak or ooze. Options no. 2 and no. 3 are important but are not specific to blood loss. Option no. 4 is irrelevant. A/O, AS, PS

6. no. 4. With a negative thoracentesis and an elevated central venous pressure (CVP), the only reasonable conclusion is that cardiac tamponade is the cause. Bleeding into the pericardial sac causes both decreased blood pressure and increased CVP. Options no. 1, no. 2, and no. 3 tend to have no effect on CVP. Normal CVP is 5 to 10 cm H_2O when a water manometer is used to obtain the reading. A/O, AN, PS

7. no. 3. When the systolic blood pressure falls below 80 mm Hg, circulation to the vital organs is severely compromised. A/O, AS, PS

8. no. 1. Increased levels of angiotensin and renin result in vasoconstriction of the peripheral vessels; thus blood is more available for the brain, heart, and kidneys. Options no. 3 and no. 4 are incorrect; these substances do not affect the respiratory center. A/O, AN, PS

9. no. 4. Although dopamine is a potent vasopressor, kidney perfusion can be maintained in the mild to moderate dosage range. In low doses (2 to 5 µg/kg/min), dopamine dilates renal, cerebral, and coronary blood vessels. In moderate doses (5 to 10 µg/kg/min), dopamine increases myocardial contractility. In high-dose ranges (over 10 µg/kg/min), dopamine constricts renal vessels. Untoward effects include dysrhythmias, angina, and pulmonary congestion. A/O, AN, PS

10. no. 3. A urine output of 30 ml/hr indicates that there is adequate kidney perfusion. In selected cases, systolic pressure of 90 or 100 mm Hg would not ensure adequate renal perfusion. The minimum for adequate urine output is 30 ml/hr. A/O, AS, PS

11. no. 1. The most precise measurement of hemodynamic status would be used, particularly in an older client. These two factors reflect fluid volume adequate enough to perfuse the body. Central venous pressure readings would best and more quickly reflect response

to treatment with CVP readings being maintained around 10 cm H$_2$O. Recommended urine output is 30 ml/hr for at least 2 consecutive hours. A/O, EV, PS

12. no. 2. As sympathomimetics, adrenergic agents cause vasoconstriction. Options no. 1 and no. 3 are incorrect and not desirable for the client in shock. Option no. 4 has no relationship to adrenergic agents. A/O, AN, PS

13. no. 1. Adrenalin is a potent cardiac stimulant that increases rate and contractility. It does not cause any of the effects listed in the other options. A/O, AN, PS

14. no. 3. As sympathomimetics, adrenergics can cause overstimulation of the heart and dysrhythmias. The other side effects listed are not considered serious. A/O, AS, PS

15. no. 1. These values indicate metabolic acidosis, as evidenced by low pH, normal Pco$_2$, and low bicarbonate level (<22 mEq/L), which indicates a metabolic disturbance. The Po$_2$ level has no bearing on determining the type of acidosis or alkalosis. A/O, AN, PS

16. no. 1. Any extreme in pH will inhibit enzyme activity with resulting loss of total body functioning. A/O, AN, PS

17. no. 4. The blood buffers (oxyhemoglobin, phosphates, carbonates) are the first line of defense. These tend to be quicker responses. Retention of bicarbonate by the kidneys is a slow process; it usually takes at least 24 hours to be effective. A/O, AN, PS

18. no. 1. A client receiving chronic steroid therapy is prone to a relative insufficiency when stressed because the adrenals cannot produce extra amounts of cortisol as required. Addison's disease is a primary adrenocortical insufficiency. Azotemia is the condition of abnormally high levels of nitrogenous wastes as measured by blood urea nitrogen. A/NM, AN, PS

19. no. 3. A client with massive trauma is at risk for the development of disseminated intravascular coagulation (DIC). Oozing of blood at the IV site is commonly one of the first assessment findings. The other findings are also typically found with DIC. A/O, AN, PS

20. no. 4. This client has deficiency of glucocorticoids and mineralocorticoids, especially when under stress. Replacement drugs are required. A/NM, AN, PS

21. no. 1. Although hemorrhage is a symptom seen in disseminated intravascular coagulation, the problem is really one of microcoagulation. Heparin would be used cautiously because it blocks the subsequent formation of microemboli by inhibiting thrombin activity. Packed red blood cells will replace the lost red blood cells. A/O, AN, PS

22. no. 2. The first phase of disseminated intravascular coagulation (DIC), hypercoagulation, results in the formation of microthrombi. Renal failure can result from thrombosis of the microcirculation of the kidneys. Options no. 1, no. 3, and no. 4 have no relationship to DIC. A/O, AN, PS

23. no. 4. Remove hypothermia equipment when the client is 1° above the recommended temperature. An additional temperature drop may occur after discontinuance of the treatment. A/O, IM, PS

24. no. 2. Decreasing pain is the most important priority at this time. As long as the pain is present, there is the danger of damage to myocardial tissue. Starting an IV is a second action, especially if the medication is ordered IV. Note that nitroglycerine SL may be ordered first to rule out severe angina. A/O, IM, PS

25. no. 2. An infarction results in anoxia of the involved tissue. This anoxia results in ischemic tissue with irritation of the nerve endings in the infarcted area. Pain in the left arm and neck is commonly the clinical presentation of referred pain. A/O, AN, PS

26. no. 3. The left ventricle of the heart, which contributes most to contraction, is most frequently the site of a myocardial infarction. Because of this, the nurse more commonly monitors myocardial infarction clients for left-sided congestive heart failure. A/O, AN, PS

27. no. 3. Keeping family and significant others informed of the client's progress is of paramount importance and is most therapeutic for the client. A/O, IM, H

28. no. 3. Denial is the most common reason for not seeking medical attention. The client may fear the consequences and thus uses denial as a defense mechanism. There is not enough information in the stem to select responses 1, 2, or 4. A/O, AN, PC

29. no. 2. Establishing an airway is the primary objective and action in any emergency, especially in a cardiopulmonary arrest. Initiating cardiac massage and calling a physician follow next in order of priority. A/O, IM, PS

30. no. 3. Presence of a carotid pulse represents adequate vascular perfusion and myocardial oxygenation. Options no. 1 and no. 2 indicate adequate perfusion to the pupils and periphery. Option no. 4 is an abnormal response that may be a manifestation of a pyramidal tract lesion, an upper motor neuron defect. A/O, EV, PS

31. no. 2. Chest pain in an acute myocardial infarction is intense and severe and is not relieved by nitroglycerin or rest. Nitroglycerin, the drug of choice for angina pectoris, relieves anginal pain. A/O, AS, PS

32. no. 1. Morphine sulfate is the drug of choice in this situation because it has a rapid action, is potent, has a diuretic effect, results in slight collateral coronary vasodilation, and is helpful to decrease anxiety. These are all particularly beneficial outcomes for the myocardial infarction client. Options no. 3 and no. 4 are not usually used for chest pain. Codiene is commonly used to suppress the cough reflex. Dilaudid is commonly used for severe pain in terminal conditions. Meperidine (Demerol) tends to lower the blood pressure with a vagal type of activity and clammy, pale skin. A/O, AN, PS

33. no. 3. With an infarction, anoxia of the myocardium occurs. Administration of oxygen will help relieve dyspnea and cyanosis associated with the pain, but the primary purpose is to increase oxygen concentration in the injured tissue of the myocardium. A/O, AN, PS

34. no. 1. The first 24 to 48 hours is a dangerous period because of the extreme irritability and instability of the heart muscle. The irritability comes from the isch-

emic area surrounding the infarcted dead-tissue area. A/O, AN, PS

35. no. 2. The heart is extremely irritable at this time, and ventricular dysrhythmias are most common and serious. The other options listed are serious but are not as commonly associated with myocardial infarction as dysrhythmias are. A/O, AN, PS

36. no. 3. The mortality rate is 80% for all clients who go into cardiogenic shock. Even sophisticated drugs and intraaortic balloon pumping may not be able to help the client who has lost the pumping action of the heart. A/O, AN, PS

37. no. 3. Whenever there is tissue death, certain enzymes are released. Creatine kinase-MB isoenzyme (CK-MB) and lactic dehydrogenase (LDH_1) isoenzymes are specific for cardiac muscle; typically, the higher the level of enzyme elevation, the greater the damage to the muscle. A 12-lead electrocardiogram is used to determine the location of a myocardial infarction. A/O, AN, PS

38. no. 3. Lidocaine decreases ventricular irritability and thereby reduces premature ventricular contractions. Procainamide is a second-choice drug if lidocaine is ineffective. Diltiazem, a calcium channel blocker, is typically administered IV push slowly, and then a drip is hung for 24 hours for the treatment of atrial fibrillation in clients after cardiac surgery. Digoxin is used to slow the heart rate and increase contractility. It is given IV push slowly and not given in an IV solution or by drip method. A/O, AN, PS

39. no. 4. Confusion is a more common initial toxic effect of lidocaine. A/O, AS, PS

40. no. 1. Administration of laxatives can prevent straining on defecation. Straining results in Valsalva's maneuver. Options no. 2 and no. 4 may stimulate Valsalva's maneuver. Liquids at room temperature neither prevent nor stimulate Valsalva's maneuver. A/O, IM, PS

41. no. 4. There is a high probability that her husband may die, and she needs to prepare for that. Actions in options no. 1, no. 2, and no. 3 would tend to facilitate movement through the grief experience. Letting her know the nurses are competent may reassure her, but it will not help with anticipatory grieving. A/O, IM, H

42. no. 4. Allowing the client to express his concerns is the initial priority. A one-on-one teaching approach is advisable for this delicate subject. When he feels comfortable, a teaching session with significant others may be planned. A/O, PL, H

43. no. 4. Liver is an organ meat high in cholesterol; tuna fish and shellfish have minimal cholesterol. Rice has the lowest amount. A/O, AN, H

44. no. 4. Taking aspirin daily prevents platelet aggregation and may decrease the risk of myocardial infarction. Family history of cardiovascular disease, diabetes, and smoking increase the risk. A/O, AS, PS

45. no. 3. This represents the most reasonable amount of activity. Walking up stairs significantly increases the workload of the heart. The physician will determine how and when the client can undertake this activity. A/O, IM, H

46. no. 1. Congestive left-sided heart failure results in a pulmonary circulatory congestion, and the characteristic finding is dyspnea. Bronchi are not obstructed by mucoid secretions. Secretions are watery and voluminous. It is unlikely that the heart will dilate to the point of lung-tissue compression severe enough to cause dyspnea. Ascites is a manifestation of right-sided heart failure, which causes portal hypertension with liver enlargement and eventually failure. A/O, AN, PS

47. no. 3. Venous pressure increases and stasis occurs, promoting the extravasation of fluid from the vascular space into the interstitial tissue. Diffusion results when solid particles in solution move from an area of higher concentration to lower concentration; osmosis is fluid moving from an area of lower solute concentration to higher concentration. Neither of these describes the cause of edema. The capillary bed does dilate, but it is the increased venous pressure that causes the edema. A/O, AN, PS

48. no. 2. Because of gravity, dependent edema, especially in the feet, occurs in right-sided cardiac failure. The edema is pitting and nonpainful in nature. Periorbital edema usually occurs as a result of head trauma or renal failure. A/O, AS, PS

49. no. 1. *Left-sided* heart failure produces pulmonary findings such as increased shortness of breath and a dry or congested cough. The other symptoms listed are systemic ones associated with *right-sided* congestive heart failure. A/O, AS, PS

50. no. 3. Potassium affects neuromuscular activity. Hyperkalemia (serum potassium greater than 5.5 mEq/L) often results in ventricular fibrillation, leading to death. A/O, AN, PS

51. no. 1. Respirations in congestive heart failure are rapid and shallow. Cheyne-Stokes respirations are seen in the terminal stages of congestive heart failure and in head-injured clients with increased intracranial pressure. Stridor is heard only with the narrowing of a large airway. A/O, AS, PS

52. no. 2. The client with congestive heart failure can breathe more easily in a Fowler's or semi-Fowler's position because gravity promotes pooling of blood in the extremities. This decreases the preload, which helps decrease the workload of the heart. Also, maximal lung expansion is permitted with less pressure being exerted from the abdominal organs, and the cough reflex is stronger in an upright position. A/O, IM, PS

53. no. 1. Overall the entire body's circulation is decreased in congestive heart failure. Thus drug absorption and distribution are slowed when drugs are given in the oral or IM route. A/O, AN, PS

54. no. 3. Furosemide (Lasix) causes a loss of potassium. Digitalis may cause a loss of magnesium. Hypokalemia and hypomagnesemia increase the effect of digoxin and increase the risk of digitalis toxicity. A/O, PL, PS

55. no. 3. Chemical agents are effective by vasodilation, which pools the blood in the peripheral areas. In turn, preload is decreased with a decrease in the workload of the heart and a decrease in the congestion. A/O, AN, PS

56. no. 4. The best action to check for postural hypotension is to check blood pressure with the client in a lying and a standing position, especially before each dose of medication, when dosage adjustments are being done to find the best dose for the client. Response 3 may be done with clients who are unable to stand; it is not the best evaluation action. A/O, IM, E

57. no. 2. Canned tuna is highly salted (628 mg sodium per 3¼ oz). Unsalted nuts are not contraindicated on a sodium-restricted diet. Whole milk and eggs are not allowed on a low-cholesterol, low-polysaturated-fat diet, but they are allowed on a 2000 mg sodium diet. Low-sodium milk is used only on a *severely* sodium-restricted diet (200 to 500 mg sodium). A/O, IM, H

58. no. 4. Breads and cereals contain almost no potassium. A/O, IM, H

59. no. 4. Thrombophlebitis is the occlusion of a vein with inflammation and thrombus formation. It results in such findings as a positive Homans' sign, history of leg pain, redness, and unilateral swelling. Pallor of the legs and shiny atrophic skin are signs of decreased arterial circulation to the extremity. A/O, AS, PS

60. no. 2. To prevent emboli, the dislodgment of a thrombus in a client with thrombophlebitis, the therapeutic interventions are usually to maintain bed rest for 5 to 10 days, elevate the legs, apply warm, moist packs to the involved site, and provide range-of-motion exercises to the *unaffected* extremity at least two times per shift. A/O, PL, PS

61. no. 2. Heparin prevents the conversion of fibrinogen to fibrin and prothrombin to thrombin by enhancing the inhibitory effects of antithrombin III. Neither parenteral nor oral anticoagulants affect existing thrombi. A/O, AN, PS

62. no. 2. Monitor the activated partial thromboplastin time (APTT) when clients are receiving parenteral anticoagulants. Prothrombin times are monitored when a client is given enteral anticoagulants such as warfarin (Coumadin) or dicumarol. A/O, IM, PS

63. no. 2. A positive Homans' sign is pain in the calf when the foot is dorsiflexed. It is a sign of phlebitis. The other responses are indicative of too much heparin, which results in bleeding. A/O, AS, PS

64. no. 3. Protamine sulfate is the antidote for heparin sodium; vitamin K (AquaMEPHYTON) is the antidote for warfarin (Coumadin). A/O, AN, PS

65. no. 2. The client should avoid using any product that increases anticoagulation (e.g., aspirin) or causes trauma to the tissues (e.g., a hard toothbrush). The client should notify the physician at once of any findings of bleeding such as easy bruising or hematuria. Melena would be difficult to monitor for because the client is on iron preparations that make the stool dark and tarlike. A/O, IM, E

66. no. 1. Hyperventilation and lowered Pco_2 are common after a pulmonary embolus. The bicarbonate is normal. O_2 and O_2 saturation are not used to evaluate the acid-base status of a client. A/O, AN, PS

67. no. 1. With results of respiratory acidosis on the arterial blood gases the client would have slow, shallow breathing or else have severe congestion in the lungs with problems such as pneumonia or noncardiogenic pulmonary edema, also known as adult respiratory distress syndrome (ARDS). The nursing action would be to get the client to breathe deeply and more rapidly. Responses 3 and 4 are typically hyperventilation situations that are found in head-injured clients. A/O, AS, PS

68. no. 3. Central cyanosis would indicate a serious drop in the Po_2. It is the most significant sign of hypoxia. Resonance is a normal finding. Increased tactile fremitus suggests lung consolidation or congestion, not hypoxia. A/O, AS, PS

69. no. 2. The ratio is 1 part of carbonic acid (Pco_2) to 20 parts of base bicarbonate (HCO_3). A/O, AN, PS

70. no. 3. Cor pulmonale is a complication of conditions causing chronic pulmonary hypertension such as pulmonary fibrosis. Hypertrophy of the right side of the heart results from chronic pulmonary hypertension and causes the signs and symptoms of right-sided heart failure. A/O, AN, PS

71. no. 3. For clients with a long-standing history of chronic obstructive pulmonary disease, hypoxemia, a $Po_2 < 80$ mm Hg, is the major stimulus to breathing. If oxygen is administered in high concentrations until the $Po_2 > 80$ mm Hg, it will eliminate the hypoxic drive with a reduction in the rate and depth of respirations. A/O, IM, PS

72. no. 1. Pursed-lip breathing prevents bronchiolar collapse, which results in air trapping and overinflated alveoli. A/O, AN, PS

73. no. 1. Hemoptysis indicates bleeding, and percussion could exacerbate this condition. The conditions indicated in options no. 2, no. 3, and no. 4 would benefit from percussion because there is the possibility of retained secretions in these situations. A/O, AN, PS

74. no. 2. Hyperkalemia always occurs with acidemia. A/O, AS, PS

75. no. 3. Anginal pain is not usually influenced by coughing or associated with a productive cough. A/O, AN, PS

76. no. 4. The pneumococcal bacteria account for the majority of pneumonia cases, and the resulting infection is characterized by rust-colored sputum. Sputum color varies with different types of organisms. A/O, AS, PS

77. no. 1. Egophony (a change in voice sound) indicates that fluid or consolidation of the lung is present. The middle lobe is correctly located in response 1. Respirations are usually rapid and shallow in pneumonia with pain on deep inspiration. Breath sounds would be diminished but not in the locations given in responses 2 and 3. A pleural friction rub, not a pericardial rub, would be auscultated. A/O, AS, PS

78. no. 3. Dullness is of medium-intensity pitch and is elicited over areas of mixed solid and lung tissues, as with the consolidated lung tissue in pneumonia. Tympanic sounds are drumlike, as heard when a gas-filled bowel is percussed. Resonance is the normal sound heard when normal lung tissue is percussed. Hyperresonance is heard over an emphysematous lung or an area with a pneumothorax. A/O, AS, PS

79. no. 2. Splinting occurs when the chest is held rigid to prevent pain on respiratory movement. A/O, AS, PS

80. no. 3. Increased fluids are needed to help liquefy secretions; no history of cardiac problems has been given that would contraindicate this action. Analgesics (although not necessarily narcotics) are given so the discomfort associated with coughing, deep breathing, percussion, and postural drainage every 2 to 4 hours can be tolerated. A/O, PL, E

81. no. 2. Venturi masks can control oxygen delivery at 24%, 28%, 31%, 35%, and 40% with a great deal of accuracy. A/O, AN, PS

82. no. 1. Gentamicin is classified as an aminoglycoside. This group of antibiotics is nephrotoxic. Blood urea nitrogen and creatinine must be monitored to assess for any decrease in renal function as shown by an increase in BUN and creatinine. However, the creatinine elevation is most specific to kidney failure. A/O, AS, PS

83. no. 4. Atelectasis is a complication of pneumonia or any other conditions with hypoventilation. It is treated with tracheal suctioning, effective coughing, and deep breathing. It is prevented mainly by deep breathing frequently. A/O, AN, PS

84. no. 3. Measures to prevent hypoxemia during suctioning include preoxygenation and limiting each suctioning to 10 to 15 seconds. Responses 1, 2, and 4 are correct actions. A/O, IM, E

85. no. 1. Tuberculosis is an infectious disease caused by the bacteria *Mycobacterium tuberculosis.* A/O, AN, E

86. no. 4. The purified protein derivative (PPD) skin test is specific for tuberculosis and is considered positive when there is induration or wheal, a raised area, of 10 mm or larger. Erythema is a redness or inflammation of the skin or mucous membranes that is the result of a dilation and congestion of the superficial capillaries. A PPD skin test may be considered positive at less than 10 mm if the client is already immunosuppressed. The general public, who have no significant risk factors and who have no contact with a patient population, would require a 15 mm induration for a positive skin test. A/O, AS, PS

87. no. 2. The PPD skin test is used to determine presence of tuberculous antibodies; it indicates, when positive, that a person has been exposed to *Mycobacterium tuberculosis* and that the body has produced tuberculosis antibodies. Further studies are needed to determine the presence of an active infection. A/O, AN, PS

88. no. 4. In the treatment of tuberculosis, drugs are often given in combination with other drugs to delay development of resistance and to increase tuberculostatic effects. A/O, AN, PS

89. no. 2. Jaundice indicates liver malfunction. Purpura is any of several bleeding disorders characterized by hemorrhage into the tissues, particularly beneath the skin or mucous membranes, producing ecchymoses or petechiae. A/O, AS, PS

90. no. 4. The peripheral neuritis that commonly occurs with isoniazid therapy can be controlled with the administration of vitamin B₆ (pyridoxine) because the neuritis is a result of pyridoxine deficiency. A/O, AN, PS

91. no. 1. Rifampin (Rimactane) will color all body fluids (including tears) orange. A/O, IM, H

92. no. 3. Isoniazid (INH) is used as preventive therapy in household members of newly diagnosed clients. It is effective and inexpensive and is given orally. A/O, AN, PS

93. no. 2. Because tuberculosis drugs, especially isoniazid (INH), are known to cause hepatitis in some persons, liver function tests are commonly done before the client begins the drug therapy and then sometimes weekly or monthly throughout the therapy. A/O, AS, PS

94. no. 3. Histoplasmosis has many of the same symptoms as tuberculosis but is caused by a fungus. A/O, AN, PS

95. no. 2. The fungus is responsive to amphotericin B, not to the other drugs listed. A/O, AN, PS

96. no. 2. This position promotes maximal ventilation of the affected lung. Positioning on the operative side would inhibit thoracic excursion and therefore ventilation. Fowler's position increases the intrathoracic space, which allows maximal ventilation. A/O, PL, PS

97. no. 2. Continuous bubbling could indicate an air leak in the system. Bubbling should be intermittent, and it indicates the expulsion of air from the pleural space. There should be fluctuation in the water-seal tube with respiration. Suction is not used in the water-seal chamber on a three-chamber or bottle system; suction is applied to the suction control chamber, which is typically the third chamber farthest from the patient. Blood is collected in the collection chamber, which is the first chamber closest to the client. A/O, AS, PS

98. no. 2. Water-seal drainage means that the chest tube is under a water seal to prevent air from entering the chest cavity. Chest-tube drainage setups must be kept below chest level at all times. The chest tube must not be attached to any tube or drainage bottle that would be open to air. A/O, AN, PS

99. no. 1. The fluid in the tube oscillates with inspiration and expiration when the water-seal apparatus is functioning properly. On inspiration the fluid will rise; on expiration the fluid will fall. A/O, AN, PS

100. no. 4. The most common symptom of bronchogenic carcinoma is the development of a cough or change in the severity of a chronic cough. There are no early signs of lung cancer. A/O, AS, PS

101. no. 1. The client will be kept NPO until the gag reflex returns in 2 to 4 hours. A/O, PL, PS

102. no. 3. The less pain the client experiences, the more effectively the client can cough and deep breathe. The other options are good but cannot be effective unless the client's postoperative pain is controlled. A/O, IM, PS

103. no. 4. The long tube submerged 3 to 5 cm below the fluid level acts as a one-way valve, permitting air and fluid to drain out of the pleural space while preventing influx of air. A/O, AN, PS

104. no. 2. Continuous bubbling in the water-seal chamber during inspiration and expiration may indicate an air

leak in the system. Bubbling should be intermittent in the water-seal chamber if there is an air leak in the lung. A/O, AN, PS

105. no. 2. After a specimen is obtained form an arterial site, application of pressure to the site for 5 minutes prevents bleeding and hematoma formation. If blood specimens are obtained from a vein, pressure to the site is typically held for 1 to 2 minutes. A/O, IM, E

106. no. 4. Normal values are as follows: pH 7.35 to 7.45, Po_2 80 to 100 mm Hg, Pco_2 35 to 45 mm Hg, oxygen saturation 95% to 98%. A/O, AS, PS

107. no. 2. The client should be less confused. Confusion usually results when the Po_2 falls below 50. A/O, EV, PS

108. no. 2. Effects of gravity are lost when lying or bending, and gastric reflux occurs more easily. Increased stress may increase stomach acid; however, position changes along with this increased acid would result in a report of symptoms being worse. Position changes that counteract the effects of gravity are a priority. A/NM, AS, PS

109. no. 3. Esophagus-sphincter pressure is increased by gastrin in the stomach and decreased by fatty foods, peppermint, alcohol, nicotine, secretin, and cholecystokinin from the small intestine. A/NM, AS, PS

110. no. 2. Smoking and alcohol aggravate and contribute to the condition. The head of the bed should be raised. Increased weight, especially in the abdominal area, may aggravate the symptoms by pushing on the esophageal sphincter. Exercise that involves bending or increased intraabdominal pressure may aggravate gastroesophageal reflux. A/NM, PL, H

111. no. 2. The late development of symptoms coupled with early lymphatic spread means that metastasis has probably occurred by the time the disease is diagnosed. Thus prognosis is poor at the time of diagnosis. Aspiration does not commonly occur in esophageal cancer; regurgitation of blood-flecked esophageal contents is more common. The most common symptoms are dysphagia and pain that increases with swallowing. A/NM, AN, PS

112. no. 1. Clients are advised to eat small meals to prevent excessive gastric distention and to avoid eating before going to bed or lying down. Swallowing air and belching tend to increase gastric regurgitation. A/NM, IM, H

113. no. 2. A local anesthetic is given to deaden the gag reflex. Do not give oral fluids until this reflex returns. Without a gag reflex, risk of aspiration is high. A/NM, IM, PS

114. no. 3. Guaiac testing is done to detect presence of occult (not visible) blood. Hydrochloric acid is tested by measuring the pH of the stomach aspirate during a gastric analysis. Options no. 2 and no. 4 are incorrect. A/NM, AN, PS

115. no. 3. Duodenal ulcer pain occurs when excess hydrochloric acid overwhelms the mucosal integrity. Nighttime pain is common with duodenal ulcers. Typically, pain with a gastric ulcer usually occurs after the ingestion of food; options no. 1, no. 2, and no. 4 would apply. A/NM, AS, PS

116. no. 2. Nicotine stimulates the secretory cells and increases gastric acidity, thus enhancing symptoms. All of the other options are incorrect. A/NM, IM, H

117. no. 2. Coffee, even when decaffeinated, is thought to stimulate gastric acidity. Coffee may increase systolic pressure; however, option no. 4 is not specific to the question. A/NM, IM, H

118. no. 4. A subtotal gastrectomy (Billroth I or II) involves removal of one half to two thirds of the lower stomach, including the antrum and pylorus. This area is the gastric-producing portion of the stomach. A Billroth I is a gastroduodenostomy; Billroth II is a gastrojejunostomy. A/NM, AN, E

119. no. 1. The vagus nerve stimulates secretion of hydrochloric acid. A vagotomy would eliminate the stimulus of hydrochloric acid and gastrin hormone secretion. The other options do not describe functions of the vagus nerve. A/NM, AN, PS

120. no. 2. The secretion of bile is blocked if the duodenum is removed. A/NM, AN, PS

121. no. 2. The high incision causes pain that, in turn, limits chest expansion. Options no. 1, no. 3, and no. 4 are incorrect. A/NM, AN, PS

122. no. 3. When bowel sounds return to normal, peristalsis has returned, and the nasogastric tube can be removed. Passage of numerous liquid stools may indicate a hyperactive bowel or other problems. Passage of flatus along with the return of bowel sounds after the procedure indicates a safe time to remove the nasogastric tube. A/NM, AN, PS

123. no. 4. After a subtotal gastrectomy, food can move quickly into the jejunum in a highly concentrated form, causing what is known as the dumping syndrome. Client teaching should include the avoidance of concentrated sweets and liquids during mealtimes to avert symptoms. Eating slowly is also recommended. Because carbohydrates leave the stomach more quickly, diet guidelines include low carbohydrates and high protein and fat. Options no. 1, no. 2, and no. 3 are incorrect. A/NM, AN, PS

124. no. 1. Aluminum hydroxide gel (Amphogel) coats the gastrointestinal mucosa, but it is not absorbed systemically. Constipation may result from the aluminum. Phosphorus excretion is enhanced; it binds the phosphorus from the serum and is lost in the stool. Both constipation and phosphorus excretion may be dose related. The other options are incorrect. A/NM, AN, PS

125. no. 2. The diet for the treatment of dumping syndrome is six small feedings with moderate protein and fat and low carbohydrates. Refined or concentrated carbohydrates should be avoided because they leave the stomach more quickly, pull fluid into the intestine, and increase insulin release. Thus the symptoms occur for dumping syndrome. A/NM, EV, PS

126. no. 2. Diarrhea with a sudden urge to defecate and borborygmi are classic symptoms of dumping syndrome. Borborygmi are noises made from gas passing through the small intestine. Other signs and symptoms include abdominal cramps, weakness, sweating, palpations, and dizziness. A/NM, EV, PS

127. no. 4. Propantheline bromide (Pro-Banthine), an anticholinergic, promotes urinary retention and inhibits gastrointestinal mobility and gastric secretions. A dry mouth is a side effect of propantheline bromide (Pro-Banthine); however, it is not dose limiting. A/NM, AN, PS

128. no. 2. A fecalith obstructs the lumen of the appendix, leading to inflammation. A/NM, AN, PS

129. no. 2. The colon is filled with bacteria that invade the peritoneal cavity after the appendix ruptures. Digestive juices are not found in the appendix. A/NM, AN, PS

130. no. 3. Vitamin C is important in the formation of granulation and collagen tissue. Vitamin E has no known special role; vitamin B_1 may have a role in antibody formation and white blood cell function; vitamin D is necessary for absorption, transport, and metabolism of calcium. A/NM, AN, PS

131. no. 2. Until the client is responsive, she should be placed in a side-lying position to prevent aspiration of secretions or vomitus. All other options are correct. A/NM, IM, E

132. no. 3. Pain is a subjective experience. Clients' reactions to pain vary widely, depending on such factors as training, culture, and previous experience. How a client exhibits pain is not always a reliable indicator of how much pain is being experienced. A/NM, AS, PS

133. no. 1. Cholecystectomy clients have an increased susceptibility to respiratory complications. Because of the subcostal incision and the discomfort associated with the incision site, they tend to breathe shallowly. Postoperative pain should be treated and controlled in a timely manner. This will facilitate coughing and deep breathing to prevent hypostatic pneumonia. Maintaining respiratory function is a priority in the early postoperative period. A/NM, PL, E

134. no. 3. An output of 30 ml or less per hour is indicative of inadequate fluid-volume replacement after surgery. Options no. 1, no. 2, and no. 4 are expected outcomes after this surgery. A/NM, AS, PS

135. no. 4. Factors that contribute to delayed wound healing in obese clients are limited vascularity of adipose tissue, dead spaces in adipose tissue left during suturing, and increased tension on sutures. A/NM, AS, H

136. no. 1. Following discharge, the client who has had abdominal surgery is usually permitted activity as tolerated. The only restriction is to avoid heavy lifting, pushing, and pulling. A low-fat diet may be required for the first few weeks after surgery; otherwise the diet is advanced as tolerated. A/NM, EV, PS

137. no. 4. Signs and symptoms consistent with a diagnosis of cholecystitis include fullness, eructation, and dyspepsia after fat ingestion; abdominal pain, usually in the right upper quadrant; and nausea and vomiting. A/NM, AS, PS

138. no. 4. The nurse would verify the order with the physician who wrote it. Meperidine (Demerol) is usually ordered because morphine tends to cause spasms of the bile ducts, which may result in increased pain. A/NM, IM, E

139. no. 4. A cholecystogram is an x-ray visualization of the gallbladder and biliary tract after oral ingestion of iodine dye. An allergy history is important. If she is allergic to any shellfish, she may be allergic to iodine. A/NM, AS, PS

140. no. 3. A T-tube is inserted whenever the common bile duct is explored. The other options describe a standard cholecystectomy, which does not require placement of a T-tube. A/NM, AN, PS

141. no. 2. The nurse would irrigate a nasogastric tube only with normal saline and as ordered to keep it patent. Using distilled water can cause electrolyte depletion in the postoperative client. In these clients the nasogastric tube should not be repositioned without a physician's order because of the risk of damage to the internal operative site. A/NM, IM, PS

142. no. 4. This answer provides the client with specific information. A/NM, IM, E

143. no. 4. The nurse would notify her physician because drainage should be 200 to 500 ml per day for the first several days. T-tubes are usually not irrigated. Continued drainage after 3 days may indicate blockage of the common bile duct. A/NM, IM, PS

144. no. 3. A T-tube is usually removed 7 to 10 days after surgery, after a T-tube cholangiogram, to determine the status of the common bile duct, which should be patent. The other options are incorrect. A/NM, AN, E

145. no. 2. Common causes associated with pancreatitis are trauma, infection, alcohol abuse, and biliary tract disease. Alcoholism and biliary tract disease are the most common factors. These disorders can cause fibrosis and edema of the pancreas, which results in inadequate digestion of fats and proteins. The pancreatic enzymes, unable to follow their normal course, build up in the ducts and eventually rupture the ducts and result in autodigestion of the pancreas. A/NM, AS, PS

146. no. 2. The exocrine function of the pancreas is to secrete three digestive enzymes—amylase, lipase, and trypsin. Secretion of insulin is an endocrine function. A/NM, AN, PS

147. no. 1. By keeping the client NPO, digestive activity is decreased and there is less pancreatic stimulation. The other options are appropriate secondary goals. A/NM, PL, PS

148. no. 3. Propantheline bromide (Pro-Banthine) is an anticholinergic drug useful as an antispasmodic to relieve pancreatic pain. Magnesium hydroxide, an antacid, is useful in mild cases. Pancreatin is given with meals to aid in digestion. A/NM, AN, PS

149. no. 1. The serum amylase is the first of the pancreatic enzymes to rise in pancreatitis, and the level is used most frequently to diagnose and to evaluate response to treatment. The AST is the former serum glutamic-oxaloacetic transaminase (SGOT) and is a liver function test. The ESR is used to determine inflammatory response. A/NM, EV, PS

150. no. 4. The serum transaminases, AST and ALT (alanine aminotransferase, formerly serum glutamic-pyruvic transaminase [SGPT]), are the first to show an elevation. Abnormal serum ammonia, bilirubin, and

prothrombin time are all indicative of more advanced, serious liver disease. A/NM, AS, PS

151. no. 2. Bed rest with bathroom privileges is recommended to promote liver regeneration. Options no. 1 and no. 3 would be appropriate but not priority. Option no. 4 is incorrect because rest is needed; however, diversional activity while on bed rest would be desirable. A/NM, PL, E

152. no. 3. Adequate calories either in the diet or through intravenous therapy are necessary for the liver to regenerate. Most clients tolerate a low-fat, high-carbohydrate diet best, with the largest meal in the morning when energy level is greatest. Liquids of 2500 to 3000 ml per day are recommended to prevent dehydration. A/NM, PL, PS

153. no. 4. In cirrhosis, the liver cells develop fatty infiltrates and degenerate by an inflammatory process. Therefore there are fewer liver cells available to accommodate the volume of blood. The inflammatory process also increases the congestion in the liver, which inhibits blood flow. This results in venous backup, causing dilation of the esophageal vessels. A/NM, AN, PS

154. no. 1. It is important for the nurse to elicit an alcohol-consumption history from the client in order to accurately observe withdrawal during hospitalization. The items in the other options may be interventions only after mutual planning with the client. A/NM, PL, E

155. no. 4. A quiet, calm environment with even lighting minimizes the chance of creating shadows and reactions such as alcoholic hallucinations. Unusual noise, restraints, or lighting may increase or stimulate agitation. Side rails that are up would be appropriate. Restraints, usually soft, might be used only if the client is in danger of harming himself. A/NM, IM, E

156. no. 2. Portal hypertension is common in cirrhosis and causes these problems. Other signs and symptoms include anorexia, weakness, fatigue, jaundice, ascites, bleeding tendencies, anemia, palmar erythema, and spider angiomas. A/NM, AS, PS

157. no. 3. Prothrombin time increases in clients with cirrhosis; it takes blood longer to clot when there is liver failure. Leukopenia is to be expected with cirrhosis. A/NM, AS, PS

158. no. 2. Portal hypertension causes blood to accumulate in the weaker vessels of the esophagus, causing them to become distended. These vessels can rupture if the distention becomes too great. The other options do not contribute to the formation of esophageal varices. A/NM, AN, PS

159. no. 2. Portal hypertension will not cause pulmonary edema. Pulmonary edema is usually caused by left-sided heart failure. A/NM, AN, PS

160. no. 1. Insertion of any tube through the esophagus traumatizes the distended vessels, making reinsertion for a faulty tube undesirable. Therefore checking the balloons for leaks before insertion is a priority. Labeling the lumens of the tube prevents confusion after the tube has been inserted. Both balloons are always inflated with air, never fluid, and are inflated after placement. A/NM, IM, E

161. no. 2. Administering a neomycin enema may be done at a later time to decrease ammonia production in the bowel and to prevent hepatic coma. The other three options are necessary before inserting the Sengstaken-Blakemore tube. A/NM, IM, E

162. no. 3. The client should be placed in a semi-Fowler's position (not supine) to promote ventilation and prevent gastric reflux and aspiration. Side lying with the head up is also acceptable. With this tube in place, the client is not able to swallow anything, including saliva. Thus actions in option no. 1 are correct. A/NM, IM, E

163. no. 3. Upward dislodgment of the esophageal balloon may result in respiratory obstruction. Upward dislodgment is more likely because tension is used with this tube to put pressure on the esophageal-gastric junction from the gastric balloon. Ulceration is not likely because the tube is used for a short time, the esophageal balloon is usually deflated every 12 hours, and the gastric balloon is usually deflated every 24 to 36 hours. If pressure on the balloons is checked periodically, esophageal rupture can be prevented. A/NM, AN, PS

164. no. 2. Vasopressin is a potent vasopressor; optimally, it results in constriction of the esophageal veins. It can be given IV or through the nasogastric tube port. A/NM, IM, PS

165. no. 4. Clients with Sengstaken-Blakemore tubes should be sedated cautiously because of the risk of aspiration and respiratory insufficiency. A/NM, PL, E

166. no. 1. This client needs a diet to correct the negative nitrogen balance and malnutrition, to promote liver regeneration, and to avoid fluid retention. The client needs a low-sodium diet to decrease ascites, which results from portal hypertension. A/NM, IM, H

167. no. 2. Hepatic encephalopathy occurs frequently in clients with severe liver disease, especially if therapy is neglected. A/NM, AN, PS

168. no. 3. In hepatic encephalopathy, the liver is unable to detoxify ammonia and convert it to urea. The ammonia levels build up and ammonia crosses the blood-brain barrier, causing decreased mentation. A/NM, AN, PS

169. no. 2. The central venous pressure will give the best and quickest indication of circulating volume. Normal is 4 to 12 cm of water pressure; less than 4 cm indicates hypovolemia, and greater than 12 cm indicates hypervolemia. A baseline reading immediately after inserting the line is a priority. This information is an indirect assessment of the adequacy of renal perfusion. A low CVP, reflecting hypovolemia, puts the client at risk for inadequate renal perfusion. A/NM, IM, PS

170. no. 4. Exophthalmos occurs primarily with hyperthyroidism; it is not a sign or symptom of hepatic encephalopathy. A/NM, AS, PS

171. no. 1. Neomycin decreases the ammonia-forming bacteria in the intestinal tract, thus decreasing the serum ammonia level. Lactulose decreases the pH of the colon, which allows ammonias to diffuse into the colon from the blood to form nonabsorbable ammonium ions. These are then eliminated in the stool. The medications in no. 3 and no. 4 are given for seizure activity. Protein-tube feeding is not given; proteins form ammonia in the process of breaking down, which is to be avoided in this case. The client will be placed on a protein restriction of 20 g per day. A/NM, AN, PS

172. no. 4. Normal bacteria found in the gastrointestinal tract cause ammonia to form. The antibacterial effect of neomycin reduces the intestinal flora; thus it decreases levels of ammonia. The client's level of consciousness will improve when serum ammonia levels are reduced. A/NM, PL, PS

173. no. 2. Proteins (amino acids) break down in the body to form ammonia; therefore a low-protein diet will help prevent the buildup of ammonia. Sodium is restricted, as well as fluid, when ascites and edema are present. A/NM, PL, E

174. no. 4. Water intake is restricted to control ascites. Options no. 1, no. 2, and no. 3 should be included in the teaching plan. A/NM, IM, H

175. no. 4. Esophageal varices are observed only with an x-ray or by direct visualization through an endoscope. A/NM, AS, PS

176. no. 3. The nutritional inadequacies are easier to correct by teaching about nutrition and diet. Long-term substance-abuse problems are difficult to control. The alcoholic client has nutritional deprivation, especially a decrease in protein intake. This deprivation results in Laënnec's cirrhosis. A/NM, AN, PS

177. no. 2. The client was admitted most likely after having vomited large quantities of vomitus or blood. Oral hygiene is most likely to make this client comfortable. A/NM, IM, E

178. no. 4. Dimenhydrinate (Dramamine) is the best selection. The other medications rely on the liver for detoxification. Caution must be taken when administering antiemetics to clients with liver damage. A/NM, PL, PS

179. no. 2. Pruritus is a result of bile salt excretion through the skin. Soap, perfumed lotion, and rubbing alcohol should be avoided because they cause further drying of the skin. Moisturizing lotions may be beneficial. Assess for scratching, which can cause subcutaneous bleeding. The skin should be patted and not rubbed during the bath. A/NM, AS, PS

180. no. 2. Weight loss or gain directly reflects water loss or gain and is the best parameter for measuring fluid balance in the body. A/NM, AS, PS

181. no. 4. Gynecomastia is an endocrine problem (estrogen excess) commonly seen in clients with cirrhosis of the liver, but it is not preventable with nursing actions. A/NM, AN, E

182. no. 2. For small tumors, an incision is made here. For larger tumors a transfrontal craniotomy may be used. Other surgical postoperative assessments include looking for signs and symptoms of meningitis, optic nerve damage, and hypopituitarism. A/NM, AS, PS

183. no. 4. Prolactin is secreted by the pituitary gland in pregnant and nursing women to produce lactation. A pituitary tumor can produce an excess of this hormone, causing galactorrhea (excessive or abnormal lactation). A/NM, AN, PS

184. no. 4. A serum calcium test will give no information about the type of tumor or size of the lesion, whereas the other studies will. Computed tomography scans help determine bone changes. Visual field testing is performed to determine if the tumor is pressing on the optic chiasm. Hormone levels would typically be elevated. A/NM, AS, PS

185. no. 2. Diabetes insipidus is a frequent temporary complication after a hypophysectomy. Large volumes of urine (up to 20 L per day) may be excreted, causing severe dehydration if not treated. The other options listed would be contraindicated because they might increase intracranial pressure or cause cerebrospinal fluid leaks into the sinuses. A/NM, PL, E

186. no. 1. Hypopituitarism is a common problem with clients who have had hypophysectomies because the anterior pituitary gland has been affected. Pituitary hormone replacements may have to be given. Cushing's disease results from excess steroid production. Acromegaly results from hyperpituitarism. A/NM, AN, PS

187. no. 3. The gonadal-stimulating hormones from the pituitary gland that affect pregnancy may be deficient, but replacements can be administered. A/NM, IM, H

188. no. 2. Tingling of the toes, fingers, or around the mouth is the first sign of hypocalcemia, which can lead to tetany. Thyroid surgery clients are at high risk for this problem because of the possibility of removal of or damage to the parathyroid gland. A/NM, AS, PS

189. no. 3. Help the client use the semi-Fowler's position with the neck supported for optimal ventilation and to avoid strain on the neck muscles. A/NM, IM, E

190. no. 3. Hypoparathyroidism leads to hypocalcemia, which causes increased neuromuscular irritability and laryngospasm. Chvostek's sign is a contraction of the facial muscles elicited in response to a light tap over the facial nerve in front of the ear. Trousseau's sign is a carpopedal spasm induced by inflating a blood pressure cuff for at least 1 minute above the client's systolic pressure. Decreased muscle tone and muscle flaccidity occur with hypercalcemia. A/NM, AS, PS

191. no. 3. Respiratory distress from edema, hemorrhage, or laryngeal nerve damage is a potential complication of a subtotal thyroidectomy, so a tracheostomy set is kept at the client's bedside. The thyroid is very vascular. A total thyroidectomy does not have as high a risk of bleeding because minimal thyroid tissue may remain. A/NM, IM, E

192. no. 2. Hypocalcemia can result from the accidental removal of one or two parathyroid glands, so calcium gluconate must be kept on hand. Calcium gluconate is more readily used than calcium chloride if given IV. Calcitonin is given in hypothyroid conditions to inhibit bone resorption (loss of calcium from the bone). Saturated solution of potassium iodine is an antithyroid drug used to treat hyperthyroidism. A/NM, AN, PS

193. no. 2. Flexing or hyperextending the neck puts excessive tension on the surgical site. Two or three pillows would strain the incision. The other options are all appropriate nursing actions. A/NM, IM, E

194. no. 2. Before instructing the client on self-care for diabetes, the nurse must establish a baseline regarding the client's knowledge of diabetes. Assessment of client knowledge is the priority before teaching. A/NM, AS, E

195. no. 3. Diabetes is a chronic disorder of carbohydrate metabolism and is one of the leading causes of death in the United States. It is not a curable illness. Diabetes responds to diet and exercise as well as to insulin. A/NM, AN, PS

196. no. 1. In diabetes, insulin deficiency results in hyperglycemia. Glucose is excreted in the urine and, acting as an osmotic diuretic, carries water and electrolytes with it. All the other options are incorrect. A/NM, AN, PS

197. no. 3. In addition, more rapid absorption can occur in unaffected sites, leading to hypoglycemia. All the other options are incorrect. A/NM, AN, H

198. no. 1. Peak hours of action for regular human insulin are 1 to 3 hours after administration. Breakfast is usually served between 8 and 9 AM. A hypoglycemic reaction would occur between 8:30 and 10:30 AM, especially if the client has not eaten much at breakfast. It is extremely important for the nurse to monitor food intake at meals when regular insulin is given before meals according to a sliding scale. A/NM, AN, PS

199. no. 4. The other options are symptoms of hyperglycemia. Other symptoms of hypoglycemia are hunger, tremor, anxiety, weakness, nausea, complaints of nightmares, and restless sleep. Major symptoms are perioral paresthesia, headache, visual changes, mental confusion, personality changes, depression, and loss of consciousness. A/NM, AS, PS

200. no. 2. Exercise is important for diabetic clients and is planned according to age and interests and in balance with the prescribed insulin and diet regimen. A client with non–insulin-dependent diabetes mellitus should have a cardiovascular evaluation before starting an exercise program. A/NM, AN, H

201. no. 4. Hunger is characteristic, but because the glucose cannot be used, weight loss occurs. A/NM, AS, PS

202. no. 1. Warm, flushed, dry skin indicates dehydration. This is the major initial problem caused by polyuria requiring treatment. Moist and cool skin is seen in hypoglycemia. A/NM, AS, PS

203. no. 3. The client has a fluid deficit of 8 to 12 L, and replacement is a priority to be carried out as rapidly as tolerated. Generally, 0.9% saline solution is used initially, then 0.45% saline and water. Regular insulin may be given via IV continuous low-dose infusions with bolus SC as needed hourly based on serum blood glucose values. A/NM, PL, PS

204. no. 4. This is the most therapeutic and most honest response. All other options do not support or address the client's comment and are incorrect. Offering false reassurance (option no. 2) is a block to therapeutic communication and will negate the client's feelings. A/NM, IM, PC

205. no. 1. Intermittent claudication is pain in the extremity with exercise, usually walking. When the energy demands exceed the oxygen supply, pain is experienced. Peripheral paresthesias reflect nerve problems and may be the result of poor circulation, but they are not classic findings. Skin may be shiny and atrophic over the ankle area in arterial insufficiency. Pain on dorsiflexion of the foot indicates venous thrombophlebitis. A/NM, AS, PS

206. no. 2. Keeping the feet covered with socks will keep the feet warm and not compromise circulation any further. Using external heat, such as hot water bottles, increases oxygen consumption and impairs arterial flow even more. Massaging the feet and flexing the toes are inappropriate actions that would do nothing for arterial circulation. A/NM, IM, PS

207. no. 3. It is important for the client to talk about any fears of body changes and loss, even if an amputation will never be needed. This response acknowledges that the nurse heard the statement, and it encourages client verbalization. A/NM, IM, PC

208. no. 4. Even though the client has non–insulin-dependent diabetes mellitus, the stress of surgery may cause the blood glucose to rise for a short time; thus it should be controlled with short-acting insulin administered according to the client's needs as determined by monitoring serum glucose levels. A/NM, IM, PS

209. no. 1. Irritability is often the first sign of hypoglycemia, particularly in the morning when the client has not had anything to eat for several hours. The nurse should also check prior glucose levels and when the last insulin was given to assess for insulin-induced hypoglycemia. A/NM, IM, PS

210. no. 4. Complex carbohydrates have much value in the diabetic diet because they are a good source of energy and keep the blood sugar more stable. The other options are incorrect. A/NM, IM, H

211. no. 3. Elevating the legs is indicated for venous, not arterial, problems of the extremities. Diabetics usually have an arterial problem. A/NM, IM, H

212. no. 2. Weakness and weight loss are symptoms of adrenocortical insufficiency. Increased skin pigmentation results because adrenal insufficiency allows melanocyte-stimulating hormone levels to increase. Option no. 4 includes the signs and symptoms of hyperthyroidism. A/NM, AS, PS

213. no. 2. Stress of any type increases the client's weakness. The client is vulnerable to stress, because she lacks the protection of the adrenal hormones—Addison's disease is hypofunction of the adrenal glands. Exertion is a type of physiologic stress. A/NM, PL, E

214. no. 4. Addison's disease is characterized by inadequate amounts of cortisol, which results in hypotension. All the other options are correct. A/NM, PL, E

215. no. 4. Critical deficiency of glucocorticoids leads to vascular collapse, hypotension, and diminished urine output. A/NM, AS, PS

216. no. 4. The client with Addison's disease can live a normal life, provided the client takes the daily medications without exception. A/NM, IM, H

217. no. 1. Clients at risk for septic shock include the very young, the very old, those with genitourinary infections who undergo cystoscopy, and those with severe gastrointestinal blood loss. A/E, AS, PS

218. no. 4. This answer gives the client an opportunity to express concerns and fears. The other options do not acknowledge the client's concerns. A/E, IM, PC

219. no. 3. Shock may be insidious in onset, and slight changes in vital signs may be the only warning. Therefore check the vital signs again in 15 minutes for any changes. A/E, IM, PS

220. no. 4. Restlessness is an early sign of septic shock. Hypotension and cool, clammy skin are late signs. In early septic shock, urinary output is slightly decreased. A/E, AS, PS

221. no. 3. Dried apricots are high in potassium and low in sodium; the other choices are high in sodium. A/E, EV, H

222. no. 3. It is important that the client with high blood pressure stop smoking. The other options are not correct statements. A/E, EV, H

223. no. 1. Forcing fluids serves as an internal irrigant, flushes the urinary tract, and decreases burning. Options no. 2 and no. 4 are important but are focused more on prevention. Option no. 1 is most important for *treating* the infection. A/E, IM, H

224. no. 4. This is a sign of possible anaphylaxis. The client should be informed about the other reactions, which are normal. A/E, AS, E

225. no. 2. Activity aids in passage of the calculus. Even though the client may need pain relief and will have to strain his urine, these do not aid in passage of stones. A/E, IM, E

226. no. 1. Calculi readily develop in immobile clients, and especially in those with multiple myeloma, because the diseased bones release calcium, leading to the formation of calculi. Options no. 2, no. 3, and no. 4 decrease the possibility of renal calculi. A/E, AN, PS

227. no. 1. The etiology of bladder cancer is related to cigarette smoking and exposure to dyes used in rubber and cable industries. A/E, AS, E

228. no. 2. Painless, gross hematuria is the most common clinical finding and the first sign in 75% of clients with carcinoma of the bladder. A/E, AS, PS

229. no. 4. Gentle acceptance of the client's anxiety and open-ended questioning allows the client the opportunity to express his feelings and concerns. The other options do not encourage the client to discuss feelings. A/E, IM, PC

230. no. 2. Instruct the client to do range-of-motion exercises for his legs, and teach him to keep his legs uncrossed. These activities decrease the risk of thrombophlebitis. A/E, IM, PS

231. no. 3. A nasogastric tube may become obstructed with mucus, sediment, or old blood. It can be checked for patency by irrigating with 30 ml of normal saline. One indicator of obstruction is nausea. Administering an antiemetic may be unnecessary if irrigating the nasogastric tube relieves the nausea. Repositioning will not help the client's nausea. A/E, IM, PS

232. no. 3. There is a risk of paralytic ileus when part of the bowel is removed. A nasogastric tube is used for 3 to 5 days or until bowel sounds return. A/E, AN, PS

233. no. 4. The urinary stoma should be dark pink to red. Dark red indicates inadequate circulation. A/E, AS, PS

234. no. 4. Morphine would be contraindicated with a blood pressure of 80/40. Intramuscular or subcutaneous injections should not be administered because of the vasoconstriction in hypotension. Medications may not be absorbed and might accumulate; then, when perfusion improves, the client could experience an overdose. A/E, IM, PS

235. no. 2. Normal potassium is 3.5 to 5.0 mEq/L. Hyperkalemia can cause lethal cardiac dysrhythmias if not promptly treated. A/E, AS, PS

236. no. 1. Fluid restriction is indicated during the oliguric phase of renal failure, when fluid overload is a problem. The sodium value in this client reflects dilution. Decreasing the fluid overload increases the sodium value. A/E, AN, PS

237. no. 3. Trousseau's sign is an indication of tetany, which results from the increased neuromuscular irritability caused by hypocalcemia. The method of eliciting this sign is to constrict the radial or brachial artery and observe the hand and fingers for spasm. The constriction can be done with a blood pressure cuff. A/E, AN, PS

238. no. 1. This is the only correct group of actions. In addition, bed rest should be maintained to reduce the buildup of lactic acid, which is released with muscle activity. Restrict fluids to reduce hypervolemia. A/E, IM, E

239. no. 3. The diuretic phase of acute renal failure causes loss of circulating volume and wide fluctuations in serum potassium and sodium. This phase is exacerbated by the buildup of urea during the oliguric phase, which acts as a natural diuretic. A/E, AS, PS

240. no. 3. The blood urea nitrogen becomes elevated because functioning nephrons are damaged and the body is unable to get rid of waste products through the kidneys. A/E, AN, PS

241. no. 1. A diet high in calories and low in protein is prescribed. The protein should be of high biologic value to prevent catabolism of body protein. A/E, IM, H

242. no. 1. Careful monitoring of the client's vital signs is imperative in evaluating the client's response to treatment. The nurse must be sure that the vital signs are accurate. A/E, PL, E

243. no. 2. These laboratory findings are consistent with renal failure. A decreased serum calcium results from both a decreased gastrointestinal absorption of calcium and an elevated serum phosphorus. The inability of the kidneys to excrete the potassium raises the potassium level, raises the hydrogen-ion level, and results in acidosis. A/E, AS, PS

244. no. 3. A likely cause of decreased serum calcium is an elevated serum phosphorus. Remember that the kidneys are unable to excrete phosphorus, and there is an inverse relationship of calcium and phosphorus.

Nutritional deficiencies would be an unlikely cause. A/E, AN, PS

245. no. 1. The kidneys are unable to excrete the hydrogen ion or reabsorb the bicarbonate ion. The result is acidosis, for which the lungs attempt to compensate by blowing off excess hydrogen ion (carbon dioxide). A/E, AN, PS

246. no. 4. Phosphorus and calcium are inversely related. Potassium levels are usually inversely related to sodium when kidney function is normal. A/E, AN, PS

247. no. 4. Aluminum hydroxide antacids bind with the phosphate ion and are then excreted in the stool. A/E, AN, PS

248. no. 3. A client treated with peritoneal dialysis may need to be dialyzed three to five times per week for 8 to 12 hours each time. Vascular access is required for hemodialysis only. Hepatitis is more problematic with hemodialysis. A/E, AN, PS

249. no. 1. Respiratory distress may indicate a fluid shift and pulmonary edema, which requires immediate attention. Hemorrhage is less likely once the catheter is in place; abdominal pain and peritonitis may also occur, but breathing is the first priority. A/E, AN, PS

250. no. 2. The life span of the shunt is 6 to 12 months. Major complications are clotting and infections, which are avoided by not using the arm for taking blood pressure or blood drawing. Daily heparinization is not common practice. Changing the Silastic tube is not possible because it would cause hemorrhage. A/E, IM, PS

251. no. 1. These are symptoms of the disequilibrium syndrome. It occurs when urea is removed more rapidly from the blood than the from the brain. The osmotic gradient caused by urea results in fluid passing to cerebral cells; thus cerebral edema occurs. A/E, IM, PS

252. no. 2. The Foley catheter is inserted to maintain urinary flow. Monitor intake and output throughout the client's preoperative and postoperative periods. A/E, PL, PS

253. no. 4. A transurethral resection is the only type of prostatic surgery not requiring an incision through the skin. A/E, IM, E

254. no. 1. If increased blood is seen, first increase the speed of the irrigation. If this is not effective, notify the physician. Do not alter the traction on the urinary catheter because its purpose is to put pressure on the prostatic bed. Manual irrigation is done mainly for clots and requires a physician's order. A/E, IM, PS

255. no. 1. The large balloon on the urinary catheter can stimulate spasms; therefore administer narcotics plus anticholinergic drugs as ordered. Providing a sitz bath and decreasing the speed of irrigation will not decrease the bladder spasms. Never decrease the traction on the urinary catheter. A/E, IM, PS

256. no. 4. Nursing strategies that can help prevent thrombophlebitis include helping with leg exercises and taking deep breaths and obtaining an order for antiembolism stockings for the client. Nursing actions cannot prevent epididymitis, osteitis pubis, or urinary incontinence. A/E, AN, PS

257. no. 1. The client should refrain from sexual inter-

course for approximately 6 weeks after surgery. In addition, he should avoid heavy lifting, straining at stool, and driving a car for approximately 6 weeks. A/E, IM, H

258. no. 2. Instruct the client to monitor his urine at home; it should be continually clear. A/E, EV, H

259. no. 1. A man with an enlarged prostate has difficulty emptying his bladder and has to strain to urinate. The stream lacks force and becomes weak, and dribbling occurs. Initiating a stream may also be a problem. A/E, AS, PS

260. no. 2. Prostatic hypertrophy can be diagnosed by rectal digital exam. Gloves and lubricant are needed. A/E, AS, E

261. no. 3. The kidneys are located in the retroperitoneum, and the bowel must be cleared of any gas or fecal material that would obscure their visualization. Additional preparation for an intravenous pyelogram includes restricting food and fluids from midnight before the exam. A/E, IM, E

262. no. 2. Continuous bladder irrigation with saline or other solutions is done to remove clotted blood from the bladder. Blood and clots are normal in the first 24 to 48 hours after transurethral resection of the prostate. A/E, PL, PS

263. no. 4. A Foley catheter can irritate the bladder mucosa, causing bladder spasms. The catheter must also be checked to ensure patency, but these sensations may be present with a patent catheter. A/E, AN, PS

264. no. 2. Temporary urinary frequency or incontinence, or both, can occur after removal of the catheter. A/E, AN, PS

265. no. 3. Race is not a factor in the client's ability to undergo surgery. It does have implications in the nursing care after surgery, especially in the assessment phase of the nursing process. A/E, AS, E

266. no. 4. There is postoperative pain with this procedure, but it can be managed with analgesics. A/E, IM, E

267. no. 2. The rectal area is less than 1 inch from the incision and prostatic bed; taking a rectal temperature could cause trauma. An air ring can cause venous stasis and edema; a hard surface may increase pain. A/E, IM, PS

268. no. 4. Sexual impotence is expected in radical perineal prostatectomies but not after transurethral resections and suprapubic and retropubic prostatectomies. However, in the immediate postoperative period, it is too early to assess this activity. A/E, IM, E

269. no. 3. This requires a physician's order. In the early postoperative period, active exercise is usually limited to leg dangling and brief ambulation. Passive exercise, however, is imperative for this client. A/E, PL, E

270. no. 1. Any invasive procedure on the urinary tract increases the risk of urinary tract infections. A/E, AN, PS

271. no. 3. After removal of the catheter, incontinence is common in the older client undergoing a prostatectomy because a Foley catheter decreases the contractility of the bladder muscle. A/E, PL, H

272. no. 1. The lower gastrointestinal tract must be clear for the exam. Cathartics are given at least 12 hours before the test, along with enemas, until the bowel is clear on the morning of the exam. A/E, IM, E

273. no. 4. The knee-chest position provides maximum exposure for the proctosigmoidoscopy. A/E, IM, E

274. no. 2. No anesthetic is given, and the client must relax, not bear down. The procedure is not painful, but it is uncomfortable. A/E, IM, E

275. no. 1. Stool samples for amoebae must be tested while they are warm and fresh, or the amoebae will die. A/E, IM, PS

276. no. 1. Ulcerative colitis is characterized by frequent diarrhea with mucus and blood, caused by inflammation of the colonic mucosa. A/E, AS, PS

277. no. 1. Vitamin K, vital to the formation of prothrombin, is normally absorbed in the colon. A/E, AN, PS

278. no. 1. Sedation and decreased bladder tone may occur, but these drugs are given to decrease gastrointestinal motility. A/E, AN, PS

279. no. 2. An ileostomy involves removal of the whole colon and formation of an ileal stoma. A/E, AN, PS

280. no. 3. An ileostomy has liquid, almost continuous drainage. Weight gain may result from newfound food tolerance. The drainage containing enzymes is irritating to the skin. A/E, AS, PS

281. no. 1. Research indicates that virtually 100% of colon polyps are premalignant and can be expected to become cancerous if not excised. Colitis and amebiasis cause chronic irritation and therefore may predispose the client to colon cancer. A/E, AS, PS

282. no. 3. Palpation is done last because it can stimulate bowel sounds. Percussion usually does not stimulate bowel sounds because the technique is superficial to the bowel. A/E, AS, PS

283. no. 4. Signs and symptoms of mechanical obstruction of the small bowel include abdominal distention, decreased flatus, and projectile vomiting. A/E, AS, PS

284. no. 3. Fluid and electrolyte deficiency is the major problem if the intestinal blood supply is not compromised. A/E, AN, PS

285. no. 2. The Miller-Abbott tube is an intestinal tube with a mercury-weighted tip that is designed to advance into the intestine. Taping it could traumatize nasal tissue and prevent further advance of the tube. A/E, IM, E

286. no. 1. Reviewing deep-breathing exercises is the priority in this situation because of the poor respiratory outcome if this teaching is not completed. The client's weight and a probable abdominal incision predispose him to postoperative pulmonary complications. A/E, IM, E

287. no. 2. Feces become increasingly firm as they progress through the colon because of water being reabsorbed back into the body. Stool in the transverse colon is mushy to semiformed, depending on the specific location. A/E, AS, PS

288. no. 3. Colostomy irrigations are usually done only once a day. A/E, IM, E

289. no. 3. The area around the stoma must be kept dry and oil free for the colostomy appliance to adhere. A/E, IM, PS

290. no. 1. Eating a balanced diet will provide proper stool consistency. A colostomy can be irrigated at any time that is convenient for the client. A/E, AN, H

291. no. 4. Gradual involvement of the client in his ostomy care is more likely to increase acceptance. A/E, PL, PC

292. no. 2. A nasogastric tube attached to suction keeps the stomach drained and decompressed. This prevents the risk of aspiration before, during, and after surgery. A/E, AN, PS

293. no. 3. Although the catheter can be used to check renal function, the proximity of the rectum and sigmoid colon to the bladder makes avoidance of injury a prime concern. A/E, AN, PS

294. no. 1. Colon tumors metastasize to other areas within the colon by direct extension. Enough colon must be removed so that the specimen margins are clear of any tumor cells. A/E, AN, PS

295. no. 3. Tube feedings circumvent swallowing, anorexia, and the gag reflex and can be administered regardless of appetite or level of consciousness, but the gastrointestinal tract distal to the feeding must be intact and functioning. A/E, AN, PS

296. no. 4. Talking to a person who has a colostomy and has it well under control can be encouraging for the new ostomate. A/E, IM, E

297. no. 3. Warm tap water causes the least irritation and stimulates evacuation of the colon. A/E, IM, PS

298. no. 4. The client must be relaxed for successful irrigation. This facilitates retention of the irrigation. A/E, AN, PS

299. no. 2. Excessive flatus is not symptomatic of colon cancer. A change in bowel habits is more common with left-sided lesions; pain and obstructive symptoms are more common with right-sided lesions. A/E, AS, PS

300. no. 3. Although the carcinoembryonic antigen has been used in recent years to aid in diagnosing colon cancer, it is not as conclusive as a biopsy of the lesion. A/E, AN, PS

301. no. 2. Neomycin is given to achieve bowel sterilization. It destroys the normal flora of the bowel and results in some loose stools. This enhances bowel cleansing and is the desired outcome. A/E, IM, PS

302. no. 1. The colostomy is permanent because the cancerous rectum will be removed. Denial or lack of understanding may be the problem. In either case, further teaching is needed. A/E, E, H

303. no. 2. Getting the client to talk about fears and concerns before the client is discharged is the priority right now. A/E, IM, PC

304. no. 2. Bone marrow depression and stomatitis are the main side effects from this drug. A decreased white blood cell count can make the client more prone to infection. A/E, AN, PS

305. no. 3. Diverticulitis is an inflammatory condition manifested by crampy lower left quadrant pain, diarrhea with blood and mucus, weakness, and anemia. Characteristic signs and symptoms of appendicitis are right lower quadrant or periumbilical pain and rebound tenderness; for cholecystitis they are nausea, vomiting, and pain and tenderness in the right subcostal region or in the epigastric region; and for pancreatitis they are vomiting and localized pain in the epigastrium or left upper quadrant with radiation of pain to the back and flanks as the pain progresses. A/E, AN, PS

306. no. 2. Diverticula often perforate. These are signs and symptoms of perforation and peritonitis. Options no. 1 and no. 3 are found in obstructive gallbladder disease. A/E, AS, PS

307. no. 1. Diverticula are usually located in the sigmoid colon. Because a diagnosis of diverticulitis has not been previously established, an x-ray examination of the entire lower gastrointestinal tract will be done, and the entire colon will be examined to rule out other abnormalities. Option no. 2 items are done for ulcer disease. Option no. 3 items are done for gallbladder disease. A Schilling test is used to assess vitamin B_{12} problems. A/E, AN, PS

308. no. 4. Clients with diverticulitis may benefit from a high-residue diet and should avoid foods that are highly refined and processed because they predispose the clients to this condition. Bulk-forming medications (e.g., psyllium hydrophilic mucilloid [Metamucil]) are helpful. Stress-management techniques are most helpful for upper-GI disturbances or colitis. A/E, IM, H

309. no. 3. Insulin shock must be ruled out as a cause when dealing with a comatose client with no signs of injury. A/SP, PL, PS

310. no. 3. A concussion is a head injury in which no actual structural damage can be identified, but the person experiences headache, a change in level of consciousness, confusion, and memory impairment. Nausea and vomiting may also occur. Altered pupil responses, nystagmus, and problems with aphasia would not be expected. The impaired consciousness can become severe after concussion, and clients must be monitored frequently to ensure that further neurologic impairment does not develop. A/SP, AS, PS

311. no. 1. Ketoacidosis will not cause unequal pupillary light reflexes. In an unconscious client, unequal pupils can result from oculomotor nerve compression, hypothalamic damage, and midbrain damage. Epidural hematoma and brain tumor both cause increasing intracranial pressure and could cause unequal and sluggish pupillary responses. A/SP, AN, PS

312. no. 1. Cheyne-Stokes respirations are initially shallow, become increasingly deep, and move steadily to a period of apnea. Option no. 4 is seen with Kussmaul's respirations. Option no. 2 is bradypnea. Option no. 3 indicates Biot's respirations. A/SP, AS, PS

313. no. 1. In decerebrate posturing there is rigid extension of both the upper and lower extremities. In decorticate posturing there is flexion of the upper extremities and extension of the lower extremities. Options no. 3 and no. 4 are not signs of neurologic posturing. A/SP, AS, PS

314. no. 2. Positioning affects intracranial pressure, and specific orders are usually written concerning permissible positioning. If an intracranial pressure monitor is in place it is critical to monitor the client's responses to position changes. Clients are usually positioned with the head of the bed elevated about 15 to 30 degrees and are not placed upright or flat. This neutral position minimizes abrupt pressure fluctuations. A/SP, IM, PS

315. no. 2. A neurologic baseline must be established so that significant postoperative changes will not be overlooked. Clients need preoperative teaching about the expected care routines, the importance of deep breathing, and the planned method of pain control, but neurologic assessment is clearly the priority issue. A/SP, PL, PS

316. no. 1. The pupil and neurologic checks are important; however, maintaining respiratory status is the highest priority. Vital signs are performed more frequently in the initial postoperative period and position changes are important, but respiratory care has the highest priority postoperatively. A/SP, PL, PS

317. no. 3. Adequate assessment of pupillary responses requires that the room be dark enough that the eyes are not already accommodating to light. Both eyes are open if the client is capable, and the light is shined into one eye at a time and the response noted. The eyes are then examined together to note the consensuality of the response. A/SP, IM, E

318. no. 2. If the pharynx is not suctioned first, the secretions will be aspirated into the trachea when the cuff is deflated. A hissing sound around the stoma, nose, or mouth indicates an air leak. Air is used to inflate a tracheostomy cuff. A/SP, IM, PS

319. no. 2. The assessment of level of consciousness is subjective and open to errors of interpretation. Therefore it is critical that every caregiver in a setting use the same tool for assessing level of consciousness and have established some detailed definitions for the use of terms such as *stuporous* or *obtunded*. The particular scale used is not as important as using the tool well, although both the Glasgow Coma scale and Rancho Los Amigos scale are excellent tools that approach the measurement slightly differently. Careful tracking of subtle changes in level of consciousness usually require more frequently monitoring than once a shift. A/SP, EV, PS

320. no. 4. Restraints will likely increase client resistance. A/SP, IM, PS

321. no. 2. Diabetes insipidus occurs when there is suppression of antidiuretic hormone (ADH), leading to uncontrolled diuresis. Syndrome of inappropriate ADH will cause the urine output to fall precipitously. Neither cerebral edema nor rising intracranial pressure directly affect urine output. A/SP, AN, PS

322. no. 2. Assessment of pain response yields important data for the neurologic assessment of unconscious clients, but it is not a risk-free procedure. Tissue trauma can result from repetitive vigorous stimulation. Neither pinprick nor sternal rubbing is recommended, and orbital pressure could result in serious eye damage. Pressure applied to the nailbeds or to the supraorbital area is currently recommended. A/SP, AS, PS

323. no. 2. Uncontrolled diuresis leads to loss of water and washout of most electrolytes. The diuresis will not increase intracranial pressure; it may even decrease it.

Diuresis is not associated with cerebral infection and retrograde amnesia. A/SP, AN, PS

324. no. 1. The two classic signs of meningeal irritation are Kernig's and Brudzinski's signs. With Kernig's sign the client is unable to fully extend the leg when it is flexed toward the abdomen. Brudzinski's sign involves involuntary flexion of the hip and knee when the neck is passively flexed toward the chest. Severe neck pain is present with all movement, but neither nystagmus nor decerebrate postures are signs of meningeal irritation. A/SP, AS, PS

325. no. 3. Tachycardia is a symptom of cardiac dysfunction. The other options are all potential symptoms of a transient ischemic attack. A/SP, AS, PS

326. no. 3. Doppler carotid studies are a safe and noninvasive method of determining whether the source of a transient ischemic attack is in the carotid arteries where treatment with endarteretomy is feasible. Neither CT nor EEG provide this kind of data, and a cerebral arteriogram is a clearly invasive test. A/SP, AN, PS

327. no. 4. Any changes in mental functioning in a head-injury client are significant and require constant monitoring. Confusion and personality changes also put the client at risk for injury, so the paramount consideration is frequent monitoring and safety interventions. The other three options may be appropriate as part of the overall plan of care but are not the best initial approach. A/SP, PL, E

328. no. 2. Emotional lability is a frequent physiologic outcome of stroke and is distressing to both the client and family. It is important for both parties to understand that this response is physiologic and not a true emotional response to events or circumstances. Distraction is one of the best methods of dealing with the problem, although it does not always work. The crucial element is realizing that the behavior is not under conscious control. A/SP, IM, H

329. no. 1. All options are important to monitor; however, adequacy of respirations always has the priority. A/SP, AS, PS

330. no. 4. Stroke affects the ability of the client to perceive food in the affected side of the mouth and effectively move it for swallowing. Therefore it has a tendency to collect among the molars, where it breaks down and can create both odor and infection. The client needs to be taught or assisted to cleanse the affected area of the mouth carefully after all meals to remove loose food debris. A/SP, IM, H

331. no. 3. Recovery from aphasia is slow and inherently frustrating for the client. Although the process is different from original language learning it still requires repetition and frequent practice to master. Therefore encouraging the client to speak and practice even when he makes mistakes is critical. Attempting to speak for the client or bypass oral communication simply slows the process and prevents the client from maximizing his residual capacities. A/SP, IM, PC

332. no. 2. A suction machine allows the nurse to maintain a patent airway. Maintaining adequate oxygenation is a basic goal for all acutely ill clients. The second priority with a client who has impaired mobility is correct positioning and protection of skin integrity. A/SP, PL, E

333. no. 2. Mouth breathing commonly occurs during a coma. Even clients who are NPO can be properly hydrated, and the risk of infection is increased if the integrity of the mucous membranes is impaired. Option no. 4 is not correct. A/SP, AN, PS

334. no. 4. Although all options are appropriate, turning the client appropriately and frequently is the best way to prevent decubitus ulcers. A/SP, IM, PS

335. no. 1. Stroke clients who are not correctly positioned and exercised tend to develop flexion contractures because flexor muscles are generally stronger than extensors. The fingers should never be tightly flexed. The footboard will not be effective in preventing a plantar flexion contracture if it is flush with the mattress. A/SP, AN, E

336. no. 3. Complete rehabilitation after major stroke is rarely possible, especially for elderly clients, but the emphasis of rehabilitation must be focused on self-care activities that enable the client to achieve an independent or assisted living situation and avoid the necessity for nursing home care. This involves adapting some self-care activities to residual functions, exploring the use of numerous assistive aids, and retraining the affected limbs and muscles where possible. Continence in particular is considered to be an achievable goal. A/SP, PL, E

337. no. 2. Hemianopia, or partial blindness, is a common outcome of stroke that may initially be overlooked. The client does not have visual perception in that area and may overlook objects that are outside his visual field. Approaching from the intact side ensures the client's attention, and teaching the client to scan enables him to move his head from side to side to safely compensate for the loss of visual field and prevent injury. A/SP, EV, E

338. no. 3. Normal cerebrospinal fluid should contain no red blood cells. The presence of less than five lymphocytes per cubic millimeter is normal. The normal color of cerebrospinal fluid is clear or colorless, and the normal glucose level is 50 to 75 mg/dl. A/SP, AS, PS

339. no. 1. Emotional lability often occurs after this type of cerebral insult. It is physiologic in nature but not fully understood. Anger and hostility may play a role as the rehabilitation proceeds, but the emotional lability is not under the client's control. Her medications do not cause these kinds of behavioral changes in the stroke client. A/SP, IM, H

340. no. 4. Movement of the head, neck, and back may cause further trauma, so it is essential that the entire spinal cord be immobilized. If the client develops acute nausea it may be necessary to turn him to prevent aspiration, but the entire head, neck, and spine will first be immobilized to prevent movement. The back will not be supported with pillows. Option no. 1 is appropriate but is not the most important consideration. A/SP, PL, E

341. no. 4. Spinal shock refers to the effects that result from spinal cord transection. It involves the suppression of

all reflex activity below the level of the injury. Tendon reflexes diminish, and temperature control and vasomotor tone are lost. Paralysis of the bladder results in urinary retention. Flaccid paralysis, not spastic paralysis, will occur. Blood pressure will be low and unstable. There is a loss of ability to perspire below the level of the injury, so the skin will feel warm, not damp, with diaphoresis. A/SP, AS, PS

342. no. 3. This is the top priority. With a C3-4 injury, paralysis of the diaphragm is likely. Options no. 1, no. 2, and no. 4 are appropriate, but maintaining the airway and adequate ventilation are the most important nursing actions. A/SP, PL, PS

343. no. 2. In early stages of injury, no reflexes will be present, and the client will have an atonic bladder. The bladder will become increasingly distended if the client is not catheterized. This alteration occurs with spinal shock. The bladder is not spastic. A/SP, AN, PS

344. no. 2. Both acute spinal cord injury and the use of a glucocorticoid to prevent further cord edema increase the client's risk of developing peptic ulcer. Dexamethasone significantly increases the outpouring of hydrochloric acid in the stomach. All secretions from the gastrointestinal tract are carefully assessed, and most clients will also be placed on prophylactic cimetidine. When the drug is administered orally it must be buffered with food or antacid. A/SP, IM, PS

345. no. 1. Injury to the spinal cord causes a massive inflammatory reaction to be initiated. Because there is such limited space for expansion in the spinal column there is a tendency for swelling to occur above and below the site of the injury, which can worsen the effects. In the cervical spine, extension upward of an injury can steadily compromise the muscles of ventilation and necessitate intubation. The client's respiratory status is monitored continuously in the early period. A/SP, EV, PS

346. no. 4. Spinal cord injury causes a loss of sympathetic stimulation to the vessels, which are then unable to constrict in response to changes in position. Clients with spinal cord injuries must be moved cautiously to prevent sudden severe drops in blood pressure. Ace bandages, antiembolism hose, and abdominal binders are all used in the attempt to support venous return to the heart during the challenge of progressive position changes. A/SP, PL, E

347. no. 3. After the resolution of spinal shock, which takes about 6 weeks, the client is likely to regain some reflex arc activity. This frequently manifests itself in the form of muscle spasms, which can become severe. Although they have occasionally been successfully used to support temporary upright posture with full braces, they cannot be brought under voluntary control and do not represent a return of function. A/SP, AN, PS

348. no. 1. The client is probably experiencing autonomic dysreflexia, which can be confirmed by finding a massively elevated blood pressure. Severe headache will also likely be present. Once the diagnosis is confirmed it would be important to sit the client up and then look for a likely cause of the episode, usually a full bladder or full bowel. Catheterization or stool removal may be necessary. A/SP, IM, PS

349. no. 4. Demineralization is a major problem with lack of stress on the long bones. Absorption and excretion of calcium are not significantly changed by the injury. A/SP, AN, H

350. no. 3. Erection can often be stimulated by stroking the genitalia or other parts of the body because it is a reflex action. Ejaculation may not be present with a complete injury but may be possible with an incomplete injury. Orgasms may occur but will be different. Fertility is typically decreased in males because the scrotum is unable to rise or lower in response to changes in environmental or body temperature. A/SP, IM, H

351. no. 2. Clients who undergo both lumbar puncture and myelogram are at risk for developing spinal headaches after the test period. The complication is theorized to be related to shifts in cerebrospinal fluid pressure and volume. Clients are encouraged to drink plenty of liquids and remain at rest after the procedures, but no effective means of preventing headache in susceptible individuals has been developed. It does not affect all clients but is debilitating when it does occur. A/SP, PL, PS

352. no. 4. The classic signs of spinal shock include bradycardia, hypotension, urinary and bowel retention, and inability to perspire below the level of the injury. Because this is a neurogenic rather than hypovolemic form of shock, the vasoconstrictive response does not occur and the skin is typically warm and dry rather than cool and clammy. A/SP, AN, PS

353. no. 4. Face and neck (approximately) 4%; anterior chest (approximately) 18%; arms and hands 18% (9% each): total = 40%. C/SP, AS, PS

354. no. 3. Options no. 1, no. 2, and no. 4 are characteristic of third-degree burns. C/SP, AS, PS

355. no. 3. Persons with burns around the head, neck, or chest are at risk of developing upper airway edema. Options no. 1, no. 2, and no. 4 are important; however, airway management always takes first priority. C/SP, PL, PS

356. no. 2. Blood volume is reduced from the burn's fluid loss, resulting in constriction of the peripheral vessels and poor drug absorption. Burn clients need effective pain relief. C/SP, AN, PS

357. no. 2. Fluid balance is a critical component of burn care. An adequate urine output is the most accurate way of evaluating the adequacy of the resuscitation efforts. The other factors contribute to understanding of fluid balance but play a supportive role. C/SP, EV, PS

358. no. 1. Sulfamylon is a carbonic anhydrase inhibitor and can lead to impairment of the renal buffering system. Options no. 2, no. 3, and no. 4 are side effects of silver nitrate. C/SP, AS, PS

359. no. 1. Dressings on the donor site are never disturbed without a specific order. C/SP, PL, PS

360. no. 4. A position of comfort often leads to a contracture because clients tend to flex joints near the burn. This includes contractures of the neck and makes the

issue of pillows important. Comfort must take a secondary position to maintenance of function. Extension is a better position. C/SP, PL, E

361. no. 4. Ingestion of a diet rich in meats and cheeses, or taking products that contain supplements of pyridoxine (vitamin B_6), can interfere with the absorption and utilization of levodopa and require dosages to be adjusted upward. A/SP, IM, H

362. no. 1. Parkinson's disease is believed to result primarily from the depletion of dopamine, an essential neurotransmitter, in the basal ganglia. Drug therapy is directed at restoring that essential balance. Parkinsonian symptoms may accompany the administration of certain neuroleptic medications, but the idiopathic disease process is the result of neurotransmitter deficits. A/SP, AS, PS

363. no. 1. There is no known cause for most cases of Parkinson's disease. Drugs and arteriosclerosis are implicated only in some cases. A/SP, AN, PS

364. no. 3. Motor function is tested by observing muscular movement, such as when the client walks. Hand grip assessment provides less complete data about motor function. Options no. 1 and no. 4 test reflex function. A/SP, AS, PS

365. no. 2. The parkinsonian gait is distinctive. The client takes quick shuffling steps and typically leans forward in a "propulsive" manner while walking. The pattern increases in speed until the client is at risk of falling. A/SP, AS, PS

366. no. 1. A decrease in rigidity and bradykinesia would indicate that the drug is having the desired effect. These are its primary effects, although the client may also experience improvement in voice strength and a decrease in tremor activity. Hypotension is a common side effect of the drug. A/SP, EV, PS

367. no. 2. Parkinson's disease classically causes slowed movements, muscle rigidity, a shuffling gait, and small rhythmic resting tremors of the hands called pill rolling. The muscles of facial expression and voice are frequently affected, creating a blank expression and soft monotone voice. The client may have difficulty controlling oral secretions. This pattern frequently leads uninformed observers to assume that the individual is cognitively impaired. A/SP, EV, PS

368. no. 2. There is no known benefit to long-term corticosteroid therapy in treating multiple sclerosis. The other options given are all true. A/SP, IM, H

369. no. 1. This will prevent head injury. Once the seizure has begun, trying to place something in the mouth is dangerous. A person having a seizure should not be moved unless there is an immediate danger. After the seizure, the person can be turned on one side to facilitate the drainage of secretions. The nurse should guide a client's movements to avoid injury, but a client should not be restrained. A/SP, IM PS

370. no. 4. Massage and stretching exercises are effective short-term strategies to use in the management of muscle spasms. Hot baths work well for other types of disease processes, but heat has been shown to exacerbate weakness in clients with multiple sclerosis and should not be employed as a strategy. Assistive

devices may help prevent injury, but they have no effect on spasms. Sleep position has no direct bearing on the problem. A/SP, AS, PS

371. no. 2. Multiple sclerosis does not respond positively to any particular dietary plan. The primary considerations involve maintaining an optimal body weight, especially if the client has limitations in strength or mobility, and supporting optimal general nutrition. Clients with multiple sclerosis appear to experience fewer disease exacerbations when they maintain good general health and nutrition and manage stress effectively. No particular nutrient balance is required. A/SP, EV, H

372. no. 1. Multiple sclerosis can affect myelinated nerves anywhere in the central or peripheral nervous system. The damaging effects occur in the myelin sheath, resulting in distinct patches of local destruction. Option no. 2 refers to the pathology of myasthenia gravis. Option no. 3 refers to the damage of Parkinson's disease. Option no. 4 can be caused by a variety of neurologic problems. A/SP, IM, H

373. no. 3. Grand mal seizures (also known as tonic-clonic seizures) are commonly preceded by a brief aura consisting of a specific movement or unnatural sensation. The three other seizure types are not characterized by auras. A/SP, AN, PS

374. no. 3. The use of Dilantin for long-term management is associated with a variety of side effects, and clients must be monitored carefully for signs of toxicity. Anorexia and nausea are frequent complaints and the drug can be taken with meals. Lethargy and drowsiness are early responses that will decrease with time. The urine has a reddish-brown coloration. Gingival hyperplasia is a common problem with long-term use. Clients need scrupulous oral hygiene, gum massage, and regular monitoring by a competent dentist. A/SP, PL, PS

375. no. 2. This test measures the electrical activity of the brain. Because epilepsy is caused by an abnormal discharge of the neurons, this test is the most specific. A/SP, AS, PS

376. no. 4. Because seizures are controlled when clients take medication, they often begin to believe they are "cured" and stop taking the drugs, at which time the seizures recur. Although the other options may precipitate a seizure in an epileptic client, particularly excess alcohol use, the effects are not consistent. A/SP, AS, PS

377. no. 3. The definition of status epilepticus is continuous seizures. Consciousness is not regained until the seizures have been controlled. A/SP, AN, PS

378. no. 3. Although some clients experience uncontrollable seizure activity that massively disrupts their lifestyle, most can expect that their seizures will be adequately controlled once the correct medication regimen has been established. Most lifestyle restrictions can be lifted at that point. Seizure disorders are rarely progressive and rarely achieve spontaneous remission. A/SP, PL, H

379. no. 3. The use of the padded tongue blade is difficult to achieve in many situations. It can only be safely

inserted before the tonic-clonic contraction phase of the seizure, and unless the client experiences a distinct and prolonged aura it may be impossible to recognize and intervene with the tongue blade in time. Attempts to insert the tongue blade once the vigorous muscle movements have begun may result in injury to the client's clenched teeth or the nurse's fingers. A/SP, EV, PS

380. no. 1. Petit mal seizures are also called absence seizures, reflecting the fact that clients typically experience a momentary loss of consciousness, which manifests itself in a blank facial expression and lack of response to the environment. Seizures are extremely brief and may recur many times throughout the day. The client may be unaware of their occurrence and simply pick up activity or conversation where it was before the seizure. A/SP, AS, PS

381. no. 2. The experience of a seizure is both disorienting and frightening to the client, who may be confused about what has occurred. The nurse should keep the client quiet and encourage rest while providing reorientation and reassurance. Frequent monitoring is not usually necessary, but the client may be extremely fatigued from the seizure and should not be pushed to be active or exercise. Rest and sleep are usually important. A/SP, IM, E

382. no. 1. The timing of Mestinon administration is important and must be carefully planned. Chewing and swallowing meals are two of the most repetitive and demanding muscle tasks that must be accomplished daily. It is critical that the medication be at peak effectiveness when a client eats to preserve the ability to chew, swallow, and protect the airway. The drug is therefore administered about 1 hour before meals. A/SP, PL, H

383. no. 1. The priority concern for a client in probable myasthenic crisis is the patency of the airway and the strength of the respiratory muscles. Therefore it is essential that suction equipment be readily available at the bedside. None of the other measures are appropriate in this situation. A/SP, PL, PS

384. no. 4. If a client is experiencing a myasthenic crisis the symptoms will respond promptly and clearly to the administration of a small dose of Tensilon, which is a short-acting anticholinesterase medication. It will have no positive effect on a cholinergic crisis and may even worsen the symptoms, but its effects can be readily counteracted with the administration of atropine. None of the other interventions is appropriate. A/SP, EV, PS

385. no. 2. The priority concerns with myasthenia gravis include compromise of the airway. Therefore it is essential to track the vital capacity volume and ensure that the client is able to protect the airway by having an intact swallowing reflex. The degree and progression of ptosis are also good bedside parameters for the status of the disease. Muscle strength evaluation in the extremities does not provide essential monitoring data because these symptoms are affected more peripherally by the disease process. A/SP, AS, PS

386. no. 2. Cholinergic drugs act in the same way as acetylcholine. A/SP, AN, PS

387. no. 4. It is impossible to tell in most situations of coma what if anything is being heard or processed by the client. Nurses should assume that the client can hear some or all of what is being said and be thoughtful about not discussing the client or situation. Instead the nurse should speak purposefully to the client, attempting to orient and stimulate, and should encourage family and friends to do likewise and not simply remain quietly at the bedside. A/SP, IM, PC

388. no. 1. The standard distance from an eye chart has been set at 20 feet. At this distance, letters of a certain size can be identified by a normal eye. Thus a person who reads the 20-feet line at a distance of 20 feet is said to have 20/20 vision. If a person can read only a line with larger letters (e.g., the 30-feet line), the visual acuity is 20/30, and so forth. A/SP, AN, PS

389. no. 4. The left occipital visual area contains fibers from the lateral half of the right retina. Thus damage to the left occipital visual area produces the pattern of blindness described in option no. 4. The reverse pattern of blindness results from damage to the right occipital visual area. A/SP, AS, PS

390. no. 3. This is the area defined as the anterior chamber. A/SP, AN, PS

391. no. 2. Presbyopia is an age-related change in which the ability to focus on objects close to the eye is lost. It usually occurs after age 40. Emmetropia is normal vision; diplopia is double vision; myopia is nearsightedness. A/SP, AN, PS

392. no. 4. Foreign bodies embedded in the eye must be removed by a physician or ophthalmologist. Rubbing the eye may abrade the corneal tissue and cause the particle to become further embedded. The eye must be protected from pressure or rubbing. After examination by the ophthalmologist, the eye may be irrigated with normal saline, not with water or boric acid. A/SP, IM, PS

393. no. 1. A sudden loss of an area of vision is associated with retinal detachment. Eye pain and a loss of peripheral vision are possible signs of acute and chronic angle glaucoma. A/SP, AN, PS

394. no. 1. Bed rest is required so that healing can occur. A/SP, PL, E

395. no. 3. This is an antiemetic, but it is specific for motion sickness and acts on the inner ear. The use of dimenhydrinate (Dramamine) is not associated with the other three options. A/SP, PL, PS

396. no. 3. The small incision to decrease pressure in the middle ear and prevent rupture of the eardrum heals quickly without accompanying hearing loss. A/SP, AN, PS

397. no. 3. Vertigo and nausea are classic signs of this syndrome. The remaining options are not characteristic of Meniére's syndrome. A/SP, AS, PS

398. no. 3. The opacity cannot be treated except by surgical removal of the lens. A/SP, AN, PS

399. no. 3. Paralytic ileus is not a complication that generally occurs after cataract extraction. How to use the call bell will be important because of postoperative positioning and eye patches. Respiratory infections must be avoided because coughing and sneezing can increase intraocular pressure. A/SP, PL, E

400. no. 1. This option correctly describes the effects of cataract lenses. The client will need time to adjust to the distortion resulting from cataract lenses; new safety measures must be learned because peripheral vision will be distorted. A/SP, AN, H

401. no. 1. Coughing increases intraocular pressure and is contraindicated for clients after eye surgery. Turning and positioning will only be allowed with the head of the bed elevated 30 degrees and with the client lying either supine or on the unoperated side to maintain intraocular pressure and to minimize swelling. Nausea and vomiting must be prevented because vomiting can increase intraocular pressure. A/SP, PL, PS

402. no. 4. Prolapse of the iris can precipitate acute glaucoma. This is the most common postoperative complication after lens extraction. A/SP, AN, E

403. no. 3. Postoperative confusion is a frequent complication of eye surgery, especially with elderly clients. The nurse should reorient the client frequently, explain all procedures, and keep the side rails up and the call light within easy reach. Restraints are contraindicated because they increase client anxiety and can increase intraocular pressure if the client strains against them. Telling the client to stay in bed is often inadequate when the client is confused. Giving a client a sedative can further increase confusion in the elderly. A/SP, IM, E

404. no. 1. There is no reason to stay in a darkened room. In fact, this combined with impaired vision can lead to injury. A/SP, PL, H

405. no. 4. Weeding requires bending, which increases intraocular pressure. The other options are all acceptable activities. A/SP, PL, H

406. no. 1. Mydriatic drugs cause dilation of the pupil. A dilated pupil can block the outflow of aqueous humor and increase intraocular pressure. A/SP, AN, PS

407. no. 4. Normal intraocular pressure, measured by a tonometer, is 12 to 20 mm Hg. Glaucoma is a disease in which the intraocular pressure increases to pathologic levels, sometimes as high as 85 to 90 mm Hg. A/SP, AS, PS

408. no. 2. The optic nerve is the sensory cranial nerve that controls visual acuity and visual fields. The olfactory nerve (I) is responsible for the sense of smell. Cranial nerve III controls pupillary reactions and external muscles of the eye. Cranial nerve IV controls external muscles of the eye. A/SP, AN, PS

409. no. 4. Lens opacity is characteristic of cataracts. In addition to options no. 1 through no. 3, optic nerve atrophy produces diminishing vision (first peripheral, then central vision). A/SP, AS, PS

410. no. 4. Atropine sulfate is an anticholinergic drug that dilates the pupil secondary to inhibition of the parasympathetic nervous system. Neostigmine, pilocarpine, and timolol are all drugs that can be used in the treatment of glaucoma. A/SP, AN, PS

411. no. 2. Routine care after eye surgery includes no coughing, no turning or turning only to the *unaffected*

side, and adequate fluid intake. The client should not experience severe eye pain. A/SP, PL, E

412. no. 1. Usually the first symptom to be noted is decreasing peripheral vision. There may be some mild aching but generally no pain. Severe pain is characteristic of *acute* glaucoma. In the late stage, the client may see halos around lights. A/SP, AS, PS

413. no. 2. The client's vision in dark places may be decreased when using miotics to control the glaucoma; for safety reasons, more light is needed. Moderate exercise is indicated to promote better circulation, but excessive exercise would be contraindicated. A/SP, PL, H

414. no. 2. Pilocarpine is the miotic that is commonly used in the medical management of glaucoma. Atropine is an anticholinergic drug that dilates the pupil secondary to inhibition of the parasympathetic nervous system. Acetazolamide (Diamox) is a carbonic anhydrase inhibitor that reduces intraocular pressure. Scopolamine is a mydriatic that is used to treat uveitis and iritis. A/SP, AN, PS

415. no. 2. Miotics constrict the pupil and contract the ciliary muscles increasing the outflow of aqueous humor, thus decreasing intraocular pressure. Mydriatics (drugs that dilate the pupil) such as atropine can precipitate an acute episode of glaucoma. A/SP, AN, PS

416. no. 1. Putting pressure on the lacrimal duct at the inner canthus of the eyes is important to prevent systemic effects of miotics. A/SP, IM, E

417. no. 1. Reduction of aqueous humor is desirable. Acetazolamide (Diamox) is the drug commonly used to do this. Carbonic anhydrase inhibitors do not dilate the pupil or affect accommodation. A/SP, AN, PS

418. no. 1. Once vision has been lost, it cannot be restored. Treatment for glaucoma is aimed at preventing the loss of vision. A/SP, PL, H

419. no. 2. A tonometry exam measures the intraocular pressure and can reveal early glaucoma. Treatment can then be initiated. Surgical procedures are avoided if possible because most of the filtering procedures can cause cataract formation. A/SP, PL, H

420. no. 4. Touching will provide stimulation and enhance the senses, one means to help prevent further regressive behaviors. Speaking in a louder voice is not necessary. Visual loss does not affect hearing. A sedative would cause further sensory deprivation. Orienting the client would be appropriate; however, frequent touch will be more effective in minimizing sensory deprivation. A/SP, IM, E

421. no. 4. Nasal packing and splinting are used to prevent postoperative edema and bleeding after a rhinoplasty. Frequent swallowing is a sign of bleeding that should be monitored frequently. Ice packs are used to control edema, but warm compresses would not be used. The head of the bed should be elevated to prevent aspiration. The gag reflex should be checked to ensure that the client will not aspirate bloody drainage. A/SP, PL, PS

422. no. 3. Initial stools may be tarry as a result of swallowed blood. Because this may also indicate hemorrhage, further assessment is in order. The physician will not be called until after the nursing assessment is completed. Options no. 2 and no. 4 are not indicated. A/SP, IM, PS

423. no. 1. Blowing the nose is contraindicated because it can cause bleeding. Increased pain and swelling are signs of infection and should be reported to the physician immediately. Rest, activity limitation, and adequate food and fluid intake help prevent infection. Aspirin should be avoided if pain relief is necessary because of its effects on coagulation. A/SP, IM, H

424. no. 1. Epinephrine is applied locally to create vasoconstriction and hemostasis. Lidocaine is an antidysrhythmic and a topical anesthetic. The remaining drugs have vasoconstrictive effects, but they are not used for local treatment. A/SP, AN, PS

425. no. 2. The sitting position and leaning forward will prevent the client from swallowing blood and secretions. A/SP, PL, E

426. no. 3. All the options are correct, but keeping the airway open is the main priority. A/SP, PL, PS

427. no. 1. Vasoconstrictive nose drops stimulate the sympathetic nervous system. This is followed by relaxation of these vessels, accompanied by nasal stuffiness. Therefore, after the nose is temporarily relieved by the nose drops, it becomes more stuffy than it was before. Phenylephrine (Neo-Synephrine) is a commonly used vasoconstrictive nasal spray. This drug may be absorbed systemically but does not cause hypotension. It does not contain cocaine and will not affect the olfactory nerve. A/SP, AN, PS

428. no. 2. The nasogastric tube prevents food and fluid from contaminating the pharyngeal and esophageal suture line. A/SP, PL, E

429. no. 2. Predisposing factors of cancer are known to be influenced by familial factors, sex differences, and environment. Long-term use of corticosteroids is associated with a higher incidence of cancer. A/CA, AS, H

430. no. 3. Guillain-Barré syndrome is characterized by progressive ascending weakness and paralysis of the muscles. It is frequently accompanied by numbness and tingling and results in loss of bladder tone and loss of independent respiratory functioning if the syndrome ascends through the chest. The client remains alert, however, and a decreased level of consciousness would not be expected. A/SP, AS, PS

431. no. 3. The exact cause of Guillain-Barré syndrome is not completely understood, but most clients can recall an episode of viral illness 4 to 6 weeks before the onset of symptoms. A/SP, AS, PS

432. no. 4. Severe cases of Guillain-Barré syndrome may ascend to involve and paralyze the diaphragm and upper respiratory muscles. A major nursing responsibility involves monitoring the client's tidal volume and vital capacity. If they fall below critical minimums, the client will be trached or intubated and placed on ventilatory support. Adequate respiratory function is therefore the priority goal, although vigorous efforts will be made to protect the skin and joints, assist the client to deal with the inevitable intense anxiety brought on by the symptoms, and support the family dynamics. A/SP, PL, PS

433. no. 2. Immediate first aid at the scene of the accident requires the fracture to be immobilized in the position in which the fracture is found to prevent further injury. Options no. 3 and no. 4 do not describe adequate splinting. A/M, IM, PS

434. no. 4. Initial assessments of any injured client with a fracture would first rule out any life-threatening injuries before dealing with the fracture. Covering open wounds, taking blood pressure, and cleaning the fracture site are all appropriate interventions, but airway and breathing always take first priority. A/M, IM, PS

435. no. 3. Increased blood pressure, confusion, and restlessness in a young adult are some of the first signs of fat emboli. Shock manifests with a decrease in blood pressure. A concussion causes signs of lethargy and possibly other signs of increased intracranial pressure. A/M, AN, PS

436. no. 3. Any malodor indicates a potential infection. A plaster cast color other than white indicates presence of drainage. The cast should not flake when dry. A plaster cast usually dries in 8 to 10 hours. It takes longer for larger casts such as long-leg or body casts. Weight bearing with short-leg plaster casts is usually possible 24 to 48 hours after application. Fiberglass casts may be different colors; they dry within minutes and can usually bear weight within 30 minutes. A/M, AS, E

437. no. 4. The other options tend to dry the cast from the outside, leaving the inside damp and crumbly with the potential of skin irritation. Options no. 1 and no. 2 risk burning the client's exposed skin. An electric fan may cause drying from the outside to the inside, resulting in too-early weight bearing when the outside is hard but the inside is soft. This creates the potential for indentations and the development of pressure sores. A/M, IM, E

438. no. 3. Rubber makes the pillow hard, which can cause dents in the cast. The other options are correct. A/M, IM, E

439. no. 2. This is a good way of assessing the amount of bleeding. As described, the bleeding is not excessive, so the physician need not be notified. With internal fixation, some slight bleeding is normal. The amount or size of bleeding should also be charted in the nurse's notes. A/M, IM, PS

440. no. 1. An infection would not be apparent on the first postoperative day. Hemorrhage would not be painful. After the first postoperative day, the cast would be almost dry; thus this pain could be from pressure. Casts are warm during the drying process but do not get hot enough to burn. A/M, AS, PS

441. no. 2. An unpleasant odor indicates infection. It need not include drainage. Temperature may not be elevated in local sites of infection. Option no. 3 is incorrect. A/M, AS, PS

442. no. 4. Cyanosis is the result of poor circulation, not nerve damage. All the other options reflect peroneal nerve palsy. A/M, AS, PS

443. no. 4. Shoe polish and alcohol might soften the cast. Shellac prevents evaporation of body moisture. A/M, IM, H

444. no. 4. Pain unrelieved by analgesics is an early sign of compartment syndrome. Clients with this problem tend to complain of severe pain on passive movements of the digits, after which they may be unable to move the digits of the affected extremity. Absence of the pulse and pallor may be present but are not reliable signs because deep circulation may still be intact. Paralysis indicates nerve damage. A/M, AS, PS

445. no. 1. Bivalving the cast (i.e., cutting it lengthwise into two equal parts) will reduce the external constriction, which is the critical problem; the other options are inappropriate. A/M, IM, PS

446. no. 2. Unrelieved pressure on nerves and vessels entering and leaving the compartments of the arm can cause paralysis and deformity of the arm and hand. Irreversible muscle damage can occur within 6 hours if untreated. Within 24 to 48 hours, permanent deformity with scarring, contractures, paralysis, and loss of sensation can occur. Impaired circulation would be detected before development of gangrene. A/M, AN, PS

447. no. 3. Fat emboli cause petechiae, usually across the chest and shoulders. When they do occur, it is within 12 to 36 hours after fracturing a long bone. Frothy sputum indicates pulmonary edema. Hypertension and coma indicate cerebral embolism. A/M, AS, PS

448. no. 4. After menopause, osteoporosis becomes a problem for many women as a result of estrogen deficiency. Additionally, calcium absorption in both men and women over age 65 declines as part of the aging process. Older women with this problem are at particular risk for fractures. A/M, AN, PS

449. no. 3. Buck's traction does not reduce the fracture; the pull is minimal, usually with less than 10 pounds. The use of Buck's traction is usually intermittent. Skeletal traction is used to reduce fractures. A/M, AN, PS

450. no. 2. The traction is applied directly to the skin, so it would irritate any existing ulcers. Other contraindications are a rash in the area to be covered, an allergy to the materials used for wrapping, and a neurovascular problem in the affected extremity (e.g., paralysis, phlebitis). The other options are not contraindications. A/M, AN, PS

451. no. 1. The traction device can cause irritation and skin breakdown if skin care is neglected. The bed acts as a splint when the client is turned on the affected side. Options no. 3 and no. 4 will cause the loss of countertraction and the effectiveness of the traction. A/M, PL, E

452. no. 4. High dietary fiber is a natural way to prevent constipation. Fluid intake should be encouraged. Medication should be used if fluids and increased fiber fail to obtain results. A/M, PL, E

453. no. 1. Total hip replacement is the treatment for avascular necrosis, which requires replacement of the femoral head. The other options are true of avascular necrosis. A/M, AN, PS

454. no. 2. The lower extremities usually rotate externally when a person is lying in bed. In addition, this client has had surgery on the thigh area, and this weakens the muscles in the extremity and further promotes external rotation. The other options are incorrect. A/M, PL, E

455. no. 2. This is the only option that will prevent external rotation. A/M, IM, E

456. no. 2. After assessment of the client, the physician should be notified of the findings. Severe pain is not normal after a hip nailing. The other options are incorrect. A/M, AS, PS

457. no. 1. The walker should always be walked into when all four legs are on the floor. The other options are incorrect. A/M, EV, E

458. no. 3. These should be prevented because both can promote dislodgment of the hip prosthesis. The affected extremity is to be abducted by the use of an abductor pillow. The other options are incorrect. A/M, IM, E

459. no. 1. The sudden onset of severe pain in the hip prosthesis site indicates dislodgment. The physician should be notified once the nurse has completed an assessment of the extremity. The other options are incorrect interventions at this time. A/M, IM, PS

460. no. 4. This is the best choice. The client probably still has the abduction pillow in place. Flexion greater than 90 degrees must be avoided to prevent prosthesis displacement. A/M, IM, E

461. no. 3. Adequate blood supply is required for tissue to heal and survive; thus the decision regarding the level of an amputation depends on the quality of vascularity of the tissue. This is best evaluated at the time of the surgery. A/M, AN, PS

462. no. 2. Firm application of an elastic bandage is necessary to prevent fluid accumulation and to continue to mold the limb if the rigid dressing comes off, at which time the physician is notified. Elevating the limb on the fifth day is contraindicated. Elevation of a lower extremity after amputation is done only for the first 24 hours postoperatively. After that, elevation promotes flexion contractures, the most common complication after amputation of lower extremities. A sterile saline dressing is used in the event of evisceration. A/M, IM, PS

463. no. 3. A "shrinker" bandage is properly applied with tighter turns around the distal end of the affected limb to promote venous return and stump molding. The other options are appropriate. A/M, IM, H

464. no. 2. The nurse should be direct and honest with the client concerning the accident and outcome of the surgery. The first step in the grieving process is acknowledgment of the loss. This option facilitates acknowledgment. Option no. 1 is not truthful and avoids the issue. Option no. 3 also avoids the issue of the loss of the arm. Option no. 4 is incorrect because phantom limb sensation is a feeling process; the sensation is related to the severing of the nerves at the amputation site. It is not a thinking process. Also, the sensation that the limb is present occurs after surgery and may last for as long as 6 months. A/M, IM, PC

465. no. 4. The client needs to identify new body boundaries by touching and reorienting to a new body. This will facilitate the rehabilitation process, especially acceptance of a changing body image. A/M, IM, PC

466. no. 4. Inflammation and systemic symptoms are characteristic of rheumatoid arthritis. Osteoarthritis is

characterized by local symptoms and usually no systemic symptoms such as fever and elevated sedimentation rate. A/M, AS, PS

467. no. 4. Clients with osteoarthritis should conserve energy when possible. This client is overweight and needs to achieve her ideal body weight in order to decrease the stress on her joints. Warm baths will decrease the discomfort and facilitate increased movement. Sliding items across the floor requires less energy than lifting and carrying them. A/M, IM, E

468. no. 2. The usual dose range of aspirin to treat inflammation is 3 to 5 g per day. Regularly scheduled intake provides a constant plasma level and increases effects. Ringing in the ears is a first sign of overdose of aspirin. Enteric-coated tablets (e.g., Ecotrin) are helpful in preventing gastrointestinal distress. A hypersensitivity reaction can occur at any time. A/M, EV, H

469. no. 1. This is the only correct option. Gout occurs in the small joints and results when urate crystals are deposited in the joints. The most common age group is 30- to 40-year-old men. Option no. 4 is characteristic of osteoarthritis. A/M, AN, PS

470. no. 4. Fluid intake is increased to prevent the precipitation of urate in the kidneys. Clients often cannot tolerate the pressure of compresses on the affected areas. Salicylates antagonize the action of some uricosuric drugs. Aspirin and other salicylates at low doses (300 to 600 mg) inhibit uric acid secretion. Acetaminophen could be substituted for simple pain relief. Deformities are rare in gout. A/M, PL, E

471. no. 1. Dietary restrictions of purine are usually initiated after the acute attack. The disease can be well controlled with dietary management and medications. Dietary management includes limiting high-purine foods and alcohol ingestion and maintaining an ideal body weight. Foods high in purine are organ meats, yeast, anchovies, sardines in oil, and meat extracts. The urine should be kept alkaline to prevent stone formation. This may be achieved by an alkaline-ash diet that includes milk, vegetables, and fruits (except for cranberries, prunes, and plums). A/M, PL, H

472. no. 4. Allopurinol (Zyloprim) is irritating to the intestinal tract. It is best to take the medication during or after the meal because medication taken on an empty stomach is more likely to cause gastrointestinal irritation. The other options are incorrect information. Fluids are usually encouraged with a minimum of 2000 ml per day. Foods with purine are usually limited or restricted but are not totally eliminated. A/M, PL, E

473. no. 2. A skin rash is the first sign of a severe hypersensitivity reaction. A/M, IM, E

474. no. 2. This is the incorrect option. Option no. 1 is the appropriate action for log rolling. Keeping the knees slightly flexed while the client is in semi-Fowler's position will decrease muscle strain in the lower back. Keeping a pillow under the head for comfort will cause no harm and will promote comfort. A/M, PL, E

475. no. 4. A thickening or lump noted in the breast is one of the signs of cancer cited by the American Cancer Society. A tumor itself does not cause pain; pain re-

sults from pressure exerted on surrounding tissue when the tumor enlarges and would be an advanced sign of cancer. Tenderness in breast tissue is more often a sign of benign fibrocystic breast disease. Options no. 1, no. 2, and no. 3 are three of the seven warning signs for cancer cited by the American Cancer Society. A/CA, AN, H

476. no. 3. According to the most recent guidelines established by the American Cancer Society, a stool guaiac slide test should be done yearly after the age of 50. A baseline mammogram should be done between the ages of 35 and 39. A Pap smear is done every 3 years after three initial negative tests that are done 1 year apart or as directed by the physician. Cancer-related checkups should be done on a yearly basis after age 50, not every 5 years. A/CA, EV, H

477. no. 1. A Pap smear is obtained to detect neoplastic cells in the cervical and vaginal secretions that have been shed by cervical and endometrial neoplastic cells. Material is collected by scraping the cervical canal and the squamocolumnar junction with a spatula or a cotton swab moistened with saline. The Pap smear does not directly evaluate the uterus, the fallopian tubes, or the cul-de-sac (the peritoneal space between the rectum and the uterus). The fallopian tubes are usually examined with a laparoscopy or culdoscopy. A/CA, AN, H

478. no. 4. A class-1 Pap smear indicates absence of atypical or abnormal cells. After three initial negative tests taken 1 year apart, Pap smears are done every 3 years or as directed by a physician. Classes 2 to 4 require more extensive evaluation to determine if a malignancy exists. Class 5 cytologic findings indicate malignancy and require treatment. After a class-1 finding, surgery, treatment, and refraining from sexual activity are not indicated. A/CA, IM, H

479. no. 1. Clients with ovarian cancer often have vague, nonspecific complaints, including changes in bowel elimination. Other symptoms include increasing abdominal girth and bloating, abdominal discomfort after meals, food intolerance, fatigue, and weight change. Postcoital bleeding is seen in cervical cancer. Dyspnea and night sweats are not associated with ovarian cancer. A/CA, AS, H

480. no. 2. Sputum samples should be collected early in the morning before the client eats or drinks. The client is not required to be NPO for 24 hours before the procedure. The client needs to be well hydrated to facilitate coughing up tenacious secretions. Using toothpaste or mouthwash should be avoided because they can affect the sample. The sample should be coughed up from deep within the lungs. Saliva should not be collected. A/CA, IM, H

481. no. 2. Small-cell lung cancer has a poor prognosis because it is rarely diagnosed in a limited and localized state. Even with treatment the client has only a 20% chance for 2-year survival. At advanced stages most clients die within 6 months. The 5-year survival rate depends on the type of lung cancer (non–small-cell cancer has a somewhat better 5-year survival rate) and stage (cancer is easier to treat in an earlier stage when

the cancer is localized). Usually by the time a lung tumor is detected on x-ray, about 75% of the disease course has elapsed. Eighty-seven percent of lung cancer clients die within 5 years. A/CA, AS, PS

482. no. 4. Options no. 1, no. 2, and no. 3 are all common systemic side effects of external radiation therapy. Dry desquamation of the skin is a common localized side effect. A/CA, AS, PS

483. no. 3. Skin markings over the treatment area should not be washed off for the duration of the therapy unless special permission is given because they are important reference marks for the radiation beams. The area should be left open to air, but sunlight should be avoided. The skin should not be massaged, and lotions, cosmetics, and powder should not be applied. These interventions will reduce the problems associated with dry desquamation of the skin. A/CA, IM, E

484. no. 4. Metoclopramide (Reglan) is a cholinergic medication used to prevent the nausea and vomiting associated with chemotherapy and delayed gastric emptying. Phentolamine mesylate (Regitine) is an alpha-adrenergic blocker used for treating hypertension. Methylcellulase (Citrucel) is a bulk laxative. Dexamethasone (Decadron) is a corticosteroid used to treat cerebral edema. A/CA, AN, PS

485. no. 2. False reassurance that everything will be all right is inappropriate. It is a block to therapeutic communication and it discounts the client's feelings. The client should understand the extent of surgery and the type and care of the ostomy. Although a cheerful, optimistic environment is important, it is essential that the client understand the proposed surgical treatment. Visitors should not be restricted. Family and friends can provide valuable social support to the client. A/CA, PL, E

486. no. 4. Testicular exams should be performed after a warm shower or bath to relax the scrotum. Testicular exams should be done by all men beginning at age 15 on a monthly basis. Reddening or darkening of the scrotum is not a normal finding and should be reported to a physician. A/CA, IM, H

487. no. 3. Colon tumors tend to spread through the lymphatics and portal vein to the liver. Although metastasis to the other sites listed is possible, the liver is most likely the first to be affected. A/CA, AN, PS

488. no. 2. 5-Fluorouracil (5-FU) is an antineoplastic, antimetabolic drug that inhibits DNA synthesis and interferes with cell replication. It is given intravenously and acts systemically. It affects all rapidly growing cells, both malignant and normal. It is used as adjuvant therapy for treating cancer of the colon, rectum, stomach, breast, and pancreas. This drug has many side effects, including bone marrow depression, anorexia, stomatitis, and nausea and vomiting. A/CA, AN, PS

489. no. 1. Bland foods of moderate temperature facilitate swallowing and decrease pain. Fluids should be encouraged to keep oral membranes moist and to decrease side effects of chemotherapy. Commercial mouthwashes should be avoided because of their alcohol content. The mouth should be rinsed with dilute H_2O_2 or normal saline solution. Lemon-glycerin

swabs should be avoided to prevent excessive drying of the oral mucosa. A/CA, PL, E

490. no. 4. Epithelial cells are extremely sensitive to chemotherapy because of their normally high rate of cell turnover. Options no. 1, no. 2, and no. 3 are not as appropriate because they do not address the client's concern. The client is requesting factual information. In addition, no. 1 negates the client's concerns. A/CA, IM, E

491. no. 3. It is important for the significant other to express feelings. Allowing the family to know the diagnosis may help him and the client through the decision-making, treatment, and follow-up care phases. No. 1 is not correct because it does not address the issue of why the husband wants the diagnoses kept from their families. The situation will be difficult to resolve unless the husband's rationale is known. Option no. 2 may be appropriate at a later time. Option no. 4 introduces new information that the husband is angry. A/CA, IM, PC

492. no. 3. Option no. 1 will detect internal occult bleeding. Options no. 2 and no. 4 will decrease the risk of bleeding. Option no. 3 is not necessary because it will not affect the risk of hemorrhage. Reverse isolation would be implemented for a granulocyte count below 2000 mm^3. A/CA, PL, PS

493. no. 2. When chemotherapy is initiated, there is a breakdown of many cancer cells. Uric acid is a cell metabolite. A/CA, AN, PS

494. no. 2. Allopurinol is an antigout drug that decreases uric acid formation. Prednisone is a corticosteroid used for immunosuppression and severe inflammation. Indomethacin inhibits prostaglandin synthesis; it is effective as an analgesic, antiinflammatory, and antipyretic agent. Hydrochlorothiazide is a thiazide diuretic that is effective in hypertension and edema. A/CA, AN, PS

495. no. 4. Thrombocytopenia is an abnormal decrease in the number of platelets, which results in bleeding tendencies. Erythrocytosis is an abnormal increase in the number of circulating red blood cells. Leukocytosis is an increase in the number of white blood cells in the blood. Polycythemia is also an excess of red blood cells and is a synonym for erythrocytosis. With chemotherapy there is a decrease in red and white blood cells, not an increase. A/CA, AS, PS

496. no. 3. Menarche before the age of 11 is a predisposing factor for breast cancer. The other three options are all considered to be risk factors for cervical cancer. Risk factors for breast cancer are late menopause (after age 50), never carrying a full-term pregnancy, carrying a first pregnancy after age 30, and presence of breast cancer in first-degree relatives. A/CA, AS, PS

497. no. 2. Many women with cervical cancer fear a loss of femininity. It is important to discuss the effects of treatment to enable the client to prepare for changes in sexual functioning. Although telling the client that she does not have to worry about pregnancy is accurate, it is not a therapeutic response. Nurses are capable of answering questions regarding sexuality. The client will need to be referred to other resources if the

client's concerns cannot be addressed by the nurse. The physician should be notified of the client's concerns, but not necessarily as a referral. A/CA, IM, PC

498. no. 1. Vaginal drainage will usually persist for 1 to 2 months after removal of a cervical implant. Diarrhea, not constipation, is usually a side effect of cervical implants. Stomatitis and xerostomia are local side effects of radiation to the mouth. A/CA, IM, PS

499. no. 3. Clients with cervical implants require a low-residue diet (and often antidiarrheal medications) to reduce the frequency of defecation. Defecation may cause accidental dislodgment of the implant from straining and sitting on a bedpan. Frequent ambulation is contraindicated because it will dislodge the implant. Bed rest in a supine or low Fowler's position should be maintained. Visitors should be limited to one 15-minute visit a day, and no pregnant women or children should be allowed because of the radiation exposure. Vaginal irrigations are contraindicated during this period of time. A/CA, IM, E

500. no. 1. Shortening and narrowing of the vagina is a distressing long-term complication of cervical implants. Women need to use a vaginal dilator twice a week to stretch the tissue. Uterine cramping is a temporary side effect that occurs only if the implant extends into the uterus. Nausea and diarrhea may occur during the initial treatment but are not long-term side effects. A/CA, AS, PS

501. no. 3. Clients who have experienced a loss need the opportunity to express their grief. It is important to allow the client to express grief (through crying or anger) over the loss of her breast. Options no. 1, no. 2, and no. 4 are all blocks to therapeutic communication and do not allow the client to verbalize her feelings. A/CA, IM, PC

502. no. 1. A significant breast cancer risk factor is a history of previous breast cancer. Breast cancer can develop bilaterally, so it is imperative that the client be instructed to perform breast self-exams on the remaining breast. A/CA, AN, H

503. no. 3. Although options no. 1 and no. 2 are technically correct, they do not address the client's feelings about her body image. The client needs to express her feelings and concerns before effective preoperative teaching can be accomplished. Option no. 4 provides false reassurance and is a block to therapeutic communication. A/CA, IM, PC

504. no. 4. Raising the side rails after premedication is an essential safety measure that must be done immediately after administration of any preoperative medication. Options no. 1, no. 2, and no. 3 should be done *before* premedicating the client. The client should be maintained on bed rest and should not get up to void because her gait may be unstable. Operative permits are not valid if obtained after administration of narcotics or consciousness-altering medications. Patient teaching must be done when client is fully awake, alert, and oriented. A/CA, IM, E

505. no. 1. Check under the client's back for drainage because gravity will draw it toward the back. A/CA, IM, PS

506. no. 1. The right axilla should not be shaved because of the risk of cutting the skin and subsequent infection development. Lymphedema after a mastectomy will increase this risk of infection. Sodium intake should not be increased because it will further increase lymphedema. A client can wear her own bra with padding after discharge or use a Reach to Recovery prosthesis. The incision should be gently cleansed with mild soap and warm water, not an antiseptic solution. A/CA, IM, H

507. no. 1. The other three options have been identified as influencing a client's adaptation to mastectomy, something that must be assessed in this case. A/CA, AS, PS

508. no. 2. Denial is often the first response to loss and grief. It is a defense against more anxiety than the client can cope with at the time. This client may experience anger, bargaining, and depression later, but her comments suggest that she is currently in the denial stage of the grief and mourning process. A/CA, AN, PC

509. no. 3. Expressions of hopelessness or despair, or both, are defining characteristics of reactive (situational) depression. P/E, AS, PC

510. no. 1. This diagnosis reflects an actual change in the structure and function of a body. Impaired verbal communication and alteration in cardiac output will not occur with an uncomplicated lumpectomy. The client may have a temporary self-care deficit with a radical mastectomy. However, this aggressive surgery is not done as frequently today. A/CA, AN, PS

511. no. 1. These measures must be instituted to promote adequate lymphatic flow in the affected arm. The other choices listed would contribute to tissue edema. A/CA, PL, E

512. no. 2. Cancer cells are generally the most rapidly dividing in the body. Healthy tissues such as bone marrow, gastrointestinal epithelium, and hair follicles are also rapidly proliferating and thus bear the brunt of the effects of many of the cytotoxic drugs. Options no. 1, no. 3, and no. 4 are incorrect. A/CA, AN, E

513. no. 3. Some women have engorgement of the breasts premenstrually, which usually disappears a few days after the onset of menstruation. Because of this possible change, it is important that the breasts be examined at the same point in the menstrual cycle each month, ideally when the hormonal influences on the breast are the smallest. CBF/W, IM, H

514. no. 3. A woman who is having a breast removed has many fears related to sexual and social acceptance, disfigurement, and death. Many women have been unable to discuss these feelings with significant others. The nurse can help the client verbalize her feelings and understand what the surgery means to her as a person. The client has a need to be understood and accepted by the nurse. The nurse can clarify any misconceptions and reduce the client's anxiety preoperatively. Sexual relations need not be altered as a result of the surgery, and a skin graft is not needed with a modified radical mastectomy. A/CA, PL, E

515. no. 3. Curling the tubing impedes free flow of the drainage and puts pressure on the skin. The skin will become irritated and could slough. In general, the wound exudate is a straw-colored fluid that is initially blood tinged. Obvious bleeding is bright red and should be immediately reported to the surgeon. To maintain suction, empty the continuous portable suction reservoir when it is half full and reestablish the negative pressure. A/CA, IM, PS

516. no. 2. Because movement of the arm is painful, the nurse should support the arm the first few times the arm is exercised. Abduct and adduct it slowly; flex and extend the elbow, wrist, and fingers. Gentle exercises help reduce muscle dysfunction. The nurse's assistance helps assure the client that movement of the arm will not cause any harm. Slings are to be avoided because they encourage immobility and an increase in lymphedema. Full range of motion cannot be achieved this early in the postoperative period. A/CA, IM, H

517. no. 4. Clients should be encouraged to resume normal activities after returning home. The nursing care goals are to strengthen self-esteem and contribute to restoring normal function with no activity restrictions after the wound is healed. A/CA, IM, H

518. no. 1. Hodgkin's disease is a malignancy of the lymphoid system that is characterized by a generalized painless lymphadenopathy. It has a 5-year survival rate of 90%. Option no. 2 refers to a multiple myeloma, no. 3 refers to AIDS, and no. 4 refers to leukemia. A/CA, AN, PS

519. no. 3. Diarrhea is not indicative of Hodgkin's disease. The other three options frequently occur with the disease. A/CA, AS, PS

520. no. 4. Lymphangiography provides an x-ray examination of the lymphatic system. A bluish contrast medium is injected into a lymphatic vessel in each foot or hand. The blue dye will give skin a bluish tinge and will discolor the stools and urine for several days.

The client must lie still during the procedure. After the procedure, the affected extremity will need to be elevated to prevent edema. Food and fluids are usually not restricted before the lymphangiography. A/CA, IM, PS

521. no. 1. Acquired immunodeficiency syndrome is characterized by a defect in cell-mediated immunity. It is believed to be caused by the human immunodeficiency virus (HIV), which is a retrovirus that destroys CD4 lymphocytes. It does not affect the lymphoid tissues. Kaposi's sarcoma is an opportunistic disease that causes multiple areas of cell proliferation in the skin and eventually in other body sites, but the disease itself is not a malignancy of the skin. Acquired immunodeficiency syndrome is not a bacterial infection; however, a number of bacterial infections occur as opportunistic diseases. A/CA, AN, PS

522. no. 2. The ELISA measures antibodies to HIV in serum or plasma and is the most widely used screening test for AIDS. The Western blot assay is a *supplemental* test conducted to validate the findings of the ELISA. Lymphangiography is a diagnostic procedure that detects disease of the lymphoid tissue. A Schilling test is used to detect vitamin B_{12} absorption. A/CA, AS, H

523. no. 4. *Pneumocystis carinii* pneumonia is a protozoal disease frequently seen in AIDS clients. The other three options are not considered opportunistic diseases of AIDS. Although non-Hodgkin's lymphoma is a cancer seen in HIV infection, Hodgkin's disease is not. A/CA, AN, PS

524. no. 4. Clients who are HIV positive should not donate blood, plasma, sperm, or body organs. They do not have to avoid casual contact with anyone and do not need to wear gloves or a mask. A/CA, EV, H

Contents

Questions *130*

Correct Answers *145*

Correct Answers with Rationales *147*

Chapter *4*

Nursing Care of the Childbearing Family

COORDINATOR

Roberta Kordish, MSN, RN

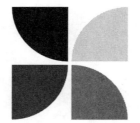

Questions

1. A woman stopped taking oral contraceptives several months ago and now suspects she is pregnant. Which of the following signs most likely suggests she is pregnant?
   ① Amenorrhea
   ② Morning sickness
   ③ Enlarged and tender breasts
   ④ A positive pregnancy test

2. A woman's last menstrual period was from November 10 to 15. She had intercourse that resulted in pregnancy on November 24. What is her expected date of delivery?
   ① July 21
   ② Aug. 17
   ③ Aug. 22
   ④ Aug. 24

3. A woman suspects that she may be pregnant and uses an over-the-counter pregnancy kit to see if this is true. Which of the following is true of these pregnancy tests done on urine samples?
   ① A positive test is based on increased estrogen excretion in the urine.
   ② The tests are 100% accurate if done 10 to 14 days after fertilization.
   ③ A positive test is based on the excretion of chorionic gonadotropin in the urine.
   ④ Home pregnancy tests are not accurate, and clients should be cautioned not to use them.

4. A primigravida is concerned about eating the proper foods during her pregnancy. Which of the following nursing actions is the most appropriate initially?
   ① Give her a list of foods to refer to in planning her meals.
   ② Emphasize the importance of limiting highly seasoned and salty foods.
   ③ Ask her to list her food intake for the last 3 days.
   ④ Instruct her to continue her usual diet because she appears to be nutritionally fit.

5. An expectant mother, gravida 3, para 2, has a hemoglobin of 11.0. Which of the following meals would indicate that she learned which foods will increase her iron intake?
   ① Ham sandwich, corn pudding, and tossed salad
   ② Fish sandwich, carrots, and fruit cup
   ③ Chicken livers, sliced tomatoes, and dried apricots
   ④ Omelet with mushrooms and green beans

6. The nurse would instruct a pregnant woman to notify the physician immediately if which of the following symptoms occurs during the pregnancy?
   ① Swelling of the face
   ② Breast tenderness and tingling
   ③ Leukorrhea
   ④ The presence of chloasma

7. A pregnant client is treated for syphilis during the first trimester with intramuscular injections of penicillin. What would her baby's diagnosis at birth most likely be?
   ① Congenital syphilis
   ② Stillborn
   ③ Normal newborn
   ④ Premature newborn

8. Constipation during pregnancy is best treated by
   ① Regular use of a mild laxative.
   ② Increased bulk and fluid in the diet.
   ③ Limiting excessive weight gain.
   ④ Regular use of bisacodyl (Dulcolax) suppositories.

9. Which of the following would be considered normal in the first trimester of pregnancy?
   ① Vaginal spotting and abdominal cramping
   ② Hematocrit of 28% and pica
   ③ Urinary frequency and trace glycosuria
   ④ Nausea and increased intractable vomiting

10. A woman has a history of a 28-day, regular menstrual cycle. At which point in her cycle is the mature ovum released from the ovarian follicle?
    ① The ovum is released on the first or second day.
    ② The ovum is released on the tenth or eleventh day.
    ③ The ovum is released on the fourteenth or fifteenth day.
    ④ Release of the ovum is unpredictable.

11. A new expectant father asks about leisure activities he can enjoy with his wife during pregnancy. Which response by the nurse best indicates an understanding of the needs of the couple during pregnancy?
    ① "Although she may tire easily, you can continue most activities you have enjoyed in the past."
    ② "You should explore more sedentary recreation now, since active exercise needs to be limited."
    ③ "You may wish to continue with your hobbies, and allow your wife to enjoy leisure activities with her friends."
    ④ "This is a time to prepare yourselves for the role of new parents, rather than thinking of yourselves."

12. The nurse teaches a pregnant woman danger signs of pregnancy. Which of the following findings reported by the woman at 32 weeks of pregnancy indicates that she has learned?
    ① Intermittent menstrual-like cramps
    ② Anxiety and insomnia
    ③ Dyspnea
    ④ Ankle edema

13. A 29-year-old woman is in the first trimester of pregnancy. The nurse instructs her about what to do if vaginal bleeding occurs. Which of the following initial actions indicates that she understands these prenatal instructions?
    ① She considers the bleeding to be normal, especially if it occurs at the time of her usual period.
    ② She records the date and amount of bleeding and reports it on her next visit.
    ③ She phones the physician to give duration and amount of bleeding.
    ④ She remains on complete bed rest until the bleeding ceases.

14. In her seventh lunar month of pregnancy, a woman who works as an assistant store manager discusses usual activities of her job with the nurse. Which of the following tasks can continue without risk to her or the baby?
    ① Working 12-hour shifts during the holiday season.
    ② Lifting 40-pound packages when unpacking merchandise.
    ③ Standing for 8 hours, ringing sales at the cash register.
    ④ Spending 20 minutes of her lunch hour taking a brisk walk.

15. A client who is in the first trimester of pregnancy calls the clinic to report her concern about contracting toxoplasmosis. In assessing the risk to this client, which factor is most critical?
    ① The client has had no direct contact with her infected sister in 5 days.
    ② The client has a cat for whom she cares.
    ③ No one in the family eats pork.
    ④ The client feels well at present.

16. A client and her husband have become vegetarians within the last year. Now that the client is in her third month of pregnancy, her physician is concerned about adequate protein intake for growth and development. He asks the nurse to discuss nutrition with the client. Considering that the client usually avoids meat and poultry, which meal would indicate planning for complementary plant proteins?
    ① Peanut butter sandwich on whole wheat bread and a glass of milk
    ② Multigrain cereal with bananas and strawberries
    ③ Spinach salad, kidney beans, and oranges
    ④ Rice, corn, and tomatoes

17. As a prenatal client approaches full term, the nurse discusses with her and her husband the antepartal classes they have attended. They tell the nurse of their participation in Lamaze classes with 10 other couples.

Which statement by this couple best indicates understanding of key concepts?
    ① "Slow deep breathing throughout labor will minimize pain."
    ② "Self-hypnosis is the key to coping."
    ③ "Avoiding touch during contractions will enhance concentration."
    ④ "We plan to continue using a wall hanging for a focal point."

18. A primipara at 39 weeks of gestation calls the prenatal clinic and states that she thinks she is in labor. Which of the following signs would indicate that she is in true labor?
    ① Walking eases her contractions.
    ② She has blood-tinged mucus from her vagina.
    ③ She thinks that the baby has dropped, and she has a persistent low backache.
    ④ Her contractions are increasing in frequency and duration.

19. One of the components of antepartal nursing care is provision of childbirth education classes in the third trimester of pregnancy. What is the main objective of most childbirth education programs in the United States today?
    ① A painless childbirth experience
    ② The participation of both parents in the birth process
    ③ The elimination of medication in labor and delivery
    ④ An emotionally satisfying birth experience

20. During the first session of a childbirth education series, one of the participants states, "I cannot relax! Just thinking of going through labor makes me tense all over." Which response is most appropriate?
    ① "Labor pains don't hurt as much as you have been led to believe. Childbirth can be a really enjoyable experience."
    ② "Once you understand the importance of natural childbirth, you will begin to relax, and your fears will disappear."
    ③ "It is quite common for women to be anxious about labor and delivery. Women can learn to relax through education and physical training."
    ④ "Fear causes tension, which results in pain. When you learn about childbirth, your fear will be eliminated, and pain will not occur."

21. In the early stage of labor, which of the following is the most appropriate strategy for the nurse to use first in teaching a couple?
    ① Assess present knowledge of the couple.
    ② Teach at the couple's level of understanding.
    ③ Use a standard teaching plan.
    ④ Reinforce key concepts as necessary.

22. A woman has been in active labor for about 14 hours. When she reaches transition, she tells her husband to leave her alone. What is the best nursing action at this time?
    ① Ask the father to leave the nurse and the client alone.
    ② Urge the client to remain quiet at this time.

③ Encourage the couple to explore their feelings for each other.

④ Accept this behavior as normal in this situation.

23. A sibling visitation program is one of the services offered by a hospital's maternity unit. A 2-year-old visiting her new baby brother seems uninterested and asks to go home. The nursing student asks the nurse if this behavior is normal. What explanation to the student would be most appropriate?

① "The parents may not have prepared the child well."

② "The little girl probably resents her mother."

③ "The social worker should assess the family situation."

④ "This behavior is common for this little girl's developmental level."

24. A child, age 2½, comes with his father to visit his mother and new baby brother on the maternity unit. Later that evening, the little boy develops a fever and is diagnosed as having rubella. Which statement by the boy's mother best indicates that she understands the implications of this infection?

① "I'll remind my mother to give my little boy aspirin for the fever."

② "My sister is 2 months pregnant; I'll ask her to stay away from our home."

③ "To prevent our new baby from contracting the infection, I'll ask the doctor to give him a vaccination now."

④ "It's good that my husband and I both had measles for 2 weeks as children."

25. The nurse is counseling a young woman about the signs of ovulation. Which of the following points should be included in the discussion?

① Ovulation comes predictably 14 days after onset of menses.

② Lower abdominal pain may be experienced at the time of rupture of the follicle.

③ The cervical mucus becomes white and less elastic when an egg is released.

④ Basal body temperature rises at ovulation and then falls about 1 degree.

26. The nurse is presenting a class on conception and childbirth at the local high school. One 14-year-old asks if a person should douche after intercourse as a precaution against pregnancy. How would the nurse respond to this question?

① "I wouldn't recommend that. It would greatly increase your chances for a vaginal infection."

② "That would be very helpful, since douching will wash the sperm from your vaginal canal."

③ "Douching is not an effective method of contraception and may even facilitate fertilization if a mature egg is available."

④ "That's a good idea, since failure rates with natural planning alone are quite high."

27. During a prenatal visit at 36 weeks, a woman comments that her husband wants her to have a tubal ligation after delivery. Which statement most indicates the need for further information about this type of contraception?

① "I know it can easily be reversed later if I change my mind."

② "The doctor tells me I can have this procedure after delivery, before I leave the hospital."

③ "I'm prepared for mild abdominal discomfort after surgery."

④ "I'm glad my hormones won't be affected by the tubal ligation."

28. The antepartal clinic receives a call from a young primigravida who has recently been diagnosed as being about 10 weeks pregnant. The sobbing woman tells the nurse, "I've started bleeding! I'm so afraid I'm losing my baby." Which one of the following would be the most appropriate initial nursing response?

① "You must be quite upset right now. Why don't you come to the clinic right away?"

② "Go to bed immediately with your feet elevated. I will call for an ambulance."

③ "It is very common for women to have some bleeding during early pregnancy."

④ "Can you describe the bleeding to me and tell me when it first began?"

29. A woman who is 8 weeks pregnant comes to the emergency department with moderate bright red vaginal bleeding. On examination, the physician finds that the client's cervix is 2 cm dilated. Which term best describes the client's condition?

① Incomplete abortion

② Inevitable abortion

③ Threatened abortion

④ Missed abortion

30. A multigravida is admitted to the hospital with a diagnosis of threatened abortion. Her initial nursing management would include which of the following?

① Examining all perineal pads for tissues and clots.

② Placing the bed in Trendelenburg's position.

③ Preparing her for a Shirodkar procedure.

④ Restricting all physical activity and fluid intake.

31. The physician tells a woman who experienced bleeding in the first trimester that she has had "a missed abortion." The woman asks the nurse to explain what this means. Which response is most appropriate?

① "It's another name for a miscarriage."

② "The baby is deformed, resulting in an abortion."

③ "The baby is no longer alive and growing, but your body hasn't expelled it yet."

④ "There was no pregnancy; your body just responded as if there was one."

32. A woman who has had repeated pregnancy losses in the fourth and fifth months of pregnancy is told that she will have a McDonald's procedure done when she is pregnant to correct an incompetent cervical os. She asks the nurse about the procedure. Which of the following statements best explains the procedure?

① "It is a suture that is put around the cervix around 24 weeks of gestation."

② "The suture around the cervix means that a cesarean delivery will be performed at term."

③ "The suture around the cervix is temporary and will be removed at term. You may be able to have a vaginal delivery if all goes well."

④ "You will have to spend most of the pregnancy in bed, but the suture will enable you to carry the baby to term."

33. After a McDonald's procedure is done for incompetent cervical os, it will be especially important for the client to receive discharge instructions regarding which one of the following?
① Abstaining from intercourse until after the suture is removed
② Reporting any signs and symptoms of labor
③ Taking prophylactic antibiotics for the remainder of pregnancy
④ Expecting a small for gestational age infant

34. A woman in her first trimester of pregnancy is seen in the antepartal clinic. An ectopic pregnancy is suspected. Which of the following symptoms would the nurse most likely expect to be present in an ectopic pregnancy?
① Spotting and unilateral pelvic pain
② Lower abdominal pain and an enlarged uterus
③ Leukorrhea and an enlarged uterus
④ Headache, profuse bleeding, and lower abdominal pain

35. In reviewing the medical records of a woman in the first trimester, which of the following findings would the nurse consider to be a risk factor for ectopic pregnancy?
① Positive Coombs' test
② Persistent glucosuria
③ Blood pressure elevations observed twice at least 6 hours apart
④ History of pelvic inflammatory disease

36. The client with a medical diagnosis of ectopic pregnancy is a high-risk client. Which of the following reasons best accounts for this?
① Surgery is required to treat this complication.
② Hemorrhage is a major problem.
③ Removal of the fallopian tube may result in sterility.
④ The ovum may abort into the abdominal cavity.

37. A pregnant woman who has completed 32 weeks of gestation calls the clinic where she has been receiving antepartal care. She tells the nurse that there is a small amount of bright-red blood coming from her vagina, but that she has no pain. Based on the information given, what cause for the bleeding would the nurse best conclude?
① Lacerated vaginal mucosa
② Premature labor
③ Ruptured vaginal varicosities
④ Low placental implantation

38. A primipara with bright-red vaginal bleeding in the third trimester of her pregnancy is hospitalized. Which of the following nursing actions is most important at this time?
① Assess the degree of cervical dilation.
② Estimate the amount of blood loss.

③ Take vital signs every 15 minutes.
④ Determine the fetal heart rate.

39. A woman in the eighth month of pregnancy has mild vaginal bleeding associated with a diagnosis of placenta previa. In caring for this client, the nurse would
① Prepare for a vaginal examination.
② Expect an emergency cesarean birth.
③ Keep the woman on bed rest.
④ Place the woman in Trendelenburg's position.

40. A woman is hospitalized with placenta previa. Which of the following is most important for the nurse to teach this client regarding her condition?
① Reduce external stimuli in the room.
② Decrease fluid intake.
③ Limit physical activity.
④ Avoid emotional upset.

41. An expectant mother, gravida 3, para 2, is admitted to the labor room in early labor with vaginal bleeding. She has a history of rapid deliveries and has had an elevated blood pressure since 28 weeks of gestation. She is slowly leaking amniotic fluid and currently has a blood pressure of 150/100 mm Hg. Which of the following predisposing factors to abruptio placentae does this client have?
① Chronic hypertension
② Pregnancy-induced hypertension
③ Precipitous delivery
④ Premature rupture of the membranes

42. In assessing the client with vaginal bleeding in the third trimester of pregnancy caused by suspected abruptio placentae, which of the following procedures would the nurse perform?
① Monitor urine output by inserting a Foley catheter.
② Perform a vaginal examination to evaluate progression of labor.
③ Check the client's vital signs every 30 minutes.
④ Conduct an abdominal examination for signs of tenderness or rigidity.

43. In providing nursing care for the woman with abruptio placentae, which of the following interventions would be most appropriate and provide the most benefit to the fetus?
① Turn the client every 30 minutes.
② Administer oxygen.
③ Estimate amount of blood loss.
④ Observe for changes in the pattern of uterine contractions.

44. The nurse is caring for a woman with a diagnosis of abruptio placentae. What complication of this condition is of most concern to the nurse?
① Disseminated intravascular coagulation syndrome
② Pulmonary embolus
③ Convulsions
④ Ruptured uterus

45. Which of the following findings would indicate that a woman might be developing complications from an abruptio placentae?
① The woman's temperature is 100°F (38.3°C).
② Fluid-filled vesicles appear in the vaginal discharge.

③ A venipuncture site continues to bleed for 15 minutes.

④ Urinary output is approximately 50 ml/hr.

46. A multipara is admitted to the labor unit in active labor. One hour later her vaginal discharge begins showing meconium staining. What would be the most appropriate initial nursing action?
① Begin preparing her for an emergency cesarean birth.
② Contact the physician immediately to report fetal distress.
③ Record a careful description of the vaginal discharge, as well as the woman's vital signs.
④ Check fetal heart tones and apply a fetal monitor, if it has not already been applied.

47. A primipara, age 40, is hospitalized for severe pregnancy-induced hypertension. Which nursing action should occur first on admission?
① Assist to cope with bed rest.
② Assess blood pressure, weight, and urine for protein.
③ Maintain a dark, quiet environment with minimal stimuli.
④ Instruct in a high-protein, low-sodium diet.

48. Which of the following nursing actions would reduce the possibility of a convulsion in a client with severe pregnancy-induced hypertension?
① Keep the side rails padded and up.
② Place the client in the room closest to the nurse's station.
③ Keep the room dimly lit.
④ Stay with the client at all times.

49. The main purpose of bed rest in a lateral position as a treatment for a woman with pregnancy-induced hypertension is to
① Reduce blood pressure and promote diuresis.
② Conserve energy in view of the impending labor.
③ Lower the incidence of headaches.
④ Limit contact with other clients.

50. The nurse administers magnesium sulfate as ordered to a woman who is hospitalized with severe pregnancy-induced hypertension. What medication would the nurse have available to counteract toxicity from the magnesium sulfate?
① Sodium chloride
② Calcium gluconate
③ Epinephrine (Adrenalin)
④ Sodium bicarbonate

51. A client is receiving magnesium sulfate to prevent possible convulsions from pregnancy-induced hypertension. The woman asks the nurse if the magnesium sulfate will affect her baby. What would be the best response?
① "No, the placenta acts as a barrier to the medication."
② "The doctor wouldn't order it if it would hurt the baby."
③ "It has a minor effect; however, the effects of a convulsion are much more severe."
④ "We don't know if this drug crosses the placental barrier."

52. A woman, gravida 2, para 0, has a medical diagnosis of class C diabetes mellitus. She is at 34 weeks of gestation. In the third trimester she asks the nurse how her baby will be delivered. Which of the following is the best response?
① "You will probably have either a cesarean delivery or have labor induced at about 37 weeks of gestation."
② "You will probably have a cesarean delivery to decrease the stress of delivery on the baby."
③ "Your pregnancy will probably be allowed to progress to term with labor occurring naturally."
④ "Your pregnancy will be carefully monitored with the time and method for delivery chosen on the basis of your status, placental function, and the baby's condition."

53. A woman who has had diabetes mellitus for 3 years becomes pregnant. On her initial prenatal visit, she asks the nurse how this pregnancy will affect her insulin requirements. Which of the following is true regarding insulin needs during pregnancy?
① Insulin needs during pregnancy will be essentially the same as before pregnancy, as long as the client maintains a well-balanced diet.
② Insulin needs will vary throughout the pregnancy and will need to be watched closely. It is not possible to predict when insulin needs will be greatest.
③ With a proper balance of nutrition and exercise, the client may not need insulin during pregnancy. This is because the baby will be producing insulin, which will be available for the mother's body to use.
④ Insulin needs will vary throughout the pregnancy. Need is likely to decrease during the first trimester and then increase throughout the remainder of the pregnancy.

54. A neonate weighs 9 pounds 6 ounces at birth. The baby's mother developed gestational diabetes in the last part of her pregnancy. Which of the following characteristics would the nurse expect to find in this newborn?
① Postmature
② Active and alert
③ Tremors
④ Low risk of hyperbilirubinemia

55. When caring for an infant in the delivery room, what is the nurse's first priority?
① Ensure proper identification.
② Establish a warm environment.
③ Maintain a patent airway.
④ Facilitate parental bonding.

56. A 23-year-old woman has insulin-dependent diabetes. Her blood sugar level has been fairly well controlled throughout pregnancy. Although her newborn is large for gestational age, he shows no signs of distress immediately after birth. Which of the following is of highest priority when caring for this woman's newborn in the nursery?
① Maintain hydration.
② Assess gestational age.

③ Initiate early feeding.
④ Monitor ketone levels.

57. A new mother with type I diabetes wants to breast-feed her baby. The nurse plans a response based on which of the following facts?
① Insulin does not pass into breast milk.
② Breast-feeding predisposes the mother to infection.
③ The breast-feeding mother has a sharply decreased caloric demand.
④ The infant of the diabetic mother is often hypoactive after birth.

58. A woman with diabetes mellitus delivered 48 hours ago. In preparing this woman for discharge, the nurse includes infant-care teaching. Which of the following is most important for this mother to know?
① Although the baby has a problem, he is normal and should be treated like any infant.
② The infant needs 24 calories per ounce of formula to counteract hypoglycemia.
③ Because the mother was diabetic during pregnancy, the baby should be seen by a pediatrician regularly throughout infancy and childhood.
④ The baby should be fed skim milk to maintain normal weight from 6 months of age.

59. Which of the following would most likely indicate potential problems for a pregnant client with a history of heart disease?
① Reduced activity tolerance
② Polyhydramnios
③ Frequent urinary tract infections
④ Frequent heartburn

60. Several years after corrective surgery for a congenital heart defect, a woman with class II cardiac disease becomes pregnant and delivers a healthy 7-pound son in a forceps-assisted delivery. The nurse notes that the woman's pulse rate is stable at 66. She received no medication in the recovery unit other than oxytocin. What is the appropriate nursing action for this woman at this time?
① Notify the physician immediately.
② Continue to assess vital signs routinely.
③ Observe for toxicity to oxytocic drugs.
④ Monitor the level of consciousness.

61. Which of the following is a priority for high-risk clients in a prenatal clinic?
① Encourage prenatal care as scheduled.
② Minimize anxiety.
③ Explain ordered diagnostic tests.
④ Refer to social service.

62. A 15-year-old primigravida registers for antepartal care at 10 weeks of gestation. This young woman is facing the psychologic task of accepting her pregnancy and "incorporating the fetus into her body image," as identified by Rubin. Which of the following behaviors best characterizes accomplishment of this task?
① Acknowledging the surprise she experiences at being in the pregnant state.
② Picturing her baby as a real human being with needs to be met.

③ Arranging a baby nursery in the home.
④ Talking about the responsibilities of motherhood.

63. During the initial antepartal appointment, which of the following nursing actions would most encourage a pregnant teenager in developing a positive response to her new, changing physical status?
① Discuss clients' rights and explain informed consent.
② Provide a description of the scope of available services.
③ Spend time with the young woman and listen to her concerns.
④ Reassure the young woman that many teenagers experience a temporary uneasiness at this time.

64. Basic nutritional counseling is an important component of prenatal care. Guidance in diet planning for pregnant teenagers differs from that of pregnant adults because of which basic consideration?
① The nutritional needs of pregnant women decline with advancing age.
② Prepregnancy weight in adolescents is not related to pregnancy outcomes, as it is in older women.
③ Older women have an increase in protein deposition.
④ Pregnant teenagers have increased nutritional needs for growth of their own bodies.

65. A pregnant teenager, 32 weeks of gestation, complains to the nurse that she seems to be tired all the time and does not have any energy. Which finding supports a diagnosis of iron-deficiency anemia?
① Hemoglobin of 8.6 g
② Hematocrit of 40%
③ Hemoglobin of 14.2 g
④ Hematocrit of 36%

66. During a nutritional counseling session a pregnant woman asks why a person needs more iron during pregnancy. The nurse answers that increased demand for iron during pregnancy is most likely caused by
① A decrease in red blood cell formation occurring in the third trimester.
② The rise in blood cell concentration occurring between 24 and 32 weeks of gestation.
③ An increase in total blood cell volume and hemoglobin mass by approximately 25% to 50% during pregnancy.
④ A decreased efficiency of iron absorption during pregnancy and fetal inability to absorb the mineral.

67. The nurse asks a pregnant woman to select foods that best meet her dietary needs for increased iron. The young woman's knowledge of foods highest in iron would be accurate if she selected which of these meals for lunch?
① A peanut butter and jelly sandwich, ½ cup cooked carrots, and 1 cup whole milk
② An 8-ounce strawberry yogurt, one banana, and 1 cup apple juice
③ Enriched macaroni, broccoli, and 1 cup orange juice
④ One-half chicken breast, split peas, and 1 cup prune juice

68. A nurse working in a prenatal clinic for pregnant teenagers is aware that these young women are at increased risk for complications during childbearing. Which of the following best describes obstetric hazards experienced by pregnant adolescents?
    ① They have an increased incidence of anemia, urinary tract infections, pregnancy-induced hypertension, prolonged labor, and compromised infants.
    ② They have decreased cognitive development, little emotional support available, and childlike behaviors, which may cause conflict.
    ③ They usually experience economic and social handicaps leading to an unsafe physical environment.
    ④ They usually have low self-esteem and a decreased ability to establish meaningful relationships.

69. A 16-year-old primigravida has completed 36 weeks of pregnancy. She has received little prenatal care and no formal prenatal education. She arrives at the hospital with complaints of uterine contractions crying, "It's time to have the baby." Which of the following nursing actions would be first?
    ① Assess her contractions.
    ② Take a nursing history.
    ③ Call the physician.
    ④ Draw blood and start an IV.

70. A primigravida is admitted to the labor unit in early labor. She has received no childbirth preparation. When will she be most receptive to learning breathing techniques?
    ① Any time between contractions
    ② During the contractions, in order to combine theory and practice
    ③ After medication, to reduce anxiety
    ④ Early, when she is most alert and comfortable

71. During a strong contraction, the laboring woman's membranes rupture. After ruling out prolapsed cord, what nursing assessment is most important at this time?
    ① Color of amniotic fluid
    ② Extent of cervical dilation
    ③ Change in baseline maternal vital signs
    ④ The woman's psychologic response to this event

72. A 15-year-old client delivers a 5-pound daughter after a difficult labor. Since delivery she has been trying to decide whether or not to keep her baby and asks the nurse what she should do. Which of the following statements made by the nurse is most appropriate?
    ① "Adoption is really the best solution to your situation."
    ② "It must be difficult to be in this position."
    ③ "Was this pregnancy planned or unplanned?"
    ④ "What would your parents like you to do?"

73. A newly delivered adolescent is displaying considerable ambivalence about giving her baby up for adoption. The nursing student is concerned that during this time, the young mother insists on caring for and feeding her infant. The nurse would best respond to the nursing student's concerns by explaining that
    ① Such behavior is typical of adolescence.
    ② This mother's caregiving indicates guilt feelings.

    ③ The caregiving contributes to a healthy grieving response.
    ④ Caring for the infant delays decision making.

74. A couple has been trying to adopt a baby for nearly 4 years. A newborn finally becomes available, and the couple and their social worker visit their 5-day-old infant in the nursery. Based on an understanding of the attachment process, what would the nurse teach the adoptive parents?
    ① "Hold the infant and talk to him often."
    ② "Sleep with the baby to enhance bonding."
    ③ "Learn basic infant care skills quickly."
    ④ "It is too late to attach completely, but you'll learn to care for your new son."

75. While dressing the infant, which comment by a new father is the most positive sign of early attachment?
    ① "Look at her watch me as I talk to her!"
    ② "See how great this pink sweater looks on her!"
    ③ "Her eyes don't look much like anyone in the family."
    ④ "I read that hiccoughs are normal for a newborn."

76. A 26-year-old primigravida at 40 weeks of gestation is admitted to the labor area. She states that her membranes ruptured in the car on the way to the hospital. Which of the following initial nursing assessments would be most important during her admission?
    ① Type of anesthesia requested for delivery
    ② Location, rate, and rhythm of fetal heart tones
    ③ Maternal vital signs
    ④ Onset, duration, and frequency of contractions

77. A pregnant woman at 40 weeks of gestation arrives at the birthing center in labor. The admitting vaginal exam reveals that the woman's cervix is 6 cm dilated and 100% effaced. The fetus is at 1+ station and left occiput anterior. The woman is having difficulty coping with her contractions, which are occurring every 3 minutes. Which of these nursing actions is most appropriate during her next contraction?
    ① Encourage her to bear down with the contraction.
    ② Check the perineum for crowning.
    ③ Provide direct coaching using chest-abdominal breathing techniques.
    ④ Show her husband how to apply firm pressure to her sacral area.

78. The nurse knows that a laboring woman is most likely in the transition phase of labor when she
    ① Begins accelerated breathing.
    ② Requests pain medication.
    ③ Becomes irritable and frightened.
    ④ Complains of rectal pressure.

79. A labor client, gravida 2, para 1, is in the transitional phase of labor. She begins to grunt and says she has to push. Upon vaginal exam, the nurse finds that her cervix is dilated 9 cm. What is the most appropriate immediate nursing action?
    ① Roll her on her side and tell her to breathe slowly.
    ② Tell her to blow out until the urge passes.
    ③ Explain in careful detail that pushing will cause the cervix to swell and delay dilation.
    ④ Tell her to push with each contraction.

80. During the course of active labor, a primigravida begins to show symptoms of hyperventilation. The nurse

instructs her to slow her breathing and breathe into her cupped hands. Which of the following would best indicate the effectiveness of this action?

① Dizziness and finger tingling decrease.

② Nausea increases.

③ Amnesia between contractions lessens.

④ The urge to push subsides.

81. After 12 hours of active labor, a primigravida has progressed to full cervical dilation and effacement without perineal bulging. The nurse would

① Prep and drape her in preparation for the birth.

② Coach her how to push effectively with contractions.

③ Allow the client and her partner to be alone together at this time.

④ Administer a narcotic analgesic.

82. A woman in the birthing room has an uneventful vaginal delivery with a midline episiotomy done under local anesthesia. During the fourth stage of labor, the nurse would include which of the following in the nursing care plan?

① Massage the fundus continuously.

② Monitor temperature every 30 minutes.

③ Palpate the uterus to check muscle tone every 15 minutes.

④ Monitor blood pressure every 5 minutes.

83. A newborn baby girl weighed 6 pounds at birth and received routine care. Her eyes were treated prophylactically with ophthalmic antibiotic ointment. This treatment is done to prevent

① Chemical conjunctivitis.

② Neonatal syphilis.

③ Herpes infection.

④ Ophthalmia neonatorum.

84. The nurse is going to care for a multigravida in the labor room. During an assessment the nurse notes a change in fetal heart rate variability on the internal monitor tracing. Previous variability was 10 to 15 beats; it is now 2 to 3 beats over several minutes. Contractions are mild. What is the best analysis of these data?

① The change is within normal limits.

② There is indication of potential hypoxia.

③ Increased fetal activity is responsible for the change in variability.

④ True variability can be assessed only with the external monitor.

85. The nurse notices that there are many variable decelerations on a laboring woman's fetal monitor strip. Variable decelerations most likely are due to

① Head compression.

② Cord compression.

③ Uteroplacental insufficiency.

④ Posterior presentation.

86. Which of the following readings on a fetal monitoring strip would be considered a normal finding?

① Late decelerations and good variability

② Early decelerations and no variability

③ Early decelerations and good variability

④ Variable decelerations and no variability

87. An expectant father is supporting his partner in labor. While watching the fetal monitor he notices that the fetal heart rate drops slightly just before his partner's contraction, then recovers at the end of the contraction. He quickly notifies the nurse of this observation. What is the most appropriate *initial* nursing action?

① Assess maternal vital signs.

② Administer oxygen.

③ Notify the physician.

④ Reassure the father that this is normal.

88. The physician orders an internal electrode for a multipara in active labor. The nurse is asked to assist in placement of the scalp electrode. Placement of an internal scalp electrode

① Is an invasive procedure.

② Is done routinely whenever an amniotomy is done.

③ Is a standard of care for all multiparous labor clients.

④ Cannot be done after membranes are ruptured.

89. A woman is in the active stage of labor. Which of the following fetal heart rate tracings would necessitate immediate action?

① Baseline fetal heart rate remains between 120 and 130.

② Fetal heart rate drops to 100 during contractions and returns to baseline of 140 to 150 when the contraction ends.

③ Baseline fetal heart rate of 130 to 140 increases to 150 just before the contraction.

④ Fetal heart rate drops to 120 during the contraction and returns to baseline of 125 to 135 1 minute after the contraction ends.

90. The nursing student asks the nurse to check the laboring client. "The baseline fetal heart rate has gradually decreased from 150 to 120. But I know that is within normal range," says the student. What is the appropriate nursing action?

① Confirm that this is within a normal heart rate range.

② Notify the physician.

③ Elevate the foot of the bed in Trendelenburg's position.

④ Take the client's blood pressure and temperature.

91. A multiparous client is admitted to the birthing unit for induction of labor. An infusion of oxytocin is started and contractions begin. After 2 hours of labor, late decelerations are observed on the fetal heart rate monitor. What would the first nursing action be?

① Turn off the oxytocin.

② Change the client to a left lateral position.

③ Administer oxygen.

④ Record the finding on the monitor strip.

92. A 41-year-old woman is admitted to the labor and delivery unit at 4 PM. While taking the history, the nurse notes the following: gravida 8, para 7; 41 weeks of completed gestation; membranes ruptured at 10 AM this morning; contractions occurring every 3 minutes; strong intensity with a duration of 60 seconds. What nursing action would take highest priority at this time?

① Get blood and urine samples.

② Do a nitrazine test on the vaginal fluid.

③ Attach monitors to client.

④ Determine extent of cervical dilation.

93. A woman in active labor receives an epidural anesthetic. What is the most important assessment for the nurse to make immediately after the epidural is started?
    ① Maternal blood pressure
    ② Maternal pulse
    ③ Level of consciousness
    ④ Cervical dilation

94. Which of the following findings on a newly delivered woman's chart would indicate that she is at risk for developing postpartal hemorrhage?
    ① Grand multiparity
    ② Premature rupture of membranes
    ③ Postterm delivery
    ④ Epidural anesthesia

95. A postpartum client is being discharged 24 hours after delivery. Which planned action by the mother indicates that she has learned what the nurse taught her regarding newborn care?
    ① She will expose the infant to sunlight a few hours each day to prevent neonatal jaundice.
    ② She will remove any yellow patches forming on the circumcised glans penis to prevent infection.
    ③ She will have the infant tested for phenylketonuria to prevent retardation.
    ④ She will apply vaseline to the cord stump daily until detachment to prevent adherence to clothing.

96. A nurse is summoned to the home of a neighbor, a multigravida, during a severe snowstorm. The neighbor appears to be in active labor. Both the pregnant woman and her husband are very apprehensive. The initial nursing action would be to
    ① Call the hospital for an ambulance.
    ② Calm both parents.
    ③ Prepare a clean delivery field.
    ④ Assess the mother's status.

97. A newly admitted labor client activates her call light for the nurse. As the nurse enters the room the client says, "I think my baby is coming now!" Nursing assessment reveals that the infant is in a vertex presentation, crowning. As the nurse assists in the delivery of the head, which would be the most appropriate instruction to the mother?
    ① Inhale during the contraction to aid in delivery.
    ② Pant during contractions to avoid forceful expulsion.
    ③ Bear down continuously to assist the abdominal muscles.
    ④ Breathe slowly and deeply to ensure proper oxygenation of the fetus.

98. While on a shopping trip at the local mall, the nurse is called on to help in the unexpected delivery of a multipara in a large department store. Before help arrives, it appears that the newly delivered mother is bleeding excessively. What nursing action is most appropriate at this time?
    ① Put the infant to the breast.
    ② Apply continuous firm pressure on the fundus with a closed fist.
    ③ Pack the vagina with a towel.
    ④ Elevate the mother's hips.

99. A primigravida is admitted for an elective cesarean delivery because of an extremely narrow pelvic outlet. Which of the following would be included in preparation for this elective cesarean delivery?
    ① Insert a nasogastric tube.
    ② Administer a cleansing vaginal douche.
    ③ Insert an internal fetal monitor.
    ④ Make sure the woman is not left alone.

100. After a scheduled cesarean delivery, a new mother will need the usual postoperative care as well as the usual postpartum care. Which of the following is true in this regard?
    ① Fundal height should not be checked because of the location of the abdominal incision.
    ② When epidural anesthesia is used, ambulation will be delayed 48 hours.
    ③ Perineal checks are not done because there should not have been any perineal trauma.
    ④ A Foley catheter will be kept in place for 3 to 4 days after delivery in order to accurately determine urinary output.

101. After a cesarean delivery, a new mother indicates that she wants to breast-feed her newborn but is uncertain if she can. The nurse's response would include which of the following?
    ① The mother's limited oral intake during the first 2 days will inhibit the production of milk.
    ② Necessary separation of the mother from the infant during postoperative recovery will delay initiation until discharge.
    ③ Breast-feeding is not dependent on method of birth and will be most successful if initiated early.
    ④ The abdominal incision will make it impossible for her to assume an appropriate position for breast-feeding.

102. A 31-year-old multipara is admitted for a planned repeat cesarean birth under regional anesthesia. Reviewing the prenatal record, the nurse notes each of the following on the woman's chart. Which would be reported to the anesthesiologist before delivery?
    ① Corrective surgery for scoliosis at age 14
    ② Trace of glucose in urine throughout pregnancy
    ③ Hemoglobin 12 g; hematocrit 39%
    ④ Acute episode of herpes type II before pregnancy

103. The physician orders an IV of 5% dextrose in normal saline to be infused over 8 hours after a cesarean birth. The IV infuses more rapidly than ordered. What assessments are most essential when IV fluids are administered too rapidly?
    ① Temperature and blood glucose
    ② Blood pressure and urinary output
    ③ Respirations and pulse rate
    ④ Level of consciousness and hematocrit

104. A woman gives birth to a 6-pound son by cesarean delivery because of abruptio placentae. General anesthetic is used for the surgery. In the postanesthesia recovery unit, which of the following assessments is most significant?
    ① Blood pressure is stable at 100/72 mm Hg.
    ② Respirations are 12 and shallow.
    ③ Temperature is constant at 99.8°F (37.6°C) orally.
    ④ Pulse is 68 and regular.

105. On the first postoperative day after cesarean delivery, a 24-year-old multipara asks to have her infant room-in with her. In planning for her comfort and for the safety of the newborn, which nursing action is most appropriate?
① Suggest that she delay breast-feeding.
② Ask that the woman's husband room-in with her and the new baby.
③ Inform her that the nurse is available to assist her.
④ Require that she maintain bed rest when the baby is in the room.

106. Before hospital discharge, a postpartum client tells the nurse that she is afraid her 3-year-old son will be jealous of the new baby. The nurse would suggest that the client take which of the following actions?
① "Ignore him; he will outgrow his jealousy."
② "Tell your son that he will learn to love the new baby."
③ "Leave your son with his grandparents until the new baby is settled at home."
④ "Bring your son a baby doll at the time the baby is taken home."

107. An excited young couple are the proud parents of a new son. As they inspect their baby they notice a dark-pigmented area on the infant's lower back and buttocks. Which notation on the chart will best explain this observation?
① Rh-negative blood type
② Positive Coombs' test
③ Ethnic background: African American
④ Maternal history of sickle cell trait.

108. A husband and wife are both sickle cell carriers. The woman asks the nurse the probability of their expected baby inheriting sickle cell disease. What response would be most appropriate to give?
① "It is not possible to predict."
② "There is a 25% probability."
③ "There is no risk with two carriers."
④ "Fifty percent of your children will have the disease."

109. On the first postpartum day, the nurse observes a new mother and her newborn during feeding. The nurse notices that the infant nurses at the breast for 15 minutes, then falls asleep. What other assessments are indicated?
① Measure abdominal circumference.
② Note the skin turgor.
③ Weigh the baby after feeding.
④ Assess frequency of feedings and infant satisfaction between feedings.

110. A 22-year-old labor client who is HIV positive is admitted to the labor unit. The nurse is aware that her risk of getting this infection from the client will be reduced by
① Wearing a mask.
② Recapping syringes carefully.
③ Receiving a prophylactic gammaglobulin injection.
④ Wearing gloves to handle the neonate in the delivery room.

111. A 35-year-old woman had a repeat cesarean birth because of a classical incision in the uterus with the first delivery. Spinal anesthesia was used for the surgery. To prevent the occurrence of a postpartal spinal headache, what intervention would the nurse implement during the first 8 hours postoperatively?
① Maintain an indwelling catheter.
② Ambulate the woman as soon as she is alert.
③ Administer analgesics and antiemetics.
④ Maintain bed rest in a flat position.

112. A multipara is admitted for induction of labor. The physician elects to rupture the membranes artificially. Subsequently, fetal heartbeat is stable at 144. Amniotic fluid is clear. A short time later, the woman experiences sudden onset of dyspnea, cyanosis, and severe apprehension. This is followed by severe chest pain. Which of the following conditions is suggested by these data?
① Acute myocardial infarction
② Pulmonary embolus
③ Hysterical reaction
④ Massive infection

113. A pregnant woman, 36 weeks of gestation, learns that she is HIV positive. She asks the clinic nurse how this will affect her unborn baby. The nurse responds
① "A cesarean delivery will prevent your baby from being infected."
② "There is about a 50% chance that your baby will be infected."
③ "Because your pregnancy is past the first trimester, the baby will not be infected."
④ "If you are symptom free when you deliver, your baby will not be infected."

114. Shortly after the delivery of her second child, a new mother begins hemorrhaging. The physician orders immediate transfusions, but the woman's husband refuses to permit the transfusions on religious grounds. Which action by the nurse is most appropriate at this time?
① Emphasize that religious values are not as important as saving lives.
② Call in the family's clergy (religious representative) to speak with the father.
③ Repeat to the couple the physician's treatment plans.
④ Tell the father that he needs to consult with his wife's family.

115. After an uneventful pregnancy, at 35 weeks of gestation a 27-year-old multipara has an abruption of the placenta. In spite of extraordinary emergency efforts, the newborn dies. Which statement would be the most appropriate for the nurse to make to the grieving mother?
① "I am so sorry."
② "Try not to feel guilty."
③ "It must be very difficult for you."
④ "At least you have other children at home."

116. A 14-year-old newly delivered primipara with a history of pregnancy-induced hypertension has just been admitted to her postpartum room with an IV infusing to which 10 ml of oxytocin (Pitocin) has been added. The rationale for administering oxytocin after delivery of the placenta is to
① Shorten the third stage of labor.
② Control postpartal bleeding.

③ Stabilize the mother's blood pressure.
④ Inhibit lactation in the bottle-feeding mother.

117. A 20-year-old primipara delivered a 7-pound baby boy with the use of low spinal anesthesia. Two hours postpartum, the woman states that her bladder feels full and that she needs to void but cannot. The nurse would first
① Walk her to the bathroom and encourage her to try to void.
② Insert a Foley catheter to prevent postpartum cystitis.
③ Administer ergonovine maleate (Ergotrate) as ordered.
④ Place her on a bedpan and run water in the bathroom loud enough for her to hear.

118. A 23-year-old woman delivers her first baby in the birthing room. Shortly after delivery, the woman begins to tremble and shake. She states that she is cold and cannot control her shaking. Nursing actions would include which of the following?
① Cover her with a warm blanket.
② Notify the physician immediately.
③ Administer a tranquilizer.
④ Discontinue the IV that contains oxytocin.

119. On the second postpartum day, a new mother complains of perineal pain. Observing her midline episiotomy, the nurse sees that it is edematous but without other signs of infection. Which of the following interventions should the nurse suggest?
① Apply pure lanolin to the perineal area.
② Assist to take warm or cool sitz baths twice a day.
③ Administer ritrodrine hydrochloride (Yutopar) as ordered.
④ Teach relaxation of gluteal muscles when sitting down.

120. A nursing student is helping a new mother start breast-feeding. The woman asks the student what causes her body to begin making milk. The student's response is based on the knowledge that milk production after delivery is a direct result of
① A decrease in estrogen and progesterone.
② An increase in insulin and glucocorticoids.
③ A decrease in oxytocin.
④ An increase in prolactin.

121. A primipara is trying to breast-feed her infant for the first time. Which of the following would be most helpful to assist this woman?
① Use a breast pump to stimulate milk production before starting to feed.
② Help the mother to gently compress her breast with fingers touching the areola so that the nipple becomes erect and graspable.
③ Instruct the mother to stroke the baby's lower lip with her nipple to stimulate the rooting reflex.
④ Assist the mother to place the tip of the nipple in the infant's slightly open mouth.

122. On the second postpartum day, a breast-feeding mother asks which type of contraceptive is acceptable to use before her first postpartal check. The nurse would advise which of the following?
① Abstinence during the fertile period based on the calendar method

② Intrauterine device
③ Condoms and contraceptive foam
④ Diaphragm and jelly

123. A 20-year-old woman delivered at the birthing center 12 hours ago and is preparing to be discharged with her new baby. Which of the following statements by the woman would indicate that she may need more teaching before her discharge?
① "I will position my baby on the side or back for sleep to reduce the risk of SIDS."
② "I know that if my lochia becomes bright red, I will need to rest and call my doctor."
③ "I need to increase my daily intake by about 500 calories because I am breast-feeding."
④ "I can resume my prepregnancy activity level in about a week."

124. A multipara has just delivered her second child, a 10-pound girl. In assessing this client immediately after delivery, which of the following would the nurse most likely find?
① Fundus located 1 to 2 cm below the umbilicus; lochia rubra
② Fundus displaced to the right and 3 cm above the umbilicus; lochia serosa
③ Fundus located 1 to 2 cm above the umbilicus; lochia rubra
④ Fundus located 3 cm below the umbilicus; lochia serosa

125. After the delivery of a large for gestational age infant, a new mother is noted to have bright-red blood continuously trickling from the vagina. Her fundus is firm and in the midline. What is the most likely cause of this bleeding?
① Lacerations
② Subinvolution
③ Uterine atony
④ Retained placental fragments

126. Which of the following conditions places a client at risk for a postpartal hemorrhage?
① Twin pregnancy
② Breech presentation
③ Prolonged rupture of membranes
④ Cesarean birth

127. Twenty-four hours after delivery, a postpartum client develops a temperature of 100°F (37.8°C), has voided 2000 ml since delivery, and is diaphoretic. Nursing actions would include which of the following?
① Notify the physician of the findings.
② Notify the nursery to feed the baby in the nursery because the mother has a fever.
③ Explain to the client that these symptoms are normal for a woman who has just delivered.
④ Suspect a postpartal infection, and isolate mother and newborn.

128. A 19-year-old woman delivered her first baby 18 hours ago. She tells the nurse that her sister has warned her to expect afterpains. The nurse's teaching is based on the knowledge that the most likely candidate for afterpains is the
① Primipara who is bottle-feeding.
② Grand multipara who is breast-feeding.

③ Woman who delivers prematurely and who is pumping her breasts.

④ Adolescent with pregnancy-induced hypertension who is breast-feeding.

129. A newly delivered woman plans to bottle-feed her baby. She asks the nurse when she should expect her first menses. The appropriate response would be

① "It usually takes at least 6 months before menstruation resumes after delivery."

② "Women who bottle-feed can expect menses 6 to 12 weeks after delivery."

③ "Your prolactin will reach a prepregnant level in about 2 weeks, triggering menstruation 2 to 4 weeks after delivery."

④ "Your doctor can tell you after drawing your blood for follicle-stimulating hormone level at your postpartum office visit."

130. A pregnant woman, gravida 6, para 5, is in the fourth stage of labor after delivering a 9-pound 14-ounce baby. The nurse has been checking her blood pressure, pulse, fundus, lochia, and perineum every 15 minutes for the past 45 minutes. As the nurse approaches for the fourth check, she notices some large new bloodstains on the top sheet. The nurse immediately removes the top sheet and blanket to discover the woman lying in a pool of blood that covers the protective bed pad. The fundus is above the umbilicus and boggy. What would the nurse's first action be?

① Take her blood pressure.

② Start an IV.

③ Give oxygen through a mask at 7 L.

④ Massage the uterus.

131. How much blood must be lost to be considered postpartal hemorrhage?

① 200 ml

② 300 ml

③ 400 ml

④ 500 ml

132. A postpartum client with a hemoglobin of 8.5 g/dl and a hematocrit of 25% has a medical diagnosis of anemia secondary to postpartum hemorrhage. Which of the following would be included in discharge planning and teaching?

① Eat a high-carbohydrate, low-fat diet.

② Take ferrous sulfate tablets with milk at each meal.

③ Stop breast-feeding the infant until the anemia is gone.

④ Expect to feel tired for possibly 2 to 4 months.

133. A primipara who is Rh-negative has delivered an Rh-positive daughter. The new mother is to receive $Rho(D)$ immune globulin (RhoGAM). Which action is essential before administration?

① Determine if the woman's Coombs' test result is negative.

② Reverify the baby's blood type.

③ Assess the paternal Rh factor.

④ Determine if the medication was given in the prenatal period.

134. A pregnant woman who is Rh-negative is to receive RhoGAM prophylactically at 28 weeks of gestation. Before receiving the medication, she asks the nurse how the drug works. Which of the following best describes how RhoGAM acts in the expectant mother's body?

① RhoGAM attaches to maternal anti-Rh antibodies and directly destroys them.

② RhoGAM limits the production of maternal antibodies.

③ RhoGAM destroys fetal Rh-positive red blood cells in the maternal circulation before sensitization occurs.

④ RhoGAM prevents fetal-maternal bleeding episodes from occurring at the placenta site.

135. A postpartum Rh-negative woman has just received RhoGAM. She asks if there is a danger of a problem occurring in future pregnancies. Which of these understandings about Rh incompatibility is most important for the nurse to communicate to this client?

① Administration of RhoGAM will provide lifelong immunity against fetal Rh disease.

② If she delivers another Rh-positive infant, she will require another dose of RhoGAM.

③ The protective antibodies formed during this pregnancy increase the risk of hemolytic disease in future infants.

④ It is safe to assume that future infants have a 50% chance of being Rh-negative.

136. A 21-year-old primipara is admitted in active labor. Prenatal history indicates that she has taken heroin regularly during the past 3 years. Initial observations on admission include jaundiced sclera and skin. Lab data confirm a diagnosis of hepatitis B secondary to substance abuse. A priority of nursing care for this client focuses on

① Maintaining strict respiratory isolation.

② Using gown and gloves during care.

③ Obtaining an order for vaccination.

④ Preparing the client for cesarean delivery.

137. Which of the following signs would be indicative of drug withdrawal in a neonate whose mother used heroin throughout pregnancy?

① Dyspnea, bradycardia, and restlessness

② Hyperactivity, irritability, and tremors

③ Pallor, subnormal temperature, and weak cry

④ Petechiae, limpness, and high-pitched cry

138. A baby is born to a heroin-addicted mother diagnosed with hepatitis B infection. The pediatrician plans to discharge the infant to his grandmother. What assessment of the family system is most important at this time?

① Does the grandmother express an interest in the mother and infant?

② Has the cause of substance abuse been identified for this mother?

③ Is the infant's father involved in plans for care?

④ Does the home situation appear to be adequate and safe for the infant?

139. With heroin addiction in the newborn, signs of withdrawal are most likely to

① Appear within the first 4 hours after birth.

② Occur 1 to 2 days after delivery.

③ Be delayed up to 5 days postnatally.

④ Be eliminated or greatly reduced if the newborn

receives a narcotic antagonist such as naloxone immediately after delivery.

140. A woman who delivered 3 weeks ago calls the postpartum unit with questions about breast-feeding while she has the flu. During the conversation, she tells the nurse that her temperature is 103°F and that she has a persistent headache and feels exhausted. What additional data should the nurse collect?
① Presence of breast redness, tenderness, or discharge
② Amount of sleep and hydration
③ Character and amount of lochia
④ Presence of edema or visual changes

141. Which of the following statements concerning intervention would the nurse include when counseling a breast-feeding mother with mastitis?
① "Take antibiotics until your temperature is normal."
② "Avoid analgesics to prevent infant drowsiness from medication exposure through breast milk."
③ "Empty your breasts regularly to prevent exacerbation and abscess formation."
④ Discontinue breast-feeding and switch to formula feeding."

142. Which of the following nursing plans would most likely prevent a nursing mother from developing mastitis?
① Treatment with prophylactic antibiotics
② Decreased frequency of nursing
③ Limited nursing time at each feeding
④ Prompt attention to cracked nipples

143. The nurse conducts a physical assessment of the neonate as the initial bath is given several hours after birth. In assessing the baby's skin, which of the following observations most likely requires special attention?
① Cyanosis of the hands and feet
② Mottling
③ Desquamation
④ Jaundice

144. In comparing the head and chest measurements of a newborn delivered by cesarean birth, which of the following observations would the nurse expect to find?
① The chest circumference is approximately 1 inch smaller than the head circumference.
② The chest circumference is approximately 1 inch larger than the head circumference.
③ The head and chest circumferences are equal.
④ The chest circumference is approximately 4 inches smaller than the head circumference.

145. Which of the following would require further assessment if found on a 1-week-old infant?
① Erythema toxicum neonatorum
② "Stork bite" marks
③ Impetigo
④ Mongolian spots

146. The nurse assesses a 1-hour-old newborn's eyes. Which condition, if found, would most likely require additional assessment?
① Transient strabismus
② Subconjunctival hemorrhage
③ Lack of tears
④ Opacity of a pupil

147. The nurse assessing a neonate's trunk shortly after birth makes the following observations. Which one would alert the nurse to the need for further assessment?
① Breast engorgement
② Audible bowel sounds
③ Palpable liver and kidneys
④ Umbilical cord with one artery and one vein

148. Which of the following assessments would the nurse report to the physician concerning a 1-hour-old infant's ears?
① The upper parts of the ears are on a plane with the angle of the eyes.
② The upper parts of the ears are well below a line extending through the inner and outer canthi of the eyes.
③ There is incurving of the pinna and instant recoil.
④ The infant responds to sound with a startle or blink.

149. The nurse observes the parents of a 3-day-old newborn interacting with their new baby. The couple is very interested in learning about their baby. The mother asks the nurse when she can "play" with the baby. Which reply shows an understanding of developmental needs in infancy?
① "When do you think it would be appropriate?"
② "After he receives his first immunizations from the physician."
③ "As soon as you feel comfortable with him, he is ready."
④ "Babies should not be played with during the first month because they have a fragile central nervous system."

150. The parents of a newborn ask the nurse how much their new baby can see. The nurse's response is based on the knowledge that the newborn's visual capacity shortly after birth is primarily
① Long-distance vision.
② Short-distance fixation.
③ Convergence of the eyes.
④ Coordinated peripheral vision.

151. What are the most appropriate stimuli for the nurse to recommend for the first parent-child play activity?
① Rattles and small stuffed toys
② Books and pictures
③ Swings and cradles
④ Human faces and black-and-white patterned objects

152. It would be most appropriate for the nurse to suggest that parents play with their newborn by
① Turning him from his abdomen to his back.
② Moving his arms and legs through the range of motion.
③ Stroking him gently from head to toe.
④ Rocking him 3 to 4 hours during the day.

153. To check the grasp reflex in the newborn, the nurse would implement which of the following actions?
① Lightly touch either corner of the baby's mouth.
② Stroke the lateral aspect of the sole upward across the ball of the foot.
③ Rotate the head to one side and then the other.
④ Exert pressure on the palm at the base of the digits.

154. To elicit the Moro's reflex, the nurse would
① Shake the infant rapidly from head to toe.
② Hold the infant in both hands and lower both hands rapidly about an inch.
③ Place the infant in the prone position and observe posture.
④ Turn the infant's head to one side while the infant is in a supine position.

155. A 10-pound 2-ounce, 38-week-gestation infant is born to a mother with class C diabetes mellitus. After spending some time with her mother in the recovery room, the baby is transferred to the nursery. Which of the following problems would the nurse be most alert for in this infant?
① Hypoglycemia
② Respiratory distress
③ Meconium aspiration
④ Generalized sepsis

156. Which of the following orders would be included when planning care for an infant of a diabetic mother?
① Limit intake to sterile water.
② Keep NPO.
③ Arrange for feeding.
④ Start infusion of insulin.

157. A 5-pound 1-ounce, 39-week-gestation infant is born to a mother who smoked heavily throughout pregnancy. The nurse determines that this neonate is
① Preterm, small for gestational age.
② Term, appropriate size for gestational age.
③ Preterm, appropriate size for gestational age.
④ Term, small for gestational age.

158. A woman developed gestational diabetes with her third pregnancy. She asks the nurse if her new baby has diabetes. What would be the nurse's best response?
① "No, we are giving your baby medication to prevent that from occurring."
② "No; however, she will probably become diabetic sometime in childhood."
③ "No, there is no connection between your diabetes and your baby."
④ "No; however, you need to make regular visits to your pediatrician."

159. On the second day of life, a neonate develops hyperbilirubinemia and is placed under phototherapy with a traditional light unit. Which of the following would be included in the nurse's plan of care for this infant?
① Keep the infant swaddled in a blanket.
② Record the type and amount of stools.
③ Maintain eye patches 24 hours per day.
④ Limit fluid intake.

160. Which of the following infants would be at *lowest* risk for hypoglycemia?
① A 2-hour-old, full-term neonate whose mother's blood-glucose level was 350 mg/dl during labor.
② A large for gestational age neonate 10 hours after birth whose Dextrostix test shows a reading of 60 mg/dl.
③ A 32-week-gestation neonate 5 hours after birth.
④ A small for gestational age neonate, 12 hours after birth, who is NPO because of respiratory distress.

161. Which of the following best indicates that a neonate may have an infection?
① Respiratory rate of 65 at rest.
② Weight increase of 3 ounces on two successive days.
③ Axillary temperature of 98.6°F (37°C).
④ Hemoglobin of 20 g/dl of blood.

162. The mother of a boy born yesterday with a cleft lip and palate is refusing to care for her infant. Which of the following is the most appropriate initial action for the nurse to take?
① Elicit the mother's feelings about her infant.
② Refer to a psychologist for maladaptive grieving.
③ Teach infant care to other family members to allow the mother time to adapt.
④ Refer to social service on discharge because of high risk for abuse or neglect.

163. A 34-week-gestation neonate in an Isolette experiences sudden apnea. The nurse would first
① Administer oxygen with positive pressure.
② Call the pediatrician.
③ Increase the humidity in the incubator.
④ Gently stimulate the infant.

164. When examining the inside of a newborn's mouth, the nurse notices a small, raised white bump on the palate; it does not come off and does not bleed when touched. Which of the following is the most likely diagnosis?
① Milia
② Thrush
③ Epstein's pearls
④ Milk curd

165. Which of the following fetal circulatory structures close and become nonfunctioning after birth?
① Ductus arteriosus, umbilical arteries, pulmonary artery, and hypogastric arteries
② Ductus venosus, foramen ovale, portal vein, and ductus arteriosus
③ Foramen ovale, pulmonary artery, ductus venosus, and umbilical vein
④ Umbilical vein, foramen ovale, ductus venosus, and ductus arteriosus

166. Neonates often "spit up" small quantities after feedings. Which of the following conditions offers the best explanation for this behavior?
① Immature cardiac sphincter
② Overfeeding by parents
③ Hyperemesis gravidarum
④ Formula intolerance

167. In examining the newborn's head during the initial physical assessment, the nurse palpates the fontanels. Which of the following would be a reportable finding?
① Anterior fontanel diamond shaped, level, and firm
② Posterior fontanel triangular, smaller than anterior
③ Anterior fontanel full and bulging
④ Posterior fontanel difficult to palpate because of diffuse swelling

168. How might the nurse best promote bonding while an infant is in an Isolette?
① Remind the mother that the staff is skillful.
② Encourage the mother to touch the infant.
③ Suggest that the mother visit the intensive care unit occasionally.
④ Inform the mother that the infant will be at home soon.

REFERENCES

Bobak I, Lowdermilk D, Jensen M, Perry S: *Maternity nursing,* ed 4, St Louis, 1995, Mosby.

Cunningham F, MacDonald P, Grant N, et al: *Williams obstetrics,* ed 19, Norwalk, Conn, 1993, Appleton & Lange.

May KA, Mahlmeister LR: *Maternal and neonatal nursing,* ed 3, Philadelphia, 1994, Lippincott.

Olds S, London M, Ladewig P: *Maternal-newborn nursing,* ed 5, Menlo Park, Calif, 1995, Addison-Wesley.

Pillitteri A: *Maternal and childhealth nursing,* Philadelphia, 1992, Lippincott.

Reeder S, Martin L: *Maternity nursing,* ed 17, Philadelphia, 1992, Lippincott.

Riordan J, Auerbach K: *Breastfeeding and human lactation,* Boston, 1993, Jones & Bartlett.

Seidel HM, Rosenstein BJ, Pathak A: *Primary care of the newborn,* St Louis, 1993, Mosby.

Sherwen LN, Scoloveno MA, Weingarten CT: *Nursing care of the childbearing family,* ed 2, Norwalk, Conn, 1995, Appleton & Lange.

Whaley L, Wong D: *Nursing care of infants and children,* ed 5, St Louis, 1995, Mosby.

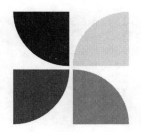

Correct Answers

1. no. 4	**49.** no. 1
2. no. 2	**50.** no. 2
3. no. 3	**51.** no. 3
4. no. 3	**52.** no. 4
5. no. 3	**53.** no. 4
6. no. 1	**54.** no. 3
7. no. 3	**55.** no. 3
8. no. 2	**56.** no. 3
9. no. 3	**57.** no. 1
10. no. 3	**58.** no. 3
11. no. 1	**59.** no. 1
12. no. 1	**60.** no. 2
13. no. 3	**61.** no. 1
14. no. 4	**62.** no. 1
15. no. 2	**63.** no. 3
16. no. 1	**64.** no. 4
17. no. 4	**65.** no. 1
18. no. 4	**66.** no. 3
19. no. 4	**67.** no. 4
20. no. 3	**68.** no. 1
21. no. 1	**69.** no. 1
22. no. 4	**70.** no. 4
23. no. 4	**71.** no. 1
24. no. 2	**72.** no. 2
25. no. 2	**73.** no. 3
26. no. 3	**74.** no. 1
27. no. 1	**75.** no. 1
28. no. 4	**76.** no. 2
29. no. 2	**77.** no. 3
30. no. 1	**78.** no. 4
31. no. 3	**79.** no. 2
32. no. 3	**80.** no. 1
33. no. 2	**81.** no. 2
34. no. 1	**82.** no. 3
35. no. 4	**83.** no. 4
36. no. 2	**84.** no. 2
37. no. 4	**85.** no. 2
38. no. 2	**86.** no. 3
39. no. 3	**87.** no. 4
40. no. 3	**88.** no. 1
41. no. 2	**89.** no. 4
42. no. 4	**90.** no. 2
43. no. 2	**91.** no. 1
44. no. 1	**92.** no. 4
45. no. 3	**93.** no. 1
46. no. 4	**94.** no. 1
47. no. 2	**95.** no. 3
48. no. 3	**96.** no. 4

97. no. 2
98. no. 1
99. no. 4
100. no. 3
101. no. 3
102. no. 1
103. no. 3
104. no. 2
105. no. 3
106. no. 4
107. no. 3
108. no. 2
109. no. 4
110. no. 4
111. no. 4
112. no. 2
113. no. 2
114. no. 2
115. no. 1
116. no. 2
117. no. 4
118. no. 1
119. no. 2
120. no. 4
121. no. 3
122. no. 3
123. no. 4
124. no. 1
125. no. 1
126. no. 1
127. no. 3
128. no. 2
129. no. 2
130. no. 4
131. no. 4
132. no. 4
133. no. 1

134. no. 3
135. no. 2
136. no. 2
137. no. 2
138. no. 4
139. no. 2
140. no. 1
141. no. 3
142. no. 4
143. no. 4
144. no. 1
145. no. 3
146. no. 4
147. no. 4
148. no. 2
149. no. 3
150. no. 2
151. no. 4
152. no. 3
153. no. 4
154. no. 2
155. no. 1
156. no. 3
157. no. 4
158. no. 4
159. no. 2
160. no. 2
161. no. 1
162. no. 1
163. no. 4
164. no. 3
165. no. 4
166. no. 1
167. no. 3
168. no. 2

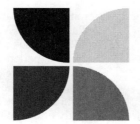

Correct Answers with Rationales

Editor's note: Three pieces of information are supplied at the end of each rationale. First, you will find a reference to a section in the *AJN/Mosby Nursing Boards Review,* where a more complete discussion of the topic may be found, should you desire more information. A second reference indicates what part of the nursing process the question addresses. The third piece of information describes the appropriate client need category.

KEY TO ABBREVIATIONS
Section of the Review Book

CBF = Childbearing Family
  W = Women's Health Care
  A = Antepartal Care
  I = Intrapartal Care
  P = Postpartal Care
  N = Newborn Care

Nursing Process Category

AS = Assessment
AN = Analysis
PL = Plan
IM = Implementation
EV = Evaluation

Client Need Category

  E = Safe, Effective Care Environment
PS = Physiologic Integrity
PC = Psychosocial Integrity
  H = Health Promotion and Maintenance

1. no. 4. A positive pregnancy test is the only probable sign; the other choices are presumptive signs. CBF/A, AS, PS

2. no. 2. Add 7 days, subtract 3 months, and add 1 year to the first day of the last menstrual period. This is Nägele's rule, which relates only to the first day of the menstrual cycle. There is no need for the client to consider the day of intercourse. CBF/A, AN, PS

3. no. 3. This is the only correct statement. Human chorionic gonadotropin in the urine confirms the pregnancy. The urine test is 95% to 97% accurate. False-positive and false-negative results are possible. Home tests are considered less accurate than lab tests, most likely because of error in use. CBF/A, AN, PS

4. no. 3. The nurse must find out the eating habits of the pregnant client before she can teach or advise her. A basic principle of the teaching-learning process is to assess the learner by obtaining a diet history. If the learner is knowledgeable, she may require reinforcement only. Providing a list of foods may be an appropriate strategy but is not an initial action. During pregnancy, nutritional needs change; however, sodium is not restricted. CBF/A, AS, H

5. no. 3. Organ meats and dried fruits are high in iron. Citrus fruit aids in absorption of iron. CBF/A, EV, H

6. no. 1. Swelling of the face is an indication of pre-eclampsia. The other symptoms are normal in pregnancy. Breast tenderness is due to increased estrogen levels. Increased vaginal discharge is the result of an increase in glandular activity. Chloasma (also called the mask of pregnancy) results from an increased activity in the adrenal glands. CBF/A, IM, PS

7. no. 3. There is a placental barrier to syphilis until the eighteenth week of pregnancy. If the mother is treated before the eighteenth week, the baby will most likely not be affected. However, titers will be positive at birth. CBF/A, AN, PS

8. no. 2. Bulk and fluid help increase peristalsis. Laxatives and suppositories should not be used routinely in pregnancy. Prevention is more desirable than treatment. CBF/A, IM, PS

9. no. 3. Urinary frequency and the spilling of sugar in the urine are normal conditions because of the pressure of the growing uterus on the bladder (frequency) and the decreased renal threshold for glucose (sugar in the urine). Vaginal bleeding and uterine cramping may indicate the possibility of a threatened spontaneous abortion. Hematocrit of 28% and pica (eating nonfoods) are associated with anemia needing correction. Intractable vomiting indicates possible hyperemesis. CBF/A, AN, PS

10. no. 3. Ovulation occurs 14 days before the start of the next menstrual cycle. CBF/A, AN, PS

11. no. 1. The couple needs to continue to enjoy recreation together, and most activities can be continued during pregnancy. New strenuous sports or activities requiring agility and balance should not be introduced at this time. CBF/A, IM, H

12. no. 1. Intermittent menstrual-like cramps are one symptom of preterm labor. Anxiety, insomnia, dyspnea, and ankle edema are normal discomforts of the third trimester. CBF/A, EV, PS

13. no. 3. This may be a sign of threatened abortion. Remaining on bed rest is appropriate after the client's condition is assessed. CBF/A, EV, PS

14. no. 4. Regular moderate activity enhances venous circulation and blood flow of oxygen and nutrients to the placenta. Long work hours, heavy lifting (>25 pounds), and prolonged standing are contraindicated in the third trimester. CBF/A, AS, E

15. no. 2. Toxoplasmosis is a protozoan infection transmitted through cat feces and undercooked meat. CBF/A, AS, E

16. no. 1. Wheat, peanuts, and milk are a complete protein. None of the other choices contain complementary proteins. CBF/A, PL, H

17. no. 4. The chief concepts of Lamaze teaching include conditioned responses to stimuli through use of a focal point. Lamaze techniques include changes in breathing as labor progresses, effleurage, and back support during contractions, but not hypnosis. CBF/A, EV, H

18. no. 4. This is the only characteristic of true labor. Option no. 1 indicates false labor; options no. 2 and no. 3 are premonitory signs of labor. Walking has a tendency to increase true labor contractions. Lightening occurs approximately 2 weeks before delivery in the primipara. CBF/I, AN, PS

19. no. 4. Childbirth classes are designed to increase clients' understanding of pregnancy and birth and to promote the optimum health of mother and baby. Through use of relaxation and other techniques, pregnant women are helped to cope better with labor and achieve an emotionally satisfying experience. The father of the baby is not always available to participate in the birth experience; successful prepared childbirth is not solely dependent on this participation. Pain-free birth and avoidance of analgesia or anesthesia are not main objectives of childbirth education. CBF/A, PL, H

20. no. 3. Fear intensifies pain in labor. Through childbirth education, pregnant women learn physiologic processes of birth and techniques to assist in relaxing and coping. Pain is subjective. Education alone will not eliminate pain. Reflecting feelings and offering coping strategies are therapeutic responses. CBF/A, IM, PC

21. no. 1. Assessment of the learners is the priority. Teaching can then be directed at the learners' level of understanding and key concepts reinforced. A standard teaching plan is not appropriate. CBF/I, IM, PC

22. no. 4. As transitional labor approaches, such behavior is common. It is not appropriate to ask the husband to leave or withdraw his support at this most crucial time. A woman in transition is not able to explore feelings. CBF/I, IM, PC

23. no. 4. Sibling rivalry is normal. Grasping the reality of a new sibling is difficult for a child at this age. CBF/P, AN, PC

24. no. 2. Any woman in the first trimester of pregnancy is at risk if exposed to rubella. Fetal defects often result from such an infection. Aspirin should be avoided because of its association with Reye's syndrome. The immune system of the newborn is immature, making antibody development for protection against future rubella infection limited. Measles (or rubeola) is a dif-

ferent infection and will not provide immunity for rubella. CBF/A, EV, PS

25. no. 2. Mittelschmerz (pain associated with ovulation) may be experienced at the time of ovulation. Ovulation occurs approximately 14 days before the onset of menstruation. The cervical mucus becomes thin, clear, and more stretchable at ovulation. Temperature drops slightly at ovulation and then rises about 1 degree after ovulation. CBF/A, IM, H

26. no. 3. Douching is an ineffective method of contraception and may even facilitate conception by forcing sperm higher up into the female genital tract. CBF/A, IM, H

27. no. 1. Although it is possible to reverse a tubal ligation in some cases (a 15% success rate), it is generally considered to be permanent sterilization. The other options are true. CBF/A, EV, H

28. no. 4. Bleeding during pregnancy is considered abnormal, but clients often overestimate the quantity of blood loss because of fear and lack of knowledge. The nurse should expand her database by obtaining more specific information about the bleeding episode. After analysis, a plan of care can be developed. CBF/A, AS, PS

29. no. 2. The term *inevitable abortion* is used to describe pregnancies complicated by bleeding, cramping, and cervical dilation (abortion is imminent). In an incomplete abortion the fetus is expelled, but parts are retained. The term *threatened abortion* means the pregnancy is jeopardized by bleeding and cramping, but the cervix is closed. In a missed abortion the fetus dies but is retained. CBF/A, AN, PS

30. no. 1. Because spontaneous abortion is threatening, all perineal pads must be inspected for the products of conception. Fluid replacement is necessary because of blood loss. There is no evidence of impending shock necessitating Trendelenburg's position. A Shirodkar procedure is done for an incompetent cervix, which is not the problem in this case. CBF/A, IM, PS

31. no. 3. This is the definition of a missed abortion. Findings in a missed abortion include spotting and a uterus that is smaller than expected for the length of pregnancy. If spontaneous evacuation of the uterus does not occur within 1 month, a suction evacuation or dilation and curettage will be done to remove the products of conception. CBF/A, IM, H

32. no. 3. McDonald's procedure is application of a temporary suture at 14 to 18 weeks of gestation. The suture is removed at term. Vaginal delivery may be possible if all else stays well. A Shirodkar procedure is the application of a permanent suture necessitating cesarean delivery. Bed rest may be used by some physicians as a treatment instead of surgical intervention. CBF/A, IM, H

33. no. 2. A woman with a suture in place for incompetent cervix must especially be aware of the signs and symptoms of labor. When labor begins, the physician will remove the suture to avoid possible complications. The other options are incorrect. CBF/A, IM, E

34. no. 1. These findings are consistent with an ectopic pregnancy. Extensive vaginal bleeding is not evident,

nor is the uterus enlarged because the pregnancy is not implanted in the uterus. Blood from a ruptured tube does not expand the uterus or flow out the vagina to any great extent. CBF/A, AS, PS

35. no. 4. A history of infection, producing tubal scarring, is a consistent finding in an ectopic pregnancy. A positive Coombs' test is indicative of antibody formation in blood incompatibilities. Glucosuria might indicate gestational diabetes, and blood pressure elevations could indicate pregnancy-induced hypertension (although this is usually in late pregnancy.) CBF/A, AS, PS

36. no. 2. Surgical intervention will be required; however, hemorrhage is the major life-threatening concern. If the tube ruptures in ectopic pregnancy, vascular collapse and hypovolemic shock may follow. The possibility of the ovum aborting into the abdominal cavity with a resulting abdominal pregnancy is rare. CBF/A, AN, PS

37. no. 4. Painless bright-red bleeding occurring in the third trimester is a cardinal sign of placenta previa, a condition in which the placenta is implanted low in the uterus. CBF/A, AN, PS

38. no. 2. Persistent vaginal bleeding may seriously threaten the mother. Monitoring vital signs and fetal heart tones is important; however, significant changes may not occur until profound bleeding is present. Vaginal examination to assess cervical dilation is never done when the woman has vaginal bleeding until the position of the placenta has been determined. CBF/A, IM, PS

39. no. 3. Bed rest might help prevent further separation of the placenta in the woman with placenta previa. Option no. 1 will cause further bleeding. Because she is in her eighth month and is bleeding only a small amount, this client will most probably be kept under observation. Trendelenburg's position is not recommended in pregnancy because this position pushes the gravid uterus against the diaphragm, impeding respiration. CBF/A, IM, E

40. no. 3. Physical activity may increase bleeding. Decreasing anxiety is advisable, but bed rest is essential to limit the chances of her condition worsening. Reducing external stimuli is more important for preventing convulsions when the client has such conditions as pregnancy-induced hypertension. There is no rationale for restricting fluids. CBF/A, IM, E

41. no. 2. Pregnancy-induced hypertension, which occurs after 24 weeks, is the primary predisposing factor for abruptio placentae. Vasoconstriction in the placenta causes placental separation. No evidence of chronic hypertension exists. Other options are not related. CBF/A, AN, PS

42. no. 4. Abdominal tenderness or rigidity or both are cardinal signs of abruptio placentae. A vaginal exam is definitely contraindicated. Options no. 1 and no. 3 are not specific for abruptio placentae. CBF/A, AS, PS

43. no. 2. The primary purpose of administering oxygen in this situation would be to increase the circulating oxygen in the mother to provide better oxygenation of the fetus. Although changing the mother's position in an attempt to improve uteroplacental circulation might be helpful, regular turning every 30 minutes would not be beneficial. Options no. 3 and no. 4 are not interventions; they are additional assessments. CBF/I, IM, E

44. no. 1. The hemorrhaging associated with abruptio placentae may deplete the woman's reserve of blood fibrinogen in the body's efforts to achieve clotting. Disseminated intravascular coagulation syndrome occurs when fibrinogen levels have been depleted. Other options are not associated with abruption. CBF/A, AN, PS

45. no. 3. Women with abruptio placentae are at risk for developing disseminated intravascular coagulation, an abnormal overstimulation of the coagulation process that ultimately leaves the woman with poorly clotting blood. Delayed clot formation at a venipuncture site is one manifestation of this condition. Fluid-filled vesicles passed vaginally are diagnostic of hydatidiform mole. The temperature and urine output given are in the normal range. CBF/I, AN, PS

46. no. 4. Meconium-stained fluid may indicate fetal hypoxia requiring further assessment but is not necessarily an indication for emergency action. For example, meconium passage is expected if the fetus is in a breech presentation. CBF/I, AS, PS

47. no. 2. Hypertension, edema, and proteinuria are cardinal signs and symptoms of pregnancy-induced hypertension. Baseline assessment of the client is a priority before designing a plan of care. CBF/A, AN, PS

48. no. 3. A loud noise or bright light may be enough to precipitate a convulsion because of the hyperactive nervous system. Keeping the side rails padded and up will protect the client, and careful monitoring of the client is in order; however, neither of these measures will reduce the possibility of convulsions. CBF/A, IM, E

49. no. 1. The client on bed rest has decreased blood pressure. There is also an increase in renal filtration rate. These physiologic changes improve uteroplacental blood flow and fetal well-being. CBF/A, PL, E

50. no. 2. Magnesium sulfate is a central nervous system depressant. It circulates freely and is excreted by the kidneys. Because a woman with severe pregnancy-induced hypertension can have compromised kidney function, magnesium toxicity can develop and manifest as loss of knee-jerk reflexes, respiratory depression, oliguria, respiratory arrest, and cardiac arrest. Calcium gluconate is the antidote for magnesium sulfate and should be kept at the bedside for emergency intervention when indicated. CBF/A, IM, E

51. no. 3. Magnesium sulfate is an excellent anticonvulsant and vasodilator that lowers blood pressure; it readily passes through the placenta. Therapeutic doses of this drug are generally well tolerated by the fetus, although some respiratory depression may result after birth. Option no. 2 does not answer the client's question. Option no. 4 is false. CBF/A, IM, H

52. no. 4. Although a cesarean delivery at 37 weeks of gestation used to be common for diabetic mothers,

current practice is to try achieving delivery at the optimum time for mother and infant. Stress for the infant is greater during a cesarean birth than during a vaginal delivery. Option no. 3 is not necessarily true. If tests indicate compromised placental circulation, delivery may be artificially brought about for the safety of the fetus. Tests of placental function and of fetal maturity help determine the prognosis of the fetus at any given time. CBF/A, PL, E

53. no. 4. Insulin needs vary throughout pregnancy with progressive insulin resistance common. The greatest incidence of insulin coma during pregnancy occurs during the second and third months; the greatest incidence of diabetic coma during pregnancy occurs around the sixth month. CBF/A, PL, PS

54. no. 3. Newborn infants of diabetic mothers tend to be immature, lethargic, and hyperbilirubinemic and tend to have latent tetany, tremors, or neuromuscular irritability. These problems can be attributed to early delivery, hypoglycemia, and hypocalcemia. CBF/N, AN, PS

55. no. 3. Although all are correct, the priority is establishing and maintaining a patent airway. CBF/N, PL, PS

56. no. 3. Excessive insulin may lead to hypoglycemia. Brain damage will result if not corrected. CBF/N, PL, E

57. no. 1. Because insulin does not pass into the breast milk, breast-feeding is not contraindicated for the mother with diabetes. Breast-feeding is encouraged; it decreases the insulin requirements for insulin-dependent clients. Breast-feeding does not increase the risk of maternal infection; it leads to an increased caloric demand. Infants of diabetic mothers often display jitteriness in response to hypoglycemia after birth. CBF/N, AN, PS

58. no. 3. This infant has an increased risk related to heredity for diabetes and should be seen regularly during childhood. CBF/N, IM, H

59. no. 1. Reduced activity tolerance is differentiated from the normal fatigue of pregnancy; it may be an early sign of congestive heart failure, a condition to which the cardiac client is highly predisposed. CBF/A, AN, PS

60. no. 2. This is a normal pulse rate for a newly delivered mother; continued routine assessments are all that is indicated. CBF/P, IM, PS

61. no. 1. Outcomes for the high-risk client and infant can be improved with regular prenatal care leading to early detection of and intervention for complications. Keeping scheduled appointments is a prerequisite to psychosocial support, teaching, or referral. CBF/A, PL, E

62. no. 1. During the first trimester, women question the reality of their condition and are often disbelieving and ambivalent. This may be expressed by surprised questions such as "Now?" or "Who, me?" Option no. 2 is associated with developmental tasks of the second trimester. Options no. 3 and no. 4 are associated with developmental tasks of the third trimester. CBF/A, AN, PC

63. no. 3. It is most important for the nurse initially to establish rapport with the client by demonstrating a concerned and accepting attitude. CBF/A, P, PC

64. no. 4. Adolescence is a time of great physical growth and development; to meet these needs as well as pregnancy needs, substantial nutritious intake is required. CBF/A, AN, PS

65. no. 1. The diagnosis of iron-deficiency anemia is made on the basis of a hemoglobin concentration value of 10 g/dl blood or less and a hematocrit value of 35% or less. CBF/A, AN, PS

66. no. 3. To meet increased circulatory needs, especially to the uterus, fetus, and placenta, the blood volume increases starting at about 3 months of gestation. Beginning at about 6 months of gestation, the total red blood cell volume and hemoglobin mass increase. Iron is necessary for red blood cell formation. CBF/A, AN, PS

67. no. 4. Food sources of iron include meat, legumes, dried fruits, enriched grains, leafy vegetables, and nuts. The iron content of prune juice is 10.5 mg per cup, and the iron content of split peas is 4.2 mg per cup; ½ breast of chicken contains 1.3 mg of iron. Of the options presented, this combination is the highest in iron content. CBF/A, EV, PS

68. no. 1. The adolescent is prone to many complications during pregnancy. This can be attributed to lack of early prenatal care and poor nutrition. The other options do not generally apply to the adolescent population. CBF/A, AN, H

69. no. 1. Assessment of the general situation is the first priority. What is important to know is how close the delivery is and how much time is available for preparation. Taking a nursing history, calling the physician, and starting an IV may follow assessment of contractions and labor. CBF/I, AS, H

70. no. 4. In early labor, motivation is high and readiness to learn is enhanced. As labor progresses, concentration becomes more difficult to maintain. CBF/I, AN, H

71. no. 1. Meconium-stained amniotic fluid can indicate fetal distress. CBF/I, AS, PS

72. no. 2. This therapeutic communication fosters open expression of feelings. The nurse can only offer alternatives. The ultimate decision lies with the client. CBF/P, IM, PC

73. no. 3. Considering crisis theory and the knowledge of the grieving process, allowing the relinquishing mother to provide care is considered healthy adaptation. CBF/P, AN, PC

74. no. 1. Adoptive parents, or any parent separated from the newborn in the period immediately after delivery, can still form a strong attachment to the infant. Encouragement and reinforcement of claiming behaviors enhance such bonding. CBF/P, IM, H

75. no. 1. This option indicates that the father is alert to cues and responds to them. This is the only option that demonstrates interaction between infant and parent. CBF/N, EV, PC

76. no. 2. After rupture of membranes it would be important to assess fetal heart tones as an indicator of fetal

well-being. Other options are part of admission assessment but not priorities. CBF/I, AS, PS

77. no. 3. Breathing techniques can help the laboring woman maintain control during contractions. The client should not bear down until she is completely dilated. Crowning will not occur until complete dilation. Sacral pressure is a comfort measure used if the fetus is in a posterior position. CBF/I, IM, PS

78. no. 4. During transition, as dilation nears completion, there is increased rectal pressure from the fetal presenting part. Accelerated breathing, irritability, fear, and the need for medication may occur at any time in active labor. CBF/I, AN, PS

79. no. 2. If the client blows, she will not be able to push, which is contraindicated at this point. Option no. 1 will not be effective in managing behavior. Option no. 3 is correct information, but it is not appropriate to explain things in detail to a client in transition. She needs direction because of her pain and emotional status during that phase of labor. Option no. 4 is incorrect. CBF/I, IM, PS

80. no. 1. This action should reverse the initial symptoms of hyperventilation or carbon dioxide insufficiency (dizziness, tingling in the hands, or circumoral numbness) by enabling the client to rebreathe carbon dioxide and replace the bicarbonate ion. Other options are not related. CBF/I, EV, PS

81. no. 2. It is now safe to assist the client with effective pushing techniques to bring the baby down to the perineum. Before complete dilation, pushing results in cervical edema and increases the danger of cervical lacerations and fetal head trauma. It is too early to prepare her for birth. Narcotics should not be given after full dilation. The client now requires constant support and monitoring by the nurse. CBF/I, IM, E

82. no. 3. The uterus must be assessed every 15 minutes to ensure that it is well contracted, thus preventing hemorrhage. The fundus should not be massaged unless it is relaxed. Constant massaging would tire the uterine muscle, contributing to hemorrhage. Blood pressure is monitored every 15 minutes and temperature every hour unless there are significant changes. CBF/P, IM, PS

83. no. 4. This treatment is to prevent gonorrheal ophthalmia neonatorum and chlamydia infection, both of which can lead to blindness. Chemical conjunctivitis may result when a 1% solution of silver nitrate is used as treatment. Neonatal syphilis must be treated with penicillin. There is no cure for herpes. CBF/N, AN, PS

84. no. 2. Absent variability is an ominous sign. Decreased or absent fluctuations indicate central nervous system depression. True variability can be determined only with internal monitoring. CBF/I, AN, PS

85. no. 2. Variable decelerations are the result of cord compression. Early decelerations result from head compression. Late decelerations result from uteroplacental insufficiency. Posterior positions should not affect fetal heart rate. CBF/I, AN, PS

86. no. 3. Early deceleration occurs in response to compression of the fetal head and does not necessarily indicate fetal distress. Lack of variability is considered a sign of possible fetal jeopardy. Fluctuations are caused by interplay of the parasympathetic and sympathetic components of the autonomic nervous system. When decreased variability is noted, the nurse must suspect compromise of these mechanisms. Variable decelerations result from cord compression and late decelerations result from uteroplacental insufficiency, both of which are abnormal. CBF/I, AN, PS

87. no. 4. Early deceleration is often caused by head compression; no action is needed. CBF/I, IM, PS

88. no. 1. This is an invasive technique requiring a written consent. Because internal monitoring is invasive, there is approximately a 17% chance of infection. Although placement of internal monitoring equipment requires ruptured membranes, it is neither routine after amniotomy nor a standard of care for all multiparas during labor. CBF/I, AN, PS

89. no. 4. This signifies late decelerations, an ominous sign that indicates uteroplacental insufficiency. Stable baseline fetal heart rates, accelerations, and early decelerations are reassuring patterns. CBF/I, AS, PS

90. no. 2. Even though the fetal heart rate is still within a normal range, the change is significant and must be reported. Progressive decrease in baseline fetal heart rate is a nonreassuring pattern. CBF/I, IM, PS

91. no. 1. Excessive oxytocin results in tetanic contractions that interfere with the fetal blood supply. It is necessary to stop the infusion to relax the uterine muscle. After turning off the oxytocin, changing the client's position and administering oxygen will help improve uteroplacental insufficiency. CBF/I, IM, PS

92. no. 4. Contractions that are strong, last 50 to 70 seconds, and occur every 2 to 3 minutes usually signal the second stage of labor. In light of this client's pregnancy history, assessment for the nearness of delivery is in order. CBF/I, IM, PS

93. no. 1. Epidural anesthesia can cause maternal hypotension because of vasodilation. Other parameters are not immediately affected by the epidural. CBF/I, IM, PS

94. no. 1. Uterine atony frequently occurs with older grand multiparas after spontaneous deliveries of full-term infants. Lack of muscle tone in the grand multipara predisposes to uterine relaxation. CBF/P, AN, PS

95. no. 3. Phenylketonuria tests are not performed with accuracy within the first 24 hours. The infant must have ingested formula or breast milk before the test results can be considered accurate. Phenylketonuria is an inborn error of metabolism caused by autosomal recessive genes. These infants have a deficiency in the liver enzyme phenylalanine hydroxylase, which is required to convert the amino acid phenylalanine to tyrosine. When the converting ability is lacking, phenylalanine accumulates, leading to progressive mental retardation. Other options are incorrect. CBF/N, E, H

96. no. 4. Before taking any other action, assessment is a priority. The reaction of the mother is not necessarily reflective of the stage of labor she is in. CBF/I, AS, E

97. no. 2. The priority at this time is to prevent a precipitous delivery that may result in damage to the fetus and a perineal tear. The mother will experience the urge to push during the contraction, but panting will prevent her from doing so. It is important to deliver the baby between contractions. CBF/I, IM, PS

98. no. 1. The sucking of the infant triggers the release of oxytocin, which contracts the uterus. Fundal massage, but not continuous pressure, is also an important nursing action to stimulate contraction of the uterus. CBF/P, IM, PS

99. no. 4. To promote safety and psychologic comfort especially if regional anesthesia has been started, the woman should not be left alone. There is no indication that the woman's membranes are ruptured or that the cervix is dilated, both of which are necessary conditions for internal monitoring. If fetal monitoring is desired, an external monitor will be employed. Nasogastric tube insertion and vaginal douches are not a part of routine cesarean preoperative care. CBF/I, IM, E

100. no. 3. This is the only true statement. Checking fundal height is an important nursing action after a cesarean delivery. Ambulation is permitted and encouraged in the first 24 hours postsurgery. The Foley catheter is ordinarily removed 24 hours after cesarean delivery. CBF/P, PL, E

101. no. 3. A cesarean delivery is not a contraindication to breast-feeding. Early and frequent feeding is the priority. Intravenous fluids will be given until oral intake is established. Mothers with cesarean births do not need to be separated from their infants. Certain adjustments in position may be necessary, but these should not limit breast-feeding. CBF/P, PL, H

102. no. 1. Regional anesthesia may be contraindicated based on this history because of changed spinal anatomy. Blood and urine findings are normal. Active herpes before pregnancy is not relative. CBF/I, AN, E

103. no. 3. Rapid infusion of intravenous fluids may result in pulmonary edema if the heart is unable to adapt to the circulatory overload. CBF/P, AS, PS

104. no. 2. The respiratory assessment indicates potential compromise after general anesthesia and should be reported immediately. Other findings are within normal limits. CBF/P, AS, PS

105. no. 3. Although this may be early for rooming-in after a cesarean birth, with nursing assistance it can be safe and desirable. Asking the father to remain around-the-clock and requiring bed rest are not realistic or therapeutic options. CBF/P, IM, E

106. no. 4. To help a 3-year-old adjust to a new sibling, a symbolic toy such as a baby doll may be provided. This can allow him to express jealous feelings through symbolic play with this toy. Other options will not meet the sibling's needs. CBF/P, IM, PC

107. no. 3. Parents of specific ethnic backgrounds (e.g., African American, Asian, Mediterranean, Native American) often note mongolian spots on their newborn. These are clusters of pigment cells, of no consequence, that generally disappear by school age. CBF/N, AN, PS

108. no. 2. Parents who are both carriers have a one-in-four chance of delivering a child with sickle cell disease; they should be made aware of the genetic implications. A carrier of sickle cell disease is heterozygous (Pp). A person with the disease is homozygous recessive (pp). Referral to a genetic counselor is appropriate. CBF/N, IM, H

109. no. 4. This behavior is normal for an infant in the first days of life. If the infant is breast-feeding 8 to 12 times in 24 hours and seems satisfied after feeding, sufficient intake is probably being obtained with nursing. Number of wet diapers and stools the infant has per day is also an indication of adequate intake but is not listed as an option here. CBF/N, AN, PS

110. no. 4. Protective barriers such as latex gloves should be used to prevent exposure to the client's body fluids, such as amniotic fluid. The pathogen in this disease is not spread through airborne methods. Sharps should be disposed of properly without recapping to avoid accidental needle sticks. CBF/I, AN, E

111. no. 4. Headache after spinal anesthesia is often attributed to the leakage of spinal fluid through the puncture site of the dura. Therefore maintaining the client in a recumbent position while the puncture hole is healing may prevent this complication. Further research, however, is still required on this issue. Option no. 1 has no effect on spinal headache occurrence; no. 3 is appropriate treatment, not prevention. CBF/P, IM, PS

112. no. 2. After rupture of membranes, an amniotic fluid embolus may occur. The symptoms suggest that the embolus traveled to the lung. CBF/I, AN, PS

113. no. 2. Although transmission rates of HIV infection from mother to infant range from 30% to 75%, professionals estimate the actual transmission rate at about 40% to 50%. The AIDS virus is passed transplacentally, so cesarean delivery will not prevent infection of the neonate. In option no. 3, transmission from mother to fetus can occur transplacentally throughout pregnancy, through contact with the mother's blood and vaginal secretions at delivery, and through ingestion of breast milk. In option no. 4, the mother's symptom-free status at birth does not protect the baby. A newborn can be symptom free at birth and still develop AIDS. A true diagnosis of HIV infection in neonates cannot be made until around 15 months of age. A/N, IM, PS

114. no. 2. It is never appropriate to argue with the value system of an individual or family. The other options listed encourage more thoughtful consideration of the choice the husband is making without addressing the underlying belief. CBF/I, IM, PC

115. no. 1. A therapeutic response at this time is one that reflects empathy. Option no. 3 might be appropriate at some later stage of the grieving process. CBF/P, IM, PC

116. no. 2. Oxytocin is used to contract the uterus and minimize postpartal bleeding. Administration of Pitocin before delivery of the placenta is inappropriate. Pitocin has no effect on blood pressure or lactation. CBF/P, AN, PS

117. no. 4. The bedpan and running water should be tried first. Eventually, the nurse may need to insert a catheter, but not as an initial action. Because of the spinal anesthetic, it is not appropriate to get the client out of bed. Ergonovine is an oxytoxic drug used to contract the uterus. CBF/P, IM, PS

118. no. 1. Postpartum chills are a common occurrence after delivery that does not require medical intervention. Possible causes are sudden release of pressure on pelvic nerves, fetus-to-mother transfusion during placental separation, or reaction to norepinepherine production during birth. Warming the client is the appropriate nursing action. CBF/P, IM, PS

119. no. 2. Research has shown both warm and cool sitz baths to be soothing and healing. Pure lanolin is used for altered skin integrity of nipples. Ritrodrine is used to stop premature labor. Tightening gluteal muscles before sitting splints the episiotomy site and minimizes pain when sitting. CBF/P, IM, PS

120. no. 4. Prolactin is the direct cause of milk production. The decrease in estrogen and progesterone after delivery of the placenta stimulate prolactin production. Oxytocin release triggers milk letdown and uterine contractions. CBF/P, AN, PS

121. no. 3. Stroking the infant's lower lip with the mother's nipple will stimulate the infant to open his mouth wide, maximizing the amount of breast tissue he grasps. This allows compression of the lactiferous sinuses where milk collects. Compressing the breast at the areola prevents proper latch. CBF/P, IM, PS

122. no. 3. The condom is the only effective, nonprescription contraceptive to use while a woman is lactating and before there is normal uterine involution. The calendar method is not useful in the postpartum period, during lactation, when cycles are unpredictable. The intrauterine device is not inserted until the os is closed and healing takes place because of the increased risk of infection. To be effective, a diaphragm must fit over the cervix, which has not undergone involution at this time. CBF/P, IM, H

123. no. 4. This is an unrealistic and potentially dangerous goal for the first week after delivery. Realistically, 3 to 6 weeks is required to safely resume prepregnant activities. All other options are correct. CBF/P, EV, H

124. no. 1. Immediately after delivery, the fundus will be about 1 to 2 cm below the umbilicus. About 12 hours after birth, the fundus is about 1 cm above the umbilicus, then begins to descend 1 cm each postpartum day. Large babies are associated with delayed involution. Expect lochia rubra for about 3 days after delivery. The normal fundus is in the midline; deviation to the right could mean a full bladder. CBF/P, AN, PS

125. no. 1. Suspect lacerations if the client is bleeding and the fundus is firm. Subinvolution and uterine atony indicate that the uterus is not contracting properly; thus the fundus would not be firm. When placental fragments are retained, the uterus will not contract. CBF/P, AN, PS

126. no. 1. Overdistention of the uterus causes poor uterine muscle tone, which in turn causes poor uterine contractions postpartally, leading to an increased risk

of hemorrhage. Breech presentation alone does not predispose to hemorrhage. Prolonged rupture of the membranes predisposes to infection. Lochia is usually less after cesarean birth. CBF/P, AN, PS

127. no. 3. All these symptoms are expected for the first day postpartum. Maternal temperature during the first 24 hours after delivery may rise to 100.4°F (38°C) as a result of dehydration. The nurse can reassure the new mother that these symptoms are normal. CBF/P, IM, PS

128. no. 2. Afterpains are more common in the multipara and the nursing mother. Multiparas have poorer muscle tone, and the uterus has the tendency to contract and relax. Oxytocin is released during breastfeeding, causing the uterus to contract. Premature delivery and pregnancy-induced hypertension are not related. CBF/P, AN, PS

129. no. 2. Menses return in 6 to 12 weeks in the nonnursing mother. Prolactin triggers ovulation, not menstruation. Response to follicle-stimulating hormone level (which does not fluctuate) is suppressed by prolactin. CBF/P, IM, H

130. no. 4. Of the options given, the only one that directly and immediately affects the bleeding is uterine massage. It might be important to start an IV with oxytocin at a rapid rate of flow and to give oxygen through a mask at 6 to 7 L/min. However, the first action is to initiate uterine massage and compression. CBF/P, IM, PS

131. no. 4. Postpartal hemorrhage is defined as blood loss equal to or in excess of 500 ml in the first 24 hours after vaginal delivery. CBF/P, AN, PS

132. no. 4. There is no documentation in the literature that breast-feeding is contraindicated after a postpartum hemorrhage and its resultant anemia. It is important, though, to replace the lost iron stores. This is accomplished by diet and ferrous sulfate or ferrous gluconate tablets. The diet should be high in protein and iron-rich foods. Iron should be taken with foods high in vitamin C such as orange juice to increase absorption. Fatigue is a problem common in the postpartum period and is aggravated by the anemia in this case. Until the blood tests are within normal range, this client would be expected to be fatigued on exertion, light-headed when arising too quickly, and pale in appearance. CBF/P, IM, H

133. no. 1. The Rh-negative mother who has no titer (negative Coombs' test result, nonsensitized) and who has delivered an Rh-positive fetus is given an intramuscular injection of anti-Rh$_o$(D) (RHoGAM). Paternal blood type might be determined for the pregnant Rh-negative woman to help determine fetal blood type but has no bearing on the mother's need for RHoGAM. Because RHoGAM provides only temporary passive immunity, administration prenatally does not affect the need for the medication postpartum. CBF/P, AS, H

134. no. 3. RhoGAM blocks antibody production by attaching to fetal Rh-positive blood cells in the maternal circulation before an immunologic response is initiated. CBF/P, AN, PS

135. no. 2. RHoGAM must be administered to unsensitized postpartum women after the birth of each Rh-positive infant to prevent production of antibodies. RHoGAM administration blocks antibody formation at this time. If the father of future fetuses is Rh-positive heterozygous, there is a 50% chance of an Rh-negative infant; if he is Rh-positive homozygous, all infants will be Rh-positive. CBF/P, IM, H

136. no. 2. Serum hepatitis is transmitted through blood; thus the nurse should use gown and gloves to avoid exposure. Respiratory precautions are unnecessary. Vaccination is given to those in high-risk categories, *not* to those who have contracted the disease. Cesarean delivery does not prevent exposure of the neonate at delivery. CBF/I, PL, E

137. no. 2. These are signs of withdrawal in an addicted newborn. The newborn may be jittery and hyperactive. The cry is often shrill and persistent with yawning and sneezing. Tendon reflexes are increased, and Moro's reflex is decreased. CBF/N, AS, PS

138. no. 4. A home visit is essential when preparing to discharge an infant into the care of others. Other factors will be considered, but safety is the priority. CBF/N, AS, H

139. no. 2. For heroin-addicted newborns, onset of withdrawal symptoms usually occurs within the first 24 to 48 hours. For barbiturate- and cocaine-addicted infants, withdrawal occurs several days after delivery. The use of narcotic antagonists to reverse respiratory depression in the drug-addicted neonate is contraindicated because these drugs may precipitate acute withdrawal in the neonate. CBF/N, AN, PS

140. no. 1. Mastitis most frequently occurs at 2 to 4 weeks postpartum with the initial symptoms of fever, chills, headache, breast tenderness, or redness. The client may describe symptoms that are generally consistent with malaise. CBF/P, AS, PS

141. no. 3. There is controversy about whether a woman should continue breast-feeding when mastitis is present. Regular emptying of breasts will prevent complications and maintain lactation. Breast-feeding is the most effective method of doing so; however, if temporarily discontinuing breast-feeding is planned, massage or use of a breast pump to empty the breasts is an alternative. Antibiotics should be continued for the whole course of prescribed treatment, not just until afebrile. Selected analgesics pose no risk to the breast-feeding baby and relieve the mother's pain from engorgement. CBF/P, IM, H

142. no. 4. Cracked nipples provide a portal of entry for bacteria. Antibiotics are used to treat mastitis and would not be given routinely simply to prevent mastitis from occurring. Waiting too long between feedings may lead to clogged ducts, predisposing to mastitis. If the infant's latch is correct, time at breast does not affect nipple integrity and should not be limited. CBF/P, P, H

143. no. 4. Jaundice in the first 24 hours after birth is a cause for concern that requires further assessment. Possible causes of early jaundice are blood incompatibility and severe hemolytic process. Acrocyanosis of the hands and feet is normal, resulting from sluggish peripheral circulation. Mottling is a normal and transient skin discoloration on exposure to decreased temperature and is due to vasoconstriction, lack of fat, and hypoxia. Desquamation, or dry peeling of the skin, is also normal and may indicate postmaturity. CBF/N, AN, PS

144. no. 1. The head circumference is approximately 13 to 14 inches. The chest circumference is 1 inch smaller (12 to 13 inches). Options no. 2 and no. 4 may indicate a pathologic condition. Option no. 3 may be true for the first day or two if a baby is born vaginally and molding is present. CBF/N, AN, PS

145. no. 3. Impetigo is a bacterial infection caused by staphylococci or streptococci, which can lead to a generalized infection, always serious in the newborn. Erythema toxicum is a normal newborn rash that disappears without treatment. Stork bites, or telangiectasia, are clusters of small, red, localized areas of capillary dilation commonly found at the nape of the neck, upper eyelids, and on the bridge of the nose. They can be blanched with pressure of a finger and will disappear without treatment. Mongolian spots are bluish-gray areas of pigmentation found over the lower back in African American and Asian infants. The spots fade within the first year or two of life. CBF/N, AN, PS

146. no. 4. An opaque pupil indicates a congenital cataract. Transient strabismus or nystagmus is present until the third or fourth month of life. Subconjunctival hemorrhage is due to the pressure sustained during birth and will resolve without treatment. Tear ducts and lacrimal glands may not function completely until a month after birth. CBF/N, AN, PS

147. no. 4. The single artery is associated with an increased incidence of various congenital anomalies and with higher perinatal mortality. Breast engorgement may be present as the result of maternal hormones. Bowel sounds are present within 1 to 2 hours after birth. The liver is large in proportion to the rest of the body and is easily felt 1 to 2 cm below the right costal margin. Kidneys are more difficult to feel but may be palpable. CBF/N, AS, PS

148. no. 2. Ears that are set lower than usual on the head may be associated with a congenital renal disorder or autosomal chromosomal abnormality. Incurving of the pinna and instant recoil are signs of maturity. The infant hears immediately after birth, and hearing becomes acute as mucus from the middle ear is absorbed. CBF/N, AS, H

149. no. 3. During periods of alert activity, play can be initiated with young infants. In the taking-hold period, the mother is particularly receptive to instruction and assistance in learning play and other parenting skills. Age-appropriate play activity creates no risk of infection or injury. CBF/N, IM, H

150. no. 2. Fixation is present at birth. The newborn can clearly see items that are within a visual field of 17 to 20 cm (about 7 to 8 inches). CBF/N, AN, H

151. no. 4. Young infants respond well to human faces and black-and-white objects because of the visual contrast

they provide. Newborns may fixate on visual stimuli for periods of 4 to 10 seconds. CBF/N, P, H

152. no. 3. Skin-to-skin touch provides a mild tactile stimulus appropriate for the infant. It can be accomplished by stroking the infant gently from head to toe. This procedure is comforting and relaxing to the infant. CBF/N, P, H

153. no. 4. This reflex is elicited if the palm of the hand is stimulated by touch. The fingers close. Touching the mouth elicits the sucking reflex. Stroking the side of the sole elicits Babinski's reflex. Rotating the head elicits the tonic neck reflex. CBF/N, AS, PS

154. no. 2. The infant experiences a sensation of falling when held in both hands and lowered rapidly about 1 inch. This will elicit Moro's reflex—abduction and extension of arms and spreading of fingers bilaterally—in an infant with an intact central nervous system. CBF/N, AS, PS

155. no. 1. Maternal glucose crosses the placental barrier and stimulates the fetal pancreas to produce large amounts of insulin. At birth, the excess insulin and absence of excess maternal glucose cause the blood glucose level to fall rapidly. CBF/N, AN, PS

156. no. 3. Hypoglycemia may be prevented by nutritive feeding (breast milk, glucose water, formula). Oral feeding should be started as soon as the infant's condition is stable. CBF/N, IM, E

157. no. 4. A term infant is one born between 38 and 42 weeks of gestation; a weight of 5 pounds 1 ounce is below the 10th percentile, making this infant small for gestational age. CBF/N, AN, PS

158. no. 4. There is an increased risk of development of diabetes later in life. CBF/N, IM, H

159. no. 2. Stools are evaluated for green color and amount. Skin should be exposed to light to allow oxidation of bilirubin from the skin. The light may injure the delicate eye structures, particularly the retina, so the eyes are patched. However, eye patches should be removed when the mother feeds the baby to promote bonding and visual stimulation. The infant requires *additional* fluids to compensate for the increased water loss through the skin and loose stools. CBF/N, IM, E

160. no. 2. Although large for gestational age infants are often prone to hypoglycemia, the Dextrostix reading in this situation indicates an adequate blood-glucose level. The time of greatest risk for this baby is the first 3 hours after birth. All the other options indicate infants at risk for hypoglycemia. The infant who is exposed to high blood-glucose levels in utero may experience rapid and profound hypoglycemia after birth because of the cessation of a high in utero glucose load. The small for gestational age infant has used up glycogen stores as a result of intrauterine malnutrition and has blunted hepatic enzymatic response with

which to carry out gluconeogenesis. The preterm infants have not been in utero for a sufficient period to store glycogen and fat. CBF/N, PN, PS

161. no. 1. Increased respirations indicate a high metabolic rate. This happens with an infection. The other options are all within normal ranges. CBF/N, AN, PS

162. no. 1. The mother's behavior indicates that she is grieving over the infant's appearance. Expression of grief and support of feelings can allow the mother to begin resolution and acceptance of a less than perfect infant. Meeting the mother's needs can allow her to then meet the infant's needs. Other options are not indicated as initial actions. CBF/N, IM, PC

163. no. 4. Periodic apnea is common in preterm infants. Usually, gentle stimulation is sufficient to get the infant to breathe. CBF/N, IM, PS

164. no. 3. Epstein's pearls are small, white cysts on the hard palate or gums of the newborn. They are normal and will disappear shortly after birth. Milia are blocked sebaceous glands located on the chin and nose of the infant. Thrush is a fungal infection characterized by white patches that appear to be milk curd on the oral mucosa. However, the white patches are not removeable with gentle washing or wiping. They have a tendency to bleed when removal is attempted. Thrush is caused by a monilial infection in the mother. CBF/N, AN, PS

165. no. 4. During fetal life, the oxygenated blood flows up the cord through the umbilical vein; a fetal structure known as the ductus venosus shunts blood from the umbilical vein to the inferior vena cava. From the inferior vena cava, the blood flows into the right atrium and goes directly into the left atrium through the foramen ovale. It then flows into the left ventricle and out through the aorta. A fetal structure known as the ductus arteriosus provides a direct communication between the pulmonary artery and aorta. CBF/N, AN, PS

166. no. 1. At birth, the newborn's cardiac sphincter is still immature, and the nervous control of the stomach is incomplete. As a result, some regurgitation may be observed, which may be minimized by slow feedings and frequent bubbling. Other options would produce vomiting of large quantities as a symptom. CBF/N, AN, PS

167. no. 3. A full bulging fontanel is a deviation from the normal range, possibly related to a tumor, hemorrhage, or infection. As such, it is reportable. All other options are within normal limits. Fontanels may be difficult to palpate if significant molding is present. CBF/N, AN, PS

168. no. 2. Parental contact promotes bonding and the parents' feeling that this is their infant. CBF/N, IM, PC

Contents

Questions *158*

Correct Answers *175*

Correct Answers with Rationales *178*

Chapter 5

Nursing Care
of the Child

COORDINATOR

Stephen Jones, MS, RN, C, PNP

Contributors

Katherine Jones, MS, RN

Debra Jeffs, MS, RN

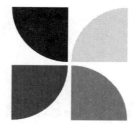

Questions

1. Mrs. Martinez brings her 7-week-old son, Ramón, in for a well-child clinic visit. Mrs. Martinez says to the nurse: "I'm concerned that my baby is sleeping a lot, a lot more than his brother or sister." The nurse's best initial response would be
   ① "How much did his brother and sister sleep?"
   ② "Why do you think this is a concern?"
   ③ "Most babies sleep a lot."
   ④ "How old are his brother and sister?"

2. What is the best advice to provide Mrs. Wong regarding her 7-month-old infant Lea and developmental milestones?
   ① Lea should be able to start using a cup to drink.
   ② Lea should be using a spoon to feed herself.
   ③ Lea should start cruising around the room shortly.
   ④ Lea can use the pincer grasp when getting objects.

3. Which of the following parameters is of most concern regarding 12-month-old Ravi's clinic visit?
   ① 50% increase in height
   ② Doubling of birth weight
   ③ Head circumference greater than chest circumference
   ④ Tripling of birth weight

4. The nurse assesses all of the following infants. Which one requires further evaluation?
   ① A 10-month-old unable to sit alone steadily
   ② A 1-month-old unable to raise his head when prone
   ③ An 8-month-old unable to sit unsupported
   ④ A 4-month-old unable to roll over completely

5. The nurse plans to work with Mrs. Eisenhower about toilet training 20-month-old John. Which of the following is the most important factor in toilet training?
   ① Mother's willingness to work at it
   ② Starting early and being consistent
   ③ Approach and attitude of mother
   ④ Developmental readiness of child

6. Kathy Jones is sitting with her 18-month-old daughter, Emily, at the well-baby clinic. She tells the nurse that Emily has been saying "no" to everything, such as this morning when Emily refused her orange juice at breakfast. The nurse explains to Mrs. Jones that Emily's negativism is normal for a toddler and that this helps her daughter meet which of the following needs?
   ① Discipline
   ② Autonomy

③ Trust
④ Consistency

7. How best can Mrs. Hernandez, mother of 20-month-old Juanita, help her toddler learn to control her own behavior?
   ① Punish her when she deserves it.
   ② Set limits and be consistent.
   ③ Allow her to learn by her mistakes.
   ④ Recognize that she is too young to be controlled.

8. Four-year-old Jason is hospitalized with multiple trauma including a fractured femur after being struck by a car. He frequently snacks on potato chips and candy and eats poorly at mealtimes. Which of the following instructions to Jason's parents would be best to improve his nutrition?
   ① "Teach him the benefit of eating a well-balanced diet."
   ② "Withhold between-meal snacks."
   ③ "Eliminate dessert if some of each food is not eaten at mealtimes."
   ④ "Offer smaller portions of each food at mealtimes and nutritious snacks."

9. The father of 4-year-old Giovanni asks the nurse how he can help Giovanni give up a night-light at bedtime. What is the nurse's best response?
   ① "Tell him that he is too old for night-lights."
   ② "Let him go to bed with the night-light, then turn it off when he's asleep."
   ③ "Give him a flashlight and tell him to use it to explore the dark room."
   ④ "Let him turn the light on and off as he wishes. He will give it up when he does not need it any more."

10. What is the nurse's best response to the parents of a 4-year-old who reportedly lies all the time?
    ① "Confront the child with this behavior, and let him know that lying is not acceptable."
    ② "The 4-year-old is old enough to tell the truth; ask him why he is not truthful."
    ③ "The 4-year-old has a vivid imagination; don't stifle his creativity by punishing him."
    ④ "Acknowledge his stories or fantasies by saying, 'What a nice story,' or, 'That's a pretend story.'"

11. Which of the following statements by the father of a 4-year-old indicates that he understood the nurse's instructions on his daughter's bed-wetting?
    ① "I'll restrict all fluids after 5 PM and remind her that she is too old to wet the bed."

② "I'll get her up to go to the bathroom at midnight, and she will be able to stay dry until morning."

③ "I'll put her in diapers at bedtime and tell her not to worry about the bed-wetting."

④ "I'll limit her fluids after dinner and make sure she urinates before going to bed."

12. Georgette, age 5, visits the pediatrician for her annual health visit. As an infant, she had the full recommended series of immunizations. Her last immunization was at 18 months. Which of the following immunizations would Georgette receive at this visit?

① DTP and OPV boosters

② Hepatitis

③ Chickenpox

④ No immunizations at this time

13. One day the mother of 5-year-old Gabriella discovers Gabriella and her cousin, Warren, age 7, undressed and curiously looking at and touching each other's bodies. What is Gabriella's mother's best initial response?

① "Warren, it's time for you to go home."

② Gabriella, we're going to have a talk when your daddy gets home."

③ "Gabriella and Warren, please put your clothes on. I'm going to wait in the kitchen for you."

④ "What are you children doing?"

14. Five-year-old Ramona asks about her grandmother's death. Which statement is most characteristic of the child between 5 and 8 years of age?

① Death is personified as a bogeyman.

② Death is considered to be reversible.

③ Death is perceived as inevitable.

④ The child recognizes that she will die.

15. An educational session on child development is conducted by the nurse for a group of parents of preschoolers at a local day care center. Which one of the following statements made by four parents at the conclusion of the session indicates a correct understanding of masturbation in young children?

① "I'll permit my child to explore his body, but explain that it is a private activity."

② "I'll say 'no' and distract him with other interests such as puzzles or books."

③ "I'll set firm limits and will not permit any bodily exploration."

④ "I'll report any masturbation by my child to the pediatrician because it could be a sign of emotional illness."

16. Which of the following nutritional guidelines is *least* appropriate for parents of school-age children?

① Have the child eat most of the meal before offering second helpings or between-meal snacks.

② Avoid forcing the child to eat or using desserts as rewards for eating disliked foods.

③ Deprive the child of a favorite food as punishment.

④ Maintain good nutrition by having only fruit, vegetables, cheese, and protein snacks available.

17. Which of the following is the *least* effective approach to teaching nutrition to school-age children?

① Discuss nutrition without reference to "right" and "wrong."

② Present consequences of eating a balanced versus an unbalanced diet.

③ Stress the importance of good table manners.

④ Encourage children to keep a journal for 3 days to monitor types of food consumed.

18. The mother of a hospitalized 2-year-old says to the nurse, "Tommy becomes more upset when I come to visit; maybe I shouldn't come to the hospital." Which one of the following is the best response by the nurse?

① "You're right. Maybe you should limit your visits to mealtimes."

② "You're right. We take care of Tommy anyway."

③ "Perhaps Tommy's father could visit instead."

④ "You should continue to stay with Tommy as much as possible."

19. The nurse plans to administer an intramuscular injection to a 9-month-old infant. Which one of the following is the correct injection site?

① Dorsogluteal

② Gluteus minimus

③ Rectus femoris

④ Vastus lateralis

20. Marilisa Conti is a 6-year-old with recurrent infection of the tonsils. Marilisa's mother was told by the surgeon that Marilisa would be scheduled for surgical removal of her tonsils and adenoids the following week. To promote Marilisa's adjustment to the hospital experience, which of these actions should the nurse take?

① Admit her early on the day of admission to meet the staff.

② Suggest that a friend schedule surgery at the same time.

③ Show diagrams of the surgical procedure.

④ Explain about the surgery a week before her admission.

21. Eight-year-old Angela is hospitalized for an appendectomy. The nurse can anticipate that Angela's greatest fear regarding surgery is related to

① Having her parents away from her.

② A loss of control.

③ Body-image changes.

④ Being admitted to a strange room.

22. Elena is a 7-year-old scheduled for surgery. Upon Elena's admission to the hospital, the laboratory technician visits her to obtain a sample of blood. Elena asks the nurse if the technician is going to hurt her. What is the nurse's best response?

① "Of course not. You won't feel a thing."

② "I don't know, but try to hold still."

③ "It will hurt a little bit, but you can squeeze my hand and count to ten."

④ "Yes, it will hurt, but we have to know your blood type if you should need a blood transfusion."

23. Which blood test is especially important preoperatively for Frank, a 6-year-old, who is scheduled for a tonsillectomy?

① Neutrophil count

② Bleeding and clotting time

③ Erythrocyte sedimentation rate

④ Serum chloride levels

24. Rachel, age 12 years, is noted to have an axillary temperature of 100.2°F an hour before surgery to correct scoliosis. What action would the nurse take first?
    ① Notify the physician immediately.
    ② Call the operating room to cancel the surgery.
    ③ Administer acetaminophen prn as ordered.
    ④ Call Rachel's parents.

25. Seven-year-old Tanya is scheduled for a tonsillectomy. Preoperatively, the nurse *must* include which of the following assessments?
    ① Observe size of the tonsils.
    ② Check for loose teeth.
    ③ Obtain a history of tonsillitis episodes.
    ④ Obtain a history of middle ear infections.

26. The nurse is preparing 9-year-old Latoya for tonsillectomy. She asks the nurse if her throat will hurt after having her tonsils out. Which of the following responses would be best for the nurse to make?
    ① "It will not hurt because you will be asleep."
    ② "It will not hurt because you are a big girl."
    ③ "It will hurt because of the incision in your throat."
    ④ "It will hurt, but we have medicine to make you feel better."

27. After tonsillectomy, the nurse monitors 8-year-old Tyler frequently for signs of hemorrhage. Which one of the following would be an early indicator of hemorrhage?
    ① Pulse rate of 95 beats per minute
    ② 25 ml of dark brown emesis
    ③ Frequent swallowing
    ④ Dried blood on Tyler's lips

28. For a child after tonsillectomy, which one of the following would be best to offer initially after the child has tolerated sips of cold water?
    ① Orange popsicle
    ② Vanilla ice cream
    ③ Cherry punch
    ④ Chocolate milk

29. The nurse is caring for 3½-year-old Christina the evening of the day she had a tonsillectomy because of chronic infections. Christina becomes restless and wants to get out of bed. Which action should the nurse take?
    ① Allow Christina's mother to hold her.
    ② Tell Christina to sit quietly in bed.
    ③ Permit Christina to walk in the halls.
    ④ Move Christina's bed near the nurse's station.

30. When the nurse does discharge teaching for a child who has undergone a tonsillectomy, which instructions should be emphasized to the parents?
    ① Monitor for bleeding during the first 10 days.
    ② Use normal saline gargles for comfort.
    ③ Remain out of school for 2 weeks.
    ④ Limit all activities for 1 month.

31. The nurse evaluates the postoperative discharge teaching plan of the parent of a 3-year-old after bilateral myringotomy with insertion of tympanostomy tubes. Which one of the following statements by the parent indicates teaching effectiveness?
    ① "I'll call the doctor immediately if the ear tubes fall out."
    ② "I'll make sure water does not get into his ears."
    ③ "I'll cleanse the inner ear canal daily with soap and water."
    ④ "I'll keep him home from nursery school until the ear tubes fall out."

32. Paul Arroyo, 10 months old, has had an elevated temperature for 48 hours. There is evidence of increasing lethargy, nausea, and vomiting. He also appears dehydrated. Meningitis is suspected. The nurse should expect which further finding related to meningitis?
    ① Weight loss of 5%
    ② Urine specific gravity of 1.007
    ③ Dry mucous membranes
    ④ Bulging fontanel

33. Five-month-old Jasmine, admitted for possible meningitis, will be having a septic workup completed. One diagnostic test is a lumbar puncture. Which of the following cerebrospinal fluid findings is highly indicative of meningitis?
    ① High glucose
    ② High protein
    ③ Low white blood cell count
    ④ Clear color

34. A 10-month-old patient has been admitted with vomiting, diarrhea, and dehydration. The physician has ordered 5% dextrose in 0.33% normal saline with 20 mEq per liter of potassium chloride to infuse at 32 cc/hr. Which of the following should be brought to the physician's attention immediately?
    ① The patient is irritable.
    ② The patient has not voided in 4 hours.
    ③ There has been one episode of vomiting.
    ④ There have been three liquid green stools.

35. In caring for a 3-year-old with meningitis, which nursing action is the least important priority during the acute stages?
    ① Monitor changes in his level of consciousness.
    ② Maintain the patency of the IV line.
    ③ Isolate him from other children.
    ④ Provide hourly tepid baths.

36. A toddler has been diagnosed with meningitis. His care plan should include which measure?
    ① Administer antibiotics as soon as they are ordered.
    ② Discourage parental participation in child's care.
    ③ Place him in isolation for 3 days.
    ④ Stimulate him every hour to keep him awake.

37. Eight-year-old Carlos has bacterial pharyngitis and is receiving oral penicillin. Which of the following statements by his mother indicates an understanding of the nurse's instructions?
    ① "I'll have him gargle with a mouthwash solution."
    ② "I'll be sure to give him all of the medicine."
    ③ "I'll give him citrus juices to drink."
    ④ "I'll keep him home from school until he finishes the medicine."

38. The mother of a 10-year-old with chickenpox (varicella) calls the nurse to ask when her child can return to school. The nurse evaluates the communicability of the child by asking the mother
    ① "Is all of the rash dry and crusted?"
    ② "Is your child coughing or sneezing?"

③ "Is your child running a temperature?"
④ "Has the rash completely faded?"

39. Trisha, 4½ years old, was admitted today for weight loss, anorexia, vaginitis, and insomnia. The night nurse observes Trisha scratching in the anal area at night. Assessing the situation, the nurse suspects that Trisha may have which one of the following conditions?
① Ulcerative colitis
② Pinworms
③ Vesicoureteral reflux
④ Scabies

40. During nap time, in the hospital, 4-year-old Darlene wets her bed. What action would the nurse take?
① Change her clothes and bed without comment.
② Call her mother for suggestions.
③ Put her in diapers and note this in the Kardex.
④ Keep the bedpan in bed at nap time.

41. Melissa Domery yells for her neighbor, who is a nurse, to come look at her daughter, 2-year-old Kirsten. The nurse finds the child sitting in the middle of the bathroom floor with several open medicine bottles strewn around the room. She is chewing on something and has white powder around her mouth. Mrs. Domery says, "Do something!" What would be the nurse's first action?
① Call the poison control center.
② Determine what Kirsten ate or drank.
③ Take Kirsten to the emergency room.
④ Observe Kirsten closely to see if any symptoms develop.

42. The mother of a 2½-year-old phones the emergency room and states that her daughter has just ingested a few acetaminophen (Tylenol) tablets and a couple of arthritis capsules. What should the nurse instruct the mother to do?
① Give her milk to coat her stomach and delay absorption.
② Keep her NPO and observe her for symptoms.
③ Give 15 ml of syrup of ipecac with 15 ml of water.
④ Administer 15 g of activated charcoal.

43. Mrs. Peckham and her toddler, Shauna, are visiting the clinic for a well-child checkup. As part of the teaching involved in anticipatory guidance, the nurse mentions how to prevent poisonous ingestions. Which of the following actions would be least appropriate?
① Label all containers.
② Lock up harmful substances.
③ Teach Shauna to avoid poisonous substances.
④ Never refer to medicine as candy.

44. Which of the following is the best indicator that parent teaching regarding poison prevention was effective?
① Parent knows the correct first aid for poisoning.
② Parents say they will teach their toddler to avoid poisons.
③ Parent memorizes the poison control center telephone number.
④ Parents verbalize the need to keep medicines out of the reach of young children.

45. The nurse will evaluate the child receiving chelation therapy, such as calcium disodium EDTA, for which of the following side effects?
① Neurotoxicity
② Ototoxicity
③ Cardiac arrhythmia
④ Nephrotoxicity

46. Which observation by the nurse best indicates that 2-year-old Lisa is at her normal developmental level?
① She undresses herself, but she needs help getting dressed.
② She points to her body parts.
③ She puts smaller objects into larger holes.
④ She builds a tower out of two blocks.

47. Mrs. White, a 24-year-old single mother and former IV drug abuser, is concerned about HIV status for both herself and her 2-month-old infant, Shaquanna. As the nurse in the clinic, you understand her concerns, and indicate that you want to assist her. The nurse's most appropriate initial action would be to
① Have her discuss this with an infectious disease practitioner.
② Send her for immediate blood work.
③ Discuss HIV and how it is transmitted.
④ Assure her that you will maintain confidentiality.

48. Vickie, a 7-year-old hemophiliac, was diagnosed as HIV-positive several months ago after repeated infections and a cold that did not get any better. Her parents have taken the news badly and are having a difficult time in accepting the diagnosis. Which initial statement best represents that the parents have started to cope with Vickie's illness?
① "I just wish it were me; she doesn't deserve it."
② "What therapies are available to help Vickie?"
③ "I really feel we need to go back to where she got her last blood transfusion and sue them."
④ "How sick will Vickie become?"

49. Janelle, a 15-year-old adolescent, asks you about sexually transmitted diseases and HIV/AIDS. After further discussion, she informs you that she has been sexually active for the past 10 months with several "older boys." What is the most appropriate advice you can provide her regarding her concerns about HIV transmission?
① The boys should come in for testing.
② She should abstain from sexual activity.
③ She should have sex only with boys she knows.
④ She should have the boys use condoms.

50. Pasquel and Linda Quinone, parents of 18-month-old, HIV-positive Luci, are concerned that their daughter is not "doing things the other children her age are doing." Luci has been on antiretroviral therapy for the past 6 months because of a worsening CD4 count. What is the most accurate information the nurse can provide to the parents regarding Luci's current development?
① There is not a lot that can be done to change Luci's current status.
② Luci should start to improve shortly.
③ The virus and medications have both contributed to Luci's present status.
④ Luci's development should continue to deteriorate.

51. Three-year-old Deborah has cerebral palsy, spastic type, with a severe motor impairment. Her mother has brought her to the clinic because she is having difficulty feeding Deborah. To improve Deborah's eating abilities, the nurse would teach her mother to
    ① Place Deborah in semi-Fowler's position with her head to one side, and allow her to suck liquids and pureed foods through a sturdy straw.
    ② Encourage Deborah to feed herself to increase her independence.
    ③ Stand behind Deborah, support her jaw with one hand, and use the other hand to handle the cup or spoon to feed Deborah.
    ④ Place Deborah in a sitting position, tilt her head slightly back, and use a Brecht feeder to give liquids and pureed foods.

52. The mother of a 5-year-old with cerebral palsy is pregnant and asks the nurse whether her second baby is likely to have cerebral palsy also. What is the nurse's best initial response?
    ① "There is a strong possibility that your next baby may have cerebral palsy."
    ② "Perhaps you were exposed to some illness or took some harmful medication when you were pregnant with your first baby."
    ③ "You're concerned that your next baby may have cerebral palsy?"
    ④ "Attending prepared childbirth classes can lessen the possibility of birth trauma and decrease the risk of cerebral palsy."

53. What would the priority nursing action be on admission of an 8-year-old with burns on his face and neck?
    ① Debride and dress the wounds.
    ② Administer antibiotics.
    ③ Observe for hoarseness, stridor, and dyspnea.
    ④ Obtain a complete history of the event.

54. Narcotics are ordered to be given intravenously to a child with second- and third-degree burns over 50% of his body. Why was the IV route selected?
    ① Fluid balance will be maintained using the IV route.
    ② Circulatory blood volume is reduced, delaying absorption from the subcutaneous and muscle tissue.
    ③ Cardiac function is enhanced by the immediate action of the drug.
    ④ Decreased metabolism increases insulin production.

55. What would be considered an *unreliable* measure of fluid loss in a 4-year-old with a burn?
    ① Hematocrit of 42
    ② Urinary output of 30 ml/hr
    ③ Change in level of consciousness
    ④ Leakage through the eschar

56. Silver sulfadiazine (Silvadene) is applied every 4 hours to a 6-year-old's burns. What side effect would the nurse be most concerned about?
    ① Metabolic acidosis
    ② Discoloration of the skin
    ③ Vomiting and diarrhea
    ④ Dehydration and electrolyte loss

57. What is the priority goal of burn wound management after the acute phase?
    ① Debride the wound of dead tissue and eschar.
    ② Limit fluid loss.
    ③ Prevent the growth of microorganisms.
    ④ Decrease formation of disfiguring scars.

58. What foods would be most appropriate for a 9-month-old child who is recovering from a burn injury?
    ① Hot dog, french fries, and cooked spinach
    ② Hamburger, raisins, and cooked beans
    ③ Omelet, mashed carrots, and crackers
    ④ Pureed chicken, cooked peas, and bananas

59. Rosalyn Greer is a newborn with Down syndrome. Her parents have been told the diagnosis and are in the process of trying to adjust. Which of the following is most appropriate to include when counseling Mr. and Mrs. Greer?
    ① Her developmental potential is greatest during infancy.
    ② She will be severely retarded.
    ③ She will have hyperreflexia.
    ④ She will be as susceptible to colds as her older brother.

60. Which of the following measures is of primary importance for parents with a young, mentally retarded child at home?
    ① Limit the amount of environmental stimulation to which the child is exposed.
    ② Have the same parent teach the child new skills.
    ③ Teach the child socially acceptable behaviors.
    ④ Maintain a consistent routine for daily activities.

61. Baby girl Rosano was born yesterday with a myelomeningocele. She is now in the special care nursery. When her father visits for the first time, he is most likely to exhibit which grief reaction?
    ① Anger
    ② Depression
    ③ Disbelief
    ④ Bargaining

62. Baby girl Garcia was born with a cleft lip. Which action by her father, Mr. Garcia, best demonstrates effective coping?
    ① Stroking and talking to his daughter.
    ② Standing silently beside the isolette.
    ③ Telling the nurse to give all information to his wife.
    ④ Asking repeatedly, "How could this happen?"

63. Preoperatively, what is the priority nursing goal for an infant with a myelomeningocele?
    ① Promote parent-infant bonding.
    ② Prevent contractures of extremities.
    ③ Protect the sac from injury.
    ④ Maintain adequate hydration.

64. Which nursing measure would be most dangerous preoperatively for an infant with myelomeningocele?
    ① Place in a prone position.
    ② Massage skin periodically with lotion.
    ③ Apply dry, sterile dressings on the sac.
    ④ Empty bladder by applying downward pressure over the suprapubic area.

65. Gail, 24 hours old, has just returned to her room from a surgical repair of a myelomeningocele. Postoperatively, it is imperative that the nurse assess for which of the following findings?
① Increased head circumference
② Congenital hip dysplasia.
③ Lower extremity movement.
④ Bladder function.

66. Baby boy Steven's IV rate is 12 ml/hr. How many drops per minute would the nurse regulate the micro-drip to infuse?
① 6
② 12
③ 24
④ 48

67. In which position should the hips of a newborn be placed who is suspected of having congenital hip dysplasia?
① Adduction
② Abduction
③ Internal rotation
④ External rotation

68. While in her crib in the hospital, Francie, age 3, begins to have a grand mal seizure with tonic and clonic movements. Which nursing measure would be implemented first?
① Place her on the floor.
② Place a small padded tongue blade between her gums.
③ Administer oxygen by mask.
④ Put a blanket between Francie and the crib rails.

69. Regina, who has seizures, will be discharged on a regimen of phenytoin. It is important to teach her parents to observe for all of the side effects. Which of the following is *not* a side effect of this drug?
① Gingival hypertrophy
② Skin rash
③ Nausea and vomiting
④ Excessive sleepiness

70. Ruth, age 1 month, is admitted after a computed tomography scan that showed developing hydrocephalus. When assessing Ruth for signs of increased intracranial pressure, the nurse observes which of the following signs that indicate the pressure is increasing?
① Absence of neonatal reflexes
② High-pitched cry
③ Pinpoint pupils
④ Sunken fontanel

71. A ventriculoperitoneal (VP) shunt is done to treat hydrocephalus. Postoperative nursing assessment and discharge teaching would be guided by the knowledge that which of the following are the most common complications of VP shunts?
① Hemorrhage and subdural hematoma
② Ascites and peritonitis
③ Obstruction and infection
④ Catheter leakage

72. What is the postoperative nursing priority for a child with a ventriculoperitoneal shunt?
① Prevent skin breakdown of the neck and abdomen.

② Help the parents cope with having a neurologically disabled child.
③ Promote adequate nutrition.
④ Prevent overhydration.

73. The nurse is caring for an infant in the clinic who had a myelomeningocele repair 10 days after birth. The child is now 5 months old. Which of the following is the best indicator of a successful outcome of care?
① Degree of attachment between child and parents
② Physical growth
③ Cognitive and motor skills
④ Temperament and social skills

74. Two-month-old Liam O'Malley has been admitted to the hospital for a febrile seizure. The nurse is explaining to the parents about febrile seizures. Which statement best explains the principal reasons for their occurrence?
① "A febrile seizure is indicative of some underlying neurologic condition."
② "A febrile seizure is usually due to a quick rise in temperature."
③ "A febrile seizure is usually due to a high temperature."
④ "A febrile seizure is usually drug induced."

75. Brendan Anthony is a 10-year-old who is admitted to the hospital for evaluation of a seizure disorder. During the history, Brendan tells the nurse that he sees stars before his eyes and then does not remember what happens afterward. The nurse would suspect that he is
① Hallucinating.
② Experiencing an aura.
③ Trying to get his parents' attention.
④ Describing a psychomotor seizure.

76. The nurse is teaching the parents of a child who has seizures about phenytoin (Dilantin). What statement indicates that the parents have *not* understood the nurse's teaching?
① "We will only use the prescribed brand of the drug."
② "The dosage may be changed during growth spurts."
③ "The medication can be discontinued if the seizures stop."
④ "Gum changes may occur after prolonged usage."

77. The night nurse is caring for the parents of an infant who has just died of sudden infant death syndrome (SIDS). The father says, "She was so healthy. I just can't understand what would have caused this. What did we do wrong?" What is the most appropriate response?
① "It sounds as though you feel responsible for what happened to your child."
② "Try not to blame yourself for her death."
③ "No one knows the cause of SIDS."
④ "Did she seem sick before bedtime?"

78. The home health nurse is visiting the Davis family, who has lost a child with sudden infant death syndrome (SIDS). What is the best indicator of their successful coping with the loss of their child?
① Moving to a new residence.
② Involving themselves in a SIDS support group.

③ Attending their church regularly.
④ Returning to work.

79. Mackenzie is a 4-month-old infant with [RSV] bronchiolitis. What sign would the nurse expect to observe when doing a physical exam?
① Shortened expiratory phase
② Dry, hacky cough
③ Drooling
④ Wheezy breath sounds

80. Why is the infant with bronchiolitis kept NPO?
① Hypoxemia reduces gastrointestinal motility.
② Oral fluids increase mucus production.
③ Tachypnea predisposes an infant to aspiration.
④ Hydration is not a concern with bronchiolitis.

81. Which of the following interventions would be inappropriate for an infant with bronchiolitis?
① Use deep suction.
② Use humidified oxygen via nasal cannula.
③ Maintain adequate hydration.
④ Monitor for cor pulmonale.

82. Baby Zabinski, age 9 weeks, is currently being treated for RSV bronchiolitis. Which of the following is least important for the nurse when planning the infant's care?
① Provide nutritional support.
② Maintain airway clearance.
③ Administer aerosolized antivirals.
④ Prevent visitation by the family.

83. When is the best time to administer chest physical therapy with postural drainage?
① Before meals
② After meals
③ Every 8 hours
④ When parents are present

84. If Lionel's weight is 3.8 kg at birth, how much would he be expected to weigh at 12 months of age?
① 7.6 kg
② 9.5 kg
③ 11.4 kg
④ 13.3 kg

85. Which of the following foods would be most appropriate for meeting a 6-month-old's developmental needs?
① Chopped egg white
② Strained vegetables
③ Animal crackers
④ Apple juice

86. Which cereal would be most appropriate for a 6-month-old?
① Oatmeal
② Rice
③ Mixed
④ Barley

87. If a 12-month-old infant's immunizations are up to date, which of the following would the infant receive next?
① Diphtheria and tetanus
② Oral polio
③ Measles, mumps, and rubella
④ Pertussis

88. Peter is admitted with airway obstruction. An endotracheal tube (ETT) is placed emergently, and Peter requires frequent suctioning. Sterile normal saline, 2 to 3 ml, is instilled into the ETT before suctioning. Which client outcome indicates that the saline was effective?
① Decreased coughing
② Loosened secretions and coughing
③ A long period of uninterrupted sleep at night
④ Improved hydration

89. Before suctioning an endotracheal tube, which of the following actions would the nurse initially perform?
① Check the ventilator's setting.
② Listen to the client's chest with a stethoscope.
③ Instill normal saline.
④ Perform postural drainage.

90. The nurse caring for Rachel, who has a tracheostomy, would know that oxygenation before suctioning is essential to
① Loosen respiratory secretions.
② Relax Rachel.
③ Restore oxygen lost during suctioning.
④ Remove sodium ions from respiratory tissue.

91. If suctioning is effective, the nurse listening to a child's chest will hear
① Coarse rhonchi.
② Increased breath sounds.
③ Fine, moist crackles.
④ Decreased breath sounds.

92. William, 12 years old, is taking ampicillin 500 mg q6h. Which of the following foods would the nurse instruct the patient's mother to include in her son's diet?
① Honey
② Yogurt
③ Bran
④ Bananas

93. Sarah, a 4-year-old, is taking amoxicillin-clavalanic acid (Augmentin) 200 mg PO q8h for an otitis media. Which statement by Sarah's parents best indicates that they understand discharge instructions related to the medication?
① "I should give Sarah the medication until the next visit."
② "If she develops a rash, I will give her some Benadryl."
③ "If Sarah has diarrhea, I will give her the BRATTS diet."
④ "I can give it to her before going to bed so as not to wake her up."

94. Which statement about cromolyn sodium (Intal) is correct?
① It stabilizes most cells.
② It is used during an acute asthmatic attack.
③ It is administered with milk PO qid.
④ It is used once a day.

95. What statement best describes the developmental level of a 10-year-old boy?
① He enjoys numbers and is able to do simple fractions.
② He is clumsy handling a pencil and pen.
③ He is interested in girls.
④ He has a huge appetite.

96. Molly, a 4½-year-old preschooler who has a history of asthma, is hospitalized with an acute episode. Which of the following nursing actions is *contraindicated* during the acute phase of Molly's illness?
① Keep Molly's room quiet.
② Provide oxygen.
③ Give Molly a cough suppressant.
④ Place Molly in a high-Fowler's position.

97. LaCreshia, age 5, has an IV that has infiltrated. When the nurse tries to apply an aqua k-pad to LaCreshia's swollen left forearm, the child begins to whine and pull away. What would the nurse say to gain LaCreshia's cooperation?
① "I'll come back in a few minutes after you calm down."
② "The doctor says this aqua k-pad will make your arm feel better."
③ "Try not to cry while I put this on."
④ "This will feel warm. I'll show you on your other arm first."

98. Which of the following aerosolized drugs would a child with an acute asthma attack most likely initially receive?
① Epinephrine
② Aminophylline
③ Cromolyn sodium
④ Albuterol

99. What assessment data best describe the respiratory status of the child early in an acute asthma attack?
① Coughing and wheezing on expiration
② Productive coughing and prolonged inspiration
③ Periods of apnea with inspiratory stridor
④ Dry, brassy cough with drooling

100. In developing a care plan for an ill, hospitalized 9-year-old girl, it is most important for the nurse to include interventions that
① Maintain psychomotor skills.
② Promote her sense of control.
③ Promote attachment to her parents.
④ Maintain her school work.

101. The parents of a 7-year-old with asthma are planning, with the nurse, measures to prevent another acute asthma attack. Which of the following is a priority activity to prevent an acute asthma attack?
① Avoid disciplinary measures.
② Avoid gym class and regular exercise.
③ Avoid overexertion and sudden exposure to cold.
④ Avoid routine immunizations.

102. The nurse evaluates her discharge teaching plan for the parent of a child with asthma as effective when the parent states
① "I'll avoid frequent dusting of rooms at home."
② "I'll be sure my daughter's immunizations and flu shots are up to date."
③ "I'll have my daughter sleep with her window open."
④ "I'll discourage my daughter's participation in any sports or physical exercise."

103. A 12-year-old is admitted to the adolescent unit with sickle cell disease. She is in vasoocclusive crisis. Her right elbow is edematous, and she states that it is very painful. In addition to pain, which of the following symptoms would she most likely manifest?
① Dactylitis
② Chronic hemolytic anemia
③ Brushfield's spots
④ Jaundice followed by pallor after a sickling crisis

104. Which of the following is least likely to cause a sickle cell crisis?
① Strenuous physical exercise
② Dehydration
③ Hot, humid weather
④ A viral infection

105. The most appropriate priority intervention for a child in vasoocclusive crisis with a painful, edematous elbow is which of the following?
① Wrap a heating pad around the child's elbow.
② Limit the child's daily fluid intake to 900 ml.
③ Handle the child gently.
④ Apply ice to the child's arms.

106. Which of the following tests is most reliable in diagnosing sickle cell disease?
① Sickledex
② Amniocentesis
③ Hemoglobin electrophoresis
④ Complete blood cell count

107. When obtaining a history from an adolescent with hemophilia, which one of the following reported manifestations would be the least cause for concern?
① Epistaxis
② Hemarthrosis
③ Hematuria
④ Platelets of 200,000

108. The father of a 10-year-old with hemophilia makes the following comment to the nurse: "My son is crazy about sports, especially football. He wants to try out for his school's football team. My wife and I are having a hard time convincing him this is not possible." Which is the best recommendation the nurse should offer?
① Allow him to try out for the team as long as he wears a helmet and body pads at all times.
② Help him start a collection of football memorabilia.
③ Encourage an interest in swimming or table tennis.
④ Suggest that he become a team coach.

109. Which of the following would be used to control an acute bleeding episode in a child with hemophilia?
① Platelets
② Fibrinogen
③ Packed cells
④ Cryoprecipitate

110. Bernard, age 16, has hemophilia. He asks the nurse if all his children will have hemophilia. Assuming that his future wife is not a carrier, what is the most accurate explanation the nurse can give?
① All Bernard's children will be carriers.
② Bernard's sons will have the disease, and his daughters will be carriers.
③ There is a 50% chance that each of Bernard's children will have hemophilia.

④ Bernard's sons will be normal, and his daughters will be carriers.

111. Which one of the following is the best indicator of a successful outcome in long-term treatment of a teenager with hemophilia?
① Bleeding episodes are prevented or treated early.
② The teen is able to keep up with peers academically.
③ Weight is maintained within age-appropriate ranges.
④ A realistic career goal is chosen.

112. Angela Rodriguez brings her 1-year-old son, Roberto, in for a well-child examination. Which of the following activities would Roberto be expected to do at this age?
① Speak with a vocabulary of 10 words.
② Walk well, forward and backward.
③ Move around solid objects.
④ Feed himself with a spoon.

113. A tuberculin test is administered to a toddler using a purified protein derivative. The site must be checked in 48 hours and 72 hours. Which of the following most accurately describes a positive reaction?
① A pruritic rash on the arm
② Fever and coughing
③ Induration of 10 mm at the site
④ A 3 mm area of erythema and swelling

114. Andrew, age 7, has tuberculosis and is being treated through the clinic. Which comment by his mother indicates that she understands discharge instructions related to his care?
① "Andrew must remain home from school until his x-rays are normal."
② "Andrew must have weekly sputum tests."
③ "Andrew should wear a mask whenever he goes out in public."
④ "Andrew must take his medication daily for at least 6 months."

115. Which instruction should be included in the teaching plan for a 6-year-old before cardiac catheterization?
① "The test will last about 15 minutes."
② "You will be told to walk around the room during the test."
③ "You will be on bed rest for two days after the test."
④ "You will have a warm feeling when the doctor puts the medicine into the tubing."

116. After cardiac catheterization, which one of the following findings in the child should the nurse immediately report to the physician?
① Temperature increase from 98.4° to 99.8°F rectally.
② One-centimeter area of brownish-red drainage on the dressing at the insertion site.
③ Irritability of the child.
④ Coldness of the affected extremity when compared with the unaffected one.

117. Mark, 28 months old, is hospitalized. His mother tells the nurse she must leave. Mark hears her and begins to cry loudly. Which action by the nurse would be best at this time?
① Ask his mother to encourage his father to stay.
② Stay with Mark and try to comfort him.
③ Ask his mother to stay until Mark goes to sleep.
④ Encourage his mother not to visit for a while.

118. Seven-year-old Eric has been admitted for cardiac tests because of increasing fainting spells. While taking Eric's vital signs, the nurse notes a sinus arrhythmia. Which of the following nursing actions would you do initially?
① Obtain a 12-lead ECG.
② Ask Eric to hold his breath while auscultating for an apical pulse.
③ Perform carotid massage.
④ Administer oxygen.

119. Calm Beldon, 3 years old, was brought by his parents to the emergency room because of respiratory distress, an elevated temperature, and nasal congestion. A loud systolic murmur was noted over the left sternal border. His diagnosis was a large ventricular septal defect. Which abnormal condition results from this defect?
① Peripheral hypoxia
② Elevated hemoglobin and hematocrit
③ Volume overload in the lungs
④ Decreased blood pressure

120. Jesse, age 18 months, has a ventricular septal defect that will be repaired when he is 3 years old. Until then, which of the following instructions to his parents would be least realistic?
① Jesse should receive a normal series of vaccines.
② No restrictions or limits are needed.
③ Jesse may experience polycythemia.
④ Jesse can set his own limits on exercise and activities.

121. Which of the following statements is true regarding congenital heart defects?
① In cyanotic defects, pressure on the right side of the heart is higher than on the left.
② In cyanotic defects, there is no mixing of oxygenated and unoxygenated blood in systemic circulation.
③ In cyanotic defects, blood is shunted from the left side of the heart to the right.
④ Acyanotic defects are usually much more complex than cyanotic defects.

122. The nurse is ready to administer digoxin to an 8-year-old girl. Her apical pulse is 60. Which action by the nurse is *most* appropriate?
① Call an emergency alert because the child is in heart block.
② Give the digoxin because the pulse is within normal range.
③ Take the radial pulse and compare it with the apical pulse.
④ Withhold the digoxin and notify the physician.

123. The nurse must administer 85 μg of digoxin bid. The

elixir comes 50 μg/ml. How many milliliters would the nurse give?

① 0.58 ml
② 1.7 ml
③ 2.55 ml
④ 3.4 ml

124. Which response would be *unexpected* from digoxin administration?

① Slower heart rate
② Greater force in myocardial contraction
③ Accelerated AV node conduction
④ Increased urinary output

125. Hypothermia is used in open-heart surgery to

① Lessen the dangers of postoperative febrile episodes.
② Stop cardiac activity.
③ Minimize respiratory action.
④ Reduce overall body metabolism.

126. For which of the following conditions would the nurse clamp off a child's thoracotomy tube?

① The appearance of large amounts of serosanguineous drainage in the tubing.
② Disconnection of the tubing.
③ Obstruction of the drainage flow because of clots.
④ Walking down the hall.

127. Richard, age 6, has had a repair of his atrial septal defect. Which of the following nursing actions would best help Richard to cough?

① Clamp off the thoracotomy tube.
② Stimulate the cough reflex with a suction catheter.
③ Support the chest with both hands.
④ Sit him in high Fowler's position.

128. The nurse notices 3-year-old Tracy sucking his thumb 2 days after cardiac surgery. Which action would be most appropriate?

① Discuss with the parents how to break this habit.
② Gently remove the thumb from his mouth while diverting his attention.
③ Recognize that his behavior is expected regression and allow him to continue.
④ Request permission to give him ice chips or sips of water by mouth.

129. Which of the following is a common finding on assessment of the infant with coarctation of the aorta?

① Presence of squatting spells
② Weak femoral pulse
③ Tachycardia during feeds
④ Clubbing of fingers and toes

130. Which of the following accurately describes the pathophysiology underlying the clinical manifestations of tetralogy of Fallot?

① Pulmonary hypertension from congested pulmonary circulation.
② Blood entering the aorta from the left side of the heart.
③ Deoxygenated and oxygenated blood mixing in the left side of the heart.
④ Deoxygenated blood recirculating without any communication with pulmonary blood flow.

131. The parents of a 2-year-old scheduled for closure of a patent ductus arteriosus are instructed that the purpose of surgery is to

① Stop unoxygenated blood from entering the systemic circulation.
② Decrease edema in the lower extremities.
③ Prevent oxygenated blood from returning to the lungs.
④ Increase the oxygenated blood in the systemic circulation.

132. To evaluate improvement in a child with rheumatic fever, the nurse would monitor which of the following tests?

① Alkaline phosphate and white blood cell count
② Throat culture
③ Antistreptolysin O (ASO) titer and erythrocyte sedimentation rate
④ Nasal smear for eosinophils and blood culture

133. The parents of a toddler share their frustration with the nurse about their son's temper tantrums. Which parental response to the tantrums would best indicate that they are handling him appropriately?

① Ignoring the tantrum.
② Reasoning with him during the tantrum.
③ Restraining him during the tantrum.
④ Placing him alone after the tantrum.

134. The nurse evaluates the pain management of a hospitalized 15-year-old in sickle cell crisis as effective by which of the following assessments?

① The child sleeps at regular intervals, is arousable and oriented, and rates pain as 2 or 3 on a scale of 1 to 10.
② The child clutches his abdomen in fetal position and moans frequently, but denies any pain.
③ The child sleeps continuously and is difficult to awaken; falls back to sleep when asked to rate pain.
④ The child cries intermittently and then falls asleep; when awake, rates pain as 4 or 5 on a scale of 1 to 10.

135. Seven-month-old Tyler has been referred to the pediatric clinic by the public health nurse because of suspected nonorganic failure-to-thrive syndrome. His mother is a 19-year-old single parent who lives alone with her son. Nursing assessment of Tyler is most likely to reveal

① Separation anxiety.
② Stiff posture when held.
③ Increased response to sensory and verbal stimuli.
④ Intense eye-to-eye contact.

136. A first-year nursing student in the clinic asks what causes nonorganic failure-to-thrive syndrome. The best reply would be that the most common cause is

① Intestinal malabsorption.
② Sensory overload.
③ Parent's limited knowledge of feeding technique.
④ Disruption in parent-infant attachment.

137. During the assessment of 1-year-old Christian, the nurse observes that he has good head control and can roll over, but he cannot sit up without support or transfer an object from one hand to another. Based on this

observation, the nurse concludes that Christian is at what developmental age?
1. 3 to 4 months
2. 5 to 6 months
3. 9 to 10 months
4. 7 to 8 months

138. A plan of care to meet the needs of an infant with failure to thrive would *not* include
1. A schedule of stimulation geared to the infant's present level of development.
2. A plan to teach the primary caregiver ways to provide stimulation.
3. A plan to have staff members pick him up and play with him whenever they can.
4. Consistency in care and caregiver.

139. Which nursing action would receive priority in the plan of care for an infant with failure to thrive?
1. Help his mother find a job.
2. Provide his mother with growth and development information.
3. Praise his mother's nurturing behaviors.
4. Encourage sibling visitation.

140. Which toys are *least* appropriate for a 7-month-old?
1. Stacking blocks
2. Large rattles
3. Colored mobiles
4. Squeeze toys

141. What is the best indication of improvement in an infant with failure to thrive?
1. Exploring the toys in his crib
2. Daily weight gain
3. Good eye contact
4. Absence of vomiting

142. Louann, 27 months old, is admitted to the pediatric unit with a 2-day history of episodic vomiting and mild diarrhea. Her weight is 15 kg, down from 16 kg. When performing an assessment of Louann, which of the following would the nurse *not* expect to find?
1. Pallor
2. Low blood pressure
3. Urine specific gravity of 1.08
4. Tachycardia

143. The physician orders an IV for a 4½-year-old boy with asthma. Based on his developmental stage, he will most likely view the starting of his IV as
1. A sign of powerlessness.
2. Necessary treatment to regain health.
3. Punishment for a previous misdeed.
4. An indicator that he is very sick.

144. The physician orders KCl 20 mEq/L to be added to the IV of a 2-year-old who is dehydrated. Before adding potassium to the child's IV, which nursing assessment would be most important?
1. Apical heart rate
2. Intake and output
3. Blood pressure
4. Heart rate

145. The nurse caring for a 14 kg 2-year-old hospitalized with dehydration is evaluating the plan of care for the past 4 hours. Which finding best indicates ineffectiveness of fluid replacement therapy and continued fluid volume deficit?
1. Urine specific gravity of 1.018
2. Urine output of 26 ml in 4 hours
3. Blood urea nitrogen of 10
4. Hematocrit of 38%

146. What acid-base imbalance occurs with frequent watery diarrhea?
1. Metabolic acidosis with slow, shallow respirations
2. Metabolic alkalosis with deep, rapid respirations
3. Metabolic alkalosis with slow, shallow respirations
4. Metabolic acidosis with deep, rapid respirations

147. Which of the following foods would *not* be acceptable to include in the diet of a child who is recovering from severe diarrhea and dehydration?
1. Applesauce
2. Yogurt
3. Saltines
4. Bananas

148. Georgette Blackman, age 22 months, is admitted to the pediatrics unit with lethargy, decreased breath sounds, and moderate dehydration. She is placed in a mist tent for humidification oxygen therapy. When monitoring Georgette, what indicates a negative response to therapy?
1. Pulse oximetry of 98%
2. Hypothermia
3. Decreasing amount of adventitious breath sounds
4. Capillary refill of less than 2 seconds

149. The nurse plans to meet the psychosocial needs of an 8-month-old during his gastrostomy tube feedings. Which one of the following actions will best meet the needs of an infant during alternative feeding methods?
1. Talking to him
2. Stroking him
3. Playing a music box
4. Giving him a pacifier

150. Michaela is to receive 375 ml of IV fluid over 8 hours. Using a microdrip, what is the desired rate of drops per minute?
1. 10
2. 23
3. 47
4. 94

151. Claudia, age 9, is receiving ampicillin for a lower respiratory tract infection. Before the nurse administers the next dose of ampicillin, Claudia informs the nurse that she has begun to have diarrhea. What should the nurse do?
1. Institute isolation precautions.
2. Change to a different antibiotic.
3. Administer the dose on time, and consult the physician.
4. Withhold the ampicillin and consult the physician about changing the antibiotic.

152. Which expected outcome would be best to evaluate the effectiveness of fluid therapy for a 6-month-old hospitalized with dehydration?
1. Blood pressure is within normal range for age.
2. Electrolytes are within normal limits.

③ Infant returns to preillness weight.
④ Urine specific gravity is above 1.030.

153. Angela, age 4, is admitted with frequent diarrhea, respiratory distress, and high fevers. How would the nurse best take her temperature?
① Oral temperatures
② Rectal temperatures
③ Axillary temperatures
④ Either oral or rectal temperatures

154. Ceftriaxone (Rocephin), 325 mg, is ordered for IM injection. The multidose vial is labeled 0.25 g/ml. How many milliliters of the medication would the patient receive?
① 0.65 ml
② 1.22 ml
③ 1.3 ml
④ 2.6 ml

155. Reginald, age 18 months, is receiving amoxicillin at home for a middle ear infection. Which of the following should the nurse include in the teaching care plan to ensure optimal absorption of the liquid form of amoxicillin?
① Administer with milk.
② Administer on an empty stomach.
③ Avoid shaking the container.
④ Store at room temperature.

156. Claudell, 2½ years old, was admitted to the hospital for the second surgical repair of his cleft palate. His mother cannot stay overnight with her son or visit because of unexpected illness. What information on admission is least important in developing a care plan for Claudell?
① His sleeping habits
② His feeding habits and ability to drink from a cup
③ His ability to drink from a cup
④ His ability to communicate

157. Sixteen-month-old Justin has been admitted to the hospital. His parents are unable to stay with him. On the morning after admission, Justin is standing in his crib crying. He refuses to be comforted and calls for his mother. The nurse approaches him to bathe him and he screams louder. She recognizes this behavior as which of the following stages of settling in?
① Protest
② Depression
③ Denial
④ Bargaining

158. What would be the most helpful nursing action when approaching a hospitalized toddler to bathe him if his mother is unavailable to help?
① Pick him up and walk him around the room.
② Sit at the bedside and spend time with him until his anxiety has decreased.
③ Be firm and begin with his bath.
④ Chart the behaviors and let the next shift bathe him.

159. After surgical repair of a cleft palate, the infant would be placed in which position?
① On his abdomen
② On his back

③ Fowler's position
④ Any position that is comfortable for him

160. To prevent an infant from damaging the surgical repair of a cleft lip, the nurse would apply which of the following?
① Mummy restraints
② Elbow restraints
③ Wrist restraints
④ Gauze wrapping on the infant's hands

161. It is 1 day after the cleft lip repair of a 16-month-old patient. Which activity is most appropriate for him?
① Play with a toy piano.
② Listen to a volunteer read a story.
③ Watch MTV.
④ Put together a puzzle with large pieces.

162. A 2-year-old has been in the hospital without his parents for 3 days. He begins to regress and lies quietly in his crib with his blanket. The nurse recognizes that he is now in which stage of separation anxiety?
① Denial
② Despair
③ Mistrust
④ Shock and disbelief

163. Clark, age 25 months, has been hospitalized for a week after surgery. He smiles easily, no longer cries when his father leaves after visiting hours, and goes to the nurses happily. He has not seen his mother since he was admitted to the hospital. What would the nurse understand about Clark's present behavior?
① He feels better physically and so is behaving better.
② He has established a routine and likes the nurses.
③ He is repressing feelings about his mother and has given up fighting separation.
④ He has forgotten about his mother.

164. A mother brings her 5-week-old infant, Mohammed, to the emergency room because she says the infant seems very hungry but has been vomiting over the past 3 days. She says that Mohammed expels the vomitus 2 to 3 feet. The diagnosis of pyloric stenosis is made. During the assessment of Mohammed, what would the nurse expect to find?
① Signs of metabolic acidosis, a palpable olive-shaped mass in the epigastric area, and scanty urination.
② Liquid green stools, dehydration, and signs of metabolic acidosis.
③ Visible peristaltic waves passing from left to right over the epigastric area, dehydration, and weight loss.
④ A palpable sausage-shaped mass in the left upper quadrant, weight loss, and signs of metabolic alkalosis.

165. A 3-week-old infant is receiving his first feeding after a pylorotomy. What position would be most appropriate for him after his feeding?
① Prone
② Semi-Fowler's on his right side
③ Flat on his right side
④ Semi-Fowler's on his left side

166. Ten-year-old Kayla is admitted to the pediatric intensive care unit in a diabetic coma. Kayla's mother is

feeling very guilty because she did not realize that her daughter could have had diabetes. She asks about the early signs of insulin-dependent diabetes in children. Which would Kayla *not* have experienced?

① Increased thirst
② Weight loss
③ Decreased appetite
④ Increased urinary frequency

167. The nurse is teaching a child and her family about the use of glucagon. They would be instructed that the purpose of this drug is to treat which of the following?

① Acidosis
② Hyperglycemia
③ Glycosuria
④ Hypoglycemia

168. Jennifer is an active, athletic 14-year-old with diabetes. What information should Jennifer understand regarding diet, exercise, and insulin?

① There is no need to adjust insulin or food intake before exercise.
② Insulin dosage should be increased before exercise.
③ Insulin dosage should be decreased before exercise.
④ Extra caloric intake should be provided before exercise.

169. The nurse evaluates consistency in the blood glucose levels of a child with diabetes by monitoring which one of the following?

① Fasting blood glucose
② Glycosylated hemoglobin (hemoglobin A_{1C})
③ Glucose tolerance test
④ Urine tests for glucose

170. A diabetic teenager is being taught about the major signs and symptoms of hypoglycemia. Which of the following would *not* be included?

① Hunger
② Tremors
③ Diaphoresis
④ Thirst

171. In planning care for a 4-year-old with diabetes, the nurse should be aware that the child's greatest fear related to her disease will most likely be

① Inability to control her diet.
② Daily insulin injections.
③ Death.
④ Rejection by her peers.

172. Sixteen-year-old Alisha has recently been diagnosed with diabetes. Which of the following situations would indicate that Alisha is at greatest risk for a hypoglycemic reaction?

① She has not taken her insulin for 3 days.
② Her urine test is positive for acetone.
③ Her urine test is negative for glucose.
④ She had an injection of NPH insulin 30 minutes ago.

173. Fourteen-year-old Adele, who has diabetes, has been invited to a slumber party. Which option indicates the most appropriate action to meet her developmental needs?

① Adjust her diet and insulin before going to the party so she does not need to eat.
② Have Adele explain to her friends that she is diabetic and will bring her own sugar-free drinks.
③ Keep Adele at home until she knows her diet restrictions.
④ Have Adele's mother call her friend's mother to explain her condition.

174. Four-year-old Benjamin was diagnosed with cystic fibrosis at 9 months of age. He has done well since then, but he is currently hospitalized for evaluation of his treatment. Which behavioral assessment is most age appropriate for Benjamin?

① He enjoys riding his bicycle.
② He has an imaginary friend named Germaine.
③ He enjoys collecting stamps.
④ He overidentifies with his peers (clothes etc.).

175. The nurse evaluates her teaching plan for the parents of a 10-month-old infant diagnosed with cystic fibrosis. The mother demonstrates an understanding of the nurses' instructions regarding pancreatic enzymes when she states:

① "I'll dilute the enzymes in a bottle of formula after each meal."
② "I'll dilute the enzymes in a bottle of water before each meal."
③ "I'll mix the enzymes in food, such as a bowl of rice cereal, during each meal."
④ "I'll mix the enzymes in a small amount of food, such as applesauce, before each meal."

176. Which one of the following statements accurately describes the pathophysiology of cystic fibrosis?

① It is a diffuse disease with formation of fibrous cysts throughout many organs of the body.
② It is a disease resulting from atrophic changes in the intestinal wall.
③ It is a genetic disease caused by an antigen-antibody immune response in the body.
④ It is an exocrine gland disease with thick, mucus secretions blocking various body organs.

177. Which problem is least likely to be present in a child with cystic fibrosis?

① Large, bulky stools
② Frequent urinary tract infections
③ Thick mucoid secretions
④ Delayed puberty

178. Which information should not be included in discharge teaching for a child with cystic fibrosis?

① The child's diet should be low in fat content.
② Restrict the child's fluids to reduce excessive sweating.
③ Encourage physical activities.
④ High-salt foods such as pretzels should be a regular part of the child's diet.

179. The parents of an infant diagnosed with cystic fibrosis are concerned about having another child because they fear any future children will also have cystic fibrosis. Which one of the following responses by the

nurse is true regarding the probability that their future children would have cystic fibrosis?
1. "All of your future children will also have cystic fibrosis."
2. "None of your future children will have cystic fibrosis."
3. "With each pregnancy, there is a 25% chance that the child will have cystic fibrosis."
4. "With each pregnancy, there is a 50% chance that the child will have cystic fibrosis."

180. Nine-month-old Brian is hospitalized with pneumonia. Because this is his third respiratory infection, cystic fibrosis is suspected. His parents should be instructed that which one of the following tests will confirm the diagnosis of cystic fibrosis?
1. Chest x-ray
2. Stool for fecal fat
3. pH analysis of gastric secretions
4. Pilocarpine iontophoresis

181. Reuben Gonzales, age 6, was admitted yesterday with acute glomerulonephritis and hematuria. He has orders for bed rest, intake and output, blood pressure q2h, sodium-restricted diet, and daily weights. What additional clinical sign would the nurse expect Reuben to exhibit?
1. Severe, generalized edema
2. Hypokalemia
3. Weight loss
4. Elevated blood pressure

182. What nursing diagnosis has the highest priority for a child with glomerulonephritis?
1. Fluid volume excess related to decreased plasma filtration.
2. Potential impaired skin integrity related to lowered body defenses.
3. Fluid volume deficit (intravascular) related to protein loss.
4. Activity intolerance related to fatigue.

183. The nurse can expect which test result to be elevated with glomerulonephritis?
1. Liver enzymes
2. Serum albumin
3. Serum antidiuretic hormone
4. Antistreptolysin O titer (ASO)

184. Eddie Lee, age 8, has just been admitted to the hospital with acute glomerulonephritis. His mother is with him. What is the primary nursing action to use when working with Eddie's mother?
1. Inform her that her son needs more independence, and encourage her to let him take care of himself.
2. Spend time at Eddie's bedside to explain hospital rules and procedures, and answer any questions that the family may have.
3. Encourage Mrs. Lee to attend the classes in family health education.
4. Teach her the basic functions of the kidneys.

185. Evidence of improvement in a 3-year-old with nephrosis includes all of the following *except*
1. Increased urine output.
2. Increased appetite.
3. Increased weight.
4. Decreased abdominal girth.

186. In planning for a child hospitalized with nephrosis, the nurse writes which one of the following expected outcomes?
1. The child will have decreased albuminemia.
2. The child will have decreased proteinuria.
3. The child will have increased urine specific gravity.
4. The child will have increased blood urea nitrogen.

187. Myra, age 13, reluctantly comes into the emergency room, brought by her mother. Myra states, "I'm OK now, my stomach doesn't hurt as much." Her mother says that Myra has been complaining of abdominal pain, has been vomiting for 8 hours, is anorexic, and has been walking with a slight limp. As they got into the car to drive to the hospital, Myra said that the pain was better. Which admitting order would the nurse question?
1. Admit for observation.
2. Give a clear-liquid diet.
3. Get a complete blood cell count.
4. Get an abdominal x-ray.

188. Kelly O'Brien, age 12, is observed lying on her back with her knees drawn up 2 days after surgery for a ruptured appendix. Her respirations are irregular, temperature is normal, and her skin is warm and dry. Her abdomen is distended. When Kelly sees the nurse, she cries, "I'm so miserable, the pain is terrible." What initial nursing action is most appropriate?
1. Check the surgical site for bleeding.
2. Calm Kelly down and reevaluate her pain in 1 hour.
3. Check patency of nasogastric drainage tube.
4. Ambulate her after administering an analgesic per physician's orders.

189. Bart, age 4, is admitted to the hospital for an appendectomy. Considering his developmental stage, which of the following would pose the greatest threat to him?
1. Surgical incision and IV
2. Separation from parents
3. Loss of independence
4. Fear of strange noises

190. Daniel Cortese, a newborn, has Hirschsprung's disease. Which is not a characteristic of this disease?
1. Refusal to take liquids
2. Failure to pass meconium within 24 to 48 hours after birth
3. Abdominal distention
4. Frequent, greenish stools

191. Which of the following is a characteristic of Hirschsprung's disease in the older infant?
1. Increased weight gain
2. Constipation
3. Bile-stained vomiting
4. Steatorrhea

192. When Hirschsprung's disease is not diagnosed in infancy, the nurse's role in later diagnostic workup would focus on which of the following?
① Bowel habits
② Disposition
③ Feeding habits
④ Skin color

193. A double-barrel colostomy is frequently performed on children with Hirschsprung's disease after resection of the affected part of the colon. The nurse accurately evaluates the functioning of this type of colostomy in which of the following ways?
① Both the proximal end and the distal end excrete feces.
② Only the proximal end excretes feces.
③ The proximal end allows for excretion of feces; the distal end excretes mucus.
④ The proximal end allows for excretion of mucus; the distal end excretes feces.

194. Initial postoperative care after colon resection does *not* include
① A clear-liquid diet.
② Nasogastric suction.
③ Frequent abdominal dressing changes.
④ IV feedings to replace electrolytes.

195. A diet low in residue is encouraged postoperatively when full bowel function returns. A low-residue diet would *not* include which of the following foods?
① Jams and preserves
② White bread
③ Vanilla ice cream
④ Spaghetti with cream sauce

196. A hospitalized 2-year-old is scheduled for a barium enema for the diagnosis and reduction of an intussusception. Which one of the following findings indicates effectiveness of this procedure?
① Passage of fewer liquid, green stools
② Increased bowel sounds
③ Passage of a brown, soft, formed stool
④ Decreased abdominal girth

197. Scoliosis can most easily be detected if the students are asked to assume which position during a school physical?
① Bend at the waist, to the right, and then to the left.
② Stand straight, and then face the nurse with arms raised overhead.
③ Bend forward at the waist with head and arms hanging freely.
④ Stand straight with back to the nurse and arms held out in front of the body.

198. Whilma DeSantis, age 9, was found to have scoliosis during her school sports physical. Whilma, also a budding gymnast, indicated that she did not want to wear a back brace. Which developmental need best explains Whilma's desire not to wear a brace?
① Change in body image
② Competency and esteem
③ Identity confusion
④ Body injury

199. Denise, age 15, was diagnosed with a 35-degree lateral curve scoliosis several months ago. Since that time, she has had numerous changes in her personality, fluctuating from moody to friendly to sullen. Which of the following is the least plausible explanation for her current behavior?
① Denise fears changes in body image.
② Denise is acting like a normal adolescent.
③ Denise is experiencing changes in hormonal activity.
④ Denise is afraid of not making the cheerleading squad.

200. When teaching a patient about what to expect when she wears a Milwaukee brace for scoliosis, the nurse would best explain that
① The brace is worn only at night.
② Frequent adjustments of the brace will be needed because of rapid growth rates during adolescence.
③ Treatment of scoliosis is long-term, but the brace will be required for only a few months.
④ A tight fit is necessary, regardless of the discomfort.

201. How does a 12-year-old girl with scoliosis probably compare in physical development to boys her age?
① She is probably 2 years behind them.
② She is developing at about the same rate.
③ She is probably 2 years ahead of most boys her age.
④ Her physical development cannot be accurately assessed because she has scoliosis.

202. Which of the following is the correct positioning for a child in Bryant's traction?
① The child's buttocks are resting on the bed and both legs are suspended at right angles to the bed.
② The child's buttocks are slightly elevated from the bed and both legs are suspended at right angles to the bed.
③ The child's buttocks are elevated on a pillow and both legs are suspended at right angles to the bed.
④ The child's buttocks and legs are flat on the bed with the pull of traction coming from the front of the bed.

203. Which of the following roommates would be least appropriate for Alisha, a 7-year-old girl with acute lymphocytic leukemia?
① Joey, a 7-year-old with a fractured femur
② Heather, a 7-year-old with cystic fibrosis
③ Josephine, a 7-year-old with a ruptured appendix
④ Janet, a 7-year-old with a brain tumor

204. Lauren, age 14, will have to undergo many diagnostic tests for possible osteogenic sarcoma. Which of the following most accurately reflects an appropriate outcome regarding Lauren's acceptance of these tests?
① The tests do not involve any risk.
② The parents should not be present at all tests.
③ Eventually the tests will become routine and tolerable.
④ Lauren and her parents need to express their feelings about the experience.

205. Which of the following solutions would be most appropriate to use initially when flushing the IV tubing after a blood transfusion?
① Salt-poor albumin
② Normal saline

③ Dextrose and water
④ Heparinized saline

206. Antonio has a reaction to a transfusion. Which behavior is *not* indicative of a reaction to a blood transfusion?
① Shivering
② Urticaria
③ Hypertension
④ Dyspnea

207. What is the initial nursing action for a patient experiencing a transfusion reaction?
① Notify the physician.
② Place in Trendelenburg's position.
③ Stop the transfusion.
④ Monitor pulse, respirations, and blood pressure.

208. Seven-year-old Bailey has acute lymphocytic leukemia and often has episodes of epistaxis. When this occurs, what would be the best initial action?
① Place her in a supine position with a small pillow under her neck.
② Place her in semi-Fowler's or high Fowler's position.
③ Administer oxygen through nasal cannula at 4 L/min.
④ Instruct her to gently blow her nose to dislodge the clot.

209. Danielle, age 4, has leukemia. While in the hospital she spikes a temperature of 103°F (39.4°C) axillary. Which of the following nursing actions would be contraindicated?
① Encourage clear fluids as tolerated.
② Monitor vital signs qh to q2h.
③ Take a rectal temperature.
④ Sponge-bathe her with tepid water.

210. Lester Brown, a 4½-year-old with advanced leukemia, has been having nightmares. Which statement least describes his thoughts regarding death?
① He identifies that death is permanent.
② He cannot verbalize his concerns.
③ He believes that he will go to sleep.
④ He will miss his parents.

211. Which side effect would *not* be expected with chemotherapy?
① Anorexia
② Alopecia
③ Stomatitis
④ Peeling skin

212. Abul is receiving methotrexate for leukemia. Which of the following is not contraindicated with methotrexate administration?
① Tetracycline
② Aspirin
③ Vitamins with folic acid
④ Antihistamines

213. Leukemic patients are sometimes given allopurinol. This drug is given to prevent which of the following?
① Hypokalemia
② Hyperkalemia
③ Hypouricemia
④ Hyperuricemia

214. The nurse would monitor which one of the following to evaluate the effectiveness of chemotherapy in an 8-year-old child with acute lymphocytic leukemia?
① Complete blood cell count
② Bleeding time
③ Blood and cerebrospinal fluid cultures
④ Blood urea nitrogen

215. Which of the following nursing actions will be most appropriate for Randi while she is receiving allopurinol for leukemia?
① Omit carbonated beverages.
② Provide foods high in protein.
③ Encourage oral fluids.
④ Monitor diet for sucrose intake.

216. Which of the following will be *contraindicated* for a leukemia patient until the disease is in remission?
① Antibiotics
② Immunizations
③ Corticosteroids
④ Bronchodilators

217. Georgianna Sokaris, age 10, is being treated for leukemia at home with vincristine. Her mother calls the clinic to say that Georgianna is complaining of weakness in her hands and feet, numbness, tingling, and jaw pain. What is the nurse's best approach?
① Recognize that Mrs. Sokaris will be very sensitive to any change in her daughter's condition.
② Tell her that this is part of the disease process and that it will disappear in 4 to 6 months.
③ Suggest that Mrs. Sokaris mention this at Georgianna's next checkup.
④ Tell her to notify the physician because these are manifestations of vincristine toxicity.

218. What is the most frequent sign of Wilms' tumor?
① Increasing abdominal girth
② Weight loss
③ Decreased urinary output
④ Hypertension

219. What is the best method of teaching the toddler about preoperative and postoperative care?
① Play using dolls
② Audiovisual devices
③ Verbal explanations
④ Using a child life specialist

220. Preoperative nursing care for the child with Wilms' tumor does *not* include
① Preparing the child and family for preoperative tests.
② Carefully monitoring blood pressure.
③ Palpating the abdomen to identify the tumor size.
④ Planning for postoperative care.

221. What is the overall goal in planning for discharge of a child with cancer?
① Decrease the effects of chemotherapy.
② Prevent nausea and vomiting.
③ Plan for psychologic support.
④ Return the child to a normal lifestyle.

222. Which of the following is most important in helping parents learn about the postoperative home care needs of a child?
① Include the parents in implementing the care plans while the child is still in the hospital.

② Give the parents informative home care literature to read.

③ Postpone teaching until discharge is imminent.

④ Allow the parents free time before teaching is begun.

REFERENCES

Bindler R, Howry L: *Pediatric drugs and nursing implications,* Newark, Conn, 1991, Appleton & Lange.

Johnson K: *The Harriett Lane handbook,* ed 13, St Louis, 1994, Mosby.

Keller L, Weir A: *The Skidmore-Roth outline series: pediatric nursing,* El Paso, Tex, 1993, Skidmore-Roth.

McKenny L, Salerno E: *Mosby's pharmacology in nursing,* St Louis, 1995, Mosby.

Parkinson C: *Study guide and workbook to accompany McCance and Huether's pathophysiology,* ed 2, St Louis, 1994, Mosby.

Pipes P, Trahms C: *Nutrition in infancy and childhood,* ed 5, St Louis, 1993, Mosby.

Smith D: *Comprehensive child and family nursing skills,* St Louis, 1991, Mosby.

Whaley L, Wong D: *Nursing care of infants and children,* ed 5, St Louis, 1995, Mosby.

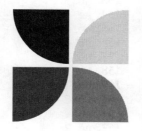

Correct Answers

1. no. 2		**47.** no. 4	
2. no. 1		**48.** no. 2	
3. no. 2		**49.** no. 2	
4. no. 1		**50.** no. 3	
5. no. 4		**51.** no. 3	
6. no. 2		**52.** no. 3	
7. no. 2		**53.** no. 3	
8. no. 4		**54.** no. 2	
9. no. 4		**55.** no. 4	
10. no. 4		**56.** no. 2	
11. no. 4		**57.** no. 3	
12. no. 1		**58.** no. 4	
13. no. 3		**59.** no. 1	
14. no. 1		**60.** no. 4	
15. no. 1		**61.** no. 3	
16. no. 3		**62.** no. 1	
17. no. 3		**63.** no. 3	
18. no. 4		**64.** no. 3	
19. no. 4		**65.** no. 1	
20. no. 4		**66.** no. 2	
21. no. 2		**67.** no. 2	
22. no. 3		**68.** no. 4	
23. no. 2		**69.** no. 4	
24. no. 1		**70.** no. 2	
25. no. 2		**71.** no. 3	
26. no. 4		**72.** no. 4	
27. no. 3		**73.** no. 3	
28. no. 1		**74.** no. 2	
29. no. 1		**75.** no. 2	
30. no. 1		**76.** no. 3	
31. no. 2		**77.** no. 1	
32. no. 4		**78.** no. 2	
33. no. 2		**79.** no. 4	
34. no. 2		**80.** no. 3	
35. no. 4		**81.** no. 1	
36. no. 1		**82.** no. 4	
37. no. 2		**83.** no. 1	
38. no. 1		**84.** no. 3	
39. no. 2		**85.** no. 3	
40. no. 1		**86.** no. 2	
41. no. 2		**87.** no. 3	
42. no. 3		**88.** no. 2	
43. no. 3		**89.** no. 2	
44. no. 4		**90.** no. 3	
45. no. 4		**91.** no. 2	
46. no. 1		**92.** no. 2	

93. no. 4
94. no. 1
95. no. 1
96. no. 3
97. no. 4
98. no. 4
99. no. 1
100. no. 2
101. no. 3
102. no. 2
103. no. 2
104. no. 3
105. no. 1
106. no. 3
107. no. 4
108. no. 4
109. no. 4
110. no. 4
111. no. 1
112. no. 3
113. no. 3
114. no. 4
115. no. 4
116. no. 4
117. no. 2
118. no. 2
119. no. 3
120. no. 2
121. no. 1
122. no. 4
123. no. 2
124. no. 3
125. no. 4
126. no. 2
127. no. 3
128. no. 3
129. no. 2
130. no. 3
131. no. 3
132. no. 3
133. no. 1
134. no. 1
135. no. 2
136. no. 4
137. no. 2
138. no. 3
139. no. 3
140. no. 1
141. no. 2
142. no. 2
143. no. 3
144. no. 2
145. no. 2
146. no. 4
147. no. 2
148. no. 2
149. no. 4
150. no. 3
151. no. 4
152. no. 3

153. no. 3
154. no. 3
155. no. 2
156. no. 4
157. no. 1
158. no. 2
159. no. 1
160. no. 2
161. no. 2
162. no. 2
163. no. 3
164. no. 3
165. no. 2
166. no. 3
167. no. 4
168. no. 4
169. no. 2
170. no. 4
171. no. 2
172. no. 2
173. no. 2
174. no. 2
175. no. 4
176. no. 4
177. no. 2
178. no. 2
179. no. 3
180. no. 4
181. no. 4
182. no. 1
183. no. 4
184. no. 2
185. no. 3
186. no. 2
187. no. 2
188. no. 3
189. no. 4
190. no. 4
191. no. 2
192. no. 1
193. no. 3
194. no. 1
195. no. 1
196. no. 3
197. no. 3
198. no. 2
199. no. 2
200. no. 2
201. no. 3
202. no. 2
203. no. 2
204. no. 4
205. no. 2
206. no. 3
207. no. 3
208. no. 2
209. no. 3
210. no. 1
211. no. 4
212. no. 4

213. no. 4
214. no. 1
215. no. 3
216. no. 2
217. no. 4

218. no. 1
219. no. 1
220. no. 3
221. no. 4
222. no. 1

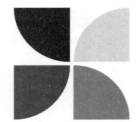

Correct Answers with Rationales

KEY TO ABBREVIATIONS

Section of the Review Book

C = Child
H = Healthy Child
I = Ill and Hospitalized Child
SPP = Sensation, Perception, and Protection
O = Oxygenation
NM = Nutrition and Metabolism
E = Elimination
M = Mobility
CA = Cellular Aberration

Nursing Process Category

AS = Assessment
AN = Analysis
PL = Plan
IM = Implementation
EV = Evaluation

Client Need Category

E = Safe, Effective Care Environment
PS = Physiologic Integrity
PC = Phychosocial Integrity
H = Health Promotion/Maintenance

1. no. 2. Open-ended questions will elicit conversation and allow the client to provide additional information. Option no. 1 could be asked later in the interview; no. 3 is more of a final statement. C/H, IM, H

2. no. 1. Lea should be able to grasp and drink from a cup between 6 and 8 months. Options no. 2, no. 3, and no. 4 are all later milestones. C/H, PL, H

3. no. 2. By 12 months of age, infants should triple their weight and increase their length by 50%, with their head circumference still greater than their chest circumference. C/H, EV, H

4. no. 1. By 2 months, the infant is able to lift his head when lying prone. The infant attempts to roll over at 4 months and turns completely over by 6 months. The

infant begins to sit alone by 6 months and sits alone steadily by 8 months. By 9 months, the infant begins to pull himself to a standing position and by 11 months stands erect with minimal support. Option no. 1 requires further evaluation because this infant is beyond the age expected for achievement of this developmental milestone. All other options include infants who are displaying expected developmental achievement. C/H, AS, EV, H

5. no. 4. Unless the child is developmentally ready, toilet training serves only to train the parent and may produce frustration. C/H, AN, H

6. no. 2. Autonomy and independence are the tasks of this age. Option no. 3 is a task of infancy; options no. 1 and no. 4 are strategies for task achievement. C/H, AN, H

7. no. 2. Setting consistent limits teaches the child self-control and provides a sense of security. Punishment by removing the child from an undesirable situation is effective only if limits are known by the child beforehand. A toddler is unable to reason and cannot readily learn from mistakes. C/H, PL

8. no. 4. Four-year-olds have a decreased appetite because their growth slows. Bone healing requires adequate nutrition, including vitamins. Small helpings of well-balanced meals and nutritious snacks should provide adequate nutrition to meet the demands of healing. C/I, NM, AN, E, PS, H

9. no. 4. Lights help decrease fears of the dark. Allowing the child to control the lights will enable him to control his fear. Exploring the room with a flashlight would increase fears at this age. Options no. 1 and no. 2 do not allow the child to get used to the dark and deal with his overactive imagination. C/H, IM, H

10. no. 4. It is important to acknowledge the child's imagination: this will be the source of creativity in later life. Options no. 1 and no. 2 are not appropriate for a 4-year-old: the child is not truly lying in an adult sense. Option no. 3 does not have the positive aspect that no. 4 has. C/H, IM, H

11. no. 4. Nighttime bladder control is achieved between 4 and 5 years of age. Option no. 4 indicates that the father has realistic expectations of his daughter without negating her self-esteem. This option is supportive and gently encouraging. Option no. 3 places all the responsibility on the child, at the same time indicating by the diapers that the child probably will not be successful. Option no. 2 sets unrealistic expecta-

tions. Option no. 1 is rigid and only emphasizes the child's "failure." C/H, E, EV, H, E

12. no. 1. According to the American Academy of Pediatrics recommended schedule, Georgette should receive DTP and OPV boosters (these should be given once between 4 and 6 years of age). Chickenpox vaccine and hepatitis are recommended to be part of routine infant-toddler immunizations. C/H, PL, PS

13. no. 3. This behavior is normal at this age and should be handled matter-of-factly. However, Gabriella's mother should take the opportunity to explain to both children that there are other, more acceptable ways they can satisfy their curiosity, such as asking their parents questions or reading age-appropriate education materials. C/H, IM, PC

14. no. 1. Most children between 5 and 8 years of age are not aware that they themselves will die; this realization comes around age 9 to 10 years, along with the awareness that death is inevitable for everyone. Option no. 2 is typical of the preschool child who perceives death as sleeping. C/H, AN, H

15. no. 1. Preschoolers need to explore their bodies, but they can begin to learn family and social limits. Option no. 1 indicates that the parent has a healthy attitude toward masturbation without conveying to the child the idea that masturbation is wrong. C/H, H, E

16. no. 3. Depriving a child of food as punishment sets up a control struggle and is unnecessary; withholding other kinds of treats or using methods relevant to the causes of behavior is more effective in teaching healthy habits. C/H, PL, H

17. no. 3. Stressing the importance of good table manners is not relevant to good nutrition. It is more effective to give information or teach the child to increase his own awareness by keeping a journal. C/H, PL, H

18. no. 4. The child is displaying typical signs of separation anxiety. The child requires consistent parental presence and support. Parents should be encouraged to room-in whenever possible and participate in the child's care. C/I, SPP, PL, PC

19. no. 4. The vastus lateralis muscle is a large, well-developed muscle removed from major nerves and blood vessels. It is easily accessible, and a tourniquet can be applied above the injection site if a hypersensitivity reaction occurs. The dorsogluteal site is contraindicated in children who have not been walking for at least 1 year because the gluteal muscles are underdeveloped. Damage to the sciatic nerve can occur with injection into this site. The gluteus minimus and rectus femoris muscles are smaller muscle masses not generally used as injection sites. C/I, PL, IM, E

20. no. 4. A 6-year-old has sufficient understanding of time to prepare cognitively for future events. The general guideline for children between ages 2 and 7 years is to tell them the number of days ahead for each year of age. The day of admission is too late to meet staff. Preadmission tours are advisable. Option no. 2 is unrealistic, and no. 3 would be too graphic and likely to increase fear. C/I, IM, PC

21. no. 2. For school-age children, loss of control and separation from peers are the major fears. Option no.

1 relates to toddlers, no. 3 to adolescents, and no. 4 to preschoolers because of their exaggerated fears and active imaginations. C/I, AN, PC

22. no. 3. This option gives the child realistic information; lying or telling the child not to complain will not help the child adjust. Suggesting that the child might get sick and need a blood transfusion is unnecessary and frightening. Straightforward, simple explanations are best. C/I, IM, E

23. no. 2. Tonsillectomy does not usually involve use of sutures, so the denuded area has the potential to bleed. The area is also highly vascular. Any bleeding dyscrasias must be checked preoperatively. Option no. 1 is elevated in allergic conditions, no. 3 is increased in chronic infections and arthritis, and no. 4 is altered in metabolic acidosis, none of which would be significant for a tonsillectomy. C/I, PL, PS

24. no. 1. Any indication of an infection, such as an elevated temperature, is a contraindication for surgery. The decision must be made by the physician. Options no. 3 and no. 4 might occur after calling the physician. C/SPP, IM, E

25. no. 2. It is imperative that before surgery the nurse assess for any loose teeth in children to prevent aspiration during anesthesia. C/I, SPP, AS, E

26. no. 4. Continuous throat pain is expected after tonsillectomy, which requires analgesia. The child should be told honestly what to expect after surgery. C/I, SPP, PL, E

27. no. 3. After tonsillectomy, hemorrhage from the excised tonsil area may cause blood to trickle down the throat and result in frequent swallowing by the child. Dark, old blood in the emesis and dried blood are common. While increased pulse is a sign of hemorrhage, a pulse rate of 95 is within normal limits for an 8-year-old. C/I, SPP, AS, E

28. no. 1. Clear, cool liquids, including water, crushed ice, and popsicles, are provided initially after tonsillectomy. Milk and milk products are avoided because they cause the child to clear the throat, which may initiate bleeding. Red and brown fluids are avoided to distinguish blood in emesis from the red or brown ingested fluids. C/I, NM, IM, PS

29. no. 1. Children in the hospital need support from parents. Quiet holding and rocking prevent crying and facilitate healing. It is best to keep Christina as quiet as possible, to prevent bleeding. C/SPP, IM, E

30. no. 1. Delayed hemorrhage occurs between the fifth and tenth postoperative day. Recovery should be complete in a week. Gargling is contraindicated. C/SPP, PL, PS

31. no. 2. After tympanostomy tube placement, care must be taken to avoid contaminated water from entering the middle ear and causing infection. The tubes fall out spontaneously within a few months. The external ear may be cleansed with sterile cotton swabs and hydrogen peroxide in the initial postoperative period if drainage is present. Restriction of attendance at school is unnecessary. C/I, SPP, EV, E, H

32. no. 4. A bulging fontanel is the most significant indication of increased intracranial pressure that would re-

sult from cerebral edema secondary to the bacterial infection. Options no. 2 and no. 4 are indicative of dehydration from the vomiting. The specific gravity is normal. C/SPP, AS, PS

33. no. 2. Abnormal cerebrospinal fluid manifests with low glucose, high white blood cell count, positive blood culture, cloudy color, and high protein. If meningitis and increasing cranial pressure are present, there is usually an increased opening pressure. C/I, AN, PS

34. no. 2. Administration of potassium in the presence of diminished renal function may lead to hyperkalemia because potassium is excreted through the kidneys. The other options are insignificant. C/SPP, AS, PS

35. no. 4. Children with meningitis are sensitive to sensory stimuli that can precipitate seizures. The activity involved in bathing could cause a seizure and would be unnecessary during the acute stage of the illness. All other options would be followed. C/SPP, PL, E

36. no. 1. Specific antibiotic therapy must be instituted immediately to prevent death and to avert residual disabilities. Isolation is only needed for 24 hours after antibiotics are begun. Options no. 4 and no. 2 are never appropriate. C/SPP, PL, PS

37. no. 2. Option no. 2 indicates his mother understands that the penicillin must be given for the entire course. Options no. 1 and no. 3 would irritate his throat and increase pain. Option no. 4 is not necessary; the child is no longer considered contagious after receiving the antibiotic for 24 hours. C/I, E, S

38. no. 1. The communicability period for chickenpox (varicella) is from 1 day before eruption of the rash (prodromal stage) to approximately 6 days after the first crop of vesicles when crusts have formed. C/I, SPP, EV, H

39. no. 2. Scratching the anal area at night and insomnia are characteristic of pinworm infestation. Option no. 4 also causes itching, but the parasite infects epidermis, not living tissue. Neither no. 1 nor no. 3 causes anal itching. C/SPP, AN, PS

40. no. 1. Children often regress to previous patterns when they are hospitalized; the 4-year-old child sleeps soundly and may sleep right through the urge to urinate. Putting a 4-year-old in diapers in the hospital is not appropriate because this encourages regression and does not help the child move to the next developmental task. C/SPP, IM, H

41. no. 2. Personnel at both the poison control center and the emergency room will need to know the substance consumed. Observing and waiting for symptoms to develop may use up too much valuable time. C/SPP, IM, PS

42. no. 3. Syrup of ipecac is an emetic. Tepid water in small amounts increases gastric irritation. Option no. 1 is appropriate for hydrocarbon ingestion. By the time symptoms appear, the substance has been absorbed and time has been wasted. Option no. 4 is given *after* an emetic to help absorb many compounds. C/SPP, IM, PS

43. no. 3. She is too young to understand or remember everything that is poisonous. It is the poorest of the four choices. The other options prevent access or condition her to respect medicine. C/SPP, PL, H

44. no. 4. This is the only option that addresses prevention. The parent has actually followed through on what she learned and provided a safe environment for her child. The other options are short term or are aimed at intervention after poisoning has occurred. C/SPP, EV, PS

45. no. 4. Nephrotoxicity is a common side effect of calcium disodium EDTA, as well as lead poisoning. C/I, E, EV, E

46. no. 1. This is characteristic of the 24-month-old child. All the other behaviors are characteristic of a younger child. C/SPP, AS, H

47. no. 4. The nurse should obtain information first before suggesting referral to any specialist or for any blood work. The client must be reassured that confidentiality and respect will be provided. C/SPP, IM, PC

48. no. 2. Her parents are seeking information on possible treatment modalities and starting to focus on the reality of the situation. Option no. 4 is a statement that may be made later in the learning and decision-making process. C/SPP, AN, H

49. no. 2. The only 100% accurate method of preventing the spread of HIV is abstinence. C/SPP, PL, H

50. no. 3. Unfortunately, both the virus and the medications used to counter the advance of HIV can cause many side effects, one of which is developmental delays. Because each child is different, it is difficult to determine whether her condition will improve or deteriorate. C/SPP, EV, PS

51. no. 3. Deborah needs assistance with feeding because of her motor impairment. This approach is the safest while providing motor stability to improve feeding. C/SPP, IM, H

52. no. 3. Reflecting the mother's feelings opens communication for further exploration and expression of her specific concerns. C/SPP, IM, H

53. no. 3. Children with orofacial burns are at risk of developing upper airway edema. Options no. 1 and no. 2 would be done later. Option no. 4 is important information to obtain after the child is stabilized. C/SPP, PL, PS

54. no. 2. Blood volume is reduced from the fluid loss, resulting in poor peripheral absorption. The other options are not true or relevant. C/SPP, AN, PS

55. no. 4. There is no way to accurately determine fluid loss from wounds. The other options are more accurate measures. C/SPP, EV, PS

56. no. 2. Silvadene is an antiinfective agent with broad antimicrobial activity, especially against *Pseudomonas*. It is not a carbonic anhydrase inhibitor, so it does not alter acid-base balance or electrolyte balance or stain tissues, linen, or dressings. It may cause a hypersensitivity reaction or, if absorbed in excess, renal function changes, with urine being monitored for sulfa crystals. C/SPP, AS, PS

57. no. 3. The major cause of death in burn clients is infection, so this is the primary goal. The other options are important secondary goals. C/SPP, PL, PS

58. no. 4. By 9 months, a child can eat ground or pureed

meats. This child needs protein sources that are easily digestible. Options no. 1 and no. 2 contain foods that can cause choking (raisins and hot dogs). Option no. 3 contains egg whites (omelet), which should not be introduced until 1 year of age. C/SPP, EV, H

59. no. 1. Children with Down syndrome are hypotonic, not spastic, and usually only moderately retarded. This decreased muscle tone compromises respiratory excursion, making the child more prone to respiratory infections. Hypotonicity may also delay achievement of motor skills, but developmental potential is greatest during infancy. What to expect must be reinforced with parents because they may see their child developing along a somewhat normal developmental curve and thus come to have unrealistic expectations of the final potential. C/SPP, IM, H

60. no. 4. Although teaching socially acceptable behaviors is important in "normalizing" the child, mentally retarded children need consistency and structure in their daily routines to foster learning and promote security. Limiting stimulation will not promote the mentally retarded child's optimal development. Having the same parent always work with the child to learn new skills is unrealistic. C/SPP, PL, E

61. no. 3. The initial phase of grief is shock and disbelief. C/SPP, AN, PC

62. no. 1. Option no. 1 indicates that Mr. Garcia is beginning to develop an attachment to his baby daughter and recognizes her first as a baby with the usual infant needs. The other options indicate that he has not yet accepted the defect and is still grieving. C/I, SPP, EV, PC

63. no. 3. Rupture of the sac can cause leakage of cerebrospinal fluid and lead to central nervous system infection with permanent brain damage. C/SPP, PL, E

64. no. 3. If a dressing is ordered, it must be kept moist to prevent damage to the fragile covering of the myelomeningocele. C/SPP, IM, E

65. no. 1. The most common complication after surgical closure of a myelomeningocele is hydrocephalus. Daily measurement of the head circumference is essential for early detection and treatment of this complication. C/SPP, AS, PS

66. no. 2. The number of drops per minute is equal to the number of milliliters per hour when a microdrip is used. C/SPP, IM, PS

67. no. 2. Keeping her hips abducted encourages the hip joints to develop normally, decreasing the probability of congenital hip dysplasia. C/SPP, PL, PS

68. no. 4. The first priority is to prevent Francie from injuring herself on the crib rails during the seizure. Tongue blades are never used for seizures. Oxygen would be given only for a prolonged seizure. A patient should not be moved during a seizure. C/SPP, IM, PS

69. no. 4. Although phenytoin may cause malaise, it does not cause excessive sleepiness in children (as phenobarbital may) and is often selected as the drug of choice for this reason. C/SPP, IM, PS

70. no. 2. A high-pitched cry is one of the key manifestations of increased intracranial pressure in infants.

Other signs include bulging fontanel and dilated pupils. Reflexes are not affected. C/SPP, AS, PS

71. no. 3. The shunt may become obstructed with cells or tissue debris. Infection is also a common complication of shunt insertion. C/SPP, AN, PS

72. no. 4. Overhydration can cause an increase in intracranial pressure and thus interfere with shunt functioning or cause damage to brain cells. C/SPP, PL, PS

73. no. 3. The major goal of treatment is to prevent neurologic damage. This is best evaluated by appraising the child's neurologic functioning using cognitive and motor development as indicators. C/SPP, EV, H

74. no. 2. Febrile temperatures usually occur because of a transient disorder; the principle, "it's not how hot the child gets, it's how quickly the child becomes hot," is a good rule to remember and relates to the body's ability to alter its set point with increasing temperature. I/SPP, AS, PS

75. no. 2. An aura is a sensory clue that often precedes a generalized tonic-clonic seizure. Absence seizures do not have an aura. C/SPP, AS, PS

76. no. 3. Sudden withdrawal of medication can precipitate status epilepticus. All other options are correct. C/SPP, EV, H

77. no. 1. The nurse is reflecting what she perceives the father is saying as a way to help him identify his feelings. Guilt is a normal response to SIDS. Options no. 2 and no. 4 are not helpful. Option no. 3 does not respond to the feelings expressed. C/O, IM, PC

78. no. 2. Involvement in a parents' support group indicates the family's willingness to face and deal openly with their daughter's death. C/O, EV, PC

79. no. 4. Wheezy and diminished breath sounds occur because of bronchiolitic obstruction. If a cough were present, it would be moist, not dry. Option no. 3 indicates upper respiratory problems. Expirations are long because air is trapped in the lower field. C/O, AS, PS

80. no. 3. An infant with fast respirations barely has a chance to swallow before he must take another breath, thus making aspiration a real possibility. Hydration is a major concern because the infant loses fluid with each respiration. Options no. 1 and no. 2 are false. C/O, AN, PS

81. no. 1. Accumulation of mucus occurs at the bronchiolar level; therefore suctioning would not be effective. C/O, PL, E

82. no. 4. It is important to provide oxygen as needed, provide adequate nutrition and fluids, monitor output, and provide antiviral (Virazole) medications. Visitors may visit, as long as they, too, follow contact secretion precautions. C/O, PL, E/H

83. no. 1. Performing chest physical therapy before meals minimizes the possibility of vomiting. Every 8 hours is too long an interval. C/O, PL, PS

84. no. 3. An infant's birth weight should double by 5 to 6 months and triple at 1 year (3.8 kg × 3 = 11.4 kg). C/H, AS, H

85. no. 3. Voluntary grasping and improved eye-hand coordination enable the infant to begin picking up finger foods. Options no. 2 and no. 4 would meet his

nutritional needs rather than his developmental needs. Egg whites are not given until after 1 year of age. C/H, PL, H

86. no. 2. Rice cereal is hypoallergenic and is easily digested. The other options have a higher propensity for causing allergy. C/H, PL, H

87. no. 3. Measles, mumps, and rubella will be given at 15 months; the others are given at 18 months. Tuberculin testing provides systematic screening of the population; it is usually done before the measles, mumps, and rubella vaccination. C/O, PL, PS

88. no. 2. Instillation of several milliliters of sterile saline loosens thick secretions and mechanically stimulates the cough reflex. It has nothing to do with sleep patterns, nor is saline a source for fluid intake. The saline instillation makes suctioning more effective. I/O, EV, PS

89. no. 2. The chest should always be auscultated before performing any therapy. Normal saline is not usually instilled every time a child is suctioned, and the child may not tolerate postural drainage. I/O, IM, PS

90. no. 3. The act of suctioning mechanically removes oxygen directly from the airway. Presuction oxygenation replaces that oxygen so that the child does not become hypoxic. Oxygen will not directly relax, but the lack of oxygen will cause her to become agitated. A/O, AN, PS

91. no. 2. Suctioning will improve respiratory exchange; therefore breath sounds will be improved. Options no. 2, no. 3, and no. 4 are evidence of continued respiratory problems. A/O, EV, PS

92. no. 2. Ampicillin destroys the normal flora of the gastrointestinal tract; yogurt will help promote its return. C/O, PL, H

93. no. 4. This indicates that parents understand the time to give Sarah the antibiotic, and need validation of a good idea. Options no. 2 and 3 are not appropriate because side effects could be occurring. There is no telling how long it will be before the next visit, and the parents would need a definite time period for medication administration. C/I, SPP, EV, H

94. no. 1. Cromolyn sodium is a mast cell stabilizer that suppresses histamine release. It is used prophylactically, usually requiring bid or tid dosing. It is not used for acute exacerbations of an asthmatic attack. C/O, AN, PS

95. no. 1. Ten-year-olds can understand some abstract concepts, including math. Options no. 3 and no. 4 are typical of early adolescence, and no. 2 reflects behaviors of the early school-age child. C/H, AS, H

96. no. 3. Medications that interfere with the cough reflex are contraindicated. The priority concern during an acute asthma attack is to promote effective air exchange by loosening secretions so that they can be coughed up and expectorated. C/O, IM, PS

97. no. 4. The 5-year-old is in a stage of concrete operations and needs to test new experiences firsthand. This option emphasizes how she will feel. The others do not. C/H, IM, PL

98. no. 4. Albuterol (Ventolin, Preventil) is considered a first-line medication, whereas epinephrine is no longer

recommended because of its action and side effects. If a child does not respond to albuterol and corticosteroids, hospitalization is usually required, with methylxanthines (of which aminophylline is an example) started IV. Cromolyn is used prophylactically. Penicillin would be used if concurrent infections sensitive to the drug existed. C/I, PL, PS

99. no. 1. An acute asthma attack usually begins with a dry, hacking cough caused by bronchial edema. This progresses to shortness of breath, tightness in the chest, and productive cough. Expiration is prolonged, and wheezing on expiration occurs. The child has difficulty speaking in full sentences, sits upright, sweats profusely, and is restless and apprehensive. Respiratory rate increases. Cyanosis and diminished breath sounds may occur as bronchospasm progresses. C/I, O, AS, PS

100. no. 2. The school-age child's greatest fear is loss of control. This is especially accentuated by frightening experiences such as hospitalization and an acute asthma attack. Options no. 1 and no. 4 would be of lesser priority during recuperation. Option no. 3 is appropriate for younger children. C/O, PL, E

101. no. 3. An acute asthma attack may be triggered by exposure to cold air or overexertion. Bronchospasm may result, precipitating the asthma attack. Children with asthma should be treated as normally as possible, including discipline and regular exercise. Immunizations that are maintained promote health in the child. C/I, O, PL, E, H

102. no. 2. The risk of having an asthma attack is lessened when the asthmatic child's immunizations are up to date and she has received seasonal influenza vaccines. The bedroom should be kept as dust free as possible. An open window while sleeping will permit allergens or cold air to enter; either may trigger an asthma attack. Regular physical exercise without excessive physical exertion is recommended for health maintenance and to promote normal childhood activities. C/I, O, EV, PS, E

103. no. 2. Hemolytic anemia is present throughout the life of a child with sickle cell disease; option no. 1 is a condition seen in infants, and answer no. 3 is a clinical sign common in Down syndrome. Pallor precedes jaundice by several days. C/O, AS, PS

104. no. 3. Infections are a major predisposing factor of crisis episodes, along with strenuous exertion, cold temperatures, dehydration, and environments of low oxygen concentration. C/O, AS, PS

105. no. 1. Heat increases circulation (and oxygen) to the area that needs it most. It is important to handle the child as gently as possible with any interventions. Limiting fluids will also increase the problems with sickling. Cold will enhance vasoconstriction and further occlusion. C/O, IM, E

106. no. 3. This test distinguishes between a heterozygous (trait) and homozygous (disease) genetic pattern. Usually a Sickledex is done for mass screening because it shows that Hb S is present. It does not differentiate between individuals who are heterozygous and homozygous. Option no. 2 is done prenatally to examine amniotic fluid for genetic testing. C/O, AS, H

07. no. 4. Hemarthrosis (bleeding into a joint space) is the classic sign of hemophilia. Manifestations include painful, stiff joints. Options no. 1 and no. 3 would be expected with hemophilia. Although slightly low, platelets of 200,000 are not significant. C/O, AS, PS

08. no. 4. This allows the boy to be involved with his peers and also maintain his interest in football. C/O, PL, PC

09. no. 4. Packed cells do not contain factor VIII, the needed coagulation factor. Coagulation factors are in plasma and cryoprecipitate. C/O, AN, PS

10. no. 4. Hemophilia is a sex-linked recessive disorder transmitted to offspring by female carriers. Bernard's sons will receive a normal sex chromosome from each parent. His daughters will all receive the abnormal Xr chromosome from him and thus will be carriers. C/O, AN, PS

11. no. 1. Prevention and control of bleeding episodes is the priority concern. Therefore the fewer the number of bleeding episodes the child has, the more successful the outcomes of treatment. C/O, EV, H

12. no. 3. A normally developing 1-year-old will be cruising and possibly walking. The other behaviors are accomplished in later months. C/H, AS, H

13. no. 3. The purified protein derivative skin test is interpreted in terms of induration, not erythema. Induration of 10 mm or more is considered positive. A lesion with 5 to 9 mm of induration is considered doubtful, although it may indicate tuberculosis in a child less than 2 years old. C/SPP, AS, PS

14. no. 4. Although there are several different protocols, the usual course of treatment is at least 6 months, with options for a 9- or 12-month sequence. A sputum specimen, if needed, is done only for diagnostic purposes. Children must wear a mask only if they cannot adequately control their coughing and secretions. Children can return to school almost immediately if they are feeling well. C/SPP, EV, H

15. no. 4. When the contrast medium is injected into the catheter, a warm sensation is experienced briefly. The procedure may last several hours, and the child will remain quietly on the table, often sedated. Bed rest for up to 24 hours after catheterization may be ordered. C/I, O, PL, E

16. no. 4. Coldness of the affected extremity may indicate arterial obstruction and requires intervention by the physician. The nurse is responsible for applying pressure 1 inch above the percutaneous site if bleeding occurs. C/I, O, EV, E, PS

17. no. 2. The best course of action for dealing with a hospitalized toddler going through the protest phase of separation anxiety would be to stay with the child and offer support and comfort. C/I, IM, PC

18. no. 2. A sinus arrhythmia is a normal physiologic phenomenon of childhood. The heart rate increases on inspiration and decreases on expiration. Breath holding causes the rate to remain steady, thus allowing assessment between breaths of any potentially pathologic arrhythmia. Carotid dressage is a potentially lethal in-

tervention done only as a last resort for a patient needing cardioversion. C/O, AS, PS

119. no. 3. The left-to-right shunt with a ventricular septal defect causes increased blood flow to the lungs because extra amounts of blood enter the right ventricle and are carried to the lungs through the pulmonary artery. C/O, AN, PS

120. no. 2. Most children with exercise intolerance rest when they need to do so. Option no. 3 is incorrect because a ventricular septal defect is an acyanotic problem that does not cause polycythemia. There is no contraindication to Jesse receiving his immunizations. C/O, IM, E

121. no. 1. In cyanotic defects, blood is shunted from the right to the left; the higher pressures on the right shunt unoxygenated blood to the left side of the heart, where it mixes with oxygenated blood and is pumped to the tissues. Cyanotic defects are more complex than acyanotic defects. C/O, AN, PS

122. no. 4. This is an abnormally slow pulse for an 8-year-old. Digoxin is not given if the pulse rate is below 80 to 100 beats per minute in young children. Bradycardia is a sign of digoxin toxicity. The physician should be notified, but it is not an emergency. Pulse deficit (radial pulse lower than apical) is not a sign of digoxin toxicity, but it may be present with decreased cardiac output.

123. no. 2.
$$\frac{50 \ \mu g}{1} = \frac{85 \ \mu g}{x}$$
$$50x = 85$$
$$x = \frac{85}{50}$$
$$x = 1.7$$
C/O, IM, PS

124. no. 3. Digoxin slows conduction as a result of decreased cardiac rate. It strengthens contractions, and it enhances urinary output by increasing renal perfusion. C/O, AN, PS

125. no. 4. Hypothermia reduces oxygen needs during surgery by decreasing metabolic rate. Too-low temperatures can stop cardiac functioning, an undesirable effect. Option no. 1 is unaffected. Respirations are controlled by a mechanical ventilator. C/O, AN, PS

126. no. 2. A chest drainage system will remove solids, such as fibrin or clotted blood; liquids, such as serous fluids; and gaseous materials. "Milking" the tubes prevents them from becoming plugged with clots or other material. The thoracotomy tube should be immediately clamped if it becomes disconnected to prevent air from entering the pleural cavity and causing a possible tension pneumothorax. It is not necessary to clamp simply for getting out of bed and walking. C/O, IM, PS

127. no. 3. Placement of the nurse's hands on either side of the operative site (encircling the chest) may reduce the pain associated with the coughing procedure by decreasing movement in the area. A side-lying position would encourage better drainage and may be easier for Richard to tolerate than sitting up. Option no. 2 causes a painful cough and is not done to stimulate cough. C/O, IM, PS

128. no. 2. Hospitalization and stress cause regression in toddlers and preschool-age children. Regression is best dealt with by accepting the behavior. Other choices do not convey acceptance. C/O, IM, PC

129. no. 2. Weak or absent femoral pulses result from decreased blood flow to areas of the body distal to the narrowed aorta. Blood pressure to these distal areas is decreased. Cool lower extremities and muscle cramps during exercise are additional manifestations. Elevated blood pressure and bounding pulses occur in body areas receiving blood from vessels proximal to the coarction of the aorta. C/I, AS, PS

130. no. 3. Tetralogy of Fallot is the most common cyanotic heart defect. It consists of four structural defects: ventricular septal defect, dextroposition (overriding) aorta, pulmonic stenosis, and right ventricular hypertrophy. C/I, O, I, E, PS

131. no. 3. Surgical correction of patent ductus arteriosus is recommended for all affected children. The patent ductus arteriosus shunts blood from the higher-pressure aorta to the pulmonary artery for recirculation through the pulmonic circulation and returns it to the left side of the heart. Increased workload on the left ventricle and pulmonary vascular congestion result. C/I, O, PL, E

132. no. 3. An elevated ASO titer occurs as an antibody reaction to a streptococcal infection. An elevated erythrocyte sedimentation rate indicates an inflammatory process. Both should return to normal as child recovers from rheumatic fever. C/I, SPP, EV, E

133. no. 1. Temper tantrums are best handled by ignoring them. Without the attention, toddlers will stop using this behavior. C/O, EV, H

134. no. 1. Effective pain management controls pain without causing severe side effects, such as excessive sedation. Children may deny pain because they fear injection or believe the pain is a punishment for misdeeds. C/I, CA, EV, E/PS

135. no. 2. The infant with failure to thrive avoids eye contact with others, has a flat affect, is withdrawn, and does not exhibit any stranger anxiety. When held, these infants often become stiff and try to pull away. They usually do not respond to sensory stimuli. C/NM, AS, H

136. no. 4. This syndrome usually describes infants who fail to gain weight as a result of psychosocial factors, such as interference with parent-infant attachment or environmental deprivation. Option no. 1 is a possible cause of *organic* failure to thrive. C/NM, AN, PC

137. no. 2. Head control comes at 2 months; rolling over comes at 5 months; sitting without support and transferring objects from one hand to another come at 8 months. Christian is around 5 to 6 months developmentally. C/NM, AN, E

138. no. 3. The infant with failure to thrive needs to have one primary caregiver per shift so that trust can be established; having many persons pick up the child ad lib does not help promote bonding and does not provide consistency. A schedule of stimulation geared to the infant's developmental level and given by the primary caregiver would be more helpful. C/NM, PL, E

139. no. 3. Infant and mother must be cared for as a unit. The infant can be helped most by promoting his mother's feelings of worth and confidence in her mothering role and behaviors. Option no. 2 would be a secondary goal. Once the mother feels better about herself, she will be more able to use the information. C/NM, PL, E

140. no. 1. Stacking blocks are appropriate for a toddler who has developed fine motor control. The others help promote infant development. C/NM, IM, H

141. no. 2. Weight gain reflects the nurturance that the child is receiving and is the most important measure of improvement with nonorganic failure to thrive. The other options are not valid measures of reversal of failure to thrive. C/NM, AN, H

142. no. 2. In mild dehydration, the body compensates for fluid loss with increased heart rate and peripheral vasoconstriction, which maintains a normal blood pressure. The peripheral vasoconstriction decreases blood supply to the kidneys, resulting in a decreased urine output with increased specific gravity. Low blood pressure is a finding in severe dehydration when compensatory mechanisms have failed. C/NM, AS, PS

143. no. 3. Because of their egocentrism, magical thinking, and developing superego (conscience), preschool children frequently view hospitalization and invasive procedures as punishment for previous wrongdoings. The other options reflect more mature thinking abilities. C/NM, AN, PC

144. no. 2. Potassium is excreted by the kidneys; therefore an adequate urine output is essential to prevent hyperkalemia. C/NM, AS, PS

145. no. 2. Adequate urine output for infants and children is 1 ml/kg/hr. Based on this patient's weight of 14 kg, her urine output should be at least 14 ml/hr, or 56 ml for 4 hours. Urine output of only 26 ml in 4 hours indicates fluid volume deficit and possibly impending acute renal failure. C/I, E, EV, E

146. no. 4. With diarrhea, there is a loss of bicarbonate, which results in metabolic acidosis. Compensation is by the respiratory system with hyperventilation. C/NM, AN, PS

147. no. 2. Temporary lactose intolerance is common with diarrhea because of depletion of lactase from the intestines. Therefore milk and milk products should be added last to this patient's diet. The BRATTS diet should be followed: bananas, rice, applesauce, tea, toast, and saltines. C/NM, PL, H

148. no. 2. A negative response would be Georgette's becoming chilled because of the use of cool mist. Improved pulse oximetry, breath sounds, and a quick capillary refill are signs of improvement. C/I, O, EV

149. no. 4. The infant fed through a gastrostomy tube should have sucking needs met. Sucking provides pleasure, relaxation, and exercise for jaw muscles. C/I, SPP, PL, E/PC

150. no. 3. When using the microdrip, drops/min equals ml/hr; 375 ml ÷ 8 hours = 46.87. C/NM, IM, PS

151. no. 4. Antibiotics such as ampicillin are a common

cause of diarrhea in children and sometimes must be discontinued, with the child placed on a different antibiotic. Diarrhea is a side effect of ampicillin and is usually self-limiting. Of particular concern is the fact that dehydration can be a complication of diarrhea. C/NM, IM, PS

52. no. 3. Degree of dehydration in infants is determined by fluid volume loss. The most accurate assessment of fluid loss is through body weight. C/I, PL/EV, E

53. no. 3. Take axillary temperatures to avoid irritating the anal area or increasing her respiratory distress. C/NM, PL, E

54. no. 3. 250 mg/325 mg = 1 ml/x; 250x = 325; x = 1.3 ml. C/NM, IM, E

55. no. 2. For the most reliable absorption, ampicillin should be administered on an empty stomach. All liquid antibiotics require shaking to mix the suspension adequately. They must be stored in the refrigerator. C/NM, IM, PS

56. no. 4. Claudell's ability to communicate, either verbally or nonverbally, is also essential information. Option no. 1 is important but not a priority, especially postoperatively. C/NM, AS, H

57. no. 1. The child under 5 years is most vulnerable and at psychologic risk when separated from parents, especially the mother, if she is the primary caregiver. Separation can interrupt emotional development and result in loss of trust in others. The child's initial reaction to separation anxiety is protest. C/I, AN, PC

58. no. 2. Sitting at the bedside and spending time is a way to begin to build a trusting relationship so that the toddler will want to come to the nurse. Options no. 1 and no. 3 are too aggressive. Option no. 4 passes responsibility to another. C/NM, IM, PC

59. no. 1. Prone position facilitates drainage of secretions, which may be copious after cleft palate surgery. C/NM, PL, PS

160. no. 2. Elbow restraints will prevent the infant from getting his hands and fingers into his mouth and thereby damaging his suture line. Mummy restraints are used only for procedures (such as IV insertions) requiring immobilization for a relatively brief period of time. C/NM, IM, E

161. no. 2. Listening to a story is appropriate in terms of the child's energy level postoperatively, and it promotes security through interaction with someone. This patient cannot use his arms because of the elbow restraints. The child is not developmentally or cognitively old enough to watch MTV. C/NM, IM, E

162. no. 2. Regression and inactivity are behaviors of despair when the primary caregiver, the mother, is lost. The child feels that his mother is not coming back and begins to grieve. C/I, AN, PC

163. no. 3. To survive, the child must repress feelings about the "lost" mother and bond to caregivers who are present. C/I, AN, PC

164. no. 3. With vomiting, there is loss of hydrochloric acid from the stomach, which results in metabolic *alkalosis*. Infants with pyloric stenosis are usually dehydrated and have weight loss and progressive constipation. Peristaltic waves are typically seen after a feeding as the stomach contracts in an attempt to force its contents through the narrowed pyloric lumen into the small intestines. A sausage-shaped mass is characteristic of intussusception, not pyloric stenosis. C/NM, AS, PS

165. no. 2. Placing the infant in a semi-Fowler's position on his right side would be the best position anatomically to facilitate flow of formula from the stomach. C/NM, PL, E

166. no. 3. The classic signs of insulin-dependent diabetes are polyuria (increased urine output resulting from osmotic diuresis from hyperglycemia), polydipsia (increased thirst as a result of fluid loss from increased urine output), polyphagia (increased appetite in an attempt to provide starving cells with energy), and weight loss (the result of fluid loss in combination with fat and protein breakdown). C/NM, AN, PS

167. no. 4. Glucagon stimulates the release of stored glycogen from the liver, which increases blood glucose. C/NM, AN, PS

168. no. 4. During exercise, there is increased use of glucose, which may precipitate a hypoglycemic reaction. To prevent low blood glucose, extra calories should be provided before exercise. Insulin dosage should not be reduced without testing blood sugar level. C/NM, PL, H

169. no. 2. Glycosylated hemoglobin (hemoglobin A_{1C}) shows the pattern of blood glucose levels over approximately 3 months (the life of the red blood cell). Glucose attaches itself to the hemoglobin in the red blood cells when blood glucose levels are elevated. The *pattern* of blood glucose levels is revealed rather than an isolated fasting blood glucose. Glucose tolerance tests are used for diagnostic purposes. Urine tests for glucose are unreliable and rarely used today. C/I, NM, EV, H

170. no. 4. Thirst is a symptom of hyperglycemia. In hypoglycemia, there is hunger and release of catecholamines in an attempt to increase blood glucose. This often results in diaphoresis and tremors. C/NM, AN, PS

171. no. 2. Peer acceptance is extremely important for school-age children. Because of the special dietary and health practices necessary for diabetics, these children often feel that they are different and fear rejection by their peer group. At this age, however, the fear of bodily injury and painful procedures is likely to be considered. C/NM, AN, PC

172. no. 2. Children with diabetes should not have completely negative urinary glucose because urine tests do not diagnose blood levels below 180 mg/dl. Children are advised to maintain urinary glucose levels of at least 1+. Options no. 1 and no. 3 indicate a potential for diabetic ketoacidosis. The effects of NPH do not occur for 10 to 12 hours. Hypoglycemic episodes have a quick onset; hyperglycemia occurs insidiously. C/NM, AS, PS

173. no. 2. This is evidence that Adele can assume responsibility for her care and has accepted that she has the disease. Options no. 1 and no. 3 are not advisable. C/NM, PL, H

174. no. 2. Most 4-year-olds cannot ride a bike; activities in options no. 3 and no. 4 occur at older ages, with option no. 4 characteristic of adolescence. C/H, AS, H

175. no. 4. The pancreatic enzymes should be mixed in only a small amount of food to ensure that the child will take all of the medication. The enzymes should be given before mealtime to facilitate digestion and absorption of nutrients. C/I, NM, EV, E

176. no. 4. Cystic fibrosis affects many body organs, especially the gastrointestinal and respiratory systems. Thick, tenacious mucus gland secretions block the pancreatic ducts, preventing the pancreatic enzymes from reaching the duodenum and impairing digestion and absorption of nutrients. Thick, tenacious secretions block the bronchi and bronchioles, leading to atelectasis, emphysema, and pneumonia. Chronic, progressive fibrosis of the organs occurs.

177. no. 2. Options no. 1, no. 3, and no. 4 are common problems; the type of stool (steatorrhea) results from the undigested fat in the gastrointestinal tract; most children with cystic fibrosis have good appetites. C/NM, AS, PS

178. no. 2. Because of the particular exocrine glands involved, large amounts of salt are lost and must be replaced, especially in hot weather. Fluids should never be restricted. Physical exercise improves respiratory status. The diet should be low in fat content because of malabsorption and contain higher amounts of sodium. C, NM, IM, H

179. no. 3. Cystic fibrosis is inherited as an autosomal recessive trait. Both parents are carriers of the defective, recessive gene. With each pregnancy, there is a 25% chance the child will inherit the defective gene from each parent. Because the gene is recessive, both defective genes must be inherited for the disease to occur. The gene is autosomal, so distribution between males and females is equal. C/I, PL/IM, H

180. no. 4. The quantitative sweat chloride test, or pilocarpine iontophoresis, is a reliable diagnostic tool for cystic fibrosis (CF). An increase in sodium and chloride ions is found in the sweat and saliva of children with CF. Sweat chloride values less than 40 indicate a negative test, values from 40 to 60 are suggestive of CF, and values greater than 60 are diagnostic of CF. C/I, NM, PL, IM, E

181. no. 4. Because of decreased glomerular filtration, there is a resulting increased circulatory congestion that leads to elevated blood pressure. Option no. 1 is typical of nephrotic syndrome; potassium levels tend to be elevated. Weight gain rather than loss would result from any edema that develops. Edema is only moderate in acute glomerulonephritis. C/E, AS, PS

182. no. 1. Diuresis is the priority goal. Once diuresis occurs, the child feels better and the blood pressure decreases. Options no. 2 and no. 3 are appropriate for nephrotic syndrome. Option no. 4 is applicable after diuresis occurs. C/E, AN, PS

183. no. 4. Acute glomerulonephritis is an inflammatory process in the glomeruli that is caused by a reaction to a streptococcal infection. This test measures streptococcal antibody levels, which would be elevated after a streptococcal infection. Options no. 2, no. 3 and no. 4 are not affected by the diagnosis. Antidiuretic hormone would be elevated with nephrotic syndrome. C/I, PL, PS

184. no. 2. Initial actions should be designed to orient the client and family to the hospital, offer information about immediate procedures of care, and build a trusting relationship. The other actions might be done later. C/E, IM, E

185. no. 3. Weight gain occurs in nephrosis secondary to generalized edema. Increased weight as a result of edema would indicate an exacerbation of the illness or lack of response to treatment. Increased urine output signals diuresis, a desired outcome. Increased appetite signals improvement because anorexia is a common manifestation of nephrosis. Decreased abdominal girth indicates less fluid retention. C/I, E, EV, E

186. no. 2. Massive proteinuria is the hallmark of nephrosis (minimal change nephrotic syndrome). As the glomerular membrane becomes permeable to protein, proteinuria and hypoalbumenia occur. Urine specific gravity is elevated. Elevated blood urea nitrogen may result from hemoconcentration. A goal of therapy is decreased proteinuria with resulting increase in blood albumin and decrease in urine specific gravity. C/I, E, PL, E

187. no. 2. Myra's history is strongly suggestive of a ruptured appendix. Often there is a sudden relief from pain after perforation, then a subsequent increase in pain when peritonitis occurs. If the appendix is perforated, Myra will need surgery, so she should have nothing by mouth. The white blood cell count is often elevated with appendicitis, so a complete blood cell count would be a useful diagnostic tool. C/E, PL, PS

188. no. 3. Her drainage tube may have become occluded or kinked. Additionally, the nurse should check for the return of bowel sounds. C/E, AN, PS

189. no. 4. The young school-age child fears assaults to his body, such as surgery. The toddler's greatest fear is separation from parents. Exaggerated fears of the unknown (monsters etc.) and an overactive imagination are common with preschoolers. Teens usually regard loss of independence as most difficult. C/E, EV, PS

190. no. 4. Because of the lack of distal colonic peristalsis, the infant is frequently unable to pass stools. When stool and flatus accumulate in the colon, the abdomen becomes distended, and the infant refuses fluids. These children usually show poor weight gain because the obstruction is below the ampulla of Vater. Vomiting is likely to be bile stained. C/E, AS, PS

191. no. 2. Steatorrhea (fat in the stool) indicates a problem with fat metabolism but is not a problem in Hirschsprung's disease. The infant may not want to eat because of the elimination problem. Constipation and vomiting are due to the backup of stools and flatus in the colon. C/E, AS, PS

192. no. 1. Although options no. 2, no. 3, and no. 4 are a part of the complete health history, the bowel habits pertain to this disease process. C/E, AS, PS

193. no. 3. Because the proximal end receives the stool, only mucus should be in the distal portion of the colon. C/E, EV, PS

194. no. 1. As with any bowel surgery, the client is given nothing by mouth until bowel function returns. C/E, IM, PS

195. no. 1. Jams and preserves contain portions of the fruit that provide residue (e.g., tiny seeds, skins). C/E, IM, PS

196. no. 3. Reduction of the intussusception can be successful with a barium enema through hydrostatic pressure during the first 24 hours. Passage of normal stool indicates reduction of the intussusception. C/I, E, EV, E

197. no. 3. The child bending forward at the waist with head and arms hanging freely allows the nurse to most easily detect any flank asymmetry or rib hump. C/M, AS, PS

198. no. 2. With the school-age child, the desires for accomplishment, social acceptance, and mastering of new skills are great. Options no. 1 and no. 3 relate to older children, and option no. 4 relates to a younger child. CM/AN, PC

199. no. 2. Mood swings are common in adolescence. C/M, AN, PC

200. no. 2. The other options are incorrect and would lead to inadequate bracing or skin breakdown. There is no guarantee how long the brace will be used. C/M, IM, E

201. no. 3. During early adolescence, girls are about 2 years ahead of their male counterparts in physical development. Scoliosis will not affect her physical development. C/M, AS, PS

202. no. 2. Because the child's weight provides the countertraction, the buttocks are slightly elevated off the bed. By applying the same amount of traction to both legs, equal stress is placed on the growing bones. C/I, M, EV, E

203. no. 2. Alisha will be susceptible to infection because of the process of neutropenia. Options no. 1, no. 3, and no. 4 do not have an infectious disease process associated with them, whereas most children hospitalized with cystic fibrosis have some type of respiratory or sinus infection. C/CA, PL, PS

204. no. 4. Coping with cancer and the medical regimen can best be facilitated by expressing feelings. The procedures never become routine, and each carries some risk. Parents can often be most helpful if they are out of the room during procedures but are available afterward for comfort. C/CA, EV, PC

205. no. 2. Hemolysis will occur if dextrose is used; salt-poor albumin is never used to flush an IV line, and heparinized saline is used after the normal saline when flushing a central venous line. C/O, IM, PS

206. no. 3. Hypotension; fever; pain in back, legs, or chest; and apprehension are all indicative of a reaction. C/CA, AS, PS

207. no. 3. The immediate responsibility is to stop the transfusion; then keep the line open with saline, obtain vital signs, and stay with the child while someone notifies the physician. C/CA, IM, E

208. no. 2. Semi-Fowler's and high Fowler's positions prevent choking or aspiration of blood. These positions also lessen the pressure in the vessels to the head. Option no. 4 would increase bleeding; no. 3 is a later action. C/CA, IM, PS

209. no. 3. Rectal temperatures are contraindicated in clients with leukemia because of alterations in platelets and increased chance of bleeding. C/CA, IM, PS

210. no. 1. A preschool-aged child can verbalize feelings, often believing that death is a temporary sleep and possibly punishment for something the child did or thought. C/I, AS, H

211. no. 4. Peeling skin is a side effect of radiation therapy. Options no. 1, no. 2, and no. 3 are effects of chemotherapy. C/CA, AS, PS

212. no. 4. Vitamins with folic acid interfere with the cytotoxic action of methotrexate because it is a folic acid antagonist. Methotrexate is toxic to the liver and kidneys and should not be administered with aspirin, sulfonamides, or tetracyclines. C/CA, AN, PS

213. no. 4. Uric acid is released during cell destruction and can accumulate in the renal tubules, resulting in uremia. Allopurinol interferes with the metabolic breakdown of xanthine oxidase to uric acid; therefore uric acid production is inhibited. C/CA, AN, PS

214. no. 1. Complete blood cell count (CBC) is one tool to evaluate the child's response to treatment for acute lymphocytic leukemia. The CBC results indicate the bone marrow's response to chemotherapy, such as myelosuppression. Severe myelosuppression may necessitate an alteration in chemotherapy administration. C/I, CA, EV, S

215. no. 3. Encouraging oral fluids ensures adequate excretion of the end products of metabolism. C/CA, PL, PS

216. no. 2. Immunizations are contraindicated with clients receiving immunosuppressive drugs. C/CA, AN, PS

217. no. 4. Vincristine can be neurotoxic; numbness, tingling, jaw pain, and ataxia are manifestations of vincristine toxicity. C/CA, IM, PS

218. no. 1. This is the most common sign. The child appears healthy except for increased abdominal size. Decreased output is seen only if the renal collecting system is involved in bilateral tumors. Hypertension is seen in children when there is pressure of the tumor on the renal artery (about 25% of the time). C/CA, AS, PS

219. no. 1. Dolls and puppets are familiar objects that the young child can actively manipulate, and thus they are good ways for the young child to learn. C/I, IM, H

220. no. 3. The abdomen is not palpated unless absolutely necessary, to prevent the spread of cancer cells into the surrounding abdominal areas. C/CA, PL, PS

221. no. 4. Although the other options may be objectives, the overall goal is to return the child to a normal lifestyle so that growth and development may continue along their normal course. C/CA, PL, H

222. no. 1. Including the parents in planning and implementation of care makes them feel useful, knowledgeable, and that they have an important role in the child's recovery. This increases compliance with the treatment regimen. Literature is a good teaching reinforcement but second in importance. Discharge planning begins with admission. Free time is important but not the sole factor for teaching objectives. C/CA, IM, H

Contents

Practice Test 1 190

Practice Test 2 196

Practice Test 3 203

Practice Test 4 209

Practice Test 5 216

Practice Test 6 222

Practice Test 7 229

Practice Test 8 236

Practice Test 9 242

Practice Test 10 248

Answers and Rationales 255

Answers and Rationales: Practice Test 1 256

Answers and Rationales: Practice Test 2 260

Answers and Rationales: Practice Test 3 265

Answers and Rationales: Practice Test 4 269

Answers and Rationales: Practice Test 5 273

Answers and Rationales: Practice Test 6 277

Answers and Rationales: Practice Test 7 282

Answers and Rationales: Practice Test 8 286

Answers and Rationales: Practice Test 9 290

Answers and Rationales: Practice Test 10 294

Chapter 6

Practice Tests

The questions in this section have been organized to simulate the scope of content covered on the NCLEX-RN exam.

The 750 questions have been divided into 10 practice tests. Each tests your nursing knowledge regarding care of the adult, the child, the childbearing family, and the client with psychosocial/mental health problems.

INSTRUCTIONS FOR TAKING THE TEST

1. Review the information in Chapter 1.
2. Time yourself, allowing 1½ hours per test.
3. Read each question carefully and select *one* best answer to each question.
4. Do not leave any questions blank because you will not be able to skip questions on the computerized NCLEX-RN.
5. Score your exam using the answer key.
6. Review the questions you answered incorrectly and restudy that specific material. Ask yourself two questions:
   a. Did I miss the question because I overlooked a key word, a key timeframe, or a critical piece of data? If you answer "yes," focus on stress reduction techniques before answering more test questions. You may be suffering from a high level of test anxiety.
   b. Did I miss the question because I was unfamiliar with the content? If you answer "yes," look up and review this content in the *AJN/Mosby Nursing Boards Review,* your textbooks, or other resources. You probably need to refresh your content knowledge.
7. Good luck!

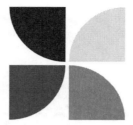

Practice Test 1

1. Jennifer Theil, a 60-year-old homemaker, is admitted to the AM admissions unit for a left total hip replacement. She states that she has had severe pain in the hip for several years and takes large doses of aspirin. She says she has no other health problems. Which lab test would normally *not* be included as part of her preoperative lab work?
   ① Blood type and crossmatch
   ② Prothrombin time
   ③ Sedimentation rate
   ④ Bence Jones protein

2. Three-and-a-half-year-old Courtney has been hospitalized with nephrosis. Which of the following manifestations would most likely be observed?
   ① Ascites
   ② Elevated blood pressure
   ③ Low urine specific gravity
   ④ Hematuria

3. A 36-year-old multipara is admitted to the labor room for induction. She is 20 days past her estimated date of delivery. Her cervix is 50% effaced and fingertip dilated. Before the induction, the woman has a contraction stress test. What does this test demonstrate?
   ① Lung maturity of the fetus
   ② The response of the fetal heart rate to fetal activity
   ③ The response of the cervix to labor
   ④ The ability of the fetus to tolerate the stress of uterine contractions

4. Mrs. Rodriguez, 43 years old, is diagnosed with a major depressive episode, recurrent. She seeks out one of the nurses she resembles in hairstyle, weight, and appearance. Additionally, she mimics the nurse's behaviors and caring mannerisms. This behavior is best defined in terms of which defense mechanism?
   ① Idealization
   ② Projection
   ③ Identification
   ④ Intellectualization

5. Because of their work commitments, 4-year-old Jason's parents are not able to stay with him while he is in the hospital. In addition to the stress created by his separation from his parents, Jason will most likely be fearful of which of the following?
   ① Intrusive procedures
   ② Unfamiliar caretakers
   ③ Dying
   ④ New roommate

6. Which action would be *inappropriate* to include preoperatively in a client's plan of care for hip replacement?
   ① Teach her to use the trapeze.
   ② Measure her for antiembolic hose.
   ③ Restrict her to bed rest until discharge.
   ④ Avoid extreme flexion and adduction of the hip.

7. Which of the following is not an expected side effect of fluoxetine (Prozac)?
   ① Sexual dysfunction
   ② Sleeplessness
   ③ Sedation
   ④ Nausea

8. An expectant mother is admitted for induction of labor. A continuous, controlled infusion of oxytocin (Pitocin) is administered, and contractions begin. Which of the following observations would be most critical at this time?
   ① Fetal heart rate and uterine contractions
   ② Uterine contractions and maternal vital signs
   ③ Fetal heart rate and maternal vital signs
   ④ Uterine contractions and maternal pain tolerance

9. A client for joint surgery is at risk for an infection developing in the operative site. Which measure will *not* prevent this complication?
   ① Scrub the leg bid before surgery with a bacteriostatic soap.
   ② Caution the client not to shave any part of the body.
   ③ Use reverse isolation for 3 days preoperatively.
   ④ Restrict in-and-out traffic in the surgical suite during the operation.

10. When planning nursing care for a preschooler, the nurse would include activities that promote a sense of
    ① Trust.
    ② Industry.
    ③ Autonomy.
    ④ Initiative.

11. An oxytocin infusion is being given to a pregnant client to induce labor. Which of the following would be most indicative of an adverse reaction to the drug?
    ① A contraction lasts over 120 seconds
    ② Deep-tendon reflexes are 2+
    ③ Urinary output is 100 ml/hr
    ④ Fetal heart accelerates with contractions

12. An order for isocarboxazid (Marplan), 30 mg PO daily, is made. The client is already taking paroxetine

(Paxil) 20 mg daily. When taking off this order, what is the most appropriate *initial* nursing action?
1. Administer the medications as ordered.
2. Check the client's blood pressure both sitting and lying down.
3. Provide the client with adequate psychoeducation about drug interactions.
4. Call the psychiatrist and question the administration of these together.

13. A client, gravida 1, para 0, is now in active labor. She expresses concern about her ability to maintain control of her behavior during the remainder of labor. Which of these nursing actions would be most supportive?
1. Reassure her of the nursing staff's competency.
2. Reassure her that medication is available.
3. Instruct her in relaxation and breathing exercises.
4. Reassure her that she will be accepted regardless of her behavior.

14. Kelly is receiving prednisone by mouth. Which of the following actions is *not* indicated?
1. Give the prednisone after meals.
2. Withhold the prednisone if Kelly's blood pressure becomes elevated.
3. Observe Kelly closely for signs of infection.
4. Provide foods high in potassium in Kelly's diet.

15. Which postoperative nursing measure would be *inappropriate* for a female client with a hip replacement?
1. Schedule active range of motion to both ankles.
2. Remind her to keep her toes pointed outward.
3. Help her to pivot on the unaffected foot.
4. Remind her not to cross her legs.

16. Ramone, age 6, has nephrosis. During the acute phase of his illness, which position is best for him to be placed in?
1. On his left side
2. On his back
3. On his abdomen
4. Semi-Fowler's position

17. Which assessment finding indicates an abnormality in a client's cardiovascular status?
1. Capillary refill: 10 seconds
2. Apical pulse rate: 74/min
3. Absence of pitting edema
4. Feet warm and pink; nonpalpable posterior tibial pulse

18. A client with a hip replacement has a wound drain connected to suction. During the first 8 hours, there was 100 ml of bright bloody drainage. The client is alert, and the vital signs are stable. Which nursing action would be most appropriate?
1. Notify the physician.
2. Apply a pressure dressing to the wound.
3. Continue to observe and record the amount of drainage.
4. Anticipate a stat order for a transfusion by ordering a unit of blood.

19. Antidepressants have various side effects. One particular antidepressant may cause a hypertensive crisis and possibly a cerebral vascular accident when combined with aged food, such as sardines, beer, cheeses, and over-the-counter cold preparations. Which drug is most likely to produce this reaction?
1. Sertraline (Zoloft)
2. Fluoxetine (Prozac)
3. Bupropion (Wellbutrin)
4. Phenelzine sulfate (Nardil)

20. A woman is in the active phase of labor. An external monitor has been applied, and a fetal heart deceleration of uniform shape is observed, beginning just as the contraction is underway and returning to the baseline at the end of the contraction. Which of the following nursing actions is most appropriate?
1. Administer O_2.
2. Turn the client on her left side.
3. Notify the physician.
4. No action is necessary.

21. Which of the following snacks would be the best choice for a child with nephrosis?
1. 1 ounce processed cheese spread, celery sticks, and Kool-Aid
2. ½ cup vanilla pudding and grape juice
3. ½ peanut butter sandwich, apple slices, and ½ cup hot cocoa
4. ½ cup corn flakes, milk, and raisins

22. Which of the following is a common sequela of a total hip replacement within the first postoperative week?
1. Urinary retention
2. Contractures
3. Weight loss
4. Incontinence, especially with coughing

23. A serious complication of a total hip replacement is displacement of the prosthesis. What is the primary sign of displacement?
1. Pain on movement and weight bearing
2. Hemorrhage
3. Affected leg 1 to 2 inches longer
4. Edema in the area of the incision

24. The fetal monitor being used to assess a primigravida's labor begins to show late decelerations. Which of the following would the nurse do first?
1. Continue to assess labor and support the mother.
2. Administer prescribed analgesia.
3. Turn her on her left side.
4. Inform the attending physician.

25. Which activity would be most appropriate for a 3-year-old hospitalized with acute nephritis?
1. Playing with other children in the playroom
2. Riding a push-pull toy in the hall
3. Having a volunteer read him a story about a child in the hospital
4. Playing with housekeeping toys in his room

26. Paula is a 32-year-old seeking evaluation and treatment of major depressive symptoms. A major nursing priority during the assessment process includes which of the following?
1. Meaning of current stressors
2. Possibility of self-harm
3. Motivation to participate in treatment
4. Presence of alcohol or other drug use

27. A client with a hip replacement has an abductor splint in place. What is the best guide to the placement of the splint?
    1. Fasten the splint firmly in place.
    2. Position the splint so that it does not interfere with the use of the bedpan.
    3. Position the strap so that it is not directly over the peroneal nerve.
    4. Position the proximal strap just above the knee.

28. Which circumstance poses the greatest risk of suicide?
    1. A history of numerous gestures
    2. A sense of hopelessness
    3. A recent loss
    4. A lack of meaningful support systems

29. Which behavior would the nurse expect a hospitalized 2-year-old to exhibit immediately after separation from her mother?
    1. Acceptance of comforting by the nursing staff
    2. Interest in the toys left by her mother
    3. Crying and calling for her mother
    4. Whining and apathetic withdrawal

30. The nurse evaluates the readiness for discharge in a client who has had a hip replacement. The client identifies which action as being *incorrect* behavior?
    1. Use a rocking chair or reclining chair when sitting for an extended time.
    2. Continue to sleep with a pillow between the knees.
    3. Take antibiotics prophylactically when dental work is being done.
    4. Hyperextend the affected leg while flexing the other one when retrieving objects from the floor.

31. Ten-year-old Jackie is admitted to the hospital with a medical diagnosis of rheumatic fever. She relates a history of "a sore throat about a month ago." Bed rest with bathroom privileges is prescribed. Which of the following nursing assessments would be given highest priority when assessing Jackie's condition?
    1. Jackie's response to being hospitalized
    2. The presence of a macular rash on her trunk
    3. Her sleeping or resting apical pulse
    4. The presence of polyarthritis and pain in her joints

32. Which group poses the least risk of suicide?
    1. Persons misusing alcohol or other drugs
    2. Older men suffering recent losses
    3. Adolescents
    4. Married men

33. Most clients are curious about the appearance and placement of the stoma of their urinary diversion. What area of the abdomen is usually used?
    1. Right side, 1 to 2 inches below the waist
    2. Superior, anterior region of the iliac crest
    3. Left side, just above the waist
    4. Area near the umbilicus

34. Gordon Isaac has cancer of the bladder. He has been admitted for a cystectomy and urinary diversion. During the critical period immediately after surgery, the nurse would be especially observant of the client's general condition. What is the most critical sign or symptom Mr. Isaac could exhibit?
    1. Absence of urinary output over a period of 1 to 2 hours

    2. Pain along the incision site
    3. Increased pulse rate to 100/min
    4. Serous drainage from the incision line

35. Which of the following is *not* a symptom of schizophrenia, paranoid type?
    1. Delusions
    2. Hallucinations
    3. Intrusiveness
    4. Ideas of reference

36. Which of the following is *not* a manifestation of Sydenham's chorea?
    1. Intellectual impairment
    2. Muscle weakness
    3. Purposeless tremors
    4. Emotional lability

37. A client has a collecting appliance fastened around the ileal conduit stoma. Select the most common problem that the nurse is trying to prevent with the use of this bag.
    1. Infection of the stoma
    2. Skin excoriation
    3. Stricture of the ileal stoma
    4. Ammonia odor from the stoma

38. What is the most important reason for attaching the ileostomy bag to gravity drainage at night?
    1. To prevent infection of the stoma resulting from urinary stasis in the bag
    2. To prevent leakage of urine around the bag on the skin that can be caused by overdistention of the bag
    3. To facilitate the normal urinary method of excretion
    4. To prevent reflux of urine into the renal pelvis

39. Which of the following is the most common defense mechanism seen in the client with schizophrenia, paranoid type?
    1. Sublimation
    2. Projection
    3. Rationalization
    4. Suppression

40. Which of the following would receive the highest priority during hospitalization of a child with rheumatic fever?
    1. Minimize cardiac damage by limiting the child to bed rest.
    2. Relieve pain by administering prescribed analgesics.
    3. Help her cope with hospitalization by providing age-appropriate activities.
    4. Prevent injury by padding the bed's side rails.

41. A 32-year-old multipara has just delivered a baby estimated to be at 43 weeks of gestation. Which of the following descriptions would best describe a postmature infant?
    1. "Wide-eyed" with downy hair
    2. Long fingernails and increased subcutaneous fat
    3. Long, coarse hair and meconium-stained skin
    4. Parchmentlike skin and a thick coating of vernix

42. A client with a new urinary diversion needs adequate teaching before his discharge. In doing discharge

teaching, which complication should be emphasized?
1. Recurrent bladder infection
2. Frequent emptying of the colon
3. Ileal stoma dilation
4. Inflammation and infection of the kidney

43. When caring for the client with schizophrenia, paranoid type, which of the following is an inappropriate treatment goal?
1. The client will demonstrate reality testing.
2. The client will dismiss internal voices.
3. The client will develop adaptive coping behaviors.
4. The client will act on impulses arising from internal voices.

44. Joseph Fenter, a 55-year-old black male, is admitted to the hospital with a diagnosis of hypertension. While taking his history, the nurse learns that he is employed as a sales manager for a large video business. His hypertension was discovered on a routine visit to the medical department at work. On admission, Mr. Fenter would most likely be expected to make which of these statements?
1. "I don't know why I am here. There is nothing wrong with me."
2. "I have been having numerous episodes of nausea and vomiting."
3. "I have been experiencing shortness of breath."
4. "I am here because I have hypertension."

45. Which activity is most appropriate for an 11-year-old who exhibits chorea during the acute phase of rheumatic fever?
1. Handheld computer games
2. Visiting other children on the unit
3. Keeping a written diary
4. Listening to records of her favorite singing groups

46. In a child with rheumatic fever, which of the following laboratory results is not relevant to this disease process?
1. Antistreptolysin-O titer
2. C-reactive protein
3. Urine protein
4. Erythrocyte sedimentation rate

47. Which of these findings would constitute a significant index of hypertension?
1. Pulse pressure of 10 mm Hg
2. Regular pulse of 90 beats/min
3. Sustained diastolic pressure greater than 90 mm Hg
4. Systolic pressure fluctuating between 135 and 140 mm Hg

48. A hypertension client is to receive a diet low in fat, sodium, and cholesterol. His knowledge of foods lowest in these elements would be good if he selected which of these menus?
1. Beans, ham, rye bread, and a carrot
2. Cold baked chicken, tomatoes, and applesauce
3. Cold cuts, salad with blue cheese dressing, and custard pie
4. Cheese sandwich, cream of mushroom soup, and chocolate pie

49. Stephanie is discharged after 3 weeks of hospitalization for rheumatic fever. Which of the following statements best indicates that Stephanie's parents have understood discharge teaching?
1. "Stephanie should lead a sedentary lifestyle for at least a year."
2. "Stephanie must take daily antibiotics for an extended time to prevent a recurrence of rheumatic fever."
3. "Stephanie should not return to her classroom but should have a home teacher the rest of the year."
4. "Stephanie may have permanent neurologic sequelae as a result of the Sydenham's chorea."

50. When teaching a client about a low-fat, low-sodium, and low-cholesterol diet, the nurse would include which of these instructions?
1. Season food with lemon juice.
2. Limit salt to 3 to 4 teaspoons per day.
3. Eat a lot of canned foods.
4. Restrict green vegetable intake.

51. May Lewis is a 25-year-old client recently diagnosed with schizophrenia, paranoid type. A treatment goal is that the client will develop a therapeutic relationship with a primary nursing staff member. Which of the following is an inappropriate intervention?
1. Permit the client to have distance in the relationship.
2. Encourage exploration and clarification of suspiciousness.
3. Provide adequate time for her to respond.
4. Permit her to isolate herself from others if she chooses.

52. A 21-year-old college student has just learned that she contracted genital herpes from her sexual partner. After completing the initial history and assessment the nurse will have data concerning areas pertinent to the disease. Which of the following would be unnecessary to include at this point?
1. Voiding patterns
2. Characteristics of lesions
3. Vaginal discharge
4. Prior history of varicella

53. The nurse administers methylergonovine (Methergine), 0.2 mg, parenterally to an intrapartal woman after completion of the third stage of labor. Which of the following would indicate that this drug has produced its desired effect?
1. A firm fundus
2. Increased duration and frequency of contractions
3. A drop in blood pressure
4. Lactation suppression

54. A client is taking the medication isosorbide dinitrate (Isordil) for symptoms of angina. Discharge teaching about isosorbide dinitrate (Isordil) would include information that this drug is which of the following?
1. A nonnitrite preparation that will not cause dilation of peripheral vessels
2. A nitrite preparation that will constrict both small and large vessels
3. A vasodilator that will cause an increase in vascular resistance
4. A nitrite preparation that will dilate both large and small vessels

55. A client takes metoprolol (Lopressor) to control his hypertension. This drug reduces blood pressure by which mechanism?
    ① Decreases cardiac output
    ② Increases cardiac output and suppresses aldosterone activity
    ③ Depletes norepinephrine from the heart and peripheral organs
    ④ Suppresses norepinephrine secretion from the medulla of the brain

56. Marty Taylor, 32 years old, is seen in the day treatment center for the first time. Her records show a diagnosis of schizophrenia, chronic undifferentiated type. Her father reports that she has had difficulty managing persistent hallucinations despite medication compliance. Which of the following is *not* useful in managing hallucinations?
    ① Encourage the client to interact with others.
    ② Focus minimally on the content of hallucinations or delusions after an initial assessment of them.
    ③ Acknowledge the client's belief in hearing voices, but inform her that they are not heard by others.
    ④ Listen attentively to the content and delusions and encourage the client to depict them.

57. Which of the following nursing diagnoses would be of highest priority in initially caring for a young woman coping with a newly diagnosed case of genital herpes?
    ① Altered sexuality patterns
    ② Impaired physical mobility
    ③ Diversional activity deficit
    ④ Disturbance in self-concept: personal identity

58. Which of the following interventions will help the client demonstrate good personal hygiene and grooming?
    ① Assess the client's self-care deficits.
    ② Disregard disheveled appearance and poor hygiene.
    ③ Urge client to participate in grooming classes.
    ④ Enhance the clients's self-care skills by performing them for the client.

59. Which of the following best describes a compound comminuted fracture?
    ① The fracture is associated with injury to surrounding tissue and structures.
    ② Bone fragments are forcibly driven into one another.
    ③ The bone is splintered into fragments that extend through the skin.
    ④ The line of the fracture forms a spiral that encircles the bone.

60. In a class on sexually transmitted diseases, a nursing student asks why these diseases have reached epidemic proportions lately. Which of the following is the best explanation of the increased incidence?
    ① Sexual permissiveness and promiscuity have continued to remain high.
    ② Medications have been found to control them.
    ③ The incidence of these diseases has increased because prostitutes transmit them.
    ④ Few people have information about how diseases are spread.

61. Fernando Cruz, age 21, sustained a compound fracture in the distal portion of the left femur while learning to ride his new motorcycle. He was placed in skeletal traction with a Thomas splint and a Pearson attachment with a 20-pound weight. A Steinman pin was inserted into the femur distal to the fracture. Mr. Cruz is admitted to the orthopedic unit. The nursing care plan would include which of the following?
    ① Ensure that the sole of the affected foot is supported against the foot of the bed.
    ② Instruct the client to move about in bed as little as possible.
    ③ Position the Thomas splint around the upper thigh without putting pressure on the groin.
    ④ Place and remove the bedpan from the affected side.

62. Ms. O'Leary, a 21-year-old graduate student, is admitted to the inpatient psychiatric unit with a diagnosis of schizophrenia, paranoid type. She approaches a staff member with hostile remarks about another client who is "trying to steal my thoughts." Which of the following is a *nontherapeutic* response to this client?
    ① Encourage the client to accept and express feelings.
    ② Define appropriate outlets for hostility with the client.
    ③ Point out the inappropriateness of her feelings.
    ④ Explain the basis of the client's hostility.

63. A 17-year-old comes to the adolescent clinic requesting a shot of penicillin to cure a case of genital herpes. He promises to continue taking medication faithfully at home. How would the nurse best respond?
    ① "I'll prepare the shot for you as long as you continue the oral medication for 10 days."
    ② "You will need to return for more penicillin if a lesion appears."
    ③ "Unfortunately, genital herpes is a lifelong disease, which at present has no cure."
    ④ "Tetracycline is the drug of choice for genital herpes."

64. Which of the following statements made by a client with a fractured leg indicates a need for further teaching or discussion?
    ① "A diet high in roughage and fiber will prevent constipation."
    ② "Maintaining a positive nitrogen balance is important."
    ③ "I need an increased calcium intake."
    ④ "The 2700-calorie diet should provide nutrients that promote healing."

65. To maintain traction, there must be countertraction. How is countertraction best applied to a client with a Thomas splint and a Pearson attachment?
    ① By raising the head of the bed to a 45-degree angle.
    ② By elevating the foot of the bed on 6-inch shock blocks.

③ By using 20 pounds of weight supported by the Steinman pin.

④ By keeping the Thomas splint in an inclined position.

66. Which of the following techniques would aid in preventing the spread of genital herpes to others?

① Careful hand washing with an antiseptic soap

② Cesarean delivery for any woman with a history of genital herpes

③ Refraining from sexual intercourse when lesions are present

④ Receiving immunization before the first sexual contact

67. Risperidone (Risperdal) is a new-generation antipsychotic that is particularly helpful in treating negative symptoms of schizophrenia. Which of the following is *not* a negative symptom of schizophrenia?

① Delusions

② Apathy

③ Social withdrawal

④ Poverty of thoughts

68. Thirty minutes after the client's delivery, the nurse makes the following assessment: fundus firm, 1 inch below the umbilicus; lochia rubra; complains of thirst; slight tremors of lower extremities. Analysis of these data is most suggestive of which of the following?

① Impending shock

② Circulatory overload

③ Subinvolution

④ Normal postpartum adjustment

69. Why is it particularly difficult to assess females for gonorrhea?

① They rarely have early distressing symptoms of the disease.

② They are less likely to seek medical attention for diseases.

③ Cultures from the cervix cannot be used for diagnostic purposes.

④ They have a lower incidence of cystitis than do males.

70. Which of the following is *not* a common side effect of risperidone (Risperdal)?

① Orthostatic hypotension

② Cognitive impairment

③ Gastrointestinal disturbances

④ Addiction

71. Because a Steinman pin has been inserted, a client is at risk of acquiring which of the following?

① Flexion contracture of the knee

② Impaired skin sensations

③ Addiction to pain medication

④ Osteomyelitis

72. Syphilis may often go undetected without a thorough sexual history. Why is this so?

① The disease is usually asymptomatic.

② Symptoms disappear after some months, even if syphilis is not treated.

③ Symptoms appear the day after sexual contact.

④ The disease first attacks internal organs.

73. One hour after delivery, a postpartum woman complains of severe perineal pain. Which nursing action would take highest priority?

① Administer prescribed pain medication.

② Apply warm compresses.

③ Inspect the perineum.

④ Instruct the client in Kegel exercises.

74. A client in skeletal traction complains that the ropes hurt his thigh. Which of the following would be the most appropriate nursing action?

① Replace the spreader bar with a wider one.

② Place padding between the thigh and the rope.

③ Employ distraction techniques.

④ Medicate with a mild analgesic.

75. What is the purpose of the Pearson attachment on skeletal traction?

① To support the lower part of the leg

② To support the upper part of the leg

③ To provide traction to the fracture

④ To prevent flexion contracture of the ankle

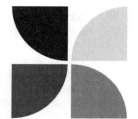

76. The nurse evaluates the rehabilitation plan of an adolescent female with an L2 spinal cord injury secondary to a motor vehicle accident as effective when which one of the following outcomes is met?
    ① The adolescent states, "I'll never be able to get pregnant and have a baby."
    ② The adolescent returns to school using lower extremity assistive devices.
    ③ The adolescent pursues summer employment as a postal carrier.
    ④ The parents of the adolescent investigate long-term institutionalization for their daughter.

77. Depression is frequently accompanied by feelings of guilt. An interdisciplinary plan of care that addresses helping the client "express guilty feeling" involves doing which of the following?
    ① Encouraging group participation
    ② Exploring feelings of hostility and anger
    ③ Analyzing circumstances that give rise to social isolation because of fears of rejection
    ④ Participating in developing activities of daily living

78. Which statement would be excluded in a teaching session about obesity and its treatment?
    ① Exercise is the most practical method of weight control.
    ② Obesity tends to run in families because of eating habits.
    ③ Food can become an individual's major source of gratification.
    ④ Obese children tend to become obese adults.

79. A 17-year-old male with a spinal cord injury at C7 suddenly develops elevated blood pressure, sweating, flushed face, and bradycardia. Which one of the following is a priority nursing intervention?
    ① Assess for bladder distention.
    ② Assess the intravenous site.
    ③ Recheck the pulse and blood pressure in 1 hour.
    ④ Obtain an axillary temperature.

80. Delusions are most likely to occur in which type of depression?
    ① Adjustment disorder, depressed mood
    ② Reactive
    ③ Major
    ④ Dysthymia

81. A client is scheduled for an upper gastrointestinal se-

ries. Which intervention would be used to prepare the client?
    ① Clear liquids for breakfast the day of the exam.
    ② A cleansing enema the morning of the exam.
    ③ Food and fluids withheld 10 to 12 hours before the exam.
    ④ Radiopaque tablets given the evening before the exam.

82. Which cluster of symptoms indicates severe depression?
    ① Crying spells and social isolation
    ② Changes in appetite, sleep, and concentration patterns
    ③ Fatigue and weakness
    ④ Negative perception of self and the future

83. The physician schedules a client for a gastric analysis with a nasogastric tube. Which nursing action would be essential when preparing a client for this gastric analysis?
    ① Force fluids for 24 hours preceding the test.
    ② Administer enemas on the preceding evening.
    ③ Withhold food the morning of the analysis.
    ④ Record the pulse rate when beginning the test.

84. Kristen Townsend is a 4-month-old admitted with a moderate degree of gastroesophageal reflux. According to her mother, "Kristen has been vomiting almost since the day she was born." In determining Kristen's readiness for discharge, which of the following statements by her mother best indicates a knowledge of gastroesophageal reflux and appropriate interventions?
    ① "I should give her antacids with each feeding."
    ② "When I make up her feeding, I should put about 1 tablespoon of rice cereal in every 4 ounces."
    ③ "After feeding Kristen, I should place her in a swing."
    ④ "I should burp her only when she's finished so I don't make her spit up more."

85. Which finding from the analysis of gastric aspirate would best support the diagnosis of a peptic ulcer?
    ① Absence of gastric secretion
    ② Increased hydrochloric acid
    ③ Lack of intrinsic factor
    ④ Decreased gastric acid

86. A noninvasive gastric analysis test is used to determine which of the following?
    ① Presence or absence of hydrochloric acid in the stomach

② Presence of gastric ulcers
③ Ability of the stomach to empty solids and liquids
④ Amount of free acid in the stomach

87. Clarence Pollard, 46 years old, is admitted to the day hospital program with a diagnosis of major depression. Which of the following statements indicates that he is clearly depressed?
① "I am never going to find another job. I am too old."
② "I am a loner and I don't need friends."
③ "My appetite is completely shot and I can't sleep."
④ "I have absolutely no energy."

88. An infant with pyloric stenosis and a history of vomiting is admitted to the hospital. Which of the following nursing actions would be implemented?
① Prepare the infant and his parents for immediate surgery.
② Monitor intravenous hydration.
③ Give diazepam (Valium) as ordered, to relax the pyloric sphincter.
④ Give small, frequent feedings.

89. A client's test results indicate a duodenal ulcer. The client is discharged with a prescription for a 1500-calorie diet with no coffee or hot spices and ranitidine (Zantac), 150 mg bid PO. What is the therapeutic effect of this drug?
① Neutralizes gastric acid
② Inhibits gastric secretions
③ Slows digestion
④ Reduces gastric motility

90. What is the most common metabolic disturbance seen in infants who have pyloric stenosis?
① Metabolic acidosis
② Metabolic alkalosis
③ Respiratory alkalosis
④ Hyperkalemia

91. Which of the following is not a manifestation of a major depressive episode?
① Alterations in appetite
② Decreased libido
③ Early-morning wakening
④ Ataxia

92. In spite of conservative treatment, a client's ulcer perforates and an emergency vagotomy and pyloroplasty are performed. What is the expected outcome after the vagotomy?
① An increase in the blood supply to the stomach
② A decrease in gastric secretions and motility
③ An increase in gastric emptying and motility
④ A decrease in the epigastric pain postoperatively

93. Depression is one of the most treatable mental disorders. It is frequently misdiagnosed or missed in the elderly. What is the greatest concern of untreated depression in the elderly?
① Suicide risk
② Social isolation
③ Loss of self-integrity
④ Increased divorce rate

94. An infant has an IV of 5% dextrose in 0.45% saline hanging. The physician has ordered potassium chloride (KCl) to be added to the IV. What important

nursing action is carried out before adding KCl to the IV?
① Check the time of last voiding.
② Look up the last serum chloride level.
③ Ensure that the IV is infusing through a large-bore needle.
④ Check skin turgor.

95. Which nursing action is inappropriate when planning postoperative nursing care for an infant with pyloric stenosis?
① Include parents in giving his feedings.
② Oral feedings will be started a few hours after surgery.
③ The infant will be NPO for days after surgery; thus sucking needs should be satisfied in other ways.
④ Monitor the infant for signs of hypoglycemia.

96. A postoperative gastric surgery client returns to the room with an IV and a nasogastric tube attached to suction. That evening the client is ambulated to the bathroom and returned to bed. Suddenly the client begins to gag and has dry heaves. What is the nurse's initial action?
① Notify the physician.
② Check the client's abdomen to see if an evisceration has occurred.
③ Check the nasogastric tube and suction equipment for kinks or malfunction.
④ Irrigate the nasogastric tube with 50 ml of normal saline.

97. Erma Olin, an 86-year-old widow, is brought to the emergency room by ambulance after suffering a fall at home. She has a history of heart problems, which require medications. When approaching Mrs. Olin, what would be the nurse's first action?
① Explain the emergency room procedures.
② Tell her that a physician will be in to examine her shortly.
③ Introduce himself or herself to the client.
④ Apply electrode patches to monitor the cardiac activity.

98. After surgical repair of the pyloric stenosis, a 4-week-old infant would be placed in which position?
① High Fowler's
② Prone
③ Right side-lying
④ Left side-lying

99. When applying electrode patches to monitor a client's cardiac activity, which of the following assessments will the nurse be unable to make?
① Level of consciousness and orientation
② Skin color and temperature
③ Muscle tension and motor activity
④ Cardiac output

100. Mr. Leggett is a 76-year-old man seeking treatment for stomach and leg pain in the ambulatory care unit. He also reports sleep and appetite disturbances over the past few months. He is informed that he is medically stable. What is the most important nursing intervention?
① Ask him about recent losses and lifestyle changes.
② Encourage him to seek a second opinion.

③ Direct him to the psychiatric nurse on duty.

④ Offer him a follow-up appointment.

101. Which of the following postoperative responses to feedings would a child with pyloric stenosis usually exhibit?

① Tolerance for clear fluids, but frequent vomiting of formula or breast milk.

② No vomiting because the infant is NPO and is on a regimen of IVs for the first 3 days.

③ Immediate tolerance of oral fluids because of release of the hypertrophied muscle.

④ Intermittent vomiting of oral fluids that diminishes over the first 24 to 48 hours.

102. A complete 12-lead ECG of a client shows a heart rate of 48 beats per minute. The client is given a diagnosis of sinus bradycardia. The most common cause of this rhythm is which of the following?

① A theophylline level of 22 μg/ml

② Pain reported at a level of 10 with a scale of 1-10

③ Digoxin level reported to be 3 ng/ml

④ Digoxin level reported to be 1.5 ng/ml

103. Which nursing observation indicates that the parents of an infant with repaired pyloric stenosis are fully prepared for his discharge?

① The infant recovers fully from surgery, and his parents express happiness.

② He retains his formula after his parents feed him.

③ His parents demonstrate the correct feeding technique.

④ He gains weight appropriate for his age.

104. When planning care for a client with a heart rate of 30, what is the primary goal for the client?

① The client will be free from further damage to the myocardium.

② The client will maintain optimal cardiac output.

③ The client will experience a decrease in environmental and emotional stimuli.

④ The client will maintain close communication with significant others.

105. The laboratory report indicates that the causes of a client's bradycardia are a drug toxicity and an acceleration of cardiac atherosclerosis. The client is to receive a permanent pacemaker. The nurse assigned to prepare the client would apply which factors?

① A planned, systematic approach to teaching a client to live with a pacemaker is a vital part of nursing care.

② The client will easily adjust to a pacemaker because the client has had a heart problem for 20 years.

③ The client probably already has some information about pacemakers from watching or listening to discussions about heart abnormalities in the media.

④ It is the physician's responsibility to teach the client about the pacemaker.

106. Which of the following indicates bladder distention after a normal vaginal delivery?

① Poor abdominal muscle tone

② Increased lochia rubra with clots

③ Uterus contracted below umbilicus

④ Uterus soft to the right of midline

107. Melanie Yelden is admitted to the hospital with diabetes mellitus. Two days later, she says to the nurse, "I don't know why I am here. I can stabilize my blood sugar at home. I need to go back to work. I feel fine." Mrs. Yelden is using which of the following defense mechanisms?

① Denial

② Rationalization

③ Sublimation

④ Suppression

108. Mrs. Yelden has begun eating a sugar-restricted diet. When her tray is served she yells at the nurse. "Do you expect me to eat this awful-tasting food?" What is the most appropriate response?

① "The food tastes awful?"

② "Mrs. Yelden, this diet will reduce your blood sugar and make it easier to stabilize your condition."

③ "I'll ask the dietitian to see you today."

④ "You sound pretty upset about the way things are going."

109. Which of the following measures is most important to ensure the safety of an infant with cloth extremity restraints?

① Avoid placing padding under the restraints because it will only increase pressure and the chance of injury.

② Fasten the restraint ties securely to the crib rails.

③ Secure all four extremities because one loose extremity can cause the child to become entangled in the restraints.

④ Frequently check how the restraints are applied and the circulation in the extremities.

110. Which intervention is inappropriate for a client in the immediate postoperative period after a permanent pacemaker insertion?

① Assess the incision q30min for bleeding.

② Monitor for dizziness, light-headedness, and chest pain.

③ Monitor the ECG for pacing spikes or pacing artifacts.

④ Use active and passive ROM exercises of both arms and shoulders.

111. Discharge planning for a client with a new pacemaker would exclude which of the following factors?

① Activity and exercise progression over the next 3 months

② Awareness of environmental hazards that might interfere with the function of the pacemaker

③ How to take a daily radial pulse

④ How to care for a permanently implanted pacemaker

112. While riding his skateboard, 14-year-old Dennis falls and fractures his elbow. Which of the following is the most severe complication of this injury?

① Fluid loss

② Pain

③ Compartment syndrome

④ Infection

113. An emergency endoscopy is performed on a client. After this procedure, what would be the nurse's primary concern?
① Urinary output
② Respiratory pattern
③ Level of consciousness
④ Gag reflex

114. Perry Lewis has been recently diagnosed with bladder cancer and has been told that his life expectancy is less than 6 months. He is 52 years old, married, and has three adolescent children. He replies, "That doctor is nuts. She thinks I am dying, but I am not really sick at all." What is the best explanation of this reply?
① It represents a common initial response to what the physician has told him.
② It suggests that he has difficulty coping with this information.
③ It suggests that he is delusional and suffers from a mental illness.
④ Further information is needed to explain this reply.

115. Jack Reynolds is a 45-year-old unemployed engineer. He was admitted to the hospital 2 days ago with acute gastrointestinal bleeding. Two years ago, cirrhosis was diagnosed; he has been a heavy drinker for many years. Although Mr. Reynolds stopped drinking several months ago, he has had two recent admissions for bleeding esophageal varices. The endoscopy reveals bleeding esophageal varices. A Sengstaken-Blakemore tube was inserted to control the bleeding. What is an important guideline to remember in caring for a client with this tube?
① The gastric outlet is attached to suction.
② Pressure on the gastric balloon can be maintained for no more than 4 hours at a time.
③ Iced saline lavages can be discontinued after the tube is inserted.
④ Traction can be discontinued when the bloody drainage is less than 50 ml/hr.

116. A child's fractured elbow is being treated with skeletal traction. Which nursing action should be implemented in caring for the child in skeletal traction?
① Encourage active range of motion for the elbow to prevent contractures.
② Remove the counterweights for relief of pain.
③ Check pin sites for bleeding, inflammation, and infection.
④ Change bed position to prevent stasis.

117. Which laboratory test is most helpful in determining the excretory function of the liver?
① Albumin/globulin ratio
② Alkaline phosphatase
③ Prothrombin time
④ Sulfobromophthalein (Bromsulphalein) test

118. What is an initial nursing goal when working with a client who has just been told that he has terminal cancer?
① The client begins to deal with imminent death.
② The client begins to accept his imminent death.

③ The client begins to say goodbye to relatives and friends.
④ The client begins to state an understanding of the disease process.

119. What physiologic effect of immobility is Shauna, a 4-year-old in traction, likely to experience?
① Hypercalcemia
② Increased vital capacity
③ Positive nitrogen balance
④ Increased metabolic rate

120. A 26-year-old woman wants to use the basal body temperature method of identifying ovulation. The nurse teaches the woman that ovulation can be identified by which of the following?
① A slight drop in temperature followed by a rise of 0.5° to 0.7°F
② A slight increase in temperature followed by a drop of 0.5° to 0.7°F
③ A steady decrease in temperature of almost 1° over 3 days followed by a return to baseline.
④ A steady increase in temperature of almost 1 degree over 3 days followed by a return to baseline.

121. An important aspect of planning the care of a dying client is which of the following?
① Point out the maladaptive nature of denial.
② Initially evade questions pertaining to death and dying.
③ Encourage expression of anger and rage.
④ Provide frequent opportunities for the client to talk.

122. The nurse assesses a client's ascites. Which of the following does *not* contribute to the formation of ascites?
① Decreased plasma proteins
② Increased portal pressure
③ Inability of liver to detoxify aldosterone
④ Inability of kidneys to handle the solute load

123. What diuretic would be ordered for a client with ascites?
① Furosemide (Lasix)
② Hydrochlorothiazide (HydroDIURIL)
③ Ethacrynic acid (Edecrin)
④ Spironolactone (Aldactone)

124. The nurse institutes pin care while caring for 9-year-old Quinn, who is in traction after breaking his leg in a skiing accident. What finding should the nurse report immediately to the physician?
① The pin moves freely through the bone.
② The skin around the pin is dry and pink.
③ Quinn has an oral temperature of 37°C.
④ The traction is pulling on the pin.

125. In addition to basal body temperature change, which of the following signs and symptoms is associated with ovulation?
① Presence of mittelschmerz
② Absence of spinnbarkeit mucus
③ Addition of 14 days to the first day of the LMP
④ Palpation of cervix as firmer and more closed

126. Mr. Lieberman had been informed that he has terminal cancer. One morning he states, "I can't

wait until this is over and I can return to work." The most therapeutic response is which of the following?

① "Your work is very important to you, isn't it?"
② "I regret to tell you that you will be unable to return to work."
③ "It sounds like things are difficult for you right now."
④ "What do you mean by this statement?"

127. A family member asks the nurse to explain the primary purpose of a portacaval shunt. Which point should the nurse include in the explanation for the primary purpose of this shunt?

① The shunt eliminates the incidence of further bleeding episodes.
② The shunt restores hepatic function.
③ The shunt reduces portal hypertension and congestion.
④ The shunt decreases further hepatic degeneration.

128. A 15-year-old will be in traction for several weeks. Which diversional activity would best meet his developmental needs?

① Reading school books
② Watching educational television
③ Receiving visits from friends
④ Building model airplanes

129. During morning care the client asks, "Am I going to die?" The most therapeutic response is which of the following?

① "This is the diagnosis your physician has given you."
② "It sounds like you think you are going to die."
③ "What made you ask that question?"
④ "This seems to bother you."

130. A woman has been unsuccessful in getting pregnant after 18 months of unprotected intercourse. Clomiphene (Clomid) is prescribed for her. Which of the following best describes how this drug works?

① It balances the estrogen-progesterone level to support ovulation.
② It increases the amount of gonadotropin secretion to stimulate maturation of the ovarian follicles.
③ It changes the pH of vaginal secretions to support sperm viability.
④ It enhances the development of the endometrium to support pregnancy.

131. A client with cirrhosis is at high risk for infection. Protection of the client from infection is a major nursing goal. To achieve this goal, the nurse would do which of the following?

① Discourage the client from ambulating in the corridor.
② Initiate cooling measures for any temperature above 100°F (37.6°C).
③ Discourage visitors from coming to see the client at this time.
④ Change the IV tubing and dressing q24-48h.

132. Newborn Audrey Trainer has a foot deformity. The deformity is diagnosed as bilateral talipes equinovarus (clubfoot). Which physical finding did the nurse document in the initial newborn assessment that supports this diagnosis?

① Manipulation of the feet seemed to induce pain.
② The feet deviated from the midline when dorsiflexed.
③ The feet were in plantar flexion.
④ The feet were not in alignment with the knees.

133. The nurse caring for a client with liver failure and a recent GI bleed assesses that the client is slightly confused and has bilateral asterixis. The nurse reports this to the physician. The nurse anticipates that the physician's orders will most likely include which of the following?

① Increased sodium by way of an IV route
② Diazepam (Valium) to decrease asterixis
③ Neomycin by mouth
④ A CT scan to rule out any neurologic complications

134. Plaster casts are applied to both feet of an infant with clubfeet to reestablish the correct alignment. Cast application is done as soon as possible after diagnosis because

① Developmental delays are prevented by early application of casts.
② The infant's rapid growth will facilitate the correction.
③ Clubfoot abnormalities cannot be corrected after the age of 6 months.
④ The skin of a newborn is less susceptible to breakdown.

135. The daughter of a client with kidney failure comes to the nurse saying, "I know Daddy is going to die. If only I'd done more to help him." The nurse's best response would be which of the following?

① "Why do you think your father is going to die?"
② "You must not feel guilty for your actions."
③ "Have you shared your feelings with your father?"
④ "I can see that you are upset. Would you like to talk?"

136. A newborn with plaster casts to correct bilateral clubfoot leaves the hospital and returns with his parents to the clinic in 3 weeks for a cast change. What observation would indicate that the nurse's instructions about cast care had not been adequately understood?

① The cast was slightly stained from urine and stool.
② The cast edges were rough.
③ The cast was covered with ink drawings.
④ The cast was wet from a bath.

137. A 35-year-old who has recently been told that she has only 6 months to live says to the nurse, "Leave me alone. You are like everyone else who is hanging around me. Get out of here and don't come back!" An appropriate response is which of the following?

① "What have I done to offend you?"
② "You sound pretty upset right now. Let's talk about it."
③ "We may be hanging around you, but we're trying to help you."
④ "I'll return later after you have cooled off."

138. It is often difficult for the nurse to help the alcoholic client explore behavioral alternatives. An effective initial step for the nurse is to do which of the following?
    ① Enlist the family's support.
    ② Assess the client's motivation.
    ③ Explore his or her own feelings and attitudes about alcohol.
    ④ Acquire knowledge about community treatment programs.

139. Mr. Ellis is a 76-year-old who has been diagnosed with cancer of the liver and has only 6 months to live. He has spent 6 weeks in the hospital and his wife wants him to come home for the remaining time of his life. What is the most therapeutic approach to this situation?
    ① Discourage her from taking him home.
    ② Encourage Mrs. Ellis to discuss this matter with the physician.
    ③ Help them deal with the seriousness of his illness.
    ④ Assist them in making realistic plans to return home.

140. Gabriella is hospitalized at the age of 4 months for corrective surgery of bilateral clubfoot. Immediate postoperative care would include
    ① Elevation of her lower extremities to decrease edema
    ② Elevation of her head to prevent feeding difficulties
    ③ Administering an oral analgesic
    ④ Positioning Gabriella in the prone position

141. Bert Arnold, age 36, is a sales representative for a large computer corporation. Three years ago, he was diagnosed as having an ulcer, and he was advised to find more time for rest and relaxation. He did not comply and, in the last month, has had more frequent epigastric pain. Which would be the most realistic short-term goal to help Mr. Arnold begin to deal with his stress?
    ① Express emotions directly
    ② Decrease workload
    ③ Use relaxation techniques daily
    ④ Decrease social commitments

142. When a client's ulcer was diagnosed 3 years ago, the physician prescribed cimetidine (Tagamet). However, on admission the client reports that the medication has not been taken as prescribed. Which approach would be *least* effective in helping the client to comply?
    ① Help the client set up a medical-reminder schedule.
    ② Educate the client about ulcer complications.
    ③ Suggest that the client enlist the help of co-workers.
    ④ Explain that taking the medication will help decrease the pain.

143. Richard Blevins, age 6 months, has had surgery to correct clubfoot. After several months of postoperative cast wearing, a brace is ordered to maintain the corrected position of Richard's feet. The nurse discusses important aspects about the brace and about Richard's care with his parents. To determine the parents' understanding of the information provided, the nurse should ask which question?
    ① "Do you have any questions?"
    ② "Could you explain to me how to apply the brace?"
    ③ "Could you show me how to apply the brace?"
    ④ "How will you apply Richard's brace?"

144. Which statement indicates that the goal for a terminally ill client was met?
    ① The client moves through the stages of grief and grieving and experiences a dignified death.
    ② The client discontinues denial and expresses anger appropriately.
    ③ The client resumes a lifestyle comparable to that before diagnosis.
    ④ The client becomes as independent as possible for the client's remaining life.

145. Perforation is a major complication of a duodenal ulcer. When this has occurred, what is the initial nursing priority?
    ① Insert a nasogastric tube.
    ② Start an IV for infusion of fluids.
    ③ Administer a high dose of an antibiotic.
    ④ Teach turning, coughing, and deep breathing.

146. A client with an ulcer is taught to check with the physician before taking any medications because there are many drugs that can aggravate the ulcer. An example of a gastrointestinal irritant drug is which of the following?
    ① Indomethacin (Indocin)
    ② Magnesium and aluminum hydroxide (Maalox)
    ③ Atropine
    ④ Acetaminophen (Tylenol)

147. Which of the following is an *inappropriate* goal of Mr. Seele, a client recently diagnosed with bipolar disorder, manic episode?
    ① Client will participate in nonstimulating activities.
    ② Client will remain injury free.
    ③ Client will experience increased sensory stimuli.
    ④ Client will render self-care measures with assistance.

148. A 20-year-old primigravida is admitted to the labor room with contractions every 10 minutes. She denies rupture of membranes. Her gestation is estimated to be at 34 weeks. Which of the following nursing actions is appropriate when caring for this woman?
    ① Prepare for a contraction stress test to determine fetal status.
    ② Prepare for the application of an internal monitor.
    ③ Prepare for evaluation of cervical dilation.
    ④ Prepare for a preterm birth.

149. The nurse instructs the parents of a toddler with a tracheostomy on home care. Which one of the following statements made by the parent indicates that further teaching is needed?
    ① "I'll allow my child to play with his playmates in play group."
    ② "I'll loosely cover the stoma with a scarf when my child plays outdoors."

③ "I'll be careful when bathing my child so water doesn't enter the stoma."

④ "I'll be sure my child wears a plastic bib at mealtimes."

150. Robert Muntz, age 35, is admitted to the hospital with complaints of nausea, vomiting, and dull, wavelike abdominal pains. He appears malnourished and has a greatly enlarged abdomen. The physician suspects cirrhosis and has ordered a liver biopsy to make a definitive diagnosis. The nurse charts the following observations on the admission physical assessment form. Which finding would *not* be associated with cirrhosis?

① Jaundiced sclerae

② Irregular pulse

③ Ascites

④ Patches of ecchymosis on the extremities

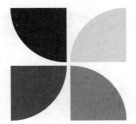

151. A client asks the nurse why, with cirrhosis, there is a tendency to bleed and have abnormal bruising. The nurse in response would include which of the following facts?
① There is inadequate vitamin K absorption.
② There is inadequate vitamin A absorption.
③ There is depressed production of platelets.
④ There is depressed production of red blood cells.

152. During tracheostomy suctioning in a child, which one of the following nursing interventions is appropriate?
① Advance the suction catheter no more than 2 cm beyond the tracheostomy tube and suction for no more than 5 to 6 seconds.
② Advance the suction catheter no more than 2 cm beyond the tracheostomy tube and suction for no more than 3 to 4 seconds.
③ Advance the suction catheter no more than 0.5 cm beyond the tracheostomy tube and suction for no more than 3 to 4 seconds.
④ Advance the suction catheter no more than 0.5 cm beyond the tracheostomy tube and suction for no more than 5 to 6 seconds.

153. What is the most appropriate nursing action for a client undergoing a liver biopsy?
① Explain to the client that the client may resume bathroom privileges after the procedure.
② Position the client in semi-Fowler's position for the procedure.
③ Turn the client to the left lateral recumbant position after the procedure.
④ Assess the client for complaints of abdominal pain after the procedure for at least 24 hours.

154. An expectant mother, 32 weeks of gestation, has a history of two previous preterm births. Which statement by this mother indicates that the nurse's teaching to prevent another preterm birth needs to be reinforced?
① "I will report regular uterine contractions if they are accompanied by pain."
② "I will drink at least 64 ounces of fluids every day and urinate every 2 hours while I am awake."
③ "I will rest on my left side for an hour every day and monitor myself for contractions."
④ "I will avoid sexual intercourse and breast manipulation until after I deliver."

155. Which of the following diets would the nurse encour- age a client with cirrhosis to select in order to best meet optimal nutritional needs?
① High protein
② High fat
③ Low calorie
④ High sodium

156. Which of the following is the most effective nursing intervention for a 58-year-old man diagnosed with bi-polar disorder, manic episode?
① Introduce him to other clients on the unit.
② Encourage him to go to his room and rest.
③ Tell him to go to the recreation room with several clients to enhance his social skills.
④ Guide him to his room and talk to him quietly.

157. What nursing action would best promote adequate respiratory function for a client with ascites?
① Instruct client to cough and deep breathe qh.
② Ambulate client frequently.
③ Maintain client in high Fowler's position in bed.
④ Provide postural drainage and percussion q2h.

158. Isu Wong, age 80, is admitted to the hospital with findings of right-sided weakness, slurred speech, dysphagia, and visual disturbances. She has a history of hypertension. The admission diagnosis is a cerebrovascular accident. What is the most probable pathophysiology of the admission findings?
① Transient ischemic attack
② Cerebral aneurysm
③ Cerebral hemorrhage
④ Meningitis

159. A 4-year-old is being prepared for correction of a mild pulmonary stenosis. He is not sure why he has to stay in the hospital. Which assessment factor is most important in deciding how much information to give him?
① Developmental age
② Desire to learn
③ Previous hospitalization history
④ Attitudes of his parents about hospitalization

160. The nurse documents that an adult client has a positive bilateral Babinski's reflex. This is indicated by which of the following?
① Dorsiflexion of the great toe with plantar stimulation
② Tremor of the foot after brisk, forceful dorsiflexion

③ Extension of the leg when the patellar tendon is struck

④ Plantar flexion of the great toe with plantar stimulation

161. A client who had a cerebral vascular accident is incontinent during the first few days of hospitalization. What would be the most satisfactory means of handling this problem?
① Insert an indwelling catheter
② Offer a bedpan q4h
③ Offer a bedpan q2h
④ Apply disposable diapers and restrict fluids

162. The nurse provides home care instruction to parents of a child with polycythemia. The nurse evaluates the teaching as effective when the parents make which of the following statements?
① "I will keep my child in bed as much as possible."
② "I will observe for any signs of bleeding or excessive bruising."
③ "I will increase my child's food intake and lessen fluid intake."
④ "I will increase my child's fluid intake."

163. While the nurse is bathing a female stroke client, she begins to mutter something unintelligible about the "plant," while pointing excitedly at a glass of water on the bedside stand. She indicates in pantomime that she wants a drink of water. This behavioral observation is most characteristic of which of the following types of aphasia?
① Visual
② Hysterical
③ Receptive
④ Expressive

164. An initial nursing action after the client with bipolar disorder manic episode has been assessed would be which of the following?
① Treat physical problems arising from the manic episode.
② Engage in increased physical activities.
③ Enhance sensory stimuli.
④ Focus on increasing self-esteem.

165. Which of the following behaviors indicates that Demerol has been effective for pain relief in a 4-year-old?
① Increased restlessness
② Respirations of 38
③ Decreased attention span
④ Apical heart rate of 90

166. Where is the speech center of the brain located?
① Medulla oblongata
② Central fissure (Broca's area)
③ Occipital lobe
④ Parietal lobe

167. A 26-year-old woman is admitted to the labor unit in preterm labor. An intravenous infusion of ritodrine hydrochloride is started. Which of the following nursing actions would be most appropriate in preventing side effects from tocolytic therapy for preterm labor?
① Maintain the laboring woman in a side-lying position, and monitor for maternal pulse greater than 140 beats/min.

② Reduce extraneous stimuli, and monitor for blood pressure greater than 140/90.
③ Use side rails, and frequently monitor for urinary output ≥ 25 cc per hour.
④ Frequently monitor maternal reflexes, and encourage fluid intake of 3000 ml or more.

168. What would be the most therapeutic nursing approach when a client's expressive aphasia is severe?
① Anticipate the client's wishes so the client will not need to talk.
② Communicate by means of questions that can be answered by the client shaking the head.
③ Keep up a steady flow of talk to minimize silence.
④ Encourage the client to speak at every possible opportunity.

169. Infusing blood components too rapidly may lead to which of the following problems?
① Hypostatic pneumonia
② Cardiac failure
③ Hemolytic anemia
④ Stress ulcer

170. A woman in preterm labor is given magnesium sulfate. The nurse understands that which of the following client findings indicates that the drug therapy is effective?
① The client does not have a convulsion.
② Contractions decrease and stop.
③ The client's blood pressure decreases.
④ The fetal heart rate shows decreased decelerations.

171. When a 75-year-old female client with a cerebral vascular accident is attempting to speak, she becomes frustrated. Her family asks how to deal with this problem. What is the best advice?
① They should continue to encourage her.
② They should realize it may be their frustration rather than the client's frustration.
③ They can help by anticipating her needs more.
④ Be patient with her, and do not expect too much progress at this time.

172. Lithium is considered a potentially dangerous drug because:
① There is a fine line between therapeutic and toxic levels.
② Lithium has addictive properties.
③ Lithium produces severe sedation and increases the risk of falls.
④ Lithium produces neuroleptic malignant syndrome.

173. A male client, age 90, has some dysphagia from his stroke, but he is beginning to eat solid foods. What is the most important aspect to prevent complications when helping him to eat?
① Use a bulb syringe when giving fluids.
② Praise him consistently if he can feed himself.
③ Keep him positioned in semi-Fowler's position.
④ Allow him to attempt to feed himself.

174. A child's cheeks are flushed and he has hives on his abdomen and lower extremities 30 minutes after a

blood transfusion is begun. Which of these actions should the nurse initially take?
① Continue to monitor for any increase in the symptoms.
② Stop the transfusion and begin an IV infusion of normal saline.
③ Check vital signs and notify the physician immediately.
④ Contact the blood bank to double-check the child's blood type.

175. A family member asks if a new cerebral vascular accident client's right arm and leg will always be paralyzed. Which of the following items is the nurse's answer primarily based on?
① Much of the initial paralysis is due to edema of brain tissue.
② Strokes are characterized by functional, rather than organic, changes.
③ New neurons will be regenerated to replace the damaged ones.
④ Future neurologic status cannot be predicted this early.

176. Lithium is a frequently used adjunct to an antipsychotic drug during the acute manic phase. Which of the following provides the best explanation for this combination?
① Antipsychotic drugs enhance the action of lithium.
② Clients with bipolar disorder also usually have schizophrenia.
③ There is an initial delay of action between administration of lithium and therapeutic effects.
④ Antipsychotic drugs enhance lithium clearance, resulting in reduced risk of toxicity.

177. Clients experiencing acute symptoms of bipolar disorder, manic episode, often refuse to take lithium. Which of the following is *not* likely to be the cause of this behavior?
① Lithium frequently produces weight gain.
② The client often finds the "high" pleasurable and desirable.
③ Lithium produces severe and permanent sexual dysfunction.
④ The client has a problem adjusting to mood changes from elation to normal mood.

178. Mrs. Smith remarks that her son, George, never had any problems with sickle cell disease until about 1 year of age. Which of the following responses best addresses Mrs. Smith's concern?
① "Infections are not a problem until 1 year of age."
② "Fetal hemoglobin levels remain high during infancy."
③ "Maternal antibodies protected George during the first year."
④ "Breast-feeding provides passive immunity for the infant."

179. Attempts to stop a client's preterm labor are unsuccessful, and her baby is born weighing 4 pounds 2 ounces. Which of the following observations of this newborn suggest a gestational age of less than 40 weeks?
① Small amounts of lanugo and vernix, testes descended, and palmar and plantar creases

② Parchmentlike skin, no lanugo, and full areolas in breasts
③ Upper pinna of ear well curved with instant recoil, small amounts of lanugo, and pink in color
④ Dark-red skin, testes undescended with few rugations, and abundant lanugo

180. Which of the following is an important difference between a preterm and term infant?
① A preterm infant will have a more efficient metabolic rate for heat production and maintenance because of its smaller size.
② The term infant will have more lanugo and more vernix than a preterm infant because of longer time in utero.
③ The term infant will be at greater risk for hypoglycemia because of larger size and greater caloric needs.
④ Heat production is low in the preterm infant because of the greater body surface related to weight and lack of subcutaneous fat.

181. What is the most common cause of sickle cell crisis?
① Acute infection
② Emotional stress
③ Strenuous activity
④ Environmental change

182. When is the best time to begin an active rehabilitation program for a new client with a cerebral vascular accident?
① When the physician orders it
② 24 hours after the critical phase of the illness
③ When the client is medically stable
④ When the entire health team can meet and decide on a comprehensive program

183. Which of the following needs would receive the highest priority while caring for a child in sickle cell crisis?
① Hydration
② Elimination
③ Mobility
④ Nutrition

184. Which one of the following would be considered most vital to the success or failure of a rehabilitation program for a stroke client?
① Physicians
② Nursing staff
③ Significant others or family members
④ Physical therapist

185. A client will be discharged on a regimen of warfarin (Coumadin), 10 mg daily. What instructions would the family receive?
① Ensure that weekly activated partial thromboplastin times are done.
② Have the client eat foods that are high in vitamin K.
③ Check the client's skin daily for bruising.
④ Expect to see pink urine for several days.

186. Gladys Witt, age 70, is undergoing hemodialysis for acute renal failure after a hysterectomy. An arteriovenous shunt has been placed in her right forearm. Which of the following is the *least* likely cause of prerenal azotemia?
① Hypovolemia
② Severe crush injuries

③ Shock

④ Poisons

187. Mr. Capelli, a client diagnosed with bipolar disorder, manic episode, yells and demands to be discharged so he can go to Fort Knox. Additionally, he is irritable, agitated, suspicious, and wearing bizarre clothing. What is the most appropriate nursing intervention at this time?

① Call the physician for a discharge order.

② Realize that the client's demands reflect sensory-perceptual disturbances, inability to cope, and intense anxiety.

③ Assess the client's abilities and limitations.

④ Encourage the client to collaborate with the nurse and plan activities of daily living.

188. What is the most important indication for hemodialysis?

① To prepare the client for renal transplant

② To control high serum potassium levels

③ To increase the life span of a client with chronic renal failure

④ To avoid diet and fluid restrictions

189. Gary, age 3, is to receive morphine, 2 mg IM q3h to q4h prn for pain. The vial reads "morphine 5 mg/ml." How much will the nurse administer?

① 0.2 ml

② 0.3 ml

③ 0.4 ml

④ 0.5 ml

190. Mrs. Lindsey is a 33-year-old demanding and angry client who is currently being treated for acute bipolar disorder, manic episode. Which of the following nursing interventions is most therapeutic in dealing with angry outbursts and emotional lability?

① Initiate measures that reduce overt aggression.

② Encourage release of action by participating in competitive sports.

③ Arrange a debate in the client government-community group to foster expression of feelings.

④ Touch the client on the shoulder and begin an active exercise program.

191. Which of the following assessments would most likely indicate respiratory distress in the preterm infant?

① Abdominal breathing with acrocyanosis

② Irregular, shallow respirations

③ Respiratory rate of 30 to 60 per minute

④ Nasal flaring

192. Roosevelt Henderson, age 7, is admitted to the pediatric unit in vasoocclusive sickle cell crisis. Mrs. Henderson is expecting her second child in 6 months and is concerned the child will have sickle cell disease. Neither Mr. nor Mrs. Henderson has the disease. What is the nurse's best response to Mrs. Henderson's concern?

① "Sickle cell disease affects every child in a family."

② "The child will have either the trait or the disease."

③ "There is a 25% chance the baby will have the disease."

④ "There is no risk of developing sickle cell disease."

193. Which of the following is inappropriate to include as a goal of hemodialysis?

① To restore fluid and electrolyte balance

② To correct acid-base imbalance

③ To replace the endocrine functions of the kidneys

④ To remove the nitrogenous by-products of protein metabolism

194. A 20-year-old client needing hemodialysis from acute renal failure after surgery asks about the need to be on the kidney machine. Which is the most appropriate response by the nurse?

① "Don't worry. I'm sure your insurance will cover the cost."

② "We can teach you to do your own treatments at home."

③ "Do you have family members who can learn to do your dialysis?"

④ "It's unlikely you'll need long-term dialysis, and we'll keep you informed about how your kidneys are recovering."

195. Which of the following behaviors does *not* indicate a reduction in symptoms of bipolar disorder, manic episode?

① The client asks for things and speaks in a calm voice.

② The client is aware of feelings and able to express them effectively.

③ The client responds effectively to limit setting.

④ The client is happy and cheerful and denies feeling depressed.

196. George Pasquel, 2½ years old, has an atrial septal defect and has been admitted for a cardiac catheterization. As the nurse prepares George for the procedure, it is most important to determine which of the following?

① Apical/radial pulse rate

② Ability to tolerate fluids

③ Capillary refill

④ Respiratory rate

197. Which of the following is the most important for nurses to understand regarding the symptoms of a conversion disorder?

① They are manifested by an underlying physical disturbance.

② They progress along motor-nerve pathways.

③ The client does not experience a primary gain from them.

④ They depict symbolic dysfunction.

198. The nurse plans to observe a hemodialysis client carefully for symptoms of disequilibrium syndrome during dialysis and immediately after. Which finding would the nurse relate to a different type of complication?

① Agitation

② Lethargy

③ Muscle twitching

④ Convulsions

199. Lee Fong, a 12½-year-old with a ventricular septal defect, is almost ready to be discharged after a cardiac catheterization. Which best demonstrates that Lee understands postprocedure care?

① "I should wait a day or so to take a shower."

② "I should leave the dressing on for at least 3 days before changing it."

③ "If I hurt, I should take two aspirin for the pain."

④ "I should be able to ride my bike tomorrow night."

200. Pulmonary stenosis most often includes which of the following cardiac pathologic conditions?
① Left-to-right shunting of blood
② Left ventricular hypertrophy
③ Right ventricular hypertrophy
④ Aortic insufficiency

201. During hemodialysis, the nurse is most concerned about observing for which of the following findings?
① A drop in urine output to 20 cc per hour
② Temperature of 99°F
③ Blood urea nitrogen change from 50 to 30
④ Heart rate change of 90 to 130

202. Preoperatively, which of the following nursing approaches is most important for a 5-year-old with a ventricular septal defect?
① Allow him to play with other children.
② Encourage him to express his feelings through play.
③ Keep him isolated to prevent exposure to infection.
④ Suggest vigorous exercise to build up his strength.

203. Theoretical causes of conversion disorders are best explained as anxiety arising from which of the following?
① A fixation at the oral stage of development, producing thoughts that are transformed into symptoms
② Repression of feelings transformed into a symptom that has special significance to the individual
③ Suppression of feelings transformed into emotional distress
④ Sublimation of feelings transformed into the presenting symptom

204. Why is regional heparinization used during the dialysis procedure?
① To retard clotting in the cannula
② To prevent clotting in the dialyzer
③ To minimize intravascular thrombosis
④ To decrease embolization of clots from the cannula

205. Which action is *inappropriate* when caring for the arteriovenous shunt?
① Palpate to assess blood flow.
② Apply a tight dressing to prevent cannula dislodgment.
③ Avoid blood pressure readings in the affected limb.
④ Apply antibiotic ointment to the shunt site.

206. Which of the following is an inappropriate goal for the client with a conversion disorder?
① The client will perform self-care activities independently.
② The client will identify and express feelings appropriately.
③ The client will form adaptive coping behaviors.
④ The client will focus on physical symptoms and express feelings.

207. Rena Klein is a 73-year-old retired telephone operator who had a hemorrhoidectomy. She has just returned from the recovery room, has an IV infusing, and is alert and oriented. What step would the nurse take after checking her vital signs?
① Auscultate her chest.
② Check the surgical site for excess bleeding.
③ Check her abdomen for distention.
④ Percuss her bladder.

208. Eight-year-old Suzanne has had a successful surgical correction of her pulmonary stenosis. In preparation of discharge and returning home, the nurse reviews numerous aspects of care. Which of the following discharge instructions should be included in her plan of care?
① Limit her physical activity in the future.
② Help Suzanne understand that she will have special needs.
③ Provide for a tutor to decrease risk of infection from classmates.
④ Treat Suzanne like a normal child.

209. Six hours after surgery, a client has not voided. What is the most appropriate nursing action to take at this time?
① Ask the client if there is a feeling of the need to urinate.
② Catheterize the client.
③ Help the client to the bathroom.
④ Run warm water over the client's fingers.

210. A 60-year-old client with a hemorrhoidectomy progresses well on the second postoperative day. What care is most appropriate at this time?
① Encourage the client to lie supine when in bed.
② Encourage the client to sit up in bed for as long as possible.
③ Have the client sit on a highly inflated rubber ring when in a chair.
④ Take the client's temperature orally.

211. Mr. Lisbon, a 25-year-old, is admitted to the unit with a diagnosis of conversion disorder. When his parents visit, they are overly concerned about their son's condition. Which of the following is most applicable to Mr. Lisbon?
① He is probably experiencing secondary gain of increased time with his parents because of his physical symptoms.
② He is getting his dependency needs met and has fewer responsibilities as long as symptoms persist.
③ A chronic illness role will evolve over time because of persistent symptoms.
④ All of the above are applicable.

212. As a goodbye gift for the nurse, 6-year-old Julian draws a multicolor picture that has as its focus a figure consisting of two circles (head and body), two stick arms, and one stick leg. What is the best response for the nurse to make?
① "Oh, what a nice picture!"
② "Tell me about your drawing."
③ "What is it?"
④ "Is that your doctor?"

213. A 70-year-old client after a hemorrhoidectomy tells the nurse that he is worried about having his first

postoperative bowel movement. What is the best response?

① "All clients with hemorrhoids are concerned about that."
② "What concerns you about it?"
③ "Are you afraid that it will be painful?"
④ "Don't worry. Your doctor has ordered medication to make it as painless as possible."

214. Which of the following instructions would be best to give a client after a hemorrhoidectomy in order to avoid postoperative infection?

① "Do perineal care with antiseptic solution after every stool, and take as many sitz baths as you need to clean the incision."
② "Do perineal care every morning and every evening, and take sitz baths as necessary to clean the incision."
③ "Do perineal care with antiseptic solution every evening, and take three sitz baths every day."
④ "Do perineal care with plain soap and water after every stool, and take a sitz bath four times a day."

215. Which of the following motor skills would the nurse be *least* likely to see a 4-year-old perform?

① Riding a tricycle
② Using scissors to cut out a favorite picture
③ Tying a bow
④ Climbing stairs like an adult

216. Which of the following is important to tell a postoperative hemorrhoidectomy client in preparation for discharge?

① "Limit your fluid intake."
② "Notify your doctor if you have increased pain when having a bowel movement."
③ "Notify your doctor when you have your first bowel movement."
④ "Stay with a low-residue, soft diet for 3 weeks."

217. Three-year-old Mark Elliot has just been admitted to the pediatric unit. Upon entering his room to begin the initial admission assessment, the nurse finds Mark sitting upright in bed, leaning forward with his mouth open. He is drooling and complaining of a sore throat. Based on these findings, the nurse should suspect that Mark has which conditions?

① Spasmodic croup
② Infectious laryngitis
③ Laryngotracheobronchitis
④ Acute epiglottitis

218. A critical aspect of caring for the client with a conversion disorder is which of the following?

① Confront the client to encourage understanding of feelings and related behaviors.
② Express empathy to promote acceptance of limitations.
③ Provide structured activities to divert attention from sick role to adaptive behaviors.
④ Administer antipsychotic agents to reduce anxiety and promote comfort.

219. A baby is born 6 weeks preterm. This newborn's hospital stay is uneventful. Which aspect of the baby's care will have the greatest permanent effect on emotional development?

① The position in which the baby is placed in the crib.
② The way in which the baby is held and touched.
③ The extent to which a quiet environment is provided.
④ The number of caretakers who provide care.

220. When a client is having external radiation for lung cancer what side effect is most likely to be experienced?

① Alopecia
② Bone marrow suppression
③ Stomatitis
④ Dyspnea

221. Nursing management of a client's irradiated skin will *not* include which of the following?

① Applying A and D Ointment prn to relieve dry skin between treatments.
② Cleansing the skin with tepid water and a soft cloth.
③ Avoiding direct exposure to the sun.
④ Redrawing the skin markings if they are accidentally removed.

222. A 25-year-old male client receiving external radiation treatments tells you that he fears he is radioactive and a danger to his family and friends. How would the nurse dispel his fears?

① Inform him that radiation machines are risk free.
② Explain that once the machine is off, radiation is no longer emitted.
③ Avoid telling him that his fears are in fact true.
④ Instruct him to spend short periods of time with his family and friends.

223. In developing a nursing care plan for a child with pneumonia, which of the following would receive the highest priority?

① Airway
② Hydration
③ Mobility
④ Elimination

224. Fatigue is part of a radiation syndrome not related to the site of therapy. How might the nurse best ensure that a client receives adequate rest?

① Schedule all the client's hospital activities early in the morning so that the client has the remainder of the day to rest.
② Encourage the client's family to carry out all activities for the client so that the client will not overexert.
③ Maintain the client's bed rest with bathroom privileges only.
④ Balance the client's daily activities with frequent rest periods.

225. The nurse assesses for findings of early cervical cancer by which of the following?

① A dark, foul-smelling vaginal discharge
② Pressure on the bladder or bowel, or both
③ Back and leg pain and weight loss
④ Vaginal discharge (leukorrhea)

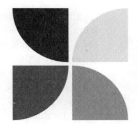

Practice Test 4

226. Carmen Lopez has become increasingly depressed and is brought to the emergency room after trying to kill herself with carbon monoxide. She is conscious and crying uncontrollably. Which of the following actions by the emergency room nurse would have the highest priority?
① Assess her mental and neurological status.
② Check her pulse, respiration, and blood pressure.
③ Sit quietly with her until she is calmer.
④ Talk with her about the problems she has been experiencing.

227. Phillip has epiglottitis. Which of the following manifestations would best indicate that Phillip's respiratory distress is increasing?
① Progressive hoarseness
② Productive cough
③ Increasing heart rate
④ Expiratory wheeze

228. Joe, age 2, has been placed on a regimen of ampicillin, 450 mg IV q6h. Which of the following nursing actions would receive the highest priority?
① Check for hypersensitivity.
② Monitor patency of the IV line.
③ Check client's name band.
④ Administer correct dose of medications.

229. A 15-year-old primigravida delivered a preterm infant 2 days ago. Provisions are made for the new mother to spend time in the premature nursery. Which of the following is the most important reason for doing this?
① To enable the mother to see nurses role model appropriate care of the newborn.
② To reassure the mother that her baby is being well cared for.
③ To provide the mother with the opportunity to handle and care for the infant in a supportive atmosphere.
④ To give the mother an opportunity to ask questions she may have concerning the infant's growth and development.

230. Shortly after Minnie is admitted to the hospital after a suicide attempt, she says, "I don't know why they saved me. I am going to do it again as soon as I get out of here. Things are never going to get better." What is the most appropriate nursing response?
① "Once you get used to the hospital things will get better."
② "It sounds like you are feeling pretty hopeless right now."

③ "You are really upset at the people who saved you."
④ "If you really wanted to kill yourself you would have."

231. A child in respiratory distress is placed in a Croupette with cool mist. What is the best rationale for this action?
① To restrict his activity
② To control his elevated fever
③ To stimulate the cough reflex
④ To reduce mucosal edema

232. Baby Girl Snow is beginning to show signs of respiratory distress. What major symptom would lead the nurse to suspect a tracheoesophageal fistula in Baby Girl Snow?
① Barrel chest
② Snorting respirations
③ Refusal of food
④ Excessive mucus

233. The nurse discusses with a client in the health care clinic the possibility of endometrial cancer. Which of the following statements is *incorrect* concerning endometrial cancer?
① Diagnosis is most frequently established by a dilation and curettage (D&C).
② Prolonged use of exogenous estrogen increases the occurrence.
③ The first and most important symptom is abnormal bleeding.
④ This malignancy tends to spread rapidly to other organs.

234. Which one of the following nursing actions is inappropriate when caring for a child in a Croupette?
① Periodically change the child's linen and pajamas.
② Frequently monitor the child's vital signs.
③ Loosely tuck the tent edges around the mattress.
④ Encourage his mother to stay with him if possible.

235. The Pap smear reveals that a client has cancer of the cervix. The mode of treatment is an abdominal hysterectomy. The client voices concern about undergoing menopause. In counseling her, which statement would be most appropriate?
① A surgical menopause will occur, and treatment with estrogen therapy will be necessary.
② The ovaries will continue to function and produce estrogen, thus preventing menopause as a result of surgery.

③ Ovarian hormone secretion ceases, but the hypothalamus will continue to secrete FSH and this prevents menopause.

④ The ovaries will cease functioning and it will be necessary to take estrogen.

236. Estrogen therapy is often prescribed to suppress the symptoms experienced by the perimenopausal client. Which symptom is inappropriate to associate with the characteristics of menopause?
① Anxiety and nervousness
② Vasomotor instability
③ Osteoporosis resulting in backache
④ Dysmenorrhea and mittelschmerz

237. What datum is crucial when caring for a client who is a high suicide risk?
① Does the client have a plan and means?
② Have other family members attempted suicide?
③ Is there history of previous suicide attempts?
④ Has the client experienced recent major stressors?

238. Which one of the following lab results would give the nurse the most information about a child's hydration status?
① White blood cell count of 12,500
② Urine specific gravity of 1.005
③ Blood Po_2 of 85 mm Hg
④ Serum potassium of 3.8 mEq/L

239. Which of the following symptoms would most likely indicate that a client is experiencing a serious complication after a hysterectomy?
① Gas pains and difficulty defecating
② Moderate amount of serosanguineous drainage on the perineal pad
③ Low-back pain, decreased urinary output
④ Incisional pain requiring narcotic administration for relief

240. What is the most appropriate room placement for a client at high risk for suicide?
① A single room on a closed psychiatric unit
② A single room on an open psychiatric unit
③ A double room on an inpatient psychiatric unit
④ Any room that permits close observation

241. In providing postoperative discharge instructions for a client after an abdominal hysterectomy, the nurse would exclude which item?
① Return to the clinic in 10 days for the removal of the vaginal packing.
② Carry out abdominal strengthening exercises.
③ Expect to experience periodic crying spells.
④ Avoid activities that increase pelvic congestion.

242. A client is seen at the health clinic with the following complaints: urgency, frequency, dysuria, suprapubic pain, and hematuria. What is the most likely cause of the urgency?
① Contracted bladder
② Inflamed bladder
③ Enlarged bladder
④ Increased vascularity in the bladder

243. The mother of a 3-year-old is concerned about his imaginary playmate. She questions the nurse about this. What would be the nurse's best response?
① Suggest that she discuss this with her pediatrician.
② Tell her that imaginary friends are normal for this age group.
③ Encourage her to spend more time with her child.
④ Discuss preschool or day care experience with her.

244. Mr. Marshall, 76 years old, is admitted with depression and a suicide attempt. He has been on paroxetine (Paxil) for several days and he is still depressed and expresses suicidal ideations. What is the reason for his persistent symptoms?
① Paxil is ineffective for this client.
② This is an adverse effect of this medication.
③ His medication must be reassessed and possibly changed.
④ Paxil takes 2 to 3 weeks to produce therapeutic effects.

245. Developmentally, a 3-year-old would be expected to perform which of the following activities?
① Tie his shoelaces
② Hop in place
③ Jump rope
④ Walk backward

246. Fluids, especially those that can aid in altering the urinary pH, should be encouraged for the client with cystitis. The client's nurse would advise the client to take liberal quantities of which of the following?
① Apple juice
② Tea and coffee
③ Vitamin C
④ Orange juice

247. The nurse plans care of a 5-year-old to reduce the stressors associated with hospitalization. Which one of the following interventions will assist the child in coping with hospitalization?
① Perform all painful procedures immediately on admission.
② Minimize intrusive genital-rectal procedures, such as rectal temperatures.
③ Encourage parents to leave the room when intrusive procedures are performed.
④ Recognize evidence of separation anxiety as abnormal.

248. The postoperative nursing care of an infant with a repaired tracheoesophageal fistula would *not* include which of the following?
① Careful monitoring of IV solutions
② Vigorous nasotracheal suctioning
③ Elevation of the head and thorax 30 degrees
④ Good skin care of gastrostomy site

249. Lisa Epstein is a 25-year-old woman admitted to the psychiatric hospital after attempting to kill her brother. Her mood is calm, and she exhibits little remorse and no close interactions with her family. Her family reports a history of running away from home and frequent job changes. Shortly after admission, she expresses feelings of affection for the male nurse assigned to her. She is seductive and cooperative and tells him, "You are the kind of man I like, and I am

glad you are my nurse." Which of the following statements best describes Miss Epstein's behavior?
1. The male nurse is someone she can really feel close to.
2. She is aware of this nurse's professional clinical skills.
3. She is skillful at meeting her needs at the expense of others.
4. She is letting the nurse know that she has insight and is willing to alter her behavior.

250. A drug that acts only on bacteria in the urine and is not absorbed systemically is which of the following?
1. Sulfisoxazole (Gantrisin)
2. Penicillin
3. Ampicillin
4. Tetracycline

251. Fourteen-year-old Susan has been prescribed a Milwaukee brace for treatment of scoliosis. At the first follow-up clinic visit her mother reports to the nurse that Susan has been refusing to wear her brace for the past week. Which one of the following is the nurse's best initial response?
1. "Susan, you know your back will not get better if you don't wear your brace."
2. "Susan, you might need surgery on your back if you won't wear your brace."
3. "Susan, you need to be in control and to decide for yourself how to proceed with the treatment."
4. "Susan, I'd like to talk with you alone for a few minutes about the brace and scoliosis."

252. In collecting data about Baby Girl Sneed, who has tracheoesophageal fistula, which finding is the nurse most likely to see in Mrs. Sneed's perinatal records?
1. Exposure to rubella in the first trimester
2. Active herpes lesions at delivery
3. Polyhydramnios in the third trimester
4. Prolonged active stage of labor

253. Which statement best describes factors that contribute to antisocial personality disorder?
1. Opportunities to form meaningful relationships existed, but the client avoided close relationships.
2. Early childhood needs for security and love were met, but later parental interactions were distant.
3. Superego development was impaired, and the client did not internalize positive identifications.
4. Below average intelligence is the basis of lifelong patterns of difficulty.

254. What organisms are sulfonamides most effective against?
1. *E. coli*
2. *Pseudomonas*
3. *Salmonella*
4. *Klebsiella*

255. Which of the following is most characteristic of rheumatoid arthritis?
1. It most often occurs in women between the ages of 40 and 80.
2. It is most commonly a nonsystemic involvement.
3. Joints are affected bilaterally and symmetrically.
4. It first occurs in a joint after a traumatic injury.

256. When working with the client with antisocial personality disorder, a primary nursing goal is which of the following?
1. Allow the client to prepare as much for treatment as often as possible.
2. Promote involvement in recreational and occupational therapies.
3. Use an interdisciplinary approach to define and set consistent limits for behavior.
4. Consistently provide sympathy and support of the client's attempts to reduce anxiety.

257. A client is seen in the obstetric clinic at 14 weeks of gestation. She complains of an intermittent, brownish-red discharge and severe nausea and vomiting. Abdominal palpation reveals the uterus to be at the level of the umbilicus. Fetal heart tones are absent. A preliminary diagnosis of a hydatidiform mole is made. Additional signs characteristic of molar pregnancy that this woman might have include which of the following?
1. Hypotension and polycythemia
2. Decreased HCG levels and bradycardia
3. Hypertension and anemia
4. Elevated WBC and tachycardia

258. Sixteen-year-old Mary Ann had surgical correction of scoliosis 6 hours ago. Which one of the following assessment findings should the nurse immediately report to the surgeon?
1. Pain rating of 3 on a scale of 1 to 10 while using patient-controlled analgesia
2. Absence of bowel sounds
3. Urine output of 30 ml for the past 2 hours through an indwelling catheter
4. Movement of toes bilaterally, pedal pulses palpable, toes cool

259. Which one of the following lab values would most likely support the diagnosis of rheumatoid arthritis?
1. Elevated sedimentation rate
2. Decreased WBC count in the synovial fluid
3. Normal hematocrit and hemoglobin
4. Absence of rheumatoid factor in the serum

260. The nurse evaluates the teaching of an adolescent after lumbar puncture as effective when the child states:
1. "I'll walk about my room to prevent a headache."
2. "I'll lie flat in bed to prevent a headache."
3. "I'll sit up in bed to prevent a headache."
4. "I'll sit up in the chair to prevent a headache."

261. Mitsu Chung, age 26, is admitted to the unit for diagnostic tests. She is 5 feet 2 inches tall and weighs 120 pounds. She appears acutely ill and complains of pain and stiffness of the joints in her hands, feet, and knees. The tentative diagnosis is rheumatoid arthritis. Which assessment finding would *not* be typical?
1. Recent weight loss and anorexia
2. Stiffness that becomes more pronounced later in the day
3. Tender, hot, and red joints
4. Low-grade fever

262. The physician suspects that a prenatal client who is 16 weeks pregnant may have a hydatidiform mole.

Which of the following diagnostic measures would be carried out to confirm a diagnosis of a hydatidiform mole?
1. Amniocentesis
2. Ultrasound
3. Laparoscopy
4. Serum estriol levels

263. Which of the following best explains common responses of clients with antisocial personality disorders?
1. Low self-esteem and poor impulse control
2. Distance and aloofness
3. Extreme guilt and dependency on others for approval
4. Selfishness and a lack of concern for others

264. Which action would be *inappropriate* to include in a plan of care for a client with arthritis?
1. Schedule the client's activities to allow for at least 8 to 10 hours of sleep every night, with naps during the day.
2. Educate the client and family to avoid quackery from health service providers.
3. Put the head of the bed in high position when helping the client out of bed.
4. Help the client to select a high-calorie, high-protein, and high-calcium diet.

265. A child with asthma begins to show signs of increasing respiratory distress. These include all of the following *except*
1. Cyanosis with tachypnea
2. Intercostal retractions
3. Increased restlessness
4. Irregular respirations

266. A primigravida is diagnosed by her obstetrician as having a hydatidiform mole. The nurse understands that this condition will most likely be treated with which of the following?
1. Dilation and curettage
2. Betamethasone therapy
3. Vacuum extraction
4. Laser treatments

267. Mr. Lipsy, a client diagnosed with antisocial personality disorder, attends family therapy with his parents. The client is frequently blamed for his parent's conflicts and cost of present hospitalization. The parents also continually seek passes and early release from the hospital. Which of the following describes the parent's beliefs and feelings?
1. They feel that he has improved and can function in the community.
2. They feel that he has been disciplined enough for his previous behavior.
3. They have ambivalent feelings about him.
4. They feel shame and responsibility for their son's behavior.

268. Prevention of deformities is a major goal for arthritics. Which nursing action would be *inappropriate* to include under this goal?
1. Place pillows under the major joints.
2. Encourage the client to lie prone several times a day.

3. Place a pillow between the legs when the client is positioned on a side.
4. Provide the client with a small pillow for the head.

269. After several weeks of hospitalization on the inpatient psychiatric unit, a 30-year-old man is diagnosed with antisocial personality disorder. He displays depression and feelings of remorse and fault. What evaluation of his progress is most pertinent?
1. He has developed a dysthymic disorder adjunct to antisocial personality disorder.
2. He is experiencing major depression in addition to antisocial personality disorder.
3. He is gaining insight into the impact of his maltreatment of others and feels depressed.
4. He recognizes that his diagnosis has a poor prognosis and feels depressed.

270. After the administration of epinephrine, the nurse would monitor a child for which sign of epinephrine toxicity?
1. Tinnitus
2. Coryza
3. Tachycardia
4. Dyspnea

271. Which of the following is an *incorrect* method to relieve pain for clients with arthritis?
1. Application of hot, moist packs to the affected joints
2. Application of cold packs to the affected joints
3. Administration of analgesics on a regular schedule every 3 to 4 hours
4. Application of massage to the joints when the client has complaints of ache in the joints

272. Which of the following nursing actions would be most appropriate for a hospitalized preschooler with asthma?
1. Position her in a supine position.
2. Limit oral fluids in order to decrease secretions.
3. Monitor intake and output and specific gravity.
4. Turn, cough, and deep breathe q2h.

273. Which of the following complications would be of greatest concern for a woman after removal of a hydatidiform mole?
1. Ectopic pregnancy
2. Choriocarcinoma
3. Pelvic inflammatory disease
4. Incompetent cervix

274. One day in the day hospital program, Mr. Linny, a client diagnosed with antisocial personality disorder, is seen helping a depressed client with a project. His attitude remains helpful and not superior. Which statement best describes his behavior?
1. He is attempting to show staff how much he has improved.
2. He is genuinely interested in helping the client complete the project.
3. His condition is improving, and his behavior reflects improved and appropriate interactions with others.
4. He is displaying apathy by doing no more than is expected of him.

275. Exercise is an important treatment modality for clients with arthritis. Which client response indicates the need for further teaching regarding physical exercise guidelines?
① "Exercise only to the point of pain, never beyond."
② "Refrain from exercising affected joints until pain and swelling subside."
③ "Isometric exercises can be done independently and without supervision."
④ "An ongoing regimen of exercise at all times for all joints is essential."

276. High-dose aspirin is prescribed for its antiinflammatory action. What nurse's instructions would be given regarding this drug?
① Take the drug 2 hours before and 2 hours after eating.
② Take the drug alternately with Tylenol.
③ Examine the stools and urine for blood.
④ The drug may need to be taken indefinitely.

277. A first grader is receiving a continuous IV drip of aminophylline. Which observation by the nurse indicates aminophylline toxicity?
① Lethargy
② Hypertension
③ Diarrhea
④ Tachycardia

278. A 39-year old male client, who has recently been diagnosed with HIV, asks the nurse for a date. What is the most therapeutic nursing response?
① "It's inappropriate for me to go out with clients."
② "Are you concerned about the impact of HIV on your life?"
③ "Are you seriously involved with anyone?"
④ "I am your nurse, not your friend."

279. Fourteen-year-old Larry Benoit is admitted to the hospital with severe injuries sustained during a motor vehicle accident in which his girlfriend had been driving. Both adolescents had been drinking, and his friend was speeding in an erratic manner. Larry suffered a third-degree burn of his right arm. Amputation remains a concern. Ten days later his condition stabilizes, and he becomes extremely demanding of the nursing staff, frequently turning on his call light and screaming for the nurse if it is not answered immediately. Larry's behavior is most likely associated with which of the following?
① Alcohol withdrawal
② Boredom
③ Psychosis
④ Adjustment disorder, depressive mood

280. Which of the following actions is expected of epinephrine?
① Relax bronchial spasms
② Liquefy respiratory secretions
③ Increase antibody formation
④ Reduce airway diameter

281. The physician may prescribe a gold preparation for arthritis clients if the present medications are not effective. What is a major *disadvantage* of gold preparations?
① They must be administered several months before benefits can be determined.
② They must be given intravenously.
③ The urine will turn green.
④ Serious adverse effects commonly occur during the first week.

282. Harlan King, age 88, sustained a left-sided cerebrovascular accident 4 weeks ago. He has been transferred to a rehabilitation unit. He is able to communicate by minimal verbal expression and gesturing that he intends to walk again and use his right arm. His wife expresses the same goals. After a comprehensive assessment and before the initiation of a rehabilitation program for Mr. King, what must all rehabilitation team members consider?
① Initial assessments will need to be modified throughout the first week or two, because the transfer to a new environment and the client's fatigue during this period will affect the accuracy of assessments.
② Try to accomplish as much as possible with this client in the first 2 weeks; after that, motivation will generally decrease and gains made thereafter will be minimal.
③ Mrs. King will need to find something to do outside the rehabilitation setting. Mr. King needs to concentrate on his rehabilitation program at this point, and too much stimulation from family members will confuse him.
④ While making ongoing diagnostic assessments, give the client as many cues as possible so that he will perform optimally.

283. Which of the following is most characteristic of asthma?
① Inspiratory stridor
② Expiratory wheezing
③ Prolonged inspiration
④ Hoarse voice

284. After removal of a hydatidiform mole, a client tells the nurse that she is very disappointed that this pregnancy did not have a successful outcome. She wonders how soon she can plan to become pregnant again. In response to this question, the nurse indicates that the recommended waiting period before the next pregnancy is
① One menstrual cycle
② Six months
③ One year
④ Five years

285. Safety precautions are an important part of poststroke care. If a client's right arm and leg have decreased sensation, along with the paresis, the client could easily be injured. Based on these data, the plan of care would include which of the following actions?
① Protect these extremities with an arm sling and bivalved leg cast.
② Instruct the client to observe the affected arm and leg frequently for positioning and to become aware of any movements that might injure them.

③ Concentrate on the positives; do not talk about the paralyzed extremities and thus depress the client.

④ Place any equipment (food tray, call light, television changer) on the client's right side so the client can safely be independent in some functions and gain self-esteem through this increase in independence.

286. The most therapeutic independent nursing approach for a client with a generalized anxiety disorder is to do which of the following?
① Administer diazepam (Valium).
② Use active-listening skills.
③ Obtain psychiatric consultation.
④ Schedule a team conference.

287. After a cerebrovascular accident, a client is having difficulty attaining sufficient nutritional intake. The client has some trouble swallowing and has choked while eating. How can eating be facilitated?
① Teach the client to eat slowly and place food in the paralyzed side of the mouth.
② Instruct the client's spouse to feed the client after ensuring that all food is cut into bite-sized pieces.
③ Help the client to a sitting position, place food in the unparalyzed side of the mouth, and have the client concentrate on chewing and swallowing.
④ Restrict the intake to liquids until chewing and swallowing capacities are fully restored.

288. Helen Jenkins, age 8, is admitted to the pediatric unit with a diagnosis of acute bronchial asthma. She has had a bad cold for several days before the attack and would awaken during the night with coughing and shortness of breath. Helen's physician has ordered epinephrine (Adrenalin) 0.03 ml stat, to be repeated in 20 minutes if no relief is obtained. What is the most common route of administration for epinephrine?
① Intramuscular
② Subcutaneous
③ Intravenous
④ Sublingual

289. One morning during the dressing change of a 17-year-old client whose arm is fractured, she asks a male nurse to go bowling with her. What best explains her behavior?
① She is acting out sexual feelings and relating to him as an adult.
② She is trying to embarrass the nurse.
③ She wants to be reassured that her arm will heal and maintain normal function.
④ Her comments are natural under the circumstances.

290. After hospitalization for the evacuation of a hydatidiform mole, a 26-year-old client is preparing to go home. Which of the following responses would best indicate to the nurse that the client has understood discharge instructions?
① "I will minimize my fluid intake and dietary iron for 1 month."
② "I will avoid the use of tampons for 1 year."
③ "I will have my blood checked for chorionic gonadotrophin monthly for 6 months."
④ "I will take prophyllactic antibiotics for 10 days."

291. It is important to minimize deformities in clients who have sustained brain damage. How is this best accomplished?
① Set up a program with the clients and let the clients be responsible for doing range-of-motion exercises on their own.
② Schedule daily visits to physical therapy while the clients are in the rehabilitation setting.
③ Remind the clients that they have flaccid paralysis of their right side and need to prevent subluxation of the right shoulder by exercise.
④ Establish a schedule to assist the clients to exercise their right side with their unaffected side.

292. The physician writes an order for Tanya, a 17-year-old whose foot was fractured in a recent motor vehicle accident, to get out of bed on crutches for the bathroom only. The nurse finds Tanya in the room of another adolescent playing a video game. The nurse confronts her, and she replies, "What difference does it make? I am going to lose my foot anyway." What is the most appropriate nursing response?
① "Where did you hear that?"
② "If you don't stay in bed you probably will."
③ "You seem upset and worried about losing your foot."
④ "I will get a wheelchair and assist you back to bed."

293. The nurse is developing a teaching plan for the parents of a 6-year-old child newly diagnosed with asthma. The nurse bases her instruction about pulmonary function tests on which one of the following?
① Pulmonary function tests reveal inspiratory difficulty and lowered oxygen saturation.
② Pulmonary function tests must be performed in an outpatient treatment center.
③ Young children can be taught to correctly perform pulmonary function tests.
④ Pulmonary function tests are difficult to interpret in children.

294. Based on knowledge of the hormonal changes of pregnancy, which hormone is necessary for a positive pregnancy test?
① Placental estrogen
② Human chorionic gonadotropin
③ Human placental lactogen
④ Luteal progesterone

295. Which behavior best typifies the client with right-sided hemiplegia?
① Unaware of limitations; plunges into activities unaware of safety factors.
② Anxious; approaches tasks in a halting, fearful way; may respond best to simple gestures.
③ Communicates with verbal directives; feels gestures and pantomime are demeaning.
④ Especially prone to spatial-perceptual problems.

296. A client recently diagnosed with vascular dementia (stroke) is in stable condition. She is restless, talkative, and asks repetitive questions. These behaviors are most indicative of which of the following?
① Confusion
② Anxiety

③ Anger
④ Suspiciousness

297. A nursing home client spends a lot of time sitting in a chair. Where do decubitus ulcers most often develop when clients spend most of their time sitting in a chair?
① Over the sacrum
② Over the coccyx
③ Over the ischial tuberosities
④ On the heels

298. The mother of child with varicella asks when the child can return to school. What would be the best response?
① "When she no longer has a fever."
② "In 2 weeks."
③ "When all her lesions have dried."
④ "When no new lesions have appeared for 24 hours."

299. A couple has been trying to conceive. The husband asks about the accuracy of home pregnancy tests. The nurse responds

① "They are about 80% accurate, with false-positives common."
② "They are about 85% accurate, with false-negatives possible."
③ "They are about 97% accurate when done carefully, according to package directions."
④ "They are unreliable because urine is tested. A blood test is needed to confirm pregnancy."

300. Lillie, a 12-year-old, is admitted to the adolescent psychiatric unit with a diagnosis of conduct disorder. She reports that she is feeling better because she has spent the night planning how to "get back" at her friend. The nurses replies, "Sounds like you are pretty upset." This is an illustration of which therapeutic communication skill?
① Acceptance
② Reflection
③ Verbalization of implied thoughts and feelings
④ Encouraging expression of feelings

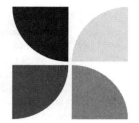

Practice Test 5

301. The nurse explains to a group of teenagers in a "family living class" that a teratogen is any factor that has an adverse effect on the developing child in utero and that the timing of exposure to such a factor is significant. The most critical period for disruption of fetal development by teratogen exposure exists during which period?
① From conception to the eighth week, during organogenesis.
② After 16 weeks, when the fetus begins swallowing amniotic fluid.
③ Beginning at 20 weeks, when the fetus is capable of producing antibodies.
④ During the third trimester, which is a period of very rapid growth.

302. What is the most therapeutic response to a demanding adolescent?
① Assign a different nursing staff daily.
② Disregard inappropriate demands.
③ Perceive the demands as manifestations of fear and anger and respond to them when possible.
④ Set firm, consistent limits on inappropriate demands.

303. Which activity is most appropriate for a 5-year-old recovering from varicella?
① Watching cartoons on television
② Talking on the telephone with friends
③ Painting with watercolors
④ Reading a book of riddles

304. What is the most important point to be included in the discharge teaching of a client who had a total endocrine gland removed?
① Meticulous skin care
② Relaxation techniques
③ Diet teaching
④ Medication administration

305. On the third postoperative day, a client shows signs and symptoms of a mild addisonian crisis. Which of the following statements best explains why this is considered a medical emergency?
① The increased cortisol levels can result in a hyperosmolar coma.
② Loss of sodium and increased potassium levels can cause life-threatening fluid and electrolyte imbalances.
③ Increased aldosterone levels can trigger cardiac failure.

The posterior pituitary gland cannot produce enough antidiuretic hormone.

306. The clinic nurse discusses adolescent development with the parent of 13-year-old Michael. Which one of the following responses by the parent indicates that additional clarification is needed by the nurse?
① "Michael needs to feel he belongs to his peer group."
② "I'll listen to Michael's concerns and try to be open to his viewpoint."
③ "Michael's rebellion against my rules only results in stricter limits."
④ "When Michael is in a bad mood, I leave him alone."

307. A client asks the nurse how her fetus' circulation is different in utero than it is once the baby is born. As a part of the explanation, the nurse describes the ductus arteriosus, the foramen ovale, and the ductus venosus, which allow the majority of fetal blood to bypass the fetal
① Kidneys and lungs
② Lungs and liver
③ Liver and spleen
④ Spleen and kidneys

308. Mary Colter, 38 years old, is brought to the emergency department in an irritable and agitated state by her brother. Her husband moved out earlier today and into a townhouse with his 22-year-old bookkeeper. He has asked for a divorce. Mrs. Colter has two sons, has completed 1 year of college, and has not worked outside of the home in 16 years. Which of the following conditions best describes this client?
① Situational crisis
② Major depressive episode
③ Psychosis
④ Bipolar disorder, manic episode

309. The most important postoperative adrenalectomy assessment would be which of the following?
① Type of nasogastric drainage
② Presence of drainage on abdominal dressing
③ Respiratory rate changes
④ Blood pressure changes

310. It is imperative to advise the mother of a child with varicella to do which of the following?
① Provide cool humidity.
② Keep the child's fingernails short and clean.
③ Apply cool compresses to the child's lesions.
④ Avoid giving the child acidic foods or fluids.

311. Preoperatively, an adrenalectomy client says to the nurse, "I want to have this operation so I will look like my old self again." What would be an appropriate response?
① "It will take several months before the changes are reversed."
② "Tell me what concerns you the most."
③ "Adjusting to body changes is never easy to do."
④ "Have you discussed this with your partner?"

312. A bilateral adrenalectomy is scheduled for a client, age 40. Client teaching should include which of the following facts?
① Lifelong replacement of corticosteroids will be required.
② Weekly ACTH injections will be done.
③ Cortisol will be required in stress situations.
④ No replacement therapy will be necessary.

313. A 6-year-old with varicella has two younger brothers. Her mother would be advised to institute which type of isolation precautions at home?
① Respiratory isolation
② Universal precautions
③ Wound and skin isolation
④ Enteric precautions

314. An important characteristic of crisis intervention is which of the following?
① It is critical to assess the cause before a solution can be determined.
② Its impact is short term unless the client achieves insight and self-awareness.
③ Appropriate solutions and options are presented to the client by the therapist.
④ It focuses primarily on helping an individual cope with the immediate crisis or problem.

315. Which of the following must be assessed when evaluating a client in crisis?
① Precipitating events, coping patterns, and available support systems
② Early childhood experiences and family interactions
③ Hallucinations, suspiciousness, and irrational thoughts
④ Past relationships with significant others

316. Which of the following would be a good choice for a high-protein, high-potassium, low-calorie, low-sodium lunch?
① Chicken, brown rice, and sliced oranges
② Tomato soup, tuna fish sandwich, and vanilla pudding
③ Macaroni and cheese, tomato salad, and baked apple
④ Broiled steak, green beans, and ice cream

317. A client with Cushing's syndrome is constantly hungry and is concerned about an inability to stop eating. This is probably occurring for which of the following reasons?
① The client is stressed, compensating by eating.
② The client is hypoglycemic, and the body compensates with hunger.
③ The client has increased cortisol levels that accelerate gluconeogenesis.

④ The client has had an increase in energy output and requires more calories.

318. Four-year-old Nancy has varicella. Her fever is 102.5° F (39.2° C). Which clinical sign would *not* be related to her diagnosis?
① Pruritus
② Lesions in four stages
③ Lymphadenopathy
④ Paroxysmal cough

319. During a childbirth education class the nurse describes fetal development and the role of the placenta in pregnancy. Which of the following is a function of the placenta?
① Produces oxytocin in increasing amounts throughout pregnancy
② Allows exchange of nutrients and waste products
③ Protects the fetus from viral infections during the first 3 months
④ Allows maternal and fetal blood to mix freely

320. What is a the first nursing priority when caring for a 38-year-old man experiencing a crisis after his wife asks for a divorce?
① Reassure him that the crisis is short.
② Assess the degree of the immediate problems and his perception of them.
③ Advise him to call his lawyer and make an appointment for the following day.
④ Call his wife and inform her of his situation.

321. After 8 years of marriage, a couple is expecting their first baby. In the seventh month of pregnancy they decide to deliver in a birthing center. The nurse conducts a tour of the suite and describes the protocols of the birth center. Which statement best indicates the couple understands the options a birthing center offers?
① "A nurse-midwife will be called in if any complications occur."
② "Use of medications in labor will be restricted."
③ "After birth the baby will be placed in a special observation area for a few hours."
④ "Use of a birthing center is limited to low-risk clients."

322. A client calls the crisis hot line and makes an appointment. As the nurse begins the interview the client begins to cry. What is the most appropriate nursing response?
① Provide the client with privacy.
② "Everything will be okay in several days."
③ Offer the client an antianxiety medication.
④ "Tell me what is troubling you."

323. What is the rationale for administering hydrocortisone (Solu-Cortef) to a child with asthma?
① It reduces anxiety.
② It diminishes inflammation.
③ It mobilizes secretions.
④ It relieves bronchospasms.

324. The physician has ordered a plasma cortisol test. The nurse plans that the blood will be drawn at
① 6 AM
② 2 PM
③ 11 AM and 8 PM
④ 8 AM and 5 PM

325. Which of the following fluid or electrolyte problems is most likely to occur with hyperadrenal function?
① Hyperkalemia
② Increased output of dilute urine
③ Sodium and H_2O retention
④ Decreased serum calcium

326. Prolonged use of steroids in children can lead to which of the following?
① Laryngeal edema
② Growth suppression
③ Grand mal seizures
④ Chronic osteoarthritis

327. Which of the following pets would be most appropriate for a child with asthma?
① Parakeet
② Dog
③ Cat
④ Fish

328. What is the most appropriate referral for a woman whose husband died several months ago and who is complaining of anxiety, weight loss, and sleep, appetite, and concentration disturbances?
① Day hospital
② Health maintanence organization (HMO)
③ Self-help group
④ Psychiatric hospitalization

329. Mr. Bernstein, whose teenage son is dying, says to the nurse, "I don't think I can go on living when my son is gone." What would be the best response?
① "Do you think your life will be over?"
② "You will find it difficult to continue your life without Tommy."
③ "Your wife will need you."
④ "I can understand how you feel."

330. Jane Johnson, age 45, is admitted to the hospital for a diagnostic workup. For the past 2 months, she has been irritable and argumentative with her boyfriend. At other times, she has been almost euphoric. She has been depressed about recent body changes. She has gained 15 pounds; her face is puffy and flushed. She has also noted numerous bruises over her body; and while her abdomen has begun to protrude, her legs have become thin. Miss Johnson is admitted with the tentative diagnosis of Cushing's syndrome. When Miss Johnson has been admitted to the hospital, the immediate nursing priority is which of the following actions?
① Decrease stress in the environment.
② Encourage liberal amounts of fluids.
③ Explain tests and procedures.
④ Provide diversional activities.

331. In planning the care of a client experiencing a crisis, which appointment scheduling is most appropriate?
① Daily session for 1 week
② Twice a week for 2 weeks
③ Three times a week for 3 weeks
④ Weekly for 6 weeks

332. A woman whose husband left her 8 weeks ago reports that she has begun working as a teacher's assistant at her son's school, has sought the services of a lawyer, and is receiving child support. This information suggests that the client is functioning at what level?
① At the same level because she is unaffected by the crisis.
② At a lower level because of the impact of the crisis.
③ At a higher level because of her personal growth.
④ At the same level because despite the crisis her level of function remains the same.

333. Roberto, who is hospitalized with a terminal illness, requests that the radio be played at night, which is against hospital rules. What would be the best course of action for the nurse?
① Gently refuse and explain the rules.
② Let him play the radio, but keep his door shut.
③ Consider the possibility of obtaining earphones for the radio.
④ Strictly enforce the rules and set limits.

334. Which of the following is incorrect to think of as a cause of Cushing's syndrome?
① Adrenal tumor
② Ectopic source of ACTH
③ Pituitary tumor
④ Adrenal atrophy

335. Which of the following test results are most indicative of Cushing's syndrome?
① Increased serum sodium and plasma free-cortisol levels
② Decreased serum potassium and BUN
③ Increased serum epinephrine and norepinephrine
④ Decreased urinary 17-ketogenic steroids and 17-hydroxycorticoids

336. Vickie, age 12, has an order for meperidine (Demerol), 50 mg with hydroxyzine (Vistaril), 25 mg IM q3h to q4h prn for pain. Which of the following is *not* an action of hydroxyzine?
① Antiemetic
② Antihistaminic
③ Central nervous system stimulant
④ Opiate and barbiturate potentiator

337. Tommy Miller is a 15-year-old with lymphoma. During the terminal phase of his illness, he is hospitalized with nausea, edema, and pruritus. His mouth is ulcerated with some infected areas visible. His parents refuse to leave him. He is becoming very restless. During the terminal stages of Tommy's illness, the nurse needs to support Mr. and Mrs. Miller. Which of the following is *not* considered supportive nursing action?
① Call their religious advisor if they request.
② Arrange an opportunity for them to talk with the physician.
③ Allow them to stay with Tommy and give them privacy.
④ Wait to be asked before providing help.

338. Chemical dependency challenges nurses to recognize symptoms of various drugs. Misty is a 23-year-old brought to the emergency department by her boyfriend, who reports that she has been extremely irritable, suspicious, and uncooperative since returning home after being out all night. During the initial as-

sessment you notice that the client has dilated pupils and increased blood pressure and pulse rate. She is also fearful and suspicious. What is the most likely cause of Misty's symptoms?
1. Cocaine withdrawal
2. Alcohol intoxication
3. Amphetamine intoxication
4. Heroin intoxication

339. A primigravida begins labor while her husband is on a business trip. When she arrives at the maternity unit, she is very upset that he cannot be with her at this time because they had prepared together for active participation in the birth. What approach can the nurse take to meet the client's needs at this time?
1. Ask if there is another individual she would like as support person.
2. Assure her that a member of the nursing staff will be with her at all times.
3. Tell her you will continue to try to locate her husband.
4. Reinforce the woman's confidence in her own abilities to cope and maintain a sense of control.

340. Misty continues to withdraw and walk away from her nurse. Which of the following is an *inappropriate* nursing action when caring for this client?
1. Touching the client on the shoulder.
2. Offering the client a prn antianxiety medication.
3. Speaking to the client in a calm and firm manner.
4. Displaying patience and empathy.

341. In assessing a client's progress during labor, which of the following observations best indicates imminent delivery?
1. Spontaneous rupture of membranes
2. 100% effacement
3. Bulging perineum
4. Strong contractions lasting 60 to 70 seconds

342. When giving mouth care to a client with cancer and with mouth ulcers, what would the nurse use?
1. A toothbrush
2. Peroxide solution
3. A mild mouthwash solution
4. Nothing; it will only annoy the client

343. Assessment findings that would commonly lead the nurse to suspect a client has Cushing's syndrome include which of the following?
1. Low blood glucose and tachycardia
2. Thickening of the skin and bruising
3. Weight loss and sodium retention
4. Delayed wound healing and osteoporosis

344. Skin care for a child with terminal cancer and pruritus would include
1. Keeping the fingernails short.
2. A daily tub bath.
3. A shower as desired.
4. A scrub with pHisoHex.

345. A couple have chosen to have their baby at a local birthing center. In accordance with the center's policies, mother and baby will be discharged 8 hours after delivery with follow-up home care. Which of the following aspects of postpartal teaching is of highest priority before discharge?
1. Discuss parent-infant bonding and cue-response behaviors.
2. Teach danger signs, temperature taking, and uterine palpation.
3. Demonstrate infant bathing and cord care.
4. Discuss alterations in postpartum sexuality.

346. Deborah Ortez, a middle-aged businesswoman, is admitted to the psychiatric unit. She tells the nurse that she came to the hospital to get away from spies on her job who are attempting to "reprogram her mind." In efforts to help this client the most important nursing intervention involves which of the following?
1. Gather more information about her job situation.
2. Confront her about the irrational nature of this story.
3. Appreciate her feelings without agreeing with them.
4. Encourage her to confront co-workers and deal with the situation realistically.

347. Which of the following is a priority goal for mother and infant during the first postpartum day?
1. Promote health during the perinatal period.
2. Teach developmental needs in the first 12 months.
3. Support maternal and neonatal thermoregulation.
4. Promote attachment.

348. Mrs. Ackers, mother of Paul, who has terminal cancer, is overheard telling another visitor that Paul will be going home soon and will be able to return to high school. Mrs. Ackers is exhibiting behavior typical of which stage of loss?
1. Denial
2. Acceptance
3. Restitution
4. Guilt

349. Charles Arden, the victim of an automobile accident, is admitted to the emergency room with a deep laceration on the right side of his head and a bleeding abrasion on his face. He is drowsy but able to respond to verbal stimuli. His vital signs are blood pressure 110/70 mm Hg, pulse 100, respirations 28. Which item would be *inappropriate* as an assessment priority for Mr. Arden?
1. Level of consciousness
2. Vital signs
3. Bladder fullness
4. Motor reflexes

350. Which drug is most likely to have a rebound effect in the treatment of cerebral edema?
1. Dexamethasone (Decadron)
2. Diazepam (Valium)
3. Mannitol (Osmitrol)
4. Prednisone (Deltasone)

351. Mrs. Ortez yells at the nurse, calling him a Martian. The most appropriate nursing response to this situation is which of the following?
1. "Do I really look like one of your co-workers?"
2. Overlook the statement.
3. "I am Mr. Porter, your nurse today."

④ "Mrs. Ortez, you are in the hospital now. There are no Martians here."

352. A 32-year-old primigravida is diagnosed to be a class I cardiac client because of uncorrected congenital heart disease. Careful assessments are particularly essential from 28 to 32 weeks of gestation because of the risk of which of the following?
① Premature delivery
② Cardiac decompensation
③ HELLP syndrome
④ Disseminated intravascular coagulation

353. Four-year-old Sean White was admitted to the hospital with burns received while playing with matches. His legs and lower abdomen are burned. In assessing Sean's hydration status, which of the following indicates less-than-adequate fluid replacement?
① Rising hematocrit and increasing urine volume
② Falling hematocrit and decreasing urine volume
③ Rising hematocrit and decreasing urine volume
④ Stable hematocrit and increasing urine volume

354. The nurse is aware that when there is injury to the right side of the brain it would be *unlikely* that the nurse would see difficulties with which of the following?
① Speech
② Perception
③ Coordination
④ Personality

355. Which of the following symptoms indicate overhydration in a burn patient after the first 24 hours?
① Elevated temperature
② Drowsiness
③ Dyspnea, moist rales
④ Diuresis

356. A 26-year-old woman has mitral stenosis as a result of repeated bouts of A beta-hemolytic streptococcal infections in childhood. She is now in her second month of pregnancy and is concerned about the effect her heart disease will have on her health and the health of her fetus. Teaching this woman the symptoms associated with congestive heart failure is important. Which of the following statements best indicates that she understands what has been taught?
① "The doctor will be able to listen to my heart and lungs at my weekly visits and see how I am doing."
② "If there is swelling of my feet and hands, I should reduce the amount of salt that I eat."
③ "When I have inadequate rest, I will have palpitations."
④ "If I have a cough or get tired more easily, I should see the doctor immediately."

357. A client with a delusional disorder refuses to eat lunch and accuses the staff of trying to poison the food. She admits that she is hungry. Because the client is hungry, what is the most appropriate nursing action?
① Explain that the staff did not prepare the food.
② Offer to taste the food.
③ Ask the dietitian to bring another tray, and explain that the food has not been poisoned.
④ Arrange to have the client's food brought up in sealed containers.

358. Antianxiety agents, such as lorazepam (Ativan), may be given with haloperidol (Haldol), an antipsychotic agent. The clearest rationale of this combination is which of the following?
① Side effects of the antianxiety agent are reduced.
② A lower dose of antipsychotic agents is required to produce therapeutic effects.
③ It reduces the risk of agranulocytosis.
④ It promotes medication compliance and increases self-care skills.

359. In caring for a 3-year-old burn patient with the "open method," which of the following is *least* appropriate?
① Place him in reverse isolation.
② Prevent him from having visitors from outside the hospital.
③ Encourage him to participate in his care.
④ Place him in a room near the nurse's station.

360. A pregnant client has class II cardiac disease. On her initial prenatal visit, the physician explains that various drugs may be needed during the antepartal period because of her cardiac status. Which is the most accurate statement about the use of drugs for cardiac conditions during pregnancy?
① Penicillin cannot be used prophylactically to prevent infections because it is not effective.
② Heparin is a safe anticoagulant because it does not cross the placenta.
③ Digitalis is contraindicated because it is a teratogen.
④ Use of diuretics will be avoided because they produce electrolyte imbalance.

361. It is determined that a client's seizures are the result of increased intracranial pressure. Which item would the nurse anticipate to be included in the initial treatment?
① Craniectomy
② Induced barbiturate coma
③ Osmotic diuretics, corticosteroids, and hyperventilation
④ Phenobarbital (Luminal) and phenytoin sodium (Dilantin)

362. Barbara Case's myasthenia gravis (MG) was diagnosed 4 years ago. The initial onset of symptoms occurred during a pregnancy. Her disease was well controlled with medication until she contracted an upper respiratory tract infection recently. Mrs. Case asks why this had to happen to her even though she is careful to always take her pyridostigmine (Mestinon) on time, 3 times every day. What explanation would be most appropriate to give Mrs. Case?
① "You have become resistant to pyridostigmine (Mestinon), but there are other medications that work just as well."
② "Symptoms of MG are often exacerbated by any kind of stress, such as infection."
③ "You need to increase your medicine to 6 times a day."
④ "Surgical excision of the thymus gland (thymectomy) often promotes better control of symptoms."

363. A woman with a medical diagnosis of mitral valve prolapse asks the nurse about the type of delivery she

will have. Which response by the nurse is the most appropriate answer for this client's question?

① "A cesarean delivery would cause the least exertion because you will not have to go through labor and delivery."

② "A vaginal delivery with forceps extraction will reduce the strain caused by pushing."

③ "A spontaneous vaginal delivery is probable because intervention is associated with risk of infection."

④ "What is important is that a regional anesthetic is used. The type of delivery is not relevant."

364. Mr. Fincher, a 53-year-old client with a history of chronic alcoholism, comes to the community mental health center with an elevated blood pressure and pulse, shakiness, and intense anxiety. He informs the nurse of his drinking history and how he has reduced his consumption over the past few days. The client must be observed for which of the following symptoms?

① Worsening withdrawal symptoms

② Possible stroke

③ Peripheral neuropathy

④ A depressive reaction

365. A 5-year-old burn patient's output through his urinary catheter is 20 ml over a 2-hour period. What would be the first nursing action?

① Check the catheter to see if it is plugged.

② Call the physician immediately.

③ Record the information on the chart.

④ Increase the intravenous fluids.

366. Which of the following would *not* be a typical finding in the physical assessment for myasthenia gravis?

① Bilateral ptosis of the eyelids

② Difficulty swallowing and chewing

③ Muscle rigidity and tremors at rest

④ Inability to raise the arms over the head

367. When 3-year-old Elena, who is severely burned, starts oral feedings, it is important that her diet have a higher than normal amount of which of the following?

① Minerals and vitamins

② Fluids and vitamins

③ Fats and carbohydrates

④ Proteins and carbohydrates

368. To prevent aspiration, what would the nurse do before offering food or fluids to a client with myasthenia gravis?

① Check to see if she is NPO for a Tensilon test.

② Question her about muscarinic effects of the pyridostigmine (Mestinon) (nausea, abdominal cramping, and diarrhea).

③ Assess cranial nerves III (oculomotor), IV (trochlear), and VI (abducens) for weakness.

④ Assess cranial nerves IX (glossopharyngeal) and X (vagus) for weakness.

369. The most common manifestation of Korsakoff's syndrome is which of the following?

① Gastrointestinal bleeding

② Paresthesias

③ Confabulation

④ Fatty liver

370. What would the nurse teach a client with myasthenia gravis about the medication regimen at discharge?

① Never use atropine sulfate as an antidote for muscarinic effects.

② Edrophonium (Tensilon) probably will be given with the pyridostigmine (Mestinon) until her infection is completely resolved.

③ Take pyridostigmine (Mestinon) on an empty stomach, 1 hour before meals.

④ Take pyridostigmine (Mestinon) with or immediately after meals.

371. To facilitate the management of myasthenia gravis, which is the most important information to discuss with a client?

① No over-the-counter medications are known to affect the action of anticholinesterase medications used in the treatment of myasthenia gravis.

② Observe for symptoms of thyroid disease because clients with myasthenia gravis also experience thyroid dysfunction.

③ Planned rest periods throughout the day will maximize strength.

④ Good body mechanics will prevent deformities.

372. What would be the best diversional activity for a 4-year-old while he is in reverse isolation?

① Lace leather wallets.

② Watch television.

③ Play with puppets.

④ Use computer word games.

373. What position will the woman with cardiac disease need to assume in labor to allow for maximum functioning of her heart?

① Supine

② Trendelenberg's

③ Dorsal recumbent

④ Semi-Fowler's

374. The most helpful nursing action needed to care for the client with chronic alcoholism is which of the following?

① Help the client manage stress using adaptive coping skills.

② Point out ways to reduce social contacts.

③ Identify ways to reduce the emotional dependency on others.

④ Suggest reality therapy as part of the discharge planning.

375. A class II cardiac client has delivered a new baby boy approximately 2 hours ago. Which of the following aspects of care would be most appropriate regarding this client's interaction with her infant?

① If the labor, delivery, and postpartum recovery are uneventful, breast-feeding is appropriate, if desired.

② Rooming-in will be possible, and the woman will be encouraged to care for herself and her baby.

③ A regular schedule will have to be arranged for the woman to visit the nursery and interact with her infant.

④ Caring for the baby will be too great a strain on the woman for at least 6 weeks, so provisions will need to be made for someone to help during this time.

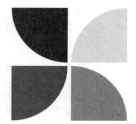

Practice Test 6

376. Five-year-old Tommy is scheduled for surgery to correct hypospadias. In hypospadias, where is the urethral opening usually located?
① Anywhere along the ventral surface of the penis
② On the dorsal surface of the penis
③ In the scrotal sac
④ Behind the scrotal sac

377. Mr. Leon is in a psychoeducation class that focuses on alcohol abstinence. Antabuse is being prescribed to assist in maintaining his sobriety. An initial teaching concern is discussing the effects of drinking while using this medication. Which of the following symptoms should he be aware of when ingesting alcohol?
① Depression, increased blood pressure, and confusion
② Headache, pallor, diarrhea, and rhinorrhea
③ Nausea and vomiting, flushed face, and decreased blood pressure
④ Slurred speech, muscle rigidity, and dilated pupils

378. A client asks whether getting pregnant again will have any effect on her myasthenia gravis. What would be the nurse's best response?
① "Pregnancy has no effect on myasthenia gravis."
② "Pregnancy may cause an exacerbation of your myasthenia gravis."
③ "What do you think?"
④ "As long as you take your medication, you have nothing to worry about."

379. A client asks, "Just what is myasthenia gravis?" What is the pathophysiologic principle on which the nurse would base a response?
① It is an autoimmune process affecting nerves and muscles.
② It is an autoimmune process affecting the myoneural junction.
③ It is a genetic defect that destroys myelin.
④ It is a "slow" viral infection that attacks skeletal muscle.

380. The primary concern of family therapy for chronic alcoholism is which of the following?
① The client's drinking problem
② The impact of the spouse's behavior on the client's alcoholism
③ Improving communication among family members to adapt healthier coping behaviors
④ Instructing family members to remain like each other

381. Which of the following assessments by the nurse would most likely indicate that a 17-year-old may have pregnancy-induced hypertension?
① A blood pressure change from 110/80 mm Hg to 120/88 mm Hg
② Complaints of swelling of fingers and eyelids
③ Weight gain of 4 pounds during the eighth month
④ Presence of 1+ glucose in the urine

382. Which of the following are highly indicative manifestations of hypospadias?
① Nausea and vomiting
② Urinary retention
③ Abnormal urinary stream direction
④ Ambiguous genitalia

383. Of the following symptoms, which does not indicate posttraumatic stress disorder?
① Recurrent sleep disturbances arising from nightmares of the traumatic incident
② Hypervigilence, startle reflex, suspiciousness, and distrust
③ Active tactile hallucinations of crawling and flying insects
④ Panic reactions triggered by recurrent memories of trauma

384. Which of the following statements best describes the pathophysiologic changes that occur in pregnancy-induced hypertension?
① There is an increase in both plasma proteins and glomerular filtration.
② There is a decrease in aldosterone production and an increase in fluid retention.
③ There is an increase in circulating blood volume and a decrease in cardiac output.
④ There is a decrease in renal and uterine circulation because of vascular constriction.

385. Mr. Arnetti seeks treatment in a community crisis center, complaining of posttraumatic stress disorder symptoms. What is the most appropriate nursing action to facilitate a therapeutic relationship?
① Create an accepting and empathic environment.
② Examine present and previous coping behaviors, and encourage formation of adaptive behaviors.
③ Teach relaxation and stress-reducing techniques.
④ Set up a couple's session so that his spouse can be more supportive.

386. When obtaining a health history for the child with hypospadias, it is most important for the nurse to include which of the following?
① Family history
② History of childhood illnesses
③ History of immunizations
④ History of toilet-training techniques

387. What is *not* necessary for the nurse to include in the preoperative teaching for a 3-year-old with hypospadias?
① Explanation to parents about the surgical procedure
② Explanation of the expected cosmetic results
③ Explanation to the child about the procedure
④ Explanation about a nephrostomy tube

388. Which action is inappropriate treatment for bacterial pneumonia?
① Auscultate the lungs q2h to q4h.
② Encourage fluids to 3 L per day.
③ Give ampicillin if the client is allergic to penicillin.
④ Encourage the client to cough by splinting the chest.

389. Innovative interventions are needed to address the complex needs of clients with posttraumatic stress disorder. Which of the following is the *least* effective nursing approach to caring for clients with posttraumatic stress disorder?
① Suggest that the client describe the traumatic event.
② Encourage the client to depict the connection between past traumatic events and present life.
③ Encourage expression of anger and rage regarding the traumatic incident.
④ Reassure the client that the nurse will assist in helping resolve presenting problems.

390. After a hypospadias repair, a 5-year-old's fears may include all of the following *except*
① Mutilation
② Punishment for misdeeds
③ Strange hospital environment
④ Loss of sexuality

391. The most likely goal of treatment for a woman with severe pregnancy-induced hypertension is which of the following?
① Stabilize her vital signs.
② Reduce the number and severity of headaches.
③ Increase urinary output.
④ Prevent convulsions.

392. Why is aspiration pneumonia more common in the right lung?
① There is an increased amount of lung tissue available for infection on the right side.
② There is an absence of ciliated mucosal lining on the right.
③ The right bronchus is shorter and wider.
④ There is enhanced conduction through the airways on the right.

393. Marie Perez, a registered nurse, has been hospitalized with a diagnosis of posttraumatic stress disorder associated with her experiences in Vietnam. She sepa-

rated from her husband several months ago. In the discharge plans, which of the following recommendations made by the nurse would be *most* beneficial?
① Encourage her to consider moving back with her husband.
② Participate in a support group of registered nurses.
③ Use lorazepam (Ativan) periodically to control symptoms.
④ Begin a job-rehabilitation program.

394. What is the best reason for encouraging a lung-congested client to increase fluid intake?
① To promote bronchial dilation
② To prevent the need for a nasogastric tube
③ To improve antibiotic therapy
④ To loosen and thin bronchial secretions

395. The school nurse is providing an educational session on personal hygiene to a group of adolescent girls. The nurse discusses measures to prevent urinary tract infections. Which one of the following statements made by four adolescents at the end of the conclusion of the session indicates that additional teaching is needed?
① "No more tub baths for me! I'm showering from now on."
② "I'll have to throw away my nylon panties and buy some cotton ones."
③ "My mother taught me about wiping from back to front, when I was 2 years old."
④ "I'll have to take time to go to the bathroom between classes more often."

396. A 32-year-old primigravida is diagnosed with mild pregnancy-induced hypertension (PIH) at 34 weeks of gestation. As the pregnancy progresses, the woman's symptoms worsen, and she is admitted to the hospital. The physician orders an IV of 200 ml magnesium sulfate diluted in 10% dextrose in water. Which of the following findings would most likely lead the nurse to discontinue magnesium sulfate and notify the physician?
① A blood pressure of 130/90
② A hyperactive knee-jerk reflex
③ A respiratory rate of 10/min
④ A urinary output of 50 ml/hr

397. Lynda Kelly, a 32-year-old pediatrician, is raped while leaving her office. The rape occurs at a nearby parking garage. A co-worker finds her lying on the ground. Speaking in a calm voice, she reports being raped. The co-worker brings her to the emergency department. Ms. Kelly suffers from physical pain, but her condition is not serious. What is the most critical action for the nurse to take?
① Inform the police.
② Consult with a psychiatric clinical specialist.
③ Provide emotional support.
④ Suggest protection from pregnancy.

398. In caring for a client with compromised pulmonary function, why must the nurse be careful to avoid over-medication with sedatives?
① They suppress bone marrow function.
② They depress the cough reflex and cause accumulation of fluids in the lung.

③ They increase the risk of superinfection.

④ They cause hypersensitivity reactions.

399. The emergency room nurse can provide the most effective emotional support to the survivor of rape by instituting which of the following?

① Presenting her with numerous questions that encourage her to depict the rape.

② Stressing the importance of talking about the rape while it is fresh in her mind.

③ Explaining the normalcy of feeling angry, fearful, and sad over time.

④ Pointing out that her initial reactions to the rape indicate that she is not coping with the situation.

400. Postoperatively, a 4-year-old develops a temperature of 101.5°F (38.6°C). What would be the priority nursing action?

① Notify the physician.

② Call the child's parents.

③ Provide a cool environment.

④ Start oral penicillin.

401. Sandra Gibson is admitted to the hospital with a diagnosis of acute bacterial pneumonia. Miss Gibson's initial symptoms are not likely to include which of the following?

① Cyanosis

② Dehydration

③ Pleuritic pain

④ Audible wheezing

402. An antepartal client is hospitalized for severe pregnancy-induced hypertension. An infusion of magnesium sulfate is started. The nurse understands that this drug mainly acts as which of the following?

① Central nervous system depressant

② Antihypertensive

③ Diuretic

④ Tranquilizer

403. One of the ambulatory care nurses tells the emergency room nurse about a survivor of rape, "She is too calm and I am sure she was not raped." An explanation for the nurse's response is illustrated by which of the following?

① She knows the nurse and knows she is not telling the truth.

② She probably knows the rapist and is trying to defend him.

③ The nurse's past rape makes her aware of her own vulnerability to rape.

④ Her views support the notion that most survivors of rape are hysterical after a rape rather than composed.

404. The nurse in the clinic instructs the mother of 4-year-old Jenny, who was recently diagnosed with a urinary tract infection, on home care. Which one of the following responses by the mother indicates that the nurse must provide further teaching?

① "Jenny should drink more fluids than usual."

② "Jenny doesn't need to return to the clinic until her next well checkup."

③ "Jenny should take all of the medicine, even if she is feeling better."

④ "Jenny shouldn't have any bubble baths."

405. Twenty-six-month-old Crystal visits the well-child clinic for a checkup. When assessing Crystal's development, the nurse would expect her to exhibit which one of the following abilities?

① Dressing herself unassisted

② Pointing to parts of her body when asked

③ Drawing a person with three to six parts

④ Speaking in four- to five-word sentences

406. After the physical, a survivor of rape requests a referral to a psychiatric clinical specialist. The psychiatric clinical specialist provides crisis intervention. The helpfulness of this form of therapy is based on which of the following reasons?

① It facilitates understanding of feelings arising from the traumatic incident.

② It helps the client relate childhood conflicts to current trauma.

③ It enables the client to benefit from long-term therapy needed to manage this traumatic event.

④ It may reduce the deleterious impact of the rape.

407. Which of the following is the *least* significant for the health care team to assess when caring for a survivor of rape?

① Identified resources, including specific support systems

② An accepting response from significant others picking her up from the emergency department

③ An ability to maintain a degree of control over her care

④ Knowledge of ways to reduce the incidence of future rape

408. Which of the following can often result from long-term corticosteroid therapy?

① Adrenal gland hypertrophy

② Adrenal insufficiency and poor response to excess stress

③ Elevated levels of corticotropin-releasing factor

④ Atrophy of the posterior pituitary gland

409. During the otoscopic examination of a toddler, she cries loudly and tries to pull away. What is the best approach?

① Explain to her why you must look into her ears.

② Postpone the ear exam until her next visit, when she will be older.

③ Say to her, "I thought you were a big girl."

④ Get someone to restrain her and proceed with the exam.

410. A pregnant woman at 40 weeks of gestation is to be induced with 10 units of oxytocin (Pitocin). After the oxytocin is started, the woman becomes very uncomfortable during contractions and states, "I don't think I'll be able to stand this pain." Vaginal examination indicates that the cervix is dilated 2 cm. What would be the most appropriate initial nursing action?

① Call the physician.

② Give an analgesic.

③ Help her try some breathing exercises.

④ Increase the rate of the IV.

411. A survivor of rape angrily explodes and tells the emergency department nurse, "You took too long. I am paying this bill and I demand better service than this!" The nurse is aware that this client has been treated kindly and supportively. Which statement best explains the basis of the client's reaction?

① She is displacing her anger about the rape onto the emergency department staff.

② She feels violated and ignored by the staff.

③ Memories of past childhood traumas are triggered by the rape.

④ She is upset at herself because she should have known better than to leave the office alone.

412. An appropriate nursing response to an angry client who is verbally attacking the nurse and the emergency department staff is which of the following?

① "Look, we have other clients and they need help too."

② "You sound pretty upset."

③ "Let's focus on the rape rather than what you don't like about the staff."

④ "Getting angry at us is not going to help you. Please lower your voice."

413. After 20 hours of labor, a client's cervix is fully dilated. The physician makes the determination that the fetus will need to be delivered with the help of forceps. Because of the need for forceps, the nurse can expect which type of anesthetic to be used?

① Saddle block

② Paracervical block

③ Pudendal block

④ Local

414. Which of the following would *not* facilitate toilet training for Emily Holly, a 2-year-old?

① Give her a toy to play with while she sits on the potty.

② Dress her in clothing with Velcro fasteners.

③ Provide her with her own potty chair.

④ Respond matter-of-factly when she has an "accident."

415. Why must corticosteroid drugs always be stopped gradually?

① Adrenocorticotropic hormone (ACTH) and corticotropin-releasing factor levels are diminished from the supplemental steroids, so no cortisol would be available with abrupt withdrawal.

② ACTH and melanocyte-stimulating hormone (MSH) levels are elevated because the negative feedback loop has been lost.

③ Ectopic ACTH syndrome could result with rapid withdrawal.

④ Poor wound healing will occur with rapid withdrawal, along with sodium retention and edema.

416. The mother of a 28-month-old says, "She just doesn't seem to eat enough; I don't know where she gets all her energy." After assessing the child's condition and finding no evidence of nutritional deficiency, the nurse's best response is which of the following?

① "You may want to increase her milk intake to be sure she gets enough calories."

② "Why don't you double her daily vitamin and mineral dose for your peace of mind?"

③ "Try giving her small portions of a variety of foods, and allow her to decide which of those foods she will eat."

④ "It's best at this age to insist that she take at least two bites of the foods you offer her to be sure she is getting enough to eat."

417. Which of the following would be most appropriate to teach a client with angina to report to the physician or clinic?

① The occurrence of pain after a business meeting

② A change in the pattern of pain

③ Pain that occurs with eating

④ The fact that nitroglycerin does not cause a tingling sensation under the tongue

418. According to the community mental health model, rape is regarded as a crisis if what circumstance exists?

① The survivor's support system buffered her against the negative impact of trauma.

② The survivor's defense mechanisms were unable to manage the present situation.

③ The stress of the rape overwhelmed the survivor and she was unable to manage it without staying with a friend.

④ Stress generated by the rape was tremendous, and the survivor's current support systems were unable to manage it.

419. A client is placed on a regimen of propranolol (Inderal) to control angina. Propranolol will be contraindicated if the client develops which of the following?

① Myocardial infarction

② Asthma

③ Cerebrovascular accident

④ Thrombophlebitis

420. Four-year-old Steffan is admitted for same-day surgery for a tonsillectomy. Preoperatively, it is most important for the nurse to check his chart for which of the following laboratory values?

① Hematocrit and hemoglobin

② Urine osmolality

③ Bleeding and clotting times

④ White blood cell count

421. An antepartum client is being induced with an oxytocin infusion because of postmaturity. Which of the following assessments would require immediate action by the nurse for this woman?

① A blood pressure increase from 110/70 to 130/80.

② Three contractions that last 90 to 95 seconds each.

③ A fetal heart rate acceleration of 10 beats per minute with a contraction.

④ A resting period of 30 to 45 seconds between contractions.

422. When preparing a child for surgery, it is especially important to check for loose teeth in which age group?

① Older infant

② Toddler-preschool

③ School-age

④ Adolescent

423. The crisis intervention approach depicts which of the following?

① Secondary prevention

② Tertiary prevention

③ Cognitive therapy

④ Reality therapy

424. When the nurse administers a beta-blocking agent such as propranolol (Inderal), it would be inappropriate to do which of the following?
① Teach the client to change positions slowly.
② Monitor for occult blood in the stool and urine.
③ Monitor the blood pressure.
④ Monitor for dyspnea and respiratory dysfunction.

425. The nurse begins diet teaching for a client with a history of cardiac dysfunction. Which of the following is inappropriate to include in the teaching plan?
① Eat smaller meals.
② Eat snacks of cheese.
③ Include more fish and chicken in the diet.
④ Limit caffeine intake.

426. Primary prevention of rape can be best accomplished by which of the following?
① Initiation of emergency measures after the rape.
② Policewomen teaching a class on rape prevention.
③ Psychiatric hospitalization for the survivor of rape.
④ A lengthy jail sentence for the rapist.

427. Which of the following best defines the meaning of hypochondriasis?
① A self-absorption with the fear of having a grave illness.
② An obsession with one's demise.
③ An underlying medical condition that causes loss of physical functioning.
④ A classification of psychosis manifested by altered sensory and motor performance.

428. A 28-year-old multipara has just delivered an 8-pound 4-ounce boy. When determining the newborn's Apgar score, the nurse assesses five areas, one of which is
① Temperature
② Blood pressure
③ Degree of head lag
④ Color

429. Which of the following best describes the nursing rationale for providing a 4-year-old with role playing as part of his preoperative preparation?
① To ensure compliant behavior
② To distract him from feelings of anxiety
③ As a means of permitting physical expression of feelings that he cannot express verbally
④ As a teaching strategy and to decrease anxiety

430. What would be *least* effective in getting a 5-year-old ready for the operating room?
① Allow him to have a visit with his 7-year-old sibling before leaving the unit.
② Allow him to take his stuffed tiger with him.
③ Allow him to wear his underwear to surgery.
④ Have a familiar nurse stay with him in the operating room until he is asleep.

431. A client with a history of cardiovascular disease wants to join a class on primary health care habits to prevent cardiovascular and respiratory disease. The client tells the nurse, "I will never quit smoking." What would be the best response to this client?
① The client cannot join unless smoking stops.
② The client can join but cannot smoke in class.

③ The client can join and can smoke in class.
④ The client can join but should not attend classes on smoking cessation.

432. Which of the following factors, being implicated in the development of colorectal cancer, should the nurse discuss with clients during a class for cancer prevention?
① Exposure to x-rays
② Low-fiber diet
③ High intake of smoked fish
④ Long history of alcohol abuse

433. The most frequently demonstrated defense mechanism of hypochondriasis is which of the following?
① Sublimation producing adaptive coping behaviors
② Repression producing physical symptoms
③ Rationalization resulting in an explanation of behavior
④ Displacement resulting in physical symptoms used to manage anxiety

434. After an angina attack, a client is discharged and referred to the outpatient clinic for a stress test and cardiac angiography. What is the rationale for the cardiac angiography?
① To dilate the coronary blood vessels
② To confirm a diagnosis of heart disease
③ To force oxygen under pressure to the myocardium
④ To bypass the diseased coronary artery

435. A client is scheduled for a lower gastrointestinal tract study. Which would be *inappropriate* to include in preparation for this test?
① Clear tea and Jell-O for breakfast the day before the test
② Castor oil or a Fleet enema, or both, the evening before the test
③ Low-cholesterol, low-fat diet the day of the test
④ Tap-water enemas until clear on the morning of the test

436. Twelve hours after 4-year-old Rebecca's tonsillectomy, the nurse would be most concerned about which one of the following clinical manifestations?
① Respirations 24/min and shallow
② Fever of 100°F (37.8°C)
③ Frequent swallowing
④ Complaint of a sore throat

437. After an uncomplicated vaginal delivery, a postpartal woman is made comfortable in the birthing/recovery room. The nurse brings the baby to the new mother to initiate breast-feeding. How can the nurse best assist the new mother?
① Assist the baby to latch.
② Give the mother privacy.
③ Explain the supply and demand nature of producing breast milk.
④ Leave written information about frequency and duration of nursing.

438. Myrtis Marcus, a 43-year-old unemployed respiratory therapist, has been admitted to the psychiatric unit with a diagnosis of hypochondriasis. Her sister accompanies her and reports that she has a chronic history of back pain for which she has been treated in numerous facilities. The most appropriate nursing action to use when caring for Miss Marcus would be which of the following?

① Encourage her to focus on her back pain because verbal expression is helpful.

② Reduce the care provided for physical symptoms in an effort to divert attention away from them.

③ Refrain from discussion of physical symptoms because more information frequently heightens her symptoms.

④ Permit her to discuss her feelings and concerns, avoiding a focus on physical symptoms.

439. Charles Woodward, a 65-year-old salesman, is admitted to the hospital with suspected cancer of the colon. A malignant rectal tumor is diagnosed, and he is scheduled for surgery. Which of the following orders for preoperative bowel preparation would the nurse question?

① Neomycin PO 1 g early in the evening; repeat in 1 hour and at bedtime

② Gastrointestinal decompression to begin 24 hours before surgery

③ Sodium polystyrene sulfonate (Kayexalate) enemas, times 2

④ Clear liquids for 2 days before the surgery

440. Tracy Goddard is a 7-year-old being seen in the clinic for the first time. While doing the physical examination, the nurse notices slight clubbing of Tracy's fingers and toes. What is the best explanation for this symptom?

① Chronic underlying respiratory infections

② Acute oxygen deprivation

③ Anemia

④ Chronic tissue hypoxemia

441. During a prenatal class on breast-feeding, one of the women asks what benefit the baby gets from colostrum before true breast milk is produced. What would be an incorrect response?

① "It provides vital antibodies for protection from infection."

② "It is concentrated nutrition in small volume to match early feeding behavior."

③ "The high carbohydrate level facilitates binding of bilirubin."

④ "The laxative action promotes early passage of meconium."

442. Letha Levin, 76 years old, is diagnosed with dementia. She is admitted to the psychiatric unit accompanied by her son. Which factor best explains the psychologic symptoms Mrs. Levin is most apt to manifest in the hospital?

① The amount of alcohol she consumed over the past 40 years

② The underlying medical condition causing the dementia

③ The level of orientation she exhibits at the time of hospitalization

④ Her premorbid personality traits

443. A client has an abdominoperineal resection and returns to the unit after surgery with a single-barreled sigmoid colostomy. Which finding would the nurse expect after this surgical procedure?

① Consistently liquid stool until the client is discharged from the hospital

② Formed stool with potential for regulation of bowel elimination

③ Sanguineous drainage from the stoma mixed with feces

④ Stool consistency that alternates between semiliquid and formed

444. The nurse is aware that certain factors may lead children to deny the existence of actual pain. Which of the following least describes these factors?

① The younger the child, the less the pain

② More easily distracted than adults

③ Lack of understanding of what "pain" means

④ Attempts to meet expectations of others

445. The nurse inspects the colostomy stoma as part of a postoperative assessment and finds that the tissue is moist with a slight bluish color. This would best be interpreted as which of the following findings?

① Early sign of necrosis

② Normal tissue from postoperative trauma

③ Early sign of infection

④ Late sign of internal hemorrhage

446. Which of the following is most helpful to the nurse in evaluating a young child's pain status?

① A verbal statement of pain

② Physiologic changes

③ Behavioral changes

④ Parental comments

447. During the first postoperative day, nursing assessments of a client who had abdominal surgery for a colostomy include which of the following?

① Rectal temperatures

② Passage of flatus

③ Tolerance of oral intake

④ Peripheral glucose checks

448. Three-month-old Tonyah has cystic fibrosis. As a neonate, she had surgery for meconium ileus. Heather's parents were told that meconium ileus was related to cystic fibrosis, but they state that they do not understand why. Which of the following explanations is most accurate?

① The bile ducts become obstructed with tenacious mucus.

② The intestinal cilia are blunted and prevent meconium from passing through the intestinal tract.

③ The small intestine is constricted, resulting in meconium impaction.

④ The pancreas is unable to secrete the enzymes necessary for digestion.

449. In assessing the orientation of the elderly client with dementia, the nurse is most likely to observe that the client is aware of which of the following?

① The day of the week

② The present location

③ Who the client is

④ Present age

450. When planning the care of the elderly, disoriented, and confused client, what is the most useful nursing action?

① Involve the client in as many structured activities as possible to reduce loneliness.

② Introduce the client to everyone on the unit as soon as possible to promote a sense of belonging.

③ Vary the client's schedule to stimulate the thinking process.

④ Maintain a consistent daily schedule to promote security and structure.

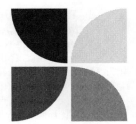

Practice Test 7

451. A client begins instruction on colostomy irrigation. Which of the following instructions would be included in the teaching?
   ① Irrigate well when diarrhea is present.
   ② Irrigate with 1500 ml to 2000 ml water.
   ③ Lubricate the catheter tip with an antibiotic ointment.
   ④ Gently insert the catheter tip with a cone until snug into the stoma.

452. Which content would be included in the teaching plan regarding common problems for the ostomate?
   ① If diarrhea occurs, eat small, high-calorie meals until normal motility returns.
   ② Prevent hard stools by taking a laxative such as milk of magnesia up to 3 times per week.
   ③ Colostomy odor can be reduced by taking charcoal and bismuth subcarbonate orally.
   ④ Abdominal cramping can be relieved by taking small sips of ginger ale.

453. Which one of the following tests is used initially to diagnose cystic fibrosis?
   ① Chromosomal studies
   ② Sweat chloride test
   ③ Chest x-ray
   ④ Stool exam for fat content

454. Mrs. Levin, a client admitted with dementia, often makes up stories when questioned. Her son reports that she has been making up stories for some time and this really bothers him. Which of the following explains Mrs. Levin's need to fill in the gaps caused by memory deficits?
   ① Amnesia
   ② Confabulation
   ③ Dissociation
   ④ Free association

455. A 3-month-old infant was admitted to the pediatric unit with a diagnosis of RSV bronchiolitis. As the nurse admitting the infant, your physical examination will most probably include which of the following symptoms?
   ① A barky, stridorous cough
   ② Conjunctivitis
   ③ A wheezy, productive cough
   ④ A low-grade temperature

456. The effectiveness of diet teaching is evaluated as a client prepares for discharge. The client demonstrates knowledge of foods *least* likely to cause intestinal gas. Which list would be selected?
   ① Canned peaches, red beets, and squash
   ② Milk, lima beans, and cheese
   ③ Steak with onions, peas, and corn
   ④ Yogurt, cola, and cheese

457. Gabriel Pacetti, a 25-year-old construction worker, is injured when his foot and ankle are crushed by a heavy, jagged tool. The foot becomes cold, black, and has absent pedal pulses. He is scheduled for a below-the-knee amputation. What instruction would the nurse give Mr. Pacetti if he is to have an introduction to quadriceps-setting exercises preoperatively?
   ① Pinch the buttocks together and then relax them.
   ② Lift the buttocks off the bed while lying flat.
   ③ Move the buttocks and both legs in order to place the feet in plantar flexion.
   ④ Move the patellas proximally, and press the popliteal spaces against the bed.

458. What would be the best short-term goal in a teaching plan for a mother who is learning to breast-feed for the first time?
   ① Client will demonstrate competence and confidence during breast-feeding.
   ② Infant will achieve a regular schedule (every 4 hours) for breast-feeding.
   ③ Client will supplement breast-feeding with formula until milk comes in and then prn.
   ④ Infant will take glucose water between feedings to prevent dehydration and constipation.

459. Ninety-year-old Mr. Ochato is visited by his daughter and son-in-law after a recent admission to an extended care facility with a diagnosis of Alzheimer's disease. He fails to recognize them. Which is the *most* appropriate nursing response?
   ① "He is confused by his new surroundings. He will recognize you tomorrow."
   ② "His memory is so bad that he will not remember you. It's a waste of time to visit him every day."
   ③ "This is a difficult time for you and him. I encourage you to visit as often as possible."
   ④ "Since he does not live with you, you might consider sending an old friend he recognizes."

460. Which of the following would be a priority to include in the plan of care for a client with a

below-the-knee amputation during the first 24 hours postoperatively?
① Apply a heating pad to the stump to relieve discomfort.
② Have a tourniquet in view at the bedside.
③ Anticipate the need for large doses of narcotic analgesics.
④ Encourage the client to look at the stump.

461. Of the following symptoms, which one is *most* likely to be exhibited by a client with dementia?
① Loss of words
② Refusal to cooperate
③ Memory loss of recent events
④ Social withdrawal

462. Ampicillin, 100 mg IV q6h, has been prescribed for an infant with a respiratory infection. The ampicillin vial contains 250 mg/1.2 ml when reconstituted. How much would be administered?
① 0.25 ml
② 0.48 ml
③ 0.75 ml
④ 2.5 ml

463. A disoriented, confused, elderly client is incontinent of stool. What is the most appropriate nursing response?
① "This is the second accident you've had today!"
② "You are too old for this, call me the next time."
③ "You need to go and change your clothes."
④ "Let me help you. I realize this is distressful to you."

464. Which is the best instruction to give a client with a below-the-knee amputation?
① Keep the stump elevated on a pillow until the wound is healed.
② Keep a pillow between the thighs when in a supine position.
③ Lie in a prone position for 30 minutes several times a day.
④ Apply lotion to the stump several times a day after the incision has healed.

465. Miss Staley, an 85-year-old with dementia, tells the nurse, "I am due in surgery in the next few minutes." Of the following responses which one shows an understanding of the client's condition?
① "Surgery has been canceled because your client's lab work is abnormal."
② "You were a surgeon, Miss Staley? Tell me about your practice."
③ "You are not doing surgery. You are in a nursing home."
④ "Another surgeon is scheduled to operate on your client."

466. An amputee client will be taught to use crutches until he can manage with a prosthesis independently. Which of the following crutch-walking instructions would be *incorrect?*
① Extend the arms while holding weights to strengthen the triceps.
② The crutches should be 16 inches less than the client's total height.
③ The axillary bars on the crutches should support the client's weight.
④ Both crutches and the affected leg are moved forward first, followed by the unaffected leg.

467. Daniel Stone, 34 years old, graduated from a local university and over the past 2 years has been employed as a social worker in a local hospital. Over the past 6 months his ability to work and communicate with others has declined. Additionally, his appearance has become increasingly disheveled. He is admitted to a local psychiatric hospital with a diagnosis of schizophrenia, paranoid type. When planning the care of Mr. Stone, the nurse recognizes which of the following as characteristic of the client with schizophrenia?
① He quickly forms meaningful relationships.
② His symptoms rapidly respond to antimanic agents.
③ He is sensitive to others' feelings.
④ He will require electroconvulsive therapy to reduce psychosis.

468. Bethany, a 4-month-old infant admitted with respiratory syncytial virus (RSV) bronchiolitis, is being treated with the antiviral drug Virazole (ribaviran). Which of the following best indicates an understanding of how this drug works?
① Kills RSV
② Prevents RSV from replicating
③ Needs to be given in conjunction with antibiotics
④ May be administered in the home

469. Which of the following nursing interventions would a priority in preventing postpartum cystitis?
① Offer the woman orange juice twice a day.
② Instruct the woman to drink up to 64 ounces of water each day.
③ Provide a nutritious diet.
④ Make sure the woman voids within the first 4 to 6 hours after delivery.

470. Seven-month-old Heather has cystic fibrosis and is receiving pancreatic enzymes to aid digestion. Which response by her parents would indicate that they understand correct administration of the enzyme?
① Mix it with water in a syringe.
② Put it in a small amount of pureed applesauce.
③ Mix it with an ounce of orange juice.
④ Add it to her formula four times a day.

471. Pancreatitis can best be described as which of the following?
① Infectious disease of the pancreas primarily seen in the African American population
② Inherited disease affecting the pancreas that is primarily seen in the African American population
③ Inflammation of the pancreas resulting in obstruction and edema
④ Outpouching of the pancreas

472. Which of the following is defined as a sensory perception without external stimuli?
① A delusion
② An illusion
③ A hallucination
④ A projection

473. The nurse knows that the pancreas is responsible for secreting which of the following?
① Sucrase, dipeptidase, lipase, and amylase
② Amylase, lactase, trypsin, and chymotrypsin
③ Amylase, lipase, pepsin, and maltase
④ Amylase, lipase, trypsin, and chymotrypsin

474. Mr. Ekpe, a 25-year-old graduate student, is admitted with a psychotic disorder. He is complaining of visual hallucinations and paranoia. His symptoms have evolved over the past 2 weeks after the treatment of peptic ulcer disease. For several weeks he was prescribed and took large doses of rantidine (Zantac). His family is concerned about his present condition and reports that he has been an ideal student and son. Which of the following best describes Mr. Ekpe's psychotic condition?
① Schizophrenia, paranoid type
② Psychosis related to an underlying medical condition
③ Bipolar disorder, manic type
④ Alcohol withdrawal, delirium tremens

475. Which would be an unlikely finding with chronic pancreatitis?
① Hypoglycemia
② Extreme epigastric pain
③ Elevated serum amylase and lipase
④ Abdominal distention

476. A client's laboratory values show hypocalcemia as a result of the inadequate metabolism of which of the following?
① Fat
② Protein
③ Starch
④ Glucose

477. Continuous focus on ideas and fantasies that have little meaning to anyone but the client represents which of the following?
① Aloofness
② Ambivalence
③ Apathy
④ Autism

478. Andrew Goll, a 56-year-old rancher, is admitted for an episode of acute pancreatitis. This is Mr. Goll's eighth admission for this disorder over the past 3 years. In planning for adequate nutrition for Mr. Goll, which action would be considered *inappropriate*?
① Administer cholinergic drugs.
② Supplement nutrition with IV fluids.
③ Give clear liquids after inflammation subsides.
④ Include a bland, low-fat diet in the teaching plan.

479. Clozapine (Clozaril) is a new-generation antipsychotic agent. What is the most serious side effect of this medication?
① Agranulocytosis
② Hypotension
③ Tolerance requiring higher doses
④ Fluid retention

480. A client with pancreatitis is complaining of severe pain. The physician has ordered meperidine (Demerol) and morphine. The nurse chooses meperidine. The best reason for selecting meperidine is that
① Meperidine depresses respirations less than morphine.
② Meperidine exerts its effects on striated muscles.
③ Morphine has a tendency to produce spasms of the sphincter of Oddi.
④ Morphine has less effect on smooth muscle.

481. What is the most common side effect of fluphenazine (Prolixin) decanoate prescribed 25 mg IM every 2 weeks?
① Extrapyramidal side effects
② Extreme sedation
③ Sexual disturbances
④ Nausea and vomiting

482. When assessing a client with a gangrenous toe, the nurse will *least* likely expect which of the following?
① Intense pain in the affected area
② Extension of the metatarsal-phalangeal joints
③ Changes in skin temperature of both feet
④ Tissue destruction greater in the distal than proximal portion

483. Clozapine (Clozaril) is absolutely contraindicated in clients with which current condition?
① Chronic obstructive lung disease
② Bone marrow suppression
③ Suicidal risk
④ Alcoholism

484. Which one of the following is the best indicator of a successful outcome of the plan of care for an infant with cystic fibrosis?
① Growth rate within normal limits.
② Achievement of development milestones.
③ Ability to digest a variety of foods.
④ Decrease in incidence of respiratory infections.

485. To determine whether a postpartum client is completely emptying her bladder, the nurse would do which of the following?
① Assess fundal height and position and percuss the bladder.
② Catheterize her for residual urine after voiding.
③ Ask the mother whether she feels perineal pressure.
④ Maintain intake and output.

486. A 21-year-old primigravida is admitted to the labor room in early labor. The nurse admitting the woman determines that her cervix is 90% effaced and dilated 2 cm. Contractions are occurring every 5 to 10 minutes, are mild to moderate in intensity, and last 15 to 30 seconds. Which type of breathing and relaxation techniques would be appropriate for this laboring woman to use at this time?
① Panting
② Modified paced breathing
③ Accelerated breathing at a rate of 1 breath every 2 seconds
④ Slow abdominal

487. Which drug is most appropriate in managing side effects of fluphenazine (Prolixin)?
① Benztropine mesylate (Cogentin) 1 mg PO bid
② Trihexyphenidyl (Artane) 15 mg PO tid

③ Buspirone (Buspar) 10 mg bid

④ Lorazepam (Ativran) 1 mg bid

488. What is the major advantage of haloperidol (Haldol) for outpatient use?

① It has less serious side effects than other phenothiazines.

② It is more effective than other antipsychotic agents.

③ It does not produce a tolerance, thus it is less addictive than other phenothiazines.

④ It is obtainable in long-acting form.

489. Ernest Washo has had diabetes mellitus for 20 years. He is admitted to the hospital with dry gangrene of the right great toe. When the nurse is working with Mr. Washo, what information is most important to ascertain?

① His age when the diabetes mellitus developed.

② His knowledge of hygienic skin measures.

③ His technique in administering insulin.

④ His willingness to look at, touch, or talk about his gangrenous foot.

490. The effectiveness of milieu therapy is based on management of the hospital climate to foster which of the following?

① Positive living and learning experiences

② Secure environment

③ Potential for enhanced socialization skills

④ Potential for learning new skills through an array of therapies

491. Bed rest is prescribed for a client with gangrene of the toes on the right foot. Which nursing care measure would be *least* therapeutic for this client?

① Heel protectors

② Footboard

③ Foot cradle

④ Sheep skin or foam pad

492. To prevent complications of the bed rest imposed on a client with gangrene, which nursing action would be *inappropriate*?

① Inspect the client's feet.

② Teach about appropriate foot care.

③ Restrict fluid intake.

④ Exercise joints and muscles.

493. Miss Landry, 19 years old, has been recently admitted to a day hospital with a diagnosis of bipolar disorder, manic episode, in remission. Family therapy has been initiated as an adjunct treatment modality. The primary goal of family therapy for a client with bipolar disorder is which of the following?

① The client will verbalize the cause of the illness.

② The family will strengthen and maintain effective communication patterns.

③ The client will deter hospitalization.

④ The client's future children will remain free of bipolar disorder.

494. The mother of Kelly, a child with cystic fibrosis, asks what the risk is of having another child with cystic fibrosis, because she and her husband are "thinking about having another baby some day." Which of the following is the best nursing response?

① "It's probably best if you don't have any more children."

② "Your next child may be a carrier but won't have the disease."

③ "You can have an amniocentesis in early pregnancy to detect whether the baby has cystic fibrosis and, if so, you may choose to have a therapeutic abortion."

④ "I'd like to refer you to the genetic counselor on our staff, who can discuss with you the probability of your second child having cystic fibrosis."

495. The nurse would perform which of the following when providing care to the skin surrounding a gangrene lesion on the toe?

① Apply an occlusive dressing.

② Dry the skin thoroughly.

③ Put lotion on the healthy tissue.

④ Soak the foot.

496. Stanley Agnew is brought to an ambulatory care clinic by his roommate. Mr. Agnew is tense, shaking, and diaphoretic. His skin is also cool and clammy. His roommate reports that Mr. Agnew has been studying for the bar exam over the past few weeks. When Mr. Agnew is asked how he is feeling, he replies, "How do you think I feel?" His eyes fill with tears and he says, "I am sorry. I am so afraid I will fail and disappoint my family." What level of anxiety is the client experiencing?

① Mild

② Moderate

③ Severe

④ Panic

497. The fetal heart rate may be accurately evaluated during labor by using a fetoscope. When is the most appropriate time to listen to fetal heart sounds in a low-risk client?

① During uterine contractions

② Between uterine contractions

③ During and for 30 seconds after uterine contractions

④ For 30 seconds before and during uterine contractions

498. The physician orders sodium hypochlorite and boric acid (Dakin's solution) for a necrotic lesion and petroleum jelly for the adjoining healthy skin. Which of the following best describes their actions?

① Dakin's solution is an antiinflammatory agent; petroleum jelly is an antiabsorbent agent.

② Dakin's solution debrides the wound; petroleum jelly protects the healthy tissue.

③ Dakin's solution dries out the lesion; petroleum jelly lubricates the surrounding tissue.

④ Dakin's solution cleanses the wound; petroleum jelly moisturizes the skin.

499. What is the most appropriate immediate nursing goal to establish for the client experiencing high levels of anxiety?

① The client will establish a trusting relationship with the nurse.

② The client will achieve insight into personal problems.

③ The client will exhibit adaptive coping behaviors.

④ The client will reduce anxiety at least one level.

500. The school nurse is asked to teach the school staff about inspecting the children for head lice. This infestation has recently become prevalent in the community. Head lice and dandruff look very similar. How can the school nurse best determine that a child has lice instead of dandruff?
① Preadolescents rarely have dandruff.
② Areas of alopecia on the nape of the neck indicate lice.
③ Children scratch more with lice than with dandruff.
④ Nits will not fall off the hair shaft when it is moved.

501. If an infection develops in a diabetic client, which effect is this most likely to have on the need for insulin?
① Undeterminable
② No effect
③ Increase the need
④ Decrease the need

502. Norvella King enters the emergency department with symptoms of an acute panic attack. She reports, "My heart started racing out of the blue, I could not breathe, and my chest felt tight." What is the most appropriate *initial* nursing action to help a client experiencing a panic attack?
① Recognize and reflect the client's feelings, and reassure the client that you will be there to help.
② Leave the client alone and encourage slow deep breaths in a paper bag.
③ Console the client and let him or her know that nothing serious is going to happen.
④ Encourage the client to express feelings and the incident that precipitated the panic attack.

503. An antepartal client, 38 weeks of gestation, is admitted to the labor unit in active labor, and the nurse determines that the fetus is in the left occiput posterior position. The client complains of severe back pain. Which nursing action would be best?
① Perform effleurage.
② Encourage her to bear down.
③ Keep her flat with a pillow under her head.
④ Encourage her to squat or to assume a hands-and-knees position.

504. A client with gangrene of the foot asks if the foot will be amputated. Which of the following approaches is the most therapeutic?
① Discuss the meaning this would have for the client.
② Explain the different types of medical management.
③ Help the client value the importance of good health.
④ Refer the question to the client's physician.

505. The school nurse is teaching day-care staff about lice. In addition to explaining how to look for the ova (nits) on the hair shafts, the nurse would instruct the staff to assess for which one of the following?
① Honey-colored vesicles
② Enlarged cervical lymph nodes
③ Alopecia
④ Ringlike lesions

506. A laboring woman's membranes rupture spontaneously when her cervix reaches 6 cm dilation. In addition to assessing the color of the fluid, what is the most important nursing action at that time?
① Call the physician.
② Take the fetal heart rate.
③ Time the contractions.
④ Prepare the woman for immediate delivery.

507. The emergency room physician sees a highly anxious client. Lorazapem 2 mg IM is ordered, and the nurse is asked to stay with the client until the client's anxiety level decreases. As the nurse approaches the client with the injection, the client says, "I don't want that dope!" What is the most appropriate nursing response?
① "The doctor would not have ordered a medication that would harm you. You need to settle down."
② "It will help calm you down, but I will not force you to take it without your approval."
③ "This is not dope! You are so distressed that you are confused."
④ "This is not dope and this shot will not harm you. Let's get this over with so you can calm down."

508. Ralph Damian is an 80-year-old client admitted to the surgical unit with complaints of left lumbosacral pain that occasionally radiates down to his groin. He reports that, a year ago, his physician told him that he had kidney stones. He also has a long history of recurrent gout. Medication for pain is listed on his admitting orders. In Mr. Damian's case, the renal stones are most likely caused by which of the following?
① Urinary stasis
② Increased excretion of calcium in the urine
③ Increased uric acid in the urine
④ A large daily intake of milk

509. Which of the following most likely indicates that the third stage of labor is coming to an end?
① Crowning of the fetal head
② Dilation of 10 cm
③ Absence of pulsation in the cord
④ A gush of blood from the vagina and a lengthening of the cord

510. Several cases of head lice are discovered in an elementary school. The nurse telephones the children's parents to inform them. Each of the infested children is treated with Kwell shampoo. What is the most important information to give their parents?
① Follow shampoo directions explicitly.
② Cut the children's hair short.
③ Prevent the children from scratching their heads.
④ Launder or disinfect the children's clothing and bedding.

511. What is the most appropriate way to initiate the assessment of a client experiencing moderate anxiety?
① "How do you normally handle anxiety?"
② "You seem pretty distressed about things on your job."
③ "Tell me what was going on when you began to feel anxious."
④ "How can I help you today?"

512. Stella Garcia, age 66, is brought to the hospital by ambulance after having suffered a fainting spell while Christmas shopping. She is accompanied by her sister, who tells the admitting physician that Mrs. Garcia recently learned she has diabetes mellitus. Before approaching Mrs. Garcia, what other information would be important to obtain from her sister?
① Is Mrs. Garcia a U.S. citizen?
② Does Mrs. Garcia speak or understand English?
③ Was the sister present when Mrs. Garcia had her fainting spell?
④ Does Mrs. Garcia have any medical insurance?

513. What is the most likely source of head lice transmission?
① Letting pets sleep with children
② Casual contact, such as play activities
③ Sharing head coverings or hair combs
④ Rolling in grassy, unmowed areas

514. A 20-year-old woman has missed two menstrual periods and has been experiencing some nausea in the mornings. She comes to the health clinic to confirm her suspicion that she might be pregnant. Which of the following physical signs might be observed on the initial examination if this client is pregnant?
① The outline of the fetus is palpated by the clinician.
② Softening of the lower uterine segment is demonstrated on bimanual examination.
③ Fetal movement is reported by the client.
④ Fetal heart rate is audible by doppler device.

515. Approximately 35 minutes after administration of lorazepam 2 mg IM injection to an anxious client, the client asks to lie down because of dizziness and lightheadedness. The most likely cause of these symptoms is which of the following?
① The client is experiencing a high level of anxiety.
② The client is withdrawing from the medication.
③ These are common adverse reactions to the medication.
④ The client has not eaten today.

516. Which assessment area would the nurse give highest priority when admitting a client to the unit?
① Mental status
② Respiratory status
③ Blood pressure
④ Heart rate

517. Parents of a child with head lice ask when the child can return to school. What would be the nurse's response?
① "After she has been shampooed three times with Kwell."
② "After shampooing with Kwell if all the nits are gone."
③ "After you cut her hair short all over."
④ "Keep her home for a few days just to be sure."

518. Thelma Tyne is a 55-year-old woman whose husband died several months ago. Recently she has experienced sleep, appetite, and concentration disturbances. She also complains of lack of energy and motivation to do her daily chores. The most likely explanation of Mrs. Tyne's symptoms is which of the following?
① Uncomplicated bereavement
② Anxiety
③ Psychosis
④ Bipolar disorder, depressed episode

519. Two siblings, Theodore, age 4, and Laura, age 2, are admitted to the hospital with a diagnosis of chronic lead poisoning. Which area of the assessment should be most detailed?
① Cardiovascular status
② Urinary output
③ Dietary habits
④ Neurologic status

520. A Spanish-speaking client's understanding of the English language is limited. What would be the best means of communicating with the client during the admission process?
① Through a hospital interpreter
② Through a close family member
③ Through a health practitioner fluent in both English and Spanish
④ Through anyone available who speaks both languages

521. What is the most appropriate goal of the client experiencing uncomplicated bereavement?
① The client will be free of fearfulness within several weeks.
② The client will reestablish activities of daily living within a month.
③ The client will be able to maintain a sense of reality within several weeks.
④ The client will be able to return to work in several weeks.

522. To best promote two preschool sibling's adaptation to being in the hospital, which nursing action would be implemented?
① Give each of them a new stuffed animal.
② Insist that one of their parents stay with them.
③ Take them to the playroom to get acquainted with the other children.
④ Place them together in the same hospital room.

523. Minnie Keyser is seen in an ambulatory care setting complaining of stomach and joint pain. After a complete physical examination with lab work, results do not support a physical basis for her complaints. She is referred to the psychiatric clinical specialist, who queries her of recent stressors. The client reports that her father died suddenly 6 months ago. She admits that she never cried or experienced grief after his death. She also states that she did not take off from her job and her family is expressing concern about her lack of emotions. Which of the following explains this client's symptoms?
① Pathologic grief reaction
② Psychotic reaction
③ Unresolved anger toward her father
④ Poor communication skills

524. During a nursing assessment, a male client with an uncomplicated bereavement begins to weep. The most

therapeutic nursing response is which of the following?

① "Don't weep. You will feel better in several days."

② Stop the assessment and ask the client to sit in the waiting room.

③ "This seems like a painful time for you."

④ Strongly encourage the client to talk and express his feelings.

525. A 58-year-old Spanish-speaking female has recently been diagnosed with diabetes mellitus by a physician.

Which of the following is an inappropriate nursing goal in the care of this client?

① The client will learn dietary principles and the role of diet.

② The client will be able to adapt her own cultural diet to meet diabetic requirements.

③ The client will safely administer the prescribed hypoglycemic agents.

④ The client will be able to adequately teach another newly diagnosed diabetic client in Spanish.

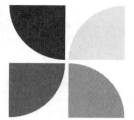

Practice Test 8

526. Which of the following observations indicate a toxic response to the drugs CaNa$_2$ EDTA and dimercaprol (BAL)?
① Seizures
② Long-bone pain
③ Oliguria
④ Anemia

527. While the nurse is taking a prenatal history, an antepartal client tells the nurse that she has been pregnant three times previously. She had a son born on her due date 6 years ago, she had twin daughters born a month early 3 years ago, and she had a miscarriage at 8 weeks of gestation last year. All three children are excited about this pregnancy. Based on this information, what obstetric history would the nurse record?
① 4, 1, 1, 1, 3
② 3, 1, 2, 1, 3
③ 3, 2, 0, 1, 2
④ 4, 1, 2, 1, 3

528. A client admitted to the acute psychiatric unit with a diagnosis of uncomplicated bereavement after his wife died states that he is feeling better the next day and requests to be discharged, saying, "I can handle things alone and the staff has been very helpful." What is the most appropriate reaction to this request?
① Communicate concerns to the health team regarding the possibility that he has decided to attempt suicide.
② Discharge the client and strongly encourage him to call back if the need arises.
③ Permit the client to go on a weekend pass to see how things go.
④ Allow him a 3-hour pass.

529. In a limited amount of time available, the nurse recognizes that which of the following is a priority in the preoperative teaching for a client with acute appendicitis?
① Leg exercises to prevent venous stasis
② Abdominal splinting for coughing and deep breathing
③ Explanation of the nasogastric tube that can be expected postoperatively
④ Explanation of drainage on the dressing

530. The nurse would prepare to administer a toddler's injection in which of the following sites?
① The gluteus medius muscle
② The deltoid muscle
③ The vastus lateralis muscle
④ The subcutaneous tissue of the abdomen

531. Michael Tortelli, a 28-year-old client who is depressed and aloof, begins to criticize the staff and the quality of care he is receiving. This behavior is best evaluated as which of the following?
① Regression
② Hostility
③ Improvement
④ Increased risk of self-harm

532. When evaluating treatment outcomes of the client with depression, the nurse would appraise which of the following?
① Ability to manage anxiety
② Ability to maintain reality testing
③ Degree of suspiciousness
④ Ability to manage activities of daily living

533. A pregnant woman asks what she can do to treat the nausea she has been having in the first few weeks of her pregnancy. Which of the following would the nurse suggest?
① "Avoid foods that are high in fiber."
② "Drink 2 glasses of water before arising."
③ "Alternate food and fluids rather than drinking with meals."
④ "Eat 3 meals per day and avoid between-meal snacks."

534. Before administering a client's preoperative medication, which nursing action is most essential?
① Report to the physician the elevated white blood cell count.
② Check to ensure that the laboratory has completed the urinalysis.
③ Ensure that the surgical consent form has been signed.
④ Provide a quiet environment.

535. As the nurse prepares to administer an injection to Raymond, age 5, he begins to cry and kick. What is the best nursing response to Raymond?
① "Raymond, your roommate is going to get an injection, too."
② "Raymond, you can cry as much as you want, but you must hold still."
③ "Be a big boy now, Raymond, and this will be over in a minute."
④ "Raymond, this will just feel like a little stick and it will be over."

536. During the eighth month of pregnancy, an expectant mother comes to the clinic for her regular prenatal visit. As part of her assessment, the nurse performs

Leopold's maneuvers. The nurse explains that this procedure

① Helps guide the fetus into the pelvis.
② Turns the baby around in the uterus.
③ Detects any fetal abnormalities.
④ Helps determine the baby's position.

537. Herbert McKay, a 36-year-old single parent, has been admitted to the orthopedic unit to assess an old knee injury. During night rounds the nurse notices that Mr. Mckay is diaphoretic, tremulous, and shaky. At 7 AM the client complains of intense agitation and nervousness and is assessed to be obviously disoriented and restless. Of the following substances, which one is most likely to be abused by this client?

① Cocaine
② Alcohol
③ Lysergic acid diethylamide (LSD)
④ Opioids

538. A client is taken to the operating room, and preparation for surgery begins. The circulating nurse's primary goal when positioning a client on the operating room table is to achieve

① A comfortable position for the client.
② A position that is acceptable to the surgeon.
③ A position that prevents exposure and promotes privacy.
④ A position that avoids circulatory impairment and protects nerve function.

539. Which of the following menus is most appropriate to serve a child with lead poisoning?

① Hamburger and bun, peas, milk, and orange slices
② Spaghetti, lettuce, grape juice, and gelatin with bananas
③ Peanut butter sandwich, raw carrots, apple juice, and vanilla pudding
④ Liver, broccoli, bread and butter, milk, and a cookie

540. A pregnant woman at 32 weeks of gestation tells the nurse that she has been having painless uterine contractions for the last week. They occur at irregular intervals and are relieved by walking. Based on this information, what would the nurse do?

① Prepare for a vaginal exam to assess cervical changes.
② Admit the woman with onset of labor.
③ Explain that these are Braxton Hicks' contractions requiring no intervention.
④ Schedule a stress test to determine fetal ability to withstand labor.

541. Mrs. Barbara Myers, 48 years old, is admitted to a medical surgical unit for unstable diabetes mellitus. She has been on this unit several times over the past 12 months. She tells one of the nurses on the evening shift, "You are the best charge nurse on this unit. You understand me better than anyone else. Nurses on the morning shift are so incompetent." Which of the following best defines the client's behavior?

① An ability to identify incompetent staff
② Ideas of grandeur
③ Difficulty forming trust with other nurses
④ An effort to manipulate the staff

542. A client receives a general anesthetic in the operating room. In order to suppress pain, general anesthesia must depress which part of the brain?

① Medulla
② Thalamus
③ Cerebellum
④ Cortex

543. Which of the following laboratory tests is *not* likely to be ordered to monitor recovery from lead poisoning?

① Blood lead level
② Hematocrit and hemoglobin
③ Urinalysis
④ Clotting and bleeding times

544. Which of the following outcomes is the best long-term indicator of successful treatment of a child with chronic lead poisoning?

① Physical growth within normal limits
② Adequate dietary intake of essential nutrients
③ Age-appropriate achievement of developmental milestones
④ Normal sleep patterns

545. Which of the following best describes behaviors seen in clients with a diagnosis of borderline personality disorder?

① Comply willingly and passively with treatment recommendations
② Readily form therapeutic relationships with staff
③ Lack concern and empathy for others
④ Have good insight into their problems

546. During a pregnant woman's checkup, the nurse listens to the fetal heart tones and determines that the rate is 96 beats per minute and the heart sound is strong. In view of these findings, what would the nurse's next action be?

① Record this rate in the mother's chart.
② Take the mother's blood pressure.
③ Take the mother's pulse.
④ Notify the physician immediately.

547. A 21-year-old male client is admitted to the postanesthesia room. The nurse obtains admitting vital signs of blood pressure 90/60 mm Hg, pulse 100, and respirations 18. Which action would be appropriate at this time?

① Recheck the vital signs in 5 minutes and get his baseline normal from the documented preoperative vital signs.
② Increase the rate of the IV slightly.
③ Place him flat and elevate his feet.
④ Cover him with a warm blanket.

548. It is now 7 hours after a male client's abdominal surgery. He complains of being unable to void, even though he has the urge. Which nursing action is most appropriate?

① Obtain an order to catheterize him.
② Help him stand at the bedside to void.
③ Wait 1 hour more before taking any action.
④ Explain to him that this is a common sensation postoperatively.

549. Amy Highlander, a very excitable and active 5-year-old, has just returned from a cardiac catheterization. Her mother suddenly calls out for the nurse to come

quickly. The nurse enters the room and sees Amy standing by the window with blood running down her leg. What would the nurse's initial action be?
① Call the physician immediately.
② Apply pressure to the site.
③ Increase Amy's IV rate.
④ Have Amy get back into bed.

550. Caring for the client with a personality disorder often generates strong emotions in the staff. Which of the following best describes staff reactions to these clients?
① Intense anger and a sense of helplessness
② The need to rescue the client from others
③ Intense concern and a positive regard
④ Social withdrawal and an absence of feelings

551. A 25-year-old primipara with type II diabetes is scheduled for a nonstress test. Which of the following is true regarding a nonstress test?
① An IV of oxytocin will be started to stimulate mild contractions.
② The test determines the gestational age of the fetus.
③ Pregnancy-induced hypertension can be diagnosed using this test.
④ The test evaluates fetal heart rates in relation to fetal movement.

552. Retained secretions in the lungs, especially postoperatively, most often result in which of the following?
① Pulmonary edema
② Fluid imbalance
③ Atelectasis and pneumonia
④ CO_2 retention

553. Which of the following newly delivered mothers is at greatest risk for a postpartal infection?
① A woman who delivered vaginally with marginal placenta previa
② A primipara who had rupture of membranes 36 hours before delivery
③ A mother who had a cesarean delivery because of cephalopelvic disproportion
④ A multigravida who delivered twins after a 10-hour labor

554. Four-month-old Emalee is brought to the clinic for a checkup and immunizations. When assessing Emalee's development, the nurse would be most concerned about which one of the following observations?
① Visually follows objects 180 degrees
② Does not attempt to transfer a toy from one hand to the other
③ Is unable to roll from back to front
④ Does not turn her head to locate sounds

555. Marshall Lindsey, 30 years old, has been diagnosed with a personality disorder. During his hospitalization he consistently tests limits and attempts to play staff against each other. Which of the following approaches is the most therapeutic for staff to manage the client's disruptive behavior?
① Give him attention when he is not manipulating others.
② Avoid intervening when the client interacts with others.

③ Respond to the client's demands as quickly as possible.
④ Provide the client with detailed instructions regarding staff expectations.

556. A postpartum mother is concerned that her 2-year-old daughter will not like the new baby. She asks the nurse what she might do. The nurse would suggest which of the following?
① "Explain to your daughter that the baby is a permanent part of your family now."
② "Expect your daughter to demand more of your attention when you bring the new baby home."
③ "Place limits on regressive behavior such as thumbsucking."
④ "Let your husband focus attention on your daughter while you focus on the new baby."

557. Abby, age 6 months, is scheduled to receive her second diphtheria/pertussis/tetanus and polio immunizations today. She has a slight cough, a runny nose, and a temperature of 100.4°F (38°C). Which of the following nursing actions is most appropriate?
① Advise parents of possible side effects of immunizations.
② Give the immunizations and recommend use of a mild analgesic as soon as they get home.
③ Postpone the immunizations.
④ Advise the parents to notify their physician.

558. Lucida Carol, age 20 months, is brought to the emergency department by her father. She has multiple facial and back bruises and a fractured skull. Child abuse is surmised. Assessing the circumstances, the nurse would determine that which information is the most pertinent?
① The parental-child interaction
② When the mishap took place
③ The number of other children living in the home
④ The age of the child's father

559. A client has a seizure. Which nursing action would be inappropriate?
① Protect the client's head.
② Restrain the client.
③ Turn the client's head or body to the side.
④ Time the seizure.

560. While caring for a 22-year-old primipara on the second postpartal day after a normal spontaneous delivery, the nurse notes that each of the following is on the chart. Which of these requires prompt notification of the physician?
① White blood cell count of 14,000
② Oral temperature of 101°F (38.3°C)
③ Profuse diaphoresis overnight
④ Hematocrit of 36%

561. The victim of an automobile accident becomes confused during the night and falls quietly asleep. The nurse takes the vital signs and finds that the blood pressure is 155/60 mm Hg, pulse is 64, and respirations are 18. The physician suspects increased intracranial pressure. Which nursing action would be first?
① Institute seizure precautions.
② Start an IV infusion.
③ Order a suction machine.
④ Start oxygen by cannula at 6 L.

562. Why is dexamethasone (Decadron) the corticosteroid drug of choice for head trauma clients?
① It is an antiinflammatory drug.
② It decreases the amount of spinal fluid secreted.
③ It crosses the blood-brain barrier.
④ It causes fewer side effects than any of the other corticosteroids.

563. During a home visit to a primipara on the third post-partum day, the visiting nurse finds the mother somewhat anxious but enthusiastic to learn more about her baby and how to care for him. She describes periodic feelings of being overwhelmed and weepy, interspersed with happiness and competence. What phase of adjustment is the mother exhibiting?
① Taking in
② Taking hold
③ Letting go
④ Bursting out

564. Which steps should be taken by hospital staff when child abuse is suspected?
① Confront the child's father.
② Notify other members of the family.
③ Inform the child protective services.
④ Remain quiet until the diagnosis is confirmed.

565. Four-month-old Elizabeth's parents state that she does not like cereal, because she always spits it out when they try to feed it to her. What is the most appropriate nursing response to the parents?
① "Discontinue cereal and try fruit instead."
② "You may need to position her differently during meals."
③ "She will outgrow this in a month or so."
④ "When she is hungry enough she will eat."

566. A 22-year-old woman delivered her first child, a boy, 24 hours ago. She had a normal vaginal delivery with a midline episiotomy and is breast-feeding her baby. Which one of the following assessments on the first postpartal day would most likely indicate normal postpartal adjustment?
① Fundus two finger breadths above the umbilicus
② Breasts engorged with red streaks
③ Moderate flow of lochia serosa
④ Lack of bowel movement since delivery

567. The father of a 4-year-old is suspected of abusing his daughter. Before the establishment of a therapeutic relationship, what is the most important initial nursing action?
① Assess family support systems.
② Recognize and manage personal negative reactions toward abusive caregivers.
③ Analyze the family's present and past coping responses to stress.
④ Determine community referrals for abusive caregivers.

568. Untreated kidney stones can dislodge and obstruct the ureter. In turn, this obstruction is the primary cause of which of the following?
① Kidney abscess
② Hydronephrosis
③ Glomerulonephritis
④ Nephrosis

569. The mother of a 2-year-old diagnosed with otitis me-

dia asks the nurse in the clinic why her child gets repeated ear infections. The nurse bases her response on which one of the following pathophysiologic understandings?
① The young child's auditory canal is straighter, shorter, and narrower.
② The young child's eustachian tube is straighter, shorter, and wider.
③ The young child lacks adequate pharyngeal lymphoid tissue.
④ The young child's temperature-regulating system is immature.

570. On the day of delivery, the nurse gives a new mother self-care instructions. Instructions regarding care of the perineal area would include which of the following?
① Wipe the perineum from back to front to prevent irritating hemorrhoids.
② Rinse the perineum after each void and elimination to prevent infection.
③ Use sterile water in a peri bottle to cleanse the perineum appropriately.
④ Avoid use of soap on perineum to prevent allergic reactions.

571. A nursing goal of abusive caregivers seeking community referral is learning about parenting skills. Which of the following suggests that an abusive parent has partially or significantly met this goal?
① The parent attends Parents Anonymous group meetings.
② The parent brings in a new toy for the hospitalized child.
③ The parent frequently calls the unit and checks on the child.
④ The child is brought in for follow-up appointments by the abusive parent.

572. One evening while in bed, a male client with a history of recurrent renal calculi complains of severe pain in the left posterior lumbar region. The first nursing responsibility would be to do which of the following?
① Strain his urine.
② Give an analgesic (e.g., morphine) as ordered.
③ Encourage movement about to facilitate excretion of the stone.
④ Encourage large fluid intake.

573. The nurse in the pediatric clinic assesses all of the following children. Which one requires further evaluation?
① A 4-year-old with recurrent episodes of otitis media who articulates poorly
② A 4-year-old recently discharged from the hospital who is awakened by nightmares
③ A 2½-year-old recently discharged from the hospital who wets the bed
④ A 2-year-old with recurrent episodes of otitis media who persists with thumbsucking

574. Which one of the following behaviors indicates that the new postpartum mother has correctly understood the nurse's instructions for preventing cracked nipples while breast-feeding?
① She uses an alcohol swab to cleanse her nipples before feeding.

② She air-dries her nipples 15 minutes after feeding.
③ She feeds in the same comfortable position at all times.
④ She keeps the areola out of the baby's mouth when feeding.

575. Which of the following behaviors is most descriptive of individuals with a diagnosis of borderline personality?
① A lack of empathy for others, poor impulse control, and difficulty managing stress
② An ability to relate to others in a meaningful manner except during stressful periods
③ Ritualistic behaviors manifested by frequent hand washing and the need to be clean
④ An intense fear of rejection, disapproval, and inability to make simple decisions

576. A urea-splitting organism such as *Streptococcus* favors the growth of inorganic renal calculi. The urea-splitting organism causes the urine to become which of the following?
① Alkaline
② Acidic
③ Neutral
④ Concentrated with sediments

577. A 33-year-old woman delivered a 7-pound 8-ounce baby girl earlier today. Which of the following behaviors would indicate that this woman is in the taking-in phase of the postpartum period?
① Talking about the details of her labor and delivery experience.
② Asking the nurse to demonstrate use of her sitz bath.
③ Performing cord care when changing the baby's diaper.
④ Planning the date for her return to work.

578. Which of the following toys and games encourages development of a 7-month-old?
① Let her throw and retrieve objects.
② Play peek-a-boo.
③ Use a crib mobile.
④ Use push-pull toys.

579. Lindsay is a 20-year-old who has recently been hospitalized for contemplating suicide using alcohol and over-the-counter medication. Over the past few days she has denied having suicidal ideations, but her mood is sad and irritable and she has become socially withdrawn. She is also experiencing appetite, sleep, and concentration disturbances. Which of the following treatments should be considered at this time?
① Administration of an antipsychotic agent
② Administration of an antidepressant
③ Electroconvulsive therapy
④ Administration of an antimanic agent

580. Nine-month-old Bradley is admitted to the pediatric unit with vomiting, colicky abdominal pain, and abdominal distention. A tentative diagnosis of intussusception is made. When assessing Bradley, which type of stool indicates a worsening of Bradley's condition?
① Fatty, bulky, and foul smelling
② Dark red and jellylike
③ Ribbonlike and dark green
④ Clay colored

581. A new mother is preparing to go home after the birth of her twin boys. She asks the nurse when it is safe to resume sexual intercourse after delivery. In response to her question, the nurse replies that intercourse can safely be resumed at which of the following times?
① As soon as she returns home
② When the physician gives approval
③ Once lochia flow has stopped
④ After the 6-week postpartum checkup

582. If the client's urine has a pH of 7.8, which of the following would most likely be given?
① Methenamine mandelate (Mandelamine)
② Vitamin C
③ Sodium bicarbonate
④ Sodium phosphate

583. Decompression drainage of the bladder is used specifically to do which of the following?
① Alleviate discomfort by providing continuous drainage.
② Prevent increased intraabdominal pressure by avoiding bladder distention.
③ Provide a means for constant irrigation of the bladder.
④ Help the muscles of the bladder to maintain their tone without overstretch.

584. During early stages of the therapeutic relationship with Mrs. Lord, who has been diagnosed with borderline personality disorder, the nurse can expect her to do which of the following?
① Experience increased feelings of suspiciousness
② Experience sensory deficits
③ Manipulate staff and other clients
④ Complain of depersonalization

585. A 28-year-old woman is suffering from metrorrhagia. The woman would be encouraged to seek medical assistance primarily because of which of the following?
① Excessive bleeding during menses may lead to anemia.
② Bleeding between periods may be the only early sign of cancer.
③ This is often symptomatic of a serious psychosomatic problem.
④ Periods that occur too frequently are usually associated with anovulation.

586. The use of bethanechol (Urecholine) in the treatment of temporary postoperative urinary retention is suggested because of its action as which of the following?
① An anticholinergic
② A cholinergic
③ An anesthetic
④ A urinary antispasmodic

587. Which description of bleeding from the abdomen is the most appropriate way for the documentation of such in the nurse's notes?
① A moderate to large amount of sanguineous drainage noted from abdominal wound
② Severe bleeding from wound over 10 minutes with saturation of 6 abdominal pads
③ Copious amounts of bright red blood coming from abdomen over 10 minutes

Sanguineous drainage from abdominal wound soaked 2 towels and 6 abdominal pads in 10 minutes

588. A 9-month-old is *not* likely to exhibit which of the following behaviors?
① Loud crying when his parents leave him
② Fear of strangers
③ Searching for hidden objects
④ Saying at least three words besides "mama" and "dada"

589. A woman is 2 days postpartum. In addition to an elevated temperature and chills, which finding would suggest she has acquired postpartal endometritis?
① Complaint of increased thirst
② Fleshy odor of lochia
③ Uterus tender when palpated abdominally
④ Diastasis recti detected on abdominal palpation

590. What is the *least* effective nursing action when the client is diagnosed with borderline personality disorder?
① Set consistent and clear limits.
② Provide an accepting and empathic environment.
③ Expect the client to maintain adequate impulse control and act in a mature manner.
④ Encourage the client to assist staff in working with regressed clients.

591. Mr. Lewis is admitted to the aftercare program with a diagnosis of borderline personality disorder. One of the treatment goals for this client is, "client will develop adaptive skills that enable him to relate to others in socially acceptable ways." The best approach to attain this goal is which of the following?
① Encourage the client to identify maladaptive behaviors and seek to change them.
② Integrate the client's assessment of social problems into treatment plan.
③ Encourage group participation with individuals with different diagnoses in an effort to learn new social skills.
④ Set consistent and firm limits with clear delineation of consequences.

592. A baby boy has just been born and appears to be normal. Erythromycin ophthalmic ointment is instilled in the baby's eyes at 1 hour of age to prevent which of the following?
① Retinopathy of prematurity
② Ophthalmia neonatorum
③ *Treponema pallidum*
④ Chemical conjunctivitis

593. Mrs. Longfellow attends a daily group that focuses on individual problems. She states, "I have never really had any problems and I am here to help others." The nurse recognizes that the client's behavior is an example of which of the following behaviors?
① Becoming a helping role model
② Poor impulse control
③ Attempting to resolve others' problems
④ Resisting working on her own problems

594. A client is admitted to the emergency room with an abdominal gunshot wound. Towels can be used to pack the gunshot wound because

① The injury is usually fatal.
② The wound is already grossly contaminated.
③ Towels absorb more than abdominal pads.
④ The client probably has minimal external bleeding.

595. Five minutes after birth, a new baby's Apgar score was 9 because of acrocyanosis. This condition in newborns is a result of which of the following?
① Retained amniotic fluid in the lungs
② Failure to breathe within the expected amount of time
③ Sluggish peripheral circulation
④ Low pulse rate

596. Preoperatively, the priority nursing goal for an infant with intussusception is to do which of the following?
① Maintain his attachment to his parents.
② Meet his needs for sucking and comfort while he is NPO.
③ Maintain adequate hydration.
④ Promote adequate rest and sleep.

597. Paula is a 22-year-old diagnosed with borderline personality disorder. One evening she returns from her weekend pass 45 minutes late and states that she forgot her appointment with her primary nurse. The most therapeutic response to this client is which of the following?
① "I am going to call your doctor because you failed to keep your appointment."
② Disregard her behavior and inquire of her interest to see someone else.
③ Ignore the forgotten appointment, and pretend it never happened.
④ Confront her about returning late and missing the appointment, and initiate identified consequences.

598. After surgery to repair intussusception, a 6-month-old returns to the unit. He is fussy and seems to be in discomfort. The nurse palpates his abdomen and notes some distention. Which action would be implemented first?
① Call the surgeon to report this observation.
② Insert a rectal tube.
③ Sit the infant upright and pat him on the back.
④ Check the nasogastric tube for patency.

599. A male client enters the emergency room with a knife protruding from his chest. The initial nursing action is to do which of the following?
① Immediately remove the knife.
② Leave the knife in until an operative setup is arranged.
③ Clean the exposed knife blade with povidone-iodine solution.
④ Cover area with a sterile towel soaked in saline.

600. Select the most correct statement about subcutaneous emphysema.
① It is caused by air sucked into the chest wall from a superficial chest wound.
② It is caused by an internal thoracic injury.
③ It can always be noted easily.
④ It is not exacerbated by coughing.

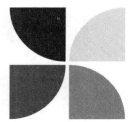

Practice Test 9

601. Which of the following statements best indicates that Mrs. Kohlberg, whose 6-year-old son Keith was bitten by a tick, understands how to prevent another occurrence?
① "I will have Keith wear a light-colored tank top."
② "I will spray Keith with insect repellent."
③ "I'll never let him into those woods again."
④ "I'll check Keith when he comes back in from playing."

602. A client with trauma to the abdomen is unable to void. A catheterization yields a small amount of bloody urine. This is most likely an indication of which of the following?
① Prostatitis
② Urethritis
③ Ruptured bladder
④ Urethral tear

603. Jesse Belden, 8 years old, has just come in from playing in the woods with his friends. His buddy Brandon notices something on Jesse's back, and both boys run to Jesse's mother. What is the best advice the nurse can provide to Mrs. Belden regarding tick removal?
① Use a sterilized needle to pry the tick loose.
② Use tweezers to grasp the tick behind the head.
③ Place vaseline around the body of the tick before pulling off.
④ Light a match and place it next to the tick.

604. When administering a blood transfusion, what is a mandatory nursing function requiring two nurses?
① Check the type and crossmatch data, numbers on the lab slips, and the information on the blood with that on the client's blood band.
② Check the type and crossmatch data, numbers on the lab slips, and the information on the blood with that on the client's chart.
③ Check for the best possible vein to ensure correct infusion.
④ Ensure that the client is rational in order to establish a baseline of behavior.

605. What is most likely to impede a 10-month-old's continued development while he is hospitalized?
① Developing mistrust of the nursing staff
② Separation from his parents
③ Restricted mobility
④ Disruption in his sleeping and eating routines

606. A client's friend volunteers to donate blood for the client. Which of these conditions would not allow the friend to donate?
① History of gonorrhea within the last year.
② History of bacterial endocarditis within the last 4 years.
③ History of hepatitis within the last 5 years.
④ History of upper respiratory tract infection within the last 6 months.

607. An infant is being breast-fed. What would this baby's stool look like at 1 week of age?
① Black and tarry
② Green and seedy
③ Light yellow and mushy
④ Bright yellow and formed

608. Which toy would be most appropriate for a 9-month-old hospitalized infant?
① An activity box for his crib
② A fuzzy stuffed animal
③ A small toy truck
④ A rattle

609. Mr. Aramis, a 32-year-old diagnosed with borderline personality disorder, informs the nurse on the night shift that he is the only one who understands his problems. He points out that the day shift is too hectic and there are not enough people on the evening shift. What is the most appropriate nursing response to this situation?
① Confront the evening shift with his complaints.
② Point out that he needs to voice his complaints to the day supervisor.
③ Gather data from each shift from other clients and share it with the client government groups.
④ Report this information at the daily staff conferences, and decide on a plan of action to deal with this client.

610. When assembling equipment to start a blood transfusion, which of the following solutions is used to flush and maintain the IV line?
① Sterile water
② Normal saline
③ 10% dextrose in water
④ Lactated Ringer's solution

611. The nurse must remain at the bedside for 15 minutes after blood is started to assess for a transfusion reaction. Which of the following, if found, would not be associated with a transfusion reaction?

① Chills, fever, and dyspnea
② Decreased blood pressure and increased pulse rate
③ Bleeding under the skin at the IV site
④ Hives and itching

612. The nurse is providing the mother of a 10-month-old infant some anticipatory guidance and instructions. All of the following are appropriate *except*

① Switch the infant from formula to 2% milk, and give him supplemental vitamins and minerals.
② Begin introducing chopped meats, egg yolk, and breads such as zwieback, one at a time, to his diet.
③ Introduce a cup for drinking juices and water.
④ Give him foods that he can feed himself using his fingers or a spoon.

613. When testing a breast-fed neonate for phenylketonuria, a false-negative result is most often the result of which condition?

① Decreased vitamin K level
② Inadequate fluid intake
③ Increased serum bilirubin
④ Insufficient protein absorption

614. What is the *least* effective strategy to cope with the client who attempts to split staff with complaints of inadequacy?

① Analyze client complaints with other staff before a plan of action is determined.
② Allow the client freedom to make rules to allay anxiety.
③ Communicate a plan of action to all staff members regarding the client's care.
④ Develop a written or computerized plan of care for consistent health care delivery.

615. Which one of the following nursing actions is best to do for a transfusion reaction?

① Notify the physician.
② Check the vital signs, and take a urine sample.
③ Stop the blood transfusion, disconnect the IV line, and infuse normal saline through a new line.
④ Stop the blood transfusion, flush the tubing with the saline from the Y-connection, and keep the vein open.

616. Donor-recipient compatibility must be assessed before renal transplant. A client with chronic renal failure waiting for a donor asks the nurse to explain tissue typing. Which statement is an *incorrect* response?

① Blood typing is the initial step in determining compatibility.
② Any natural sibling of the recipient is an ideal donor.
③ Two human leukocyte antigens (HLAs) are inherited from each parent.
④ A mixed lymphocyte culture requires 5 to 7 days to perform.

617. Sarah Rosen is a newborn with a bilateral cleft lip and a cleft palate. Sarah's parents are young but seem concerned and willing to learn about her care. The teach-

ing plan for the parents will include all of the following *except*

① Remove the nipple frequently when feeding Sarah.
② Encourage mother to breast-feed.
③ Sarah's security needs can be met in other ways besides sucking.
④ Sarah's mental functioning should be normal.

618. To determine a newborn's gestational age, the admitting nurse would assess which of the following?

① Body temperature and posture
② Amount of lanugo and plantar creases
③ Heart rate and breast tissue
④ Degree of jaundice and popliteal angle

619. Adam Bernstein, 29 years old, is admitted to an acute psychiatric unit with a diagnosis of major depression. Several months ago, he sustained second- and third-degree burns in a house fire in which his 12-month-old son and wife were killed. He was unable to attend the funeral because of severe burns. He is thin and socially withdrawn. What is the best explanation for Mr. Bernstein's behavior?

① His physical condition remains serious.
② The grief process was delayed because he was unable to attend the funeral.
③ The idea of not being able to see his child and wife is devastating.
④ He is experiencing an intense sense of isolation.

620. A client who is scheduled for an organ transplant will receive the drug azathioprine (Imuran) before surgery and after the transplant. What would the nurse teach the client about this medication?

① The drug causes immunosuppression and therefore the client should avoid crowds and contact with obviously ill people.
② The drug stimulates kidney output.
③ Frequent monitoring of blood pressure will be required.
④ An increase in the number of circulating antibodies can be anticipated.

621. Preoperatively, which of the following nursing actions is most important for a 4-week-old with a bilateral cleft lip?

① Burp him frequently during feedings.
② Offer him small, frequent feedings to avoid tiring him.
③ Hold him in a low or supine position to facilitate swallowing.
④ Thicken the feedings to increase his intake and retention.

622. Which observation is inappropriate to associate with tissue rejection in a client who has had a kidney transplant?

① Weight gain
② Decreased urine output
③ Swelling in the kidney area
④ Rising white blood cell count

623. A 1-day-old infant has a core temperature of 100.4°F (38°C). The temperature of the Isolette reads 98°F (36.6°C). The neonate's elevated tempera-

ture is most probably a result of which of the following?
1. An infection
2. The temperature of the Isolette
3. A maternal infection
4. A neonatal abnormality

624. Which of the following is inappropriate to include in the early postoperative care for a renal transplant client?
1. Irrigate the Foley catheter frequently.
2. Maintain reverse isolation.
3. Turn and reposition frequently.
4. Monitor the stool for blood.

625. Since the loss of his son and wife, Mr. Bernstein has lost 11 pounds. Which nursing action would be the most beneficial at this time?
1. Encourage him to eat with another client recovering from depression.
2. Isolate him from others during mealtimes.
3. Allow him to eat in the dining room so he can select meals that are appealing to him.
4. Consult with the dietitian to prepare special meals to maintain a proper diet.

626. Sally Burnside, age 15, is interested in donating her kidneys for transplant should she die unexpectedly. She asks if she can carry a donor card. Based on the Uniform Anatomical Gift Act, what can the nurse tell her?
1. She must wait until she is 18 because she is a minor.
2. All she needs to do is sign a card.
3. She may carry a donor card, provided her parents have cosigned the card in the presence of witnesses.
4. A donor card is not necessary, because her parents could give permission if the need arises.

627. Jorge Benton has a soft-tissue cleft palate. When he is 14 months old, he is admitted for repair of his cleft palate. What is the best reason for the palate to be repaired at this age?
1. To correct the palate before speech development
2. To prevent damaging tooth buds
3. To allow better postoperative cooperation
4. To prevent recurrent bouts of tonsillitis

628. A client returns for a follow-up visit 1 year after his renal transplant. He tells the nurse he feels so well that he has decided to stop taking his prednisone. The nurse is concerned because he may experience which of the following?
1. Infection
2. Organ rejection
3. Psychosis
4. Anemia

629. A baby who weighed 8 pounds at birth is now 3 days old and weighs 7 pounds 8 ounces. He is voiding six times a day and breast-feeds 8 to 10 times a day. Which nursing action would probably be appropriate at this time?
1. Consult with the physician about adding supplementary formula to his diet.
2. Teach parents to weigh him before and after breast-feeding.

3. Continue to support his mother's breast-feeding efforts.
4. Suggest offering glucose water between feedings to prevent dehydration.

630. Sean Collins, age 52, experiences retrosternal chest pain that radiates down his left arm when he is engaged in strenuous physical activity. A resting electrocardiogram (ECG) is normal, but a stress ECG shows ST depression. As the nurse takes a history, which of the following questions is most relevant?
1. "Can you describe the pain and the events that led up to it?"
2. "Are you taking any medications for chest pain?"
3. "How many packs of cigarettes do you smoke daily?"
4. "Did the pain radiate to your jaw or neck?"

631. Mr. Petty is having difficulty falling asleep. Which of the following measures would promote sleep in this client?
1. Permit him to exercise vigorously 20 minutes nightly at 9:30 PM.
2. Encourage him to take a cool shower and a hot cup of tea.
3. Recommend watching TV nightly until midnight.
4. Provide a back rub and a glass of warm milk.

632. An ECG primarily gives information about which of the following?
1. Excitation of the myocardium
2. Perfusion of the myocardium
3. Contractile force of the myocardium
4. Integrity of the myocardium

633. A male newborn is circumcised on the second postpartal day. Care for this baby boy within the first 4 hours after surgery would include which of the following?
1. Inspect the site every hour for signs of infection.
2. Monitor and record first voiding.
3. Withhold feeding immediately after the procedure.
4. Apply fresh, sterile gauze dressing to the penis with each diaper change.

634. Cardiac isoenzymes are drawn on a client with chest pain. Why were they ordered?
1. To identify the causative organism
2. To determine how well the blood is oxygenated
3. To rule out gas or indigestion
4. To determine the presence of tissue damage

635. Individuals diagnosed with dysthymic disorder experience varying levels of energy. What is the best time of day to schedule activities for a person with depression?
1. Morning
2. Noon
3. Late afternoon
4. Evening

636. Anginal pain can involve the left arm and jaw, in addition to the chest, because these areas are all supplied by which of the following parts of the nervous system?
1. Cranial nerve (vagus)
2. Spinal nerves
3. Autonomic nervous system
4. Spinal cord segment

637. During a discussion with a client about how anginal pain is caused by coronary insufficiency, the client asks the nurse to explain when the coronary arteries fill with blood. Which statement is most accurate to include for the explanation of when the coronary arteries fill with blood?
    ① The ventricle contracts, and the aortic valve is closed.
    ② The ventricle contracts, and the aortic valve is open.
    ③ The ventricle relaxes, and the aortic valve is closed.
    ④ The ventricle relaxes, and the aortic valve is open.

638. Which of the following are common long-term problems that might develop in a child with a cleft lip and cleft palate?
    ① Headaches and malocclusion
    ② Dental caries and emotional problems
    ③ Contractures of the mandible
    ④ Speech problems and otitis media

639. In which age group is eczema most frequently seen?
    ① Infancy
    ② Childhood
    ③ Adolescence
    ④ It is seen equally in all age groups

640. A neonate's bilirubin level rises to 18 mg, and he is treated with traditional phototherapy. Which of the following assessments would not be included in the plan of care by the nurse?
    ① Infant temperature
    ② Infant feeding
    ③ Infant elimination
    ④ Infant blood pressure

641. A client is given nitroglycerin, 0.4 mg, to take sublingually during his angina attacks. The dosage of 0.4 mg is equivalent to how many grains?
    ① 1/250 grain
    ② 1/200 grain
    ③ 1/150 grain
    ④ 1/100 grain

642. Which of the following is an indicator of grief resolution in the client with depression?
    ① The client refrains from crying.
    ② The client discusses both positive and negative aspects of the relationship with the deceased.
    ③ The client becomes more detached and infrequently speaks of the deceased.
    ④ The client begins to seek staff in efforts to talk about present stressors.

643. The initial objective of nursing care of the infant or child with eczema is which of the following?
    ① Treatment of pruritus
    ② Identification of the allergen
    ③ Giving treated baths
    ④ Education for diet regimen

644. A multipara enters the labor and delivery unit at 40 weeks of gestation. Her cervix is 4 cm dilated and 80% effaced. Her contractions are 3 to 5 minutes apart and are associated with moderate discomfort. Based on the information presented, the labor room

nurse determines that this woman is in which phase of labor?
    ① First stage, latent phase
    ② First stage, active phase
    ③ First stage, transition phase
    ④ Second stage

645. Nitroglycerin produces dilation of the coronary collateral circulation 1 to 2 minutes after being put under the tongue. The client should be instructed to
    ① Administer one tablet q2min for five doses.
    ② Administer one tablet q5min for ten doses.
    ③ Administer one tablet q5min for three doses.
    ④ Administer one tablet q10min for five doses.

646. What are common side effects of nitroglycerin therapy?
    ① Headache, hypotension, and dizziness
    ② Hypertension, flushing, and loss of consciousness
    ③ Hypotension, shock, and convulsions
    ④ Headache, hypertension, and convulsions

647. What information would the nurse give to a client about nitroglycerin?
    ① "Take the tablets with meals."
    ② "Take the tablets only for severe pain."
    ③ "A burning sensation under the tongue is normal."
    ④ "Call your doctor if you have a headache or flushing."

648. Which of the following baths would the nurse recommend for a child with eczema?
    ① Warm water and soap
    ② Cool water and soap
    ③ Tepid water only
    ④ Warm water with lipid soap

649. A primipara has progressed in her labor. She is restless and complaining of severe pain. Her cervix is 5 cm dilated and 100% effaced. The vertex is at 0 station. She requests pain medication, and the physician has ordered meperidine (Demerol). Which of the following nursing actions is most appropriate?
    ① Give her the meperidine (Demerol) because it is an optimal time to do so.
    ② Try to have her wait until her cervix is at least 6 cm dilated and the vertex is at 1+ station.
    ③ Tell her that meperidine (Demerol) will cause her baby to be "sleepy" when it is born.
    ④ Give her one half of the ordered dose of the medication.

650. Nicole Ruth, a 40-year-old aerospace engineer, has had surgery for the removal of a duodenal ulcer. She states that she has been under increasing stress in her employment and is concerned about being able to continue in her position. Which of the following statements most accurately describes Mrs. Ruth's condition?
    ① The stress of her job has contributed to a physical condition of known medical origin.
    ② Stress is not a direct cause of her physical condition.
    ③ Her personality traits play a major role in her current physical problems.

④ Genetic influences are the major important causes of her physical problem.

651. Henry Nims, age 88, is admitted with a diagnosis of chronic obstructive pulmonary disease (COPD). His orders include antibiotics and respiratory therapy, including chest physical therapy, and ultrasonic nebulizer. Mr. Nims' tidal volume is 250 cc. This is commonly considered to be which of the following?
① High
② Low
③ Normal
④ High for his age group

652. Meperidine (Demerol) 75 mg is ordered for a laboring woman. The label indicates that the vial contains 100 mg of meperidine/ml. How many milliliters will the nurse administer?
① 1.0 ml
② 0.5 ml
③ 0.75 ml
④ 1.5 ml

653. A COPD client's dead-space volume is most likely to be which of the following?
① 150 ml
② Above 150 ml
③ 100 to 150 ml
④ Below 100 ml

654. A client's vital capacity will be the greatest in which position during an acute exacerbation of asthma?
① Fowler's position
② Semi-Fowler's position
③ Fowler's position with a slight forward lean
④ Fowler's position with a slight backward lean

655. Which activity would be most appropriate for a 2-year-old with eczema?
① Playing with clay
② Naming pictures in a book or magazine
③ Building a column with plastic building blocks
④ Drawing pictures of familiar objects with crayons

656. A client's arterial blood gases on admission were pH 7.40, Po_2 60 mm Hg, Pco_2 60 mm Hg, HCO_3 30 mEq/L. These values are most indicative of which condition?
① Respiratory acidosis
② Compensated respiratory acidosis
③ Respiratory alkalosis
④ Compensated respiratory alkalosis

657. When instructing parents about skin care of eczema at home, which of the following instructions is *not* appropriate?
① Provide a cool, dry environment.
② Wear wool clothing in the winter.
③ Rinse clothes twice during washing.
④ Keep nails short.

658. Uncompensated metabolic acidosis reflected in arterial blood gases could best be considered as an expected event for which of the following?
① A client with asthma and a respiratory rate of 28
② A client with pneumonia and respiratory rate of 30
③ An emphysema client with a respiratory rate of 28

④ An emphysema client with pneumonia and a respiratory rate of 48

659. A COPD client most likely becomes adjusted to which of the following?
① Elevated Pco_2 and Po_2 levels
② Lowered Pco_2 and elevated Po_2 levels
③ Elevated Pco_2 and lowered Po_2 levels
④ Lowered Pco_2 and Po_2 levels

660. Which of the following principles accurately explains the effects on the fetus of analgesics and anesthetics administered to the mother during the intrapartum period?
① Medication effects are generally negligible if they are administered 2 or more hours before delivery.
② Medication effects are related to the duration of labor.
③ Medication effects are time, dose, and route related.
④ Medication effects are related to maternal age and weight.

661. The client suffering from a terminal illness is *least* likely to experience which of the following psychosocial reactions?
① A sense of loss
② Disturbance in self-concept
③ Anxiety
④ A sense of control

662. Which of the following responses indicates that parents of a toddler with eczema do *not* fully understand how to prevent their daughter from scratching affected areas?
① "She wears elbow restraints for short periods of time when we can't directly supervise her."
② "Sometimes she wears cotton gloves so she won't irritate her rash."
③ "We've been dressing her in one-piece outfits."
④ "She wears close-fitting clothes."

663. A client has copious amounts of thick, tenacious yellow mucus, which he cannot expectorate. The client requires suctioning, and the nurse becomes concerned that a cardiopulmonary arrest might occur during suctioning. Which of the following would *not* precipitate a cardiac arrest during suctioning?
① Depletion of oxygen to the brain
② Depletion of oxygen to the heart
③ Vagal nerve stimulation
④ Electrolyte imbalance

664. Six-month-old Leslie was admitted for dehydration caused by diarrhea. According to her parents, Leslie's diarrhea started 2 days ago and has not stopped since. Which of the following is of primary concern when determining Leslie's hydration status?
① Closed posterior fontanelle
② Urine specific gravity of 1.022
③ Serum sodium of 128 mEq/L
④ Heart rate of 136

665. Which rate of oxygen flow per cannula would most likely be ordered for a 50-year-old female with asthma?
① Rate of 2 to 3 L/min
② Rate of 4 to 6 L/min

③ Rate of 6 to 8 L/min
④ Rate of 8 to 10 L/min

666. The nurse in the clinic prepares to administer immunizations to a child who is infected with the human immunodeficiency virus (HIV). Which one of the following represents an accurate understanding of immunizations in HIV-positive children?
① The nurse will withhold the annual influenza vaccine.
② The nurse will withhold the pneumococcal vaccine.
③ The nurse will administer only diphtheria-tetanus vaccine and not the pertussis vaccine.
④ The nurse will substitute inactivated polio vaccine for the oral polio vaccine.

667. An asthma client with pneumonia begins to exhibit restlessness, combativeness, and tachycardia, but cyanosis is not evident. The nurse would expect to find the arterial Po_2 to be in which of the following ranges?
① 48 to 52 mm Hg
② 30 to 40 mm Hg
③ 60 to 70 mm Hg
④ Greater than 70 mm Hg

668. What is the primary purpose of mucomyst treatment for a congested COPD client?
① Open clogged airways.
② Loosen accumulated secretions.
③ Promote dilation of smooth muscle bands around airways.
④ Provide adequate ventilation.

669. The nurse evaluates the progression of acquired immunodeficiency syndrome (AIDS) in an 18-month-old who is positive for the human immunodeficiency virus (HIV) by monitoring which one of the following?
① Differential white blood cell count
② Prothrombin time
③ Bleeding time
④ Conjugated (direct) bilirubin

670. Which of the following findings would the nurse most likely anticipate contributing to the development of aplastic anemia?
① Vitamin B_{12} malabsorption
② Drugs
③ Folic acid deficiency
④ Genetic factors

671. The most effective approach to caring for clients with a physical disorder affected by psychologic factors is which of the following?
① Developing effective stress-reducing activities.
② Consistently expressing concerns and feelings in efforts to reduce and redirect emotional tension.
③ Returning to work to distract attention from physical symptoms.
④ Appreciating the relationship between emotions and physical reactions.

672. Which is the *least* reliable sign of adequate ventilation?
① Speaking without shortness of breath
② Chest or abdominal movement with each respiration
③ Airflow at mouth or nose
④ Skin color

673. Four-year-old Jackson is hospitalized with an upper respiratory infection and right otitis media. He is pale and lethargic and has a low-grade fever. Jackson's condition is diagnosed as acute lymphoblastic leukemia. Jackson's initial pallor and lethargy are most likely the result of which of the following?
① An accumulation of toxic wastes in body tissues caused by poor kidney functioning.
② Body tissues being deprived of oxygen because of a decrease in the number of red blood cells.
③ Excessive needs for energy because of Jackson's respiratory and ear infections.
④ A reduced blood flow to body tissues caused by a decreased heart rate.

674. Which diagnostic test would best contribute to the most conclusive diagnosis of aplastic anemia?
① Bone marrow aspiration
② Schilling's test
③ Hemogram
④ Differential blood cell count

675. Mandy, a preschooler with acute lymphoblastic leukemia, has petechiae; a 2-minute nosebleed; and bruises on various parts of his body. Which one of the laboratory findings would the nurse expect to find?
① Low serum calcium level
② Abnormal thrombin production
③ Decreased platelet count
④ Elevated partial thromboplastin time

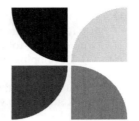

676. Sodium citrate, 30 ml, is ordered to be given to a woman before cesarean delivery. What is the primary rationale for administering an antacid before this surgery?
1. To settle the laboring mother's stomach
2. To increase digestion during labor
3. To prevent pneumonia in case of aspiration during anesthesia
4. To lower the pH of the blood in case of possible hyperventilation

677. Roderick McDowell, a 48-year-old engineer, seeks evaluation of chest pains, shortness of breath, hyperventilation, and tingling sensations in his fingers. After a complete physical examination with lab work, his physician refers him to the psychiatric clinical specialist for evaluation. His history reveals recent stressors arising from an impending divorce recently sought by his wife of 25 years and fears of losing his job because of a recent company buyout. He also admits worrying all the time even when he had few stressors. The most likely explanation of the client's symptoms is which of the following?
1. Generalized anxiety disorder
2. Agoraphobia
3. Posttraumatic stress disorder
4. Social phobia

678. When caring for a client with anemia, the most important nursing action is which of the following?
1. Teach the client about the required diet.
2. Collaborate with client to balance rest and activity.
3. Encourage the client to have some physical activity.
4. Maintain the client's fluid and electrolyte balance.

679. Which of the following nursing measures is *contraindicated* for a 7-year-old with leukemia?
1. Administer intramuscular narcotics to alleviate pain.
2. Handle his extremities with care while turning him.
3. Use stool softeners prn.
4. Provide frequent oral hygiene.

680. Ann Perry, a 45-year-old woman, is admitted to the nursing unit with the diagnosis of hyperthyroidism. The nurse anticipates that the initial assessment would include which physical findings to support this diagnosis?
1. Elevated vital signs, nervousness, and weight gain
2. Elevated vital signs, nervousness, and weight loss
3. Decreased vital signs, lethargy, and weight gain
4. Decreased vital signs, nervousness, and weight loss

681. An expectant father has been supporting his wife throughout labor. He tells the nurse that he heard someone say that the baby was ROP. The father asks the nurse what that means. What would be the nurse's best response?
1. "Your baby is fine. Those initials simply refer to the baby's position in the birth canal."
2. "ROP stands for right occiput posterior. This means your baby is head down, with the back of its head pointing toward your wife's right buttock. She may have back pain."
3. "ROP means your baby is bottom down with the head under your wife's right rib cage. This means your wife will not be able to deliver vaginally."
4. "ROP stands for right orbital presentation. This means your baby's head is extended and will need to flex before delivery can be completed."

682. The nurse would monitor a hyperthyroid client for which complication?
1. Cold intolerance
2. Sensitivity to narcotics
3. Increased tachycardia
4. Increased lethargy

683. Which statement best indicates that 11-year-old Samuel, who has acute lymphoblastic leukemia, understands the use of chemotherapy for treatment?
1. "I must be getting worse because the drugs make me so sick."
2. "I won't be able to return to school until my disease-fighting cells increase."
3. "I can tolerate the nausea, because I know the drugs will kill all the cancer cells."
4. "I don't want a wig, because boys don't lose their hair."

684. A hyperthyroid client's nursing diagnosis of sleep pattern disturbance could be aided by
1. Restricting fluid intake.
2. Administering liotrix (Thyrolar).
3. Using a private room.
4. Providing a warm environment.

685. Miss Leslie Greenbolt, a 32-year-old district attorney hospitalized with migraine headaches, informs the nurse that she is unable to attend the next stress-reduction class because of headaches. When the nurse tells her that group is part of managing the headaches,

she shouts, "Why are you putting me through these changes, you are the only one who is concerned about my participation in these groups!" This reaction is a surprise to the nurse because this client is generally quiet and cooperative. The most appropriate nursing response is which of the following?
① "Okay, I certainly do not want to upset you."
② "I don't care what other nurses do, you need to go to your class."
③ "You look pretty upset and I am unclear what this is about."
④ "Please lower your voice. I have spoken to you respectfully and I expect the same from you."

686. Allen Lane, age 14, is admitted to the hospital with end-stage leukemia. His parents decide to remain with him constantly. What is the most reasonable nursing plan?
① Be available to the Lanes for emotional support while providing most of Allen's care.
② Leave the Lanes alone with Allen to help them work through their grief.
③ Provide all meals and sleeping accommodations for the Lanes.
④ Teach the Lanes to give Allen most of the care he needs.

687. A 26-year-old multipara has been in labor for about 9 hours. After careful assessment, her fetus is discovered to be in breech presentation. In planning care for this woman, the nurse will need to take into account the typical consequences of fetal malpresentation. Which of the following consequences is most pertinent to the care of this client?
① Malpresentation frequently slows descent and the dilation of the cervix.
② There is no increase in the risk of birth trauma with breech birth.
③ Because labor is more efficient in multiparas, malpresentation does not have a significant impact on the effectiveness of the contractions.
④ Regardless of presentation or position, the cardinal movements of labor remain the same.

688. A hyperthyroid client during the euthyroid state will require which of the following diets?
① Low-fat, low-sodium, low-calorie diet
② High-protein, high-carbohydrate, high-calorie diet
③ Regular diet
④ Low-carbohydrate, high-protein diet

689. A baby girl who was born at 39 weeks of gestation has been admitted to the observation nursery. She weighs 7 pounds 1 ounce and had Apgar scores of 9 at 1 minute and 10 at 5 minutes. The nurse admitting the infant to the nursery notes a temperature of 96.8° F (36°C) on admission. Which nursing action is most appropriate at this time?
① Bathe the infant.
② Call the pediatrician to check the infant.
③ Place the infant under a radiant warmer.
④ Administer oxygen by mask.

690. A client is discharged on a levothyroxine (Synthroid) regimen after an uncomplicated, subtotal thyroidectomy. During the clinic visit several months later, the client complains of tiredness and of feeling cold. What content area during the teaching session would be most emphasized if the nursing diagnosis of knowledge deficit regarding self-management is made?
① The lack of thyroid hormones produced by the remaining thyroid tissue indicates a need for more exogenous hormone.
② The excess hormone produced by the remaining thyroid tissue indicates a need for less exogenous hormone
③ The parathyroids will grow and will be able to meet the body's needs for the hormones.
④ The parathyroids are overactive from having been disturbed during surgery, but symptoms should disappear soon.

691. Which of the following diagnostic findings would be *least* likely to be found in acute pyelonephritis?
① Cloudy, foul-smelling urine
② Bacteria and pus in the urine
③ Low serum WBC count
④ Hematuria

692. A baby boy born at 38 weeks of gestation is taken to the admitting nursery 30 minutes after birth. Five hours later the nurse notes that the baby's temperature has not risen over 96.8°F (36°C). What condition would this baby be most prone to develop?
① Metabolic acidosis
② Hypercalcemia
③ Polycythemia
④ Hyperglycemia

693. Jim Taylor, 15 months old, is admitted to the hospital with diarrhea for the past 2 days. The physician suspects the toddler has eaten something contaminated by *Salmonella*. Which of the following foods or fluids are most likely to be contaminated by salmonella?
① Water and fruits
② Eggs and poultry
③ Milk and vegetables
④ Beef and pork

694. The nurse does a complete assessment of the newborn after delivery. All of the following are noted. Which requires immediate attention?
① Cephalohematoma
② Milia
③ Acrocyanosis
④ Expiratory grunting

695. Mr. Clint Jackson II, 69 years old, is hospitalized for asthma. He is observed having difficulty making decisions. A primary goal of nursing care will need to involve which of the following?
① His wife will assume more responsibility for scheduling the client's rest periods.
② The client will adhere to the physician's orders more closely.
③ The client will collaborate with the nurse in planning his care.
④ The client will recommend to his wife when he needs to rest.

696. What is the major reason why an injection of vitamin K is given to newborns in the nursery?
① It helps conjugate bilirubin in the infant.
② It prevents Rh sensitization in the infant.
③ It reduces the possibility of hemorrhage in the infant.
④ It increases the infant's resistance to infection.

697. Phenazopyridine hydrochloride (Pyridium) is ordered for a client. This drug has which of the following classifications?
① Antibiotic
② Narcotic
③ Analgesic
④ Antipyretic

698. While performing a newborn assessment, the nurse observes the following: respiratory rate 44 and irregular, apical heart rate 148, and bluish hands and feet. How would the nurse interpret these data?
① Possible cardiovascular problem. Call the physician.
② Respiratory distress. Administer oxygen.
③ Normal newborn. Continue to observe.
④ Cold stress. Place infant in heated Isolette.

699. Julie Warner is a 28-year-old admitted on the nurse's shift with a fever of 102°F (38.9°C). Her complaints indicate dysuria, frequency, and malaise. Acute pyelonephritis is suspected. What is the priority nursing action for Mrs. Warner?
① Encourage ambulation.
② Force fluids up to 3000 ml per day.
③ Restrict protein in the diet.
④ Keep urine pH more acidic.

700. Long-term management for a female client with a kidney infection includes the prevention of reinfection. Which of the following instructions would be included in teaching?
① Void at least every 6 hours.
② Use vaginal sprays to mask the odor.
③ Empty her bladder before and after intercourse.
④ Discontinue antibiotics when the pain disappears.

701. Which of the following observations is considered normal for a full-term neonate?
① Heart rate of 90 beats per minute
② Jaundice in the first 24 hours
③ Nasal flaring
④ Uncoordinated eye movements

702. A new mother is worried because her 3 day-old infant, who weighed 7 pounds at birth, has lost 8 ounces since birth. How would the nurse respond to this mother's concern?
① "You will need to supplement breast-feeding with formula."
② "The birth weight may have been recorded incorrectly since this is a substantial loss."
③ "There is no need to worry unless the baby loses a pound."
④ "It is normal for an infant to lose up to 10% of her weight in the first few days."

703. For a 6-month-old infant, what is the most critical clinical manifestation of the degree of dehydration?
① Sunken fontanel
② Weight loss
③ Decreased urine output
④ Dry skin

704. Before administering an initial dose of phenazopyridine hydrochloride (Pyridium), what would the nurse tell a client about this drug?
① This drug causes transient nausea.
② Food interferes with the absorption.
③ This drug colors the urine red or orange.
④ Bladder spasms are a side effect.

705. The nurse observes signs of jaundice in the face and chest of a newborn with type O, Rh-positive blood on the third day of life. The baby is assessed as 38 weeks of gestation, average for gestational age, and Coombs negative. What is the most likely explanation of the jaundice?
① Liver failure
② Physiologic jaundice
③ Erythroblastosis fetalis
④ Sepsis

706. A 36-year-old woman has just had her first pregnancy confirmed. She has been married 5 years and appears excited and nervous after hearing she is pregnant. In performing an initial assessment of this woman during the first trimester, what is most appropriate for the nurse to assess?
① Pattern of weight gain
② Cervical dilation
③ Plans for childbirth preparation
④ Past medical history

707. Hypokalemia in an infant would be manifested by which of the following?
① Muscle weakness and lethargy
② Hunger
③ Hyperreflexia
④ Apnea

708. Sulfamethoxazole-trimethoprim (Bactrim DS) is a common antimicrobial agent ordered in combination with phenazopyridine hydrochloride (Pyridium). What does "DS" stand for?
① Dose specific
② Decreased symptoms
③ Double strength
④ Deficient strain

709. A 27-year-old woman is pregnant at 6 weeks of gestation for the second time. Her first baby had several severe congenital anomalies and died soon after birth. On her first prenatal visit with this pregnancy, the woman asks the nurse, "How soon can I find out if I'm carrying a normal baby?" Which response by the nurse would be most appropriate?
① "A 24-hour estriol can be done now."
② "Chorionic villus sampling can be done at 8 weeks."
③ "Glucose screening can be done at 24 weeks."
④ "Liver enzymes and platelet studies can be done at 28 weeks."

710. Five-year-old Shaquella was hospitalized after a 3-day bout of vomiting and diarrhea. Her IV was just capped off to a saline well, and it has been determined to discontinue her NPO status. Which of the following would be least appropriate to give initially?
① Gatorade
② Toast
③ Apple juice
④ Saltines

711. Methenamine mandelate (Mandelamine) is prescribed for a client's urinary tract infection. Which of the following conditions is necessary to increase the effectiveness of this drug?
① Crystalluria
② Leukocytosis
③ Alkaline urine
④ Acid urine

712. Nursing measures for a client with bacterial meningitis would exclude which action?
① Turning frequently
② Applying a thin coating of lotion to the client's skin, followed by talcum powder, which is washed off and reapplied q8h
③ Encouraging passive range-of-motion exercises
④ Coughing every 1 to 2 hours

713. In planning nursing care for a newborn with myelomeningocele, the priority outcome is which of the following?
① Promotion of drainage of cerebrospinal fluid from the sac
② Circulation of cerebrospinal fluid through the spinal cord
③ Protection of the sac from pressure, injury, and infection
④ Prevention of musculoskeletal complications in the upper extremities

714. Seven-year-old Clarence's weight is at the 95th percentile, and his height is at the 75th percentile. Based on this information, which of the following conclusions is most warranted?
① Clarence is overweight and should be referred to the dietitian for nutrition counseling.
② Clarence's weight is disproportionate to his height, and he should be counseled to reduce his caloric intake.
③ Clarence's weight and height indicate that he is growing normally.
④ Additional information should be collected before drawing conclusions.

715. The most desirable method of rewarming a client after induced hypothermia is which of the following?
① Surface rewarming
② Natural rewarming
③ Bloodstream rewarming
④ Artificial rewarming

716. A young woman comes to the clinic for an initial prenatal appointment at 10 weeks of gestation. Her history reveals that she smokes a pack of cigarettes each day. She asks the nurse what risks are associated with smoking in pregnancy. The nurse identifies all of the following *except*
① Spontaneous abortion
② Abruptio placentae
③ Intrauterine growth retardation
④ Fetal limb anomalies

717. A common complication to anticipate during the rewarming process is which of the following?
① Acidosis
② Oliguria
③ Shock
④ Cardiac irregularity

718. In addition to a brief explanation of the lumbar puncture procedure, which action is also a priority responsibility of the nurse?
① Position the client in a fetal position.
② Position the client safely and properly in a lateral recumbent position with knees flexed.
③ Prepare the suction canister with a tonsil suction if available.
④ Prepare a suture set so that it will be ready after the procedure.

719. A woman is 8 weeks pregnant. Her blood work at this prenatal visit demonstrates the following results: blood type A, Rh negative, rubella titer 1:64, hemoglobin 14 g, hematocrit 37%, serology for syphilis: nonreactive. How would the nurse interpret these data?
① Rubella vaccine should be given.
② Iron supplements are needed.
③ The father of the baby should be checked for the Rh factor.
④ Her fetus could acquire congenital syphilis.

720. During morning care, how would the nurse assist a client on bed rest in the acute phase of an illness to prevent joint complications?
① Active range of motion to all extremities
② Passive range of motion to all extremities
③ Exercises to augment motor function as it returns
④ Nerve stimulation

721. Which finding would the nurse immediately report to the physician if a client is scheduled for a lumbar puncture?
① Unequal pupils
② Lack of lateralization
③ Suspicion of meningitis
④ Nuchal rigidity

722. Prenatal teaching includes recommendations about rest and exercise. Which of the following is appropriate advice for the pregnant woman?
① Avoid swimming during pregnancy.
② Use the Kegel exercise to help relieve leg cramps.
③ Relax in a hot tub before bed to aid in better sleep.
④ Report any shortness of breath or decreased fetal activity and stop exercising if they occur to prevent any fetal damage.

723. A 9-year-old boy's vision is tested at school. The results show he has 20/30 vision in his left eye and 20/40 vision in his right eye. Corneal light reflex and cover

tests are normal. Which follow-up action is most indicated?

① Rescreen him in 1 month.
② Test him for color blindness.
③ Discuss with the physician a referral to an ophthalmologist or optometrist.
④ Counsel his mother that the findings are normal.

724. Eight-year-old Felicia is at the pediatrician's office for a precamp physical. Before today, Felicia had received the full recommended series of childhood immunizations. Which of the following would be appropriate to administer to her?

① No immunization
② A tetanus booster
③ Diphtheria (adult type) and tetanus booster
④ Measles and mumps vaccines

725. When psychologic factors influence or worsen a medical condition, such as asthma, migraine headaches, or ulcers, which of the following will not be apparent?

① Dependency concerns
② Impaired decision-making skills
③ Rigid and controlling behaviors
④ Impaired reality testing

726. Bacterial meningitis is confirmed by a cerebrospinal fluid culture. The client has been transferred to a dimly lit private room. The family asks why. The nurse's explanation should include which of the following?

① Increased stimulation such as bright lights may precipitate a seizure.
② Inappropriate secretion of antidiuretic hormone can be minimized.
③ It is easier to check the client's pupils in a darkened room.
④ Most clients with meningitis have photophobia.

727. The mother of a infant born with myelomeningocele asks the nurse whether her child will ever walk. The nurse bases her response on which one of the following statements?

① The location of the myelomeningocele along the spinal cord indicates the likelihood of ability to ambulate.
② No children born with myelomeningocele are able to ambulate.
③ After surgical repair of the myelomeningocele, development will proceed normally.
④ Neurologic deficits can only be assessed after surgical correction of the myelomeningocele.

728. Which of the following is most likely to be the cause of iron-deficiency anemia in a toddler?

① Excessive milk intake, which decreases the intake of solid foods.
② Insufficient iron stores at birth.
③ Refusal to eat iron-rich foods because of their unappealing taste.
④ A normal physiologic occurrence during the toddler years.

729. A pregnant woman at 38 weeks of gestation has active genital herpes simplex type 2. What kind of a delivery would the nurse advise her to expect if she still has active lesions when she goes into labor?

① Low-segment cesarean birth
② Vaginal delivery with low forceps
③ Vacuum extraction–assisted vaginal birth
④ Method selected by client

730. Early in the second trimester, a woman is scheduled to have an amniocentesis. Which of the following would be a reason for having an amniocentesis at this time?

① To assess fetal lung maturity
② To estimate the gestational age of the fetus
③ To determine alphafetoprotein levels
④ To evaluate placental functioning

731. During a prenatal visit in the seventh month of pregnancy, an expectant mother complains of severe leg cramps, especially at night. When the nurse is instructing her on ways of alleviating this problem, which of the following is the most appropriate action to advise?

① Walk briskly around the room.
② Lie down and immobilize the affected leg.
③ Straighten her leg, and dorsiflex her ankle.
④ Rub her leg until the pain subsides.

732. Which of the following signs and symptoms would the nurse expect assessment of an 18-month-old with iron-deficiency anemia to reveal?

① Overweight, poor activity tolerance, and flushed face
② Pallor, fatigue, and irritability
③ Pallor, average muscle tone, and accelerated growth rate
④ Activity tolerance, good muscle tone, and average growth rate

733. Two-year-old Ryan has iron-deficiency anemia. His mother has been taught how to administer Ryan's oral iron preparation at home. Which statement by his mother indicates the need for clarification by the nurse?

① "I'll give Ryan his medicine between meals with fruit or juice."
② "I'll use a straw, syringe, or dropper placed to the back of Ryan's mouth when I give him his medicine."
③ "I'll help Ryan brush his teeth after he takes the medicine to decrease the likelihood of staining his teeth."
④ "I'll expect the color of Ryan's stool to change to a dark yellow."

734. A client is admitted to the emergency room with a stiff neck and temperature of 102°F (38.8°C), heart rate 100, and respiration rate 22. The client has had an earache for 1 week but has not sought treatment for it. Twenty minutes after the start of hypothermia treatments with a blanket, what response would the nurse most likely expect to find?

① Heart rate 80, respiratory rate 18
② Heart rate 120, respiratory rate 28
③ Heart rate 100, respiratory rate 22
④ Heart rate 60, respiratory rate 12

735. Which test result indicates that treatment for iron-deficiency anemia has been successful?
① Hemoglobin: 14.2 g/dl
② Hematocrit: 28%
③ Platelets: 100,000/mm³
④ White blood cell count: 10,000 cells/mm³

736. The nurse teaches a multipara about varicose veins in pregnancy. Which of the following would indicate that this woman understands how to obtain relief from the discomfort of the varicosities in her legs?
① She plans to sit with her legs crossed at the knees.
② She plans to wear knee-high hose with stretch bands.
③ She plans to elevate her legs above her hips when lying down or sitting.
④ She plans to take a new job as a secretary and remain sedentary most of her work day.

737. A 29-year-old woman is in the thirty-fourth week of her pregnancy. At her antepartal visit, the nurse notes that the woman has gained 3 pounds since her last visit at 32 weeks and is complaining that her wedding ring is tight. Her urine shows 1+ proteinuria, and her blood pressure is increased from a baseline of 100/70 to 130/85. What is the suspected cause?
① Normal fluid retention of pregnancy
② Early cardiac decompensation
③ Asymptomatic pyelonephritis
④ Mild pregnancy-induced hypertension

738. Twelve-year-old Zachary has newly diagnosed insulin-dependent diabetes. He is on the pediatric unit. Which of the following would *not* be an expected finding in Zachary's nursing history?
① Rapid weight gain
② Drinking large amounts of fluids
③ Lethargic and tired
④ Sudden return of bed-wetting

739. A serious complication associated with hypothermic therapy is which of the following?
① Peripheral vasoconstriction
② Cold skin
③ Frostbite
④ Heat loss

740. Nine-year-old Kayla Marie is admitted with ketoacidosis. The physician orders an "insulin IV push." Which type of insulin would the nurse anticipate that the physician will order?
① Ultra Lente
② Regular
③ NPH
④ PZI

741. A primipara has decided to breast-feed her baby, and the nurse teaches her about the breast-feeding process, including the milk ejection (let-down) reflex. Which one of the following statements indicates most clearly to the nurse that the client understands the nature of the reflex?
① "I have excess milk now, but the quantity will adjust itself, depending on the baby's needs."
② "If I use a bottle often, I will stop secreting adequate milk for the baby."

③ "When milk drips from my other breast, I know that my baby is getting milk."
④ "The more the baby sucks and stimulates my breast, the more I will produce."

742. Hypothermia treatment will most likely put a client at risk for the development of which of the following?
① Emboli
② Respiratory alkalosis
③ Metabolic alkalosis
④ Excess ADH secretion

743. Gladys Irving is a 58-year-old school teacher who becomes extremely anxious when she rides the elevator. Her anxiety is manifested by shortness of breath, diaphoresis, palpitations, and an apprehension of closed spaces. These symptoms are an example of which of the following?
① Psychosis
② Phobic disorder
③ Obsessive-compulsive disorder
④ Stress disorder

744. A child with diabetes has an order for 1400-calorie, ADA diet. The nurse explains to him and his parents that this means
① He can eat what he wants as long as he avoids concentrated sweets.
② He can substitute items on one food list with other items from the same food list.
③ He can substitute any food item for any other as long as his total daily calorie intake remains the same.
④ He must carefully weigh or measure all portions of his food intake.

745. Which of the following signs indicate impending insulin shock?
① Increased urination
② Acetone breath
③ Tremors
④ Increased thirst

746. A breast-feeding mother asks how her diet should change to meet nutritional needs during lactation. What is the most appropriate response the nurse can give?
① "You need an additional 500 calories per day plus more iron and folic acid."
② "You need an additional 500 calories per day plus more protein and calcium."
③ "You need an additional 800 calories per day plus more iron and folic acid."
④ "You need an additional 800 calories per day plus more protein and calcium."

747. The temperature of a client with bacterial meningitis sharply increases. The nurse will most likely observe which of the following?
① Loss of corneal response
② Loss of gag reflex
③ IM medications taking effect quickly
④ Fading of sensorium

748. Nuchal rigidity will *not* be seen in which condition?
① Meningitis
② Intracranial mass with herniation

③ Intracranial hematoma
④ Cerebral concussion

749. When planning care for a client with ascending paralysis, which rationale explains the need for respiratory-assistance equipment to be kept immediately available?
① Respiratory failure can occur if intercostal muscles are affected.
② Intracranial pressure can exert pressure on the medulla and cause respiratory arrest.
③ High fever associated with this syndrome often disrupts the normal respiratory patterns.
④ The particular bacteria or viruses (or both) in the cerebrospinal fluid have a special affinity for the nerves that control respiration.

750. Cranial nerves can be affected by Guillain-Barré syndrome. The facial nerve is commonly involved. What would the nurse most likely observe if the motor nucleus of the facial nerve becomes dysfunctional?
① Decreased ability to distinguish tastes in the anterior two thirds of the tongue
② Pain in the distribution area of the affected nerve
③ Inability to wrinkle the forehead and smile
④ Inequality of pupils and bilateral sluggish response to light

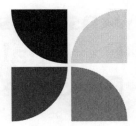

Answers and Rationales

KEY TO ABBREVIATIONS

Three abbreviations follow the rationales. The first abbreviation refers to the section of the Review book where discussion of the topic can be found. The second abbreviation refers to the step of the nursing process that the question addresses. The third abbreviation refers to the appropriate client need category.

Section of the Review Book

P = Psychosocial and Mental Health Problems
    T = Therapeutic Use of Self
    L = Loss and Death and Dying
    A = Anxious Behavior
    C = Confused Behavior
    E = Elated-Depressive Behavior
    SM = Socially Maladaptive Behavior
    SS = Suspicious Behavior
    W = Withdrawn Behavior
    SU = Substance Use Disorders
A = Adult
    H = Healthy Adult
    S = Surgery
    O = Oxygenation
    NM = Nutrition and Metabolism
    E = Elimination
    SP = Sensation and Perception
    M = Mobility
    CA = Cellular Aberration

CBF = Childbearing Family
    W = Women's Health Care
    A = Antepartal Care
    I = Intrapartal Care
    P = Postpartal Care
    N = Newborn Care
C = Child
    H = Healthy Child
    I = Ill and Hospitalized Child
    SPP = Sensation, Perception, and Protection
    O = Oxygenation
    NM = Nutrition and Metabolism
    E = Elimination
    M = Mobility
    CA = Cellular Aberration

Nursing Process Category

AS = Assessment
AN = Analysis
PL = Planning
IM = Implementation
EV = Evaluation

Client Need Category

E = Safe, Effective Care Environment
PS = Physiologic Integrity
PC = Psychosocial Integrity
H = Health Promotion and Maintenance

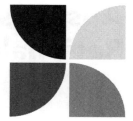

Answers and Rationales: Practice Test I

1. no. 4. The Bence Jones protein is a test for multiple myeloma. A type and crossmatch would be done because of anticipated blood loss, which is substantial in bone or joint surgery. The prothrombin time is required because she has been taking large doses of aspirin. A sedimentation rate can rule out the possibility of infection. A/SP, AS, PS

2. no. 1. The child with nephrosis usually exhibits generalized edema, ascites, an elevated urine specific gravity, yet normal blood pressure. C/E, AS, PS

3. no. 4. The purpose of a contraction stress test is to observe fetal heart rate response to uterine contractions. Fetal lung maturity is measured by the 4s ratio of amniotic fluid. Option 2 describes findings of a nonstress test. Cervical response to induction is predicted by the Bishop scale. CBF/I, AN, E

4. no. 3. Identification means that a person takes on certain qualities associated with others. Idealization is the conscious or unconscious overestimation of another's attributes. Projecting refers to attributing one's negative ideas and feelings to other people. Intellectualization refers to avoiding by substituting a superficial logical explanation. P/E, AS, PS

5. no. 1. Older toddlers and preschoolers are especially fearful of procedures that threaten their body integrity, such as rectal temperatures and injections. C/I, AN, PC

6. no. 3. The client will be maintained on bed rest for only 2 to 5 days, depending on the surgeon. Early ambulation is encouraged to decrease the risk of postoperative complications. An overhead frame and trapeze are placed on the bed to prevent flexion of the hip when the client lifts up for back care and linen changes. Extreme flexion and adduction of the hip should be avoided because this can cause dislocation. If hip dislocation occurs the client may require further surgery, traction, or a hip spica cast. Antiembolic hose or a sequential compression device will be used to promote venous return. A/SP, PL, E

7. no. 3. Sedation is not a side effect of fluoxetine (Prozac). Sleeplessness, sexual dysfunction, and gastrointestinal disturbances are common side effects of this medication. P/E, AN, PS

8. no. 1. Risks with the administration of oxytocin are related to uterine tetany and fetal distress from decreased uteroplacental blood flow. CBF/I, AS, PS

9. no. 3. Reverse isolation is not used, but the other interventions listed are done in an effort to prevent infection. A/SP, PL, E

10. no. 4. The preschooler is involved in mastering a sense of initiative vs. guilt. C/H, AN, H

11. no. 1. If contractions exceed 90 seconds in duration, there is a danger of a ruptured uterus as well as interference with placental perfusion. The remaining options are normal or expected findings. CBF/I, EV, PS

12. no. 4. Clients who take selective serotonin reuptake inhibitors (SSRIs) such as paroxetine should not be given MAO inhibitors either simultaneously or immediately after treatment. Isocarboxazid (Marplan) should be withheld until orders are clarified. P/E, AN, PS

13. no. 4. Acceptance is needed in time of stress. As labor progresses the client may have difficulty maintaining control. The client will require assurance that she will be accepted regardless of her behavior. CBF/I, IM, PC

14. no. 2. Prednisone should never be withheld, but tapered gradually, because sudden withdrawal may precipitate an adrenal crisis. C/E, IM, PS

15. no. 2. The client should keep her toes pointed toward the ceiling to prevent adduction or external rotation. Plantar and dorsiflexion of both ankles should be encouraged to promote venous return. Legs should not be crossed because this abducts the hip. The client will pivot on the unaffected leg until full weight bearing is allowed. A/SP, PL, PS

16. no. 4. Children with nephrosis often develop ascites. Semi-Fowler's position relieves the respiratory difficulties that often occur with ascites. C/E, PL, E

17. no. 1. Normal capillary refill occurs within 2 seconds. A delay of over 5 seconds is considered abnormal. An apical pulse rate of 74 is within normal limits. Pitting edema is an abnormality that indicates accumulation of excess fluid in the body tissues. A posterior tibial pulse is frequently nonpalpable; this absence is considered a normal variation if skin color and temperature are normal. A/SP, AN, PS

18. no. 3. Wound drainage of 100 ml after hip replacement over an 8-hour period is not unusual. The nurse should continue to monitor the amount of drainage. It should diminish over the first 2 postoperative days. If not, the physician must be notified. A/SP, AS, PS

19. no. 4. Phenelzine (Nardil), as well as isocarboxazid (Marplan) and tranylcypromine (Parnate), are MAO

inhibitors. When these drugs are combined with tyramine-containing foods (e.g., aged cheese and alcoholic beverages), the reaction cited in the question can occur. Side effects of tricyclic antidepressants (amitriptyline and imipramine) are usually associated with hypotension, not hypertension. Side effects of lithium are usually not associated with cardiovascular changes unless toxic levels are reached; then the changes are hypotensive. Side effects of selective serotonin reuptake inhibitors such as sertraline include restlessness and sleep disturbances, and other antidepressants such as bupropion increase the risk of seizures. P/E, IM, PC

20. no. 4. This is a normal occurrence called an early deceleration. It is most likely a result of head compression, and it requires no action. CBF/I, IM, PS

21. no. 3. Children with nephrosis need a low-sodium, high-protein, high-potassium diet to combat edema. This snack is highest in potassium and protein and low in sodium. C/E, IM, PS

22. no. 1. Urinary retention is a common problem after a total hip replacement because of the recumbent position. In the elderly male client, prostatic enlargement can also be a contributing factor. Incontinence with coughing is called *stress incontinence* and is not related to hip replacement. Weight loss and contractures normally do not occur if appropriate positioning is done and nutritional supplements are provided. A/SP, AN, PS

23. no. 1. Pain on movement and weight bearing indicates pressure on the nerves or muscles caused by the dislocation. Other symptoms of dislocation include inability to bear weight and a shortening of the affected leg. Edema is not a primary sign of displacement. A/SP, AS, PS

24. no. 3. Late decelerations are most likely a result of uteroplacental insufficiency and require prompt action. Turning the client on the left side to relieve pressure on the vena cava by the gravid uterus may correct the problem. The physician should be notified if the heart rate is not corrected by nursing actions. Options 1 and 2 will not address the problem. CBF/I, IM, PS

25. no. 3. This activity requires little energy expenditure while the child is acutely ill and also increases his sense of control and security by allowing him to project his own feelings into the story. C/I, IM, H

26. no. 2. Unless the client is first assessed for self-harm or suicide potential, the staff will not observe the necessary degree of vigilance needed in the client's environment. Physical needs are the second most critical concern with a depressive client. Though the client may be encouraged to attend group therapy as part of the treatment plan, the client's safety takes precedence. Response to medication takes time and is not an initial concern. P/E, AS, PC

27. no. 3. Pressure on the peroneal nerve places the client at risk for foot drop. The other three options are appropriate interventions for the use and placement of abductor splints. A/SP, IM, PS

28. no. 1. A sense of hopelessness poses the greatest risk of suicide. Other options also increase the risk of suicide and should be assessed thoroughly. P/E, AN, PC

29. no. 3. Separation anxiety is a common response by toddlers to separation from parents. The initial stage of separation anxiety is protest, characterized by crying, screaming for parent, and inconsolableness. C/I, AN, H

30. no. 1. Rocking chairs and recliners are difficult to get out of and cause the hip to be flexed beyond the safe limits. A/SP, EV, H

31. no. 3. The only permanent damage that may result from rheumatic fever is cardiac damage. Therefore close monitoring of cardiac status is imperative. C/O, AS, PS

32. no. 4. Specialists in suicidology have developed profiles of high-risk groups. Generally, persons cited in options no. 1 through no. 3 have a higher risk of suicide than married men. Clients with alcoholism have a high risk associated with lack of disinhibition. Women *attempt* suicide more frequently than do men (a 3 to 1 ratio), but men *commit* suicide more often than women by a 3 to 1 ratio. Suicide rates vary according to marital status, with married persons having the lowest rates, followed by the never married. Widowed or divorced persons have the highest rate. P/E, AS, PS

33. no. 1. This is the best position both anatomically (near the terminal ileum) and for the client. It will be visible for self-care but will not interfere with clothing. Inappropriate placement can make appliance management tj;1difficult for the client. The stoma should be placed on a flat surface of the abdomen, away from scars, incisions, bony prominences, indentations, skin folds, the umbilicus, and inguinal creases. The stoma should not be placed at a client's belt line. A/E, AN, PS

34. no. 1. Urine output of at least 30 ml per hour is vital to show adequate renal perfusion. Because there is no bladder, urine output becomes evident immediately. Pain and serous drainage at the incision line are expected findings. Changes in pulse rate are important to monitor; however, this is not the most critical sign. A/E, AS, PS

35. no. 3. The client with schizophrenia, paranoid type is not intrusive. These clients are socially aloof rather than intrusive. Options no. 1, no. 2, and no. 4 are characteristic manifestations of schizophrenia, paranoid type. P/W, AS, PC

36. no. 1. Sydenham's chorea does not impair intellectual functioning. Because of the symptoms, the chief problem is one of safety for the child. C/O, AS, PS

37. no. 2. Skin excoriation is caused when urine remains in contact with the skin, and the appliance prevents this contact. A/E, AN, PS

38. no. 4. Although leakage could occur, the most important reason is to prevent reflux, which predisposes the client to pyelonephritis. A/E, AN, PS

39. no. 2. The client with paranoid schizophrenia projects his fantasy world and emotions on others. Sublimation, rationalization, and suppression might be used by a paranoid schizophrenic but are not characteristically present. P/W, AS, PC

40. no. 1. This goal must have priority because permanent cardiac valvular damage may result from rheumatic fever. C/O, PL, E

41. no. 3. This best describes the postmature infant. Because of prolonged gestation, these infants are more wide-eyed, have decreased vernix, dry and peeling skin, and long fingernails. Chronic hypoxia in utero may account for the wide-eyed, alert appearance. They exhibit varying degrees of wasting and thus have decreased subcutaneous fat. Meconium staining results from a stress response to intrauterine hypoxia. CBF/N, AN, PS

42. no. 4. This is the most common long-term problem other than skin excoriation. A cystectomy involves removal of the bladder, so recurrent bladder infections are not a possibility. Because the urine does not drain into the functioning GI tract, frequent emptying of the colon does not occur; this is a complication with a ureterosigmoidostomy. Ileal stomal dilation is not a complication. A/E, PL, H

43. no. 4. Acting on auditory hallucinations does not teach the client to cope in the world of reality. Options no. 1, no. 2, and no. 3 are appropriate goals that are achievable and will incorporate the individual into the "real world." P/P, PL, E

44. no. 1. Denial of illness and fear of losing control are predominant when clients discover they have a chronic disease. Uncomplicated hypertension is usually asymptomatic, so many clients are unaware that they have a chronic illness. If symptoms do occur, they include headache, dizziness, fainting, epistaxis, and tinnitus. As the disease progresses, symptoms are related to target organ damage. Nausea, vomiting, and shortness of breath occur with inadequate cardiac perfusion. A/O, AS, PC

45. no. 4. Bed rest is prescribed, so the patient cannot visit other children on the unit. Because of the chorea, she is unable to play computer games or write in a diary. Therefore listening to records is the best activity at this time. C/O, IM, PS

46. no. 3. Rheumatic fever does not cause albuminuria. Nephrosis and nephritis cause large amounts of protein loss. C/O, AS, PS

47. no. 3. Normal blood pressure ranges from 115 to 120 mm Hg systolic over 75 to 80 mm Hg diastolic. A sustained diastolic pressure of greater than 90 mm Hg is defined as hypertension by the American Heart Association. A pulse pressure of 10 mm Hg is abnormally low (normal is 30 to 40 mm Hg). A narrowed pulse pressure may be seen in shock, pericardial effusion, aortic stenosis, and constrictive pericarditis. A widened pulse pressure is seen in hypertension. A resting pulse rate over 100 beats/min is considered abnormal in adults. A systolic blood pressure greater than 140 is considered elevated. Systolic hypertension is frequently seen in elderly clients who have atherosclerosis. A/O, AS, PS

48. no. 2. Foods low in fat, sodium, and cholesterol include baked chicken (fowl), raw vegetables, and raw fruits. Ham, cold cuts, and chocolate pie are high in sodium. Cheese, cream-based soups, and blue-cheese dressing are high in cholesterol, saturated fat, and sodium. A/O, EV, H

49. no. 2. Long-term antibiotic therapy with penicillin or erythromycin is necessary to prevent serious cardiac damage or a recurrence of rheumatic fever. C/O, EV, H

50. no. 1. Lemon juice and vinegar are acceptable to season foods when no added salt is allowed in the diet. Canned foods are high in sodium. Fruits and vegetables should be encouraged because they are low in sodium, fat, and cholesterol. One teaspoon of salt alone has 2400 mg sodium. Total sodium intake on a low-sodium diet should be below 3000 mg. A/O, IM, E

51. no. 4. Mutual withdrawal is a common staff problem when clients withdraw from staff; isolation should be avoided when treating clients with schizophrenia. Options no. 1, no. 2, and no. 3 will assist the client by allowing some control over how quickly a relationship with a staff member is formed. P/P, IM, PC

52. no. 4. The other three options list common reasons for which clients with herpes seek care. C/SPP, AS, PS

53. no. 1. Methylergonovine (Methergine) is an oxytoxic drug given to contract the uterus after a placental delivery. CBF/P, EV, PS

54. no. 4. Isosorbide dinitrate (Isordil), a nitrite preparation, dilates small and large blood vessels. A/O, IM, PS

55. no. 1. Metoprolol (Lopressor) is a beta-adrenergic blocking agent that reduces blood pressure by its action on the beta receptors in the heart. A/O, AN, PS

56. no. 4. This option would give positive reinforcement to the client's retreat from reality. It is more helpful to help the client develop adaptive behaviors. Options no. 1 and no. 2 will assist the client in focusing on reality and avoiding retreat and withdrawal. It is necessary to initially assess the content of the hallucinations to determine if the voices are directing the individual to harm herself or others. P/P, IM, PC

57. no. 1. Having herpes leads to an alteration or limitation in sexual relationships as well as alterations in achieving perceived or desired sex roles. Other nursing diagnoses listed do not have as high a priority at this time. C/SPP, AN, PS

58. no. 1. Identifying client needs for assistance is the initial step in assisting a client to be self-directing with hygiene and grooming. Group work is difficult for a client with schizophrenia, and doing hygiene makes the client more dependent. Ignoring lack of hygiene is counterproductive to the goal. P/P, IM, PC

59. no. 3. Option no. 1 describes a closed fracture; no. 2, an impacted fracture; no. 4, a spiral fracture. A/SP, AN, PS

60. no. 1. The idea underlying these social changes is that with the advent of antibiotics and the contraceptive pill, people began to lose fear of untreated disease and pregnancy, leading to increased exposure to infection. The other three options listed are not true statements. C/SPP, AN, PS

61. no. 3. The splint tends to dig into the groin, causing irritation. The foot plate is attached to the Pearson splint. Immobility is not likely to be a problem because balanced traction allows a great deal of freedom to move. Bedpan use is easier from the unaffected side. A/SP, PL, E

62. no. 3. Confronting and arguing with a client with paranoia tends to increase the hostility, paranoia, mistrust, and more intense defense of delusions. The other options are beneficial for managing hostile behavior. P/P, IM, PC

63. no. 3. Treatment for genital herpes is most often symptomatic because there is no known cure for the disease at present. C/SPP, IM, PS

64. no. 3. Calcium is lost from the bone after a fracture. Serum calcium levels are increased, and the potential for renal calculi is increased. Thus a normal or decreased calcium intake is indicated along with sufficient fluids. The U.S. Recommended Caloric Intake for an average healthy male is 2600 cal. Nutritional needs will be met if the diet is well balanced with foods from all levels of the food pyramid. A positive nitrogen balance is important in wound healing. Roughage and fiber are important in preventing constipation when bed rest is prescribed for the client. A/SP, EV, H

65. no. 2. Raising the foot of the bed enables the client's body weight to oppose the traction. The body weight is the countertraction. A/SP, PL, PS

66. no. 3. Before sexual intercourse, partners should examine themselves and each other for evidence of disease. Genital herpes is spread through sexual contact. No vaccine is available to prevent the disease. Cesarean delivery is recommended when viral cultures are positive, herpetic lesions are present, or membranes have been ruptured less than 12 hours. C/SPP, PL, PS

67. no. 1. A delusion is a positive symptom of schizophrenia. The other symptoms are negative symptoms. P/P, AS, PS

68. no. 4. These are normal observations in the immediate postpartum period. CBF/P, AN, PS

69. no. 1. Early symptoms of gonorrhea include a slight purulent discharge, a vague feeling of fullness in the pelvis, and discomfort in the abdomen. Many women disregard these vague symptoms (if they are present) and do not seek treatment. C/SPP, AN, PS

70. no. 4. Risperidone and other antipsychotic agents are not addictive. The other symptoms represent adverse reactions produced by risperidone. P/P, AS, PS

71. no. 4. The pin enters the bone and provides an opening for bacteria. The pin does not inhibit knee-joint movement or cause nerve damage. A/SP, AN, PS

72. no. 2. Although the symptoms of syphilis are similar to those of a host of other diseases, they disappear without treatment, providing false reassurance to the client that nothing is really wrong. C/SPP, AN, PS

73. no. 3. Such pain may be associated with the development of a hematoma. Further assessment is necessary before selecting an appropriate nursing action. CBF/P, AS, PS

74. no. 1. A narrow spreader bar allows the ropes to rub against the outer aspect of the thigh. Placing padding would still result in pressure on the skin. Options no. 3 and no. 4 are inappropriate because if the ropes are correctly positioned, the client will not be uncomfortable. A/SP, IM, E

75. no. 1. In option no. 2 skeletal traction with a Thomas splint provides traction and support of the upper leg. A/SP, AN, PS

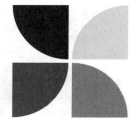

Answers and Rationales: Practice Test 2

76. no. 2. Spinal cord injury at the L2 level usually results in an ability to ambulate with assistive devices, such as braces. The lack of sensation does not prevent conception and pregnancy. Labor and delivery present special challenges. Vocational limitations are few, except for jobs requiring extensive standing or walking. Institutionalization is not necessary because there is great potential for rehabilitation. C/SPP, EV, H

77. no. 2. Anger and resentment often underlie guilt. The depressed client may attend group therapy, but talking about anger and resentment is more central to getting at guilt. When group therapy is ordered, the client may or may not deal with anger and resentment in that setting. Options no. 3 and no. 4 do not facilitate expression of guilty feelings. P/E, IM, PC

78. no. 1. Obesity is a complex, multidimensional problem with many possible causes. One cause is that there tends to be a familial predisposition; children of obese parents tend to be obese. Food can also become a source of gratification or validation. Eating food often causes a person to feel warm, relaxed, and euphoric. Many people eat to cope with life's stresses. The most comprehensive and effective treatment of obesity combines an eating plan for weight loss, exercise, behavioral change, social support, and cognitive restructuring. Although exercise is an important component of weight loss, it is not as effective as weight loss that occurs in combination with other therapies. Obesity in children tends to lead to obesity in adulthood because in children there is not only an increase in the size of fat cells, but an increase in their number as well. A/NM, AN, PS

79. no. 1. Autonomic dysreflexia is caused by visceral distention or irritation, such as distended bladder or bowel, in children with high spinal cord injuries. Prompt assessment and intervention is necessary to prevent further complications, such as shock and encephalopathy. The distended bladder is slowly drained through catheterization followed by evaluation. If symptoms persist, further causes are investigated, such as presence of impacted feces. C/SPP, IM, PS

80. no. 3. In severe major depression, the client may lose contact with reality. This may be manifested by a fixed false belief (delusion), such as paranoid ideation that evil forces will destroy the client. Reactive depression is related to grief reactions and usually does not include distortions of thought severe enough to be considered delusions. Delusions are also not characteristic of dysthymia and adjustment disorder, depressed mood. P/E, AN, PC

81. no. 3. An upper gastrointestinal series and barium swallow must be done on an empty stomach. Food and fluids are withheld for several hours. Cleansing enemas are given before large-bowel exams. Radiopaque tablets are given 10 to 12 hours before gallbladder x-rays. A/NM, PL, PS

82. no. 4. Options no. 1, no. 2, and no. 3 may apply to a number of other health care problems; no. 4 is specific to depression. P/E, AS, PC

83. no. 3. A fasting specimen of hydrochloric acid is used to obtain baseline data. Eating stimulates acid production. Because this test assesses only the pH of gastric juices, an enema is not required. The test will not cause cardiac alterations, so monitoring the pulse rate is not required. A/NM, PL, PS

84. no. 2. Infants with gastroesophageal reflux (GER) may benefit from thickened feedings, varying from 1 teaspoon to 1 tablespoon of rice cereal per ounce. Antacids are not routinely given. Option no. 3 will tend to increase the chance of GER because of compression of the lower esophageal sphincter into the abdominal cavity; infants should be bubbled and burped after every ounce. C/NM, EV, H

85. no. 2. Peptic ulcers are directly related to high levels of hydrochloric acid. Option no. 1 is too vague. Lack of intrinsic factor results in anemia. Decreased acid is not related to ulcers. A/NM, AN, PS

86. no. 1. A noninvasive or tubeless gastric analysis (Diagnex Blue Test) is done to determine the presence or absence of hydrochloric acid in the stomach. It does not indicate the amount of free acid in the stomach. The presence of gastric ulcers is best determined through direct visualization (endoscopy, gastroscopy). The rate of gastric emptying is best determined with a gastric emptying scan. A/NM, AN, PS

87. no. 1. The negative view of the self and the future are indicated by option no. 1. These cognitive changes best indicate depression. Option no. 2 indicates that the client at times feels bad; however, the client also demonstrates awareness of mood and style of coping. This is not an indication of suffering from depression. Options no. 3 and no. 4 indicate a need for further assessment but do not necessarily indicate depression. P/E, AS, PC

Key to abbreviations may be found on p. 255.

88. no. 2. An infant with pyloric stenosis often suffers from fluid and electrolyte imbalances, primarily from vomiting. These need to be corrected before surgery; a child in proper acid-base and fluid balance is a much better surgical risk. C/NM, PL, PS

89. no. 2. Ranitidine (Zantac) inhibits histamine at the H_2 receptor sites in the parietal cells. This in turn inhibits gastric acid secretion. Typically, a gastric pH > 5 is desired. Antacids (e.g., Maalox) neutralize acids in the stomach. Smooth muscle relaxants decrease motility. A/NM, AN, PS

90. no. 2. The obstruction is at the pyloric sphincter. The child becomes dehydrated from vomiting; thus metabolic alkalosis and hypokalemia are common findings. C/NM, AN, PS

91. no. 4. Options no. 1 through no. 3 are common symptoms of a major depressive episode. Ataxia, an inability to coordinate voluntary muscular movements, has not been reported in depression. P/E, AS, PC

92. no. 2. A vagotomy is done to eliminate the acid-secreting stimulus of the gastric cells. It has no effect on postoperative pain or stomach perfusion. A/NM, AN, PS

93. no. 1. Elderly clients pose the greatest risk of completed suicides. The other options may occur, but the greatest concern is suicide. P/E, AN, PS

94. no. 1. Potassium is excreted through the kidneys. If the client is not voiding and potassium is infusing, levels could rapidly become toxic. C/NM, AS, PS

95. no. 3. Feedings are usually started shortly after surgery. Parents may have become negatively conditioned to preoperative vomiting, so they need to be included in positive postoperative feeding experiences. Hypoglycemia may occur as a result of preoperative depletion of hepatic glycogen. C/NM, PL, PS

96. no. 3. Nausea and gagging may be due to kinks or a nonpatent tube, which can cause an increased volume of retained gastric secretions and pressure on the anastomosis. The risk of evisceration usually occurs later, after the sutures are removed. Option no. 4 may be a second action only if there is an order. A/NM, IM, PS

97. no. 3. This is a basic principle when approaching any client for the first time. It establishes rapport and communicates respect for the individual. The other three options would be done after the introduction is made. A/O, IM, PC

98. no. 3. This position facilitates emptying of the stomach by taking advantage of the stomach's normal curvature. C/NM, PL, PS

99. no. 4. When applying electrodes, an assessment using touch can be done concurrently to determine skin and muscle conditions. Level of consciousness and orientation are assessed in the evaluation of the client's response to the explanation of electrode application. Cardiac output is determined by actual monitoring, either noninvasively by blood pressure or invasively by an arterial line or a central line (e.g., Swan-Ganz). A/O, AS, PS

100. no. 1. Assessing the client for cause of depression is the most important nursing assessment because it can be facilitated by determining if he has experienced re-

cent losses or lifestyle changes. Older clients tend to focus on somatic complaints rather than psychosocial issues. The other options are important, but no. 1 is the most important. P/E, AS, PS

101. no. 4. The usual response after surgery for pyloric stenosis includes some vomiting for up to about 48 hours after surgery. C/NM, AS, PL

102. no. 3. Severe pain and theophylline toxicity, blood levels >20 μg/ml are causes of tachycardia. Sinus bradycardia in clients over age 65 is usually a result of medications, especially digoxin, or electrolyte imbalances of potassium or magnesium. A serum digoxin level of > 2 ng/ml is considered toxicity. A/O, AN, PS

103. no. 3. This indicates that parental learning has taken place. C/NM, EV, H

104. no. 2. Bradycardia results in a decrease in cardiac output; therefore all nursing activity would be directed at maintaining the best possible cardiac output. Options no. 1 and no. 3 are related to this primary goal and subsumed under it. Maintaining close contact with significant others is important, but it does not receive priority over maintaining cardiac output, a physiologic need that has priority over a psychosocial need. A/O, PL, E

105. no. 1. A planned, systematic approach to client teaching is essential when a major alteration in activities of daily living and lifestyle will be the outcome of an illness. Options no. 2 and no. 3 are assumptions that cannot be made. Client education is a shared responsibility. A/O, PL, E

106. no. 4. A full bladder displaces the uterus and prevents contraction. Other options are normal expectations. CBF/P, AN, PS

107. no. 1. The denial is evident. She has difficulty facing the seriousness of her situation. Rationalization is an unconscious mechanism whereby a person creates a logical, socially acceptable explanation for a thought, feeling, or behavior. Sublimation is the conscious or unconscious channeling of unacceptable drives into acceptable activities. Suppression is a conscious decision to exclude a thought or feeling. P/L, AN, PC

108. no. 4. This response indicates to the client that the anger she is expressing was heard and offers the opportunity to deal with those feelings. Restating the most provocative part of her complaint will further escalate her anger. Option no. 2 is an excellent explanation of why she needs a diet to control her blood sugar, but only after she has had an opportunity to verbalize her anger and feel understood will she be able to listen to it. Option no. 3 avoids the feeling tone of her complaint. She will only have numerous other complaints because the real issue has been avoided. P/L, IM, PC

109. no. 4. Because restraints can severely restrict circulation and injure tissue, they must be checked frequently and regularly. The padding mentioned in option no. 1 is often helpful. Restraints should never be tied to the side rails. C/NM, IM, E

110. no. 4. Excess arm movement and arm raising should be avoided for 5 weeks after the insertion of the pacemaker. The incision should be assessed q30min for bleeding. Dizziness, light-headedness, and chest pain are all signs of pacemaker failure and should be monitored. A pacing spike or artifact is a vertical line that appears on the ECG each time the pulse generator fires an impulse. This spike should be followed by a QRS complex, called capture, when there is appropriate pacemaker function. A/O, IM, PS

111. no. 4. Permanently implanted pacemakers require no physical or technical care. Teaching must focus on any adjustments to be made in activities of daily living and of recreational activities (e.g., no contact sports). A/O, PL, E

112. no. 3. Compartment syndrome is possible because this type of fracture is frequently caused by substantial force that produces neurovascular disruption. Fluid loss is not a major problem. Infection (osteomyelitis) is a potential complication of any bone trauma and not specific to elbow fracture. Severe pain is associated with compartment syndrome but is a symptom of the complication and not a complication in itself. C/M, AN, PS

113. no. 4. Local anesthesia is used for this procedure; testing for the gag reflex is necessary and a priority to prevent aspiration. Although urine output, respiratory patterns, and level of consciousness are always important to monitor, the endoscopy does not directly cause any alterations in these systems. A/NM, PL, E

114. no. 1. The first stage in dealing with a terminal illness is denial, and the client's comment is a common expression of denial. There are insufficient data to conclude that Mr. Lewis may not be able to cope with his problem or that his behavior is unusual. P/L, AN, PC

115. no. 1. The gastric outlet is attached to low intermittent suction to drain blood from the stomach. As long as there are bloody returns in the gastric aspirate, iced lavage is continued. Traction is maintained for a physician-specified time to ensure control of bleeding. If traction is maintained for more than 72 hours, esophageal necrosis may result. A/NM, PL, E

116. no. 3. Skeletal traction involves pull directly to a bone by a pin inserted through the bone distal to the fracture. The pin sites should be checked each shift for potential problems. Only skin traction can be periodically removed for rewrapping if pull to the part is maintained. The other options counteract the treatment regimen. C/M, PL, PS

117. no. 4. Of the options listed, only the sulfobromophthalein test measures liver excretory function. This is a dye-clearance study. Alkaline phosphatase (ALP) is a liver enzyme that is increased in obstructive biliary disease and liver dysfunctions. The albumin-globulin ratio measures the liver's ability to synthesize these proteins. The prothrombin time assesses the liver's ability to synthesize factor VII. A/NM, AS, PS

118. no. 1. Because the client is in the first stage of dealing with death and dying issues, the initial priority is to help clients begin dealing with their situation. The client must begin to deal with impending death before initiating goals of options no. 2 and no. 3. Option no.

4 is not the first or more important goal, and it would not necessarily help face death. P/L, PL, PC

119. no. 1. Hypercalcemia results from osteoclastic activity occurring more rapidly than does osteoblastic activity when weight bearing is diminished. Calcium is released into the bloodstream, leading to osteoporosis. The other options occur with normal mobility. C/M, AN, PS

120. no. 1. Ovulation is believed to occur just before, at, or just after the temperature drop. The fertile period extends 3 days before and after this. CBF/W, AN, H

121. no. 4. Dying clients need opportunities to talk and to progress at their own pace. Clients must not be isolated or pushed into other stages. Answer questions about death as they arise. Denial may be adaptive and normal up to a point. If the client denies the seriousness of the health threat but complies with treatment, denial can be adaptive. P/L, PL, E

122. no. 4. Increased hydrostatic pressure from portal hypertension and the diminished synthesis of albumin by the liver result in ascites. The inability of the liver to break down aldosterone also contributes to the process because increased aldosterone levels cause increased sodium reabsorption. A/NM, AN, PS

123. no. 4. Spironolactone (Aldactone) would be the first choice because its action is to block aldosterone production, which the liver cannot detoxify. In addition, spironolactone is potassium sparing. A/NM, AN, PS

124. no. 1. The pin should be secure and immobile in the bone. Options no. 2, no. 3, and no. 4 are normal. C/M, EV, PS

125. no. 1. Mittelschmerz, or lower quadrant abdominal discomfort, is caused by the ruptured ovarian follicle. At ovulation, spinnbarkheit, or stretchable cervical mucus, appears and the cervix is palpated as softer and more open. Ovulation occurs 14 days before the next menstrual period, not necessarily 14 days after the last one. CBF/W, AS, PS

126. no. 3. Respond to denial with realistic and empathic statements about the client's feelings. Do not encourage denial or try to interrupt it abruptly. Focusing on the client's job, rather than feelings, suggests avoidance by the nurse. Option no. 2 is too confronting at this point and would increase the client's high anxiety level. Option no. 4 would encourage the client's denial. P/L, IM, PC

127. no. 3. The operation diverts the blood from the portal circulation and decreases some of the portal hypertension. It cannot prevent bleeding, nor does it facilitate liver regeneration or restore function. A/NM, AN, PS

128. no. 3. Peer contact is most important for the adolescent. Removal from school and normal physical activities make it necessary that peer contacts are maintained. The other options could be healthy diversions, but they are of secondary importance. C/H, AN, PC

129. no. 2. The client should be encouraged to express feelings about death. A willingness to talk about it should be met with encouragement to do so. Option no. 1 shows insensitivity and interferes with further exploration of the client's concerns. Option no. 3 avoids the issue of death. Option no. 4 assumes the client is bothered, rather than exploring feelings about accepting the client's prognosis. P/L, IM, PC

130. no. 2. Increased amounts of gonadotropins (follicle-stimulating hormone and luteinizing hormone) stimulate the maturation of the ovarian follicle, followed by ovulation and, later, development of the functioning corpus luteum. CBF/W, P, PS

131. no. 4. Any opening in the skin is a portal of entry for bacteria. Cooling measures will do nothing to decrease or prevent infection and generally will not be initiated until the temperature has gone above 101°F (38.3°C) or 102°F (38.8°C). Only visitors who are obviously ill with an infectious disorder should be discouraged from visiting. Ambulation will reduce many postoperative complications that can lead to infection. A/NM, IM, E

132. no. 2. This is the physical finding that would indicate clubfoot. Pain is not associated with clubfoot. Newborns usually have bowed legs, and frequently the foot is not aligned with the knee. C/M, AS, PS

133. no. 3. In this client, encephalopathy has most likely developed because of the recent bleeding. Neomycin is given to decrease the ammonia production in the intestines from the breakdown of blood. Increased ammonia levels are believed to bring on symptoms of hepatic encephalopathy. Asterixis, also called liver flap or liver tremor, is a flapping tremor of the hands. Asterixis and confusion are commonly associated with hepatic encephalopathy. A CT scan is not required because the symptoms indicate a metabolic origin and not structural damage. Sodium should be restricted in clients with liver disease because of the risk of the formation of ascites. Diazepam (Valium), metabolized by the liver, is contraindicated because with liver dysfunction the medication levels will remain high and hinder accurate evaluation of the client's mental status. A/NM, AN, PS

134. no. 2. This is the basis for the treatment regimen. Temporary developmental delay may actually be caused by treatment. After the age of 6 months, clubfoot can be corrected but requires longer and more invasive treatment than if it were detected at birth. A newborn's skin is thin and fragile and has potential for breakdown. C/M, AN, PS

135. no. 4. The daughter needs an opportunity to express feelings and receive some support. Eventually she will need to discuss things with her father. Options no. 1 and no. 2 do not give the daughter an opportunity to express her thoughts and feelings. A/NM, IM, PC

136. no. 4. A plaster cast should not be allowed to become wet because it will soften and lose its effectiveness. Cleaning should be done with a nonchlorine cleanser. Rough edges can occur but only present a problem if the skin underneath becomes excoriated. With an infant in a cast, urine and stool soiling cannot be completely prevented. C/M, EV, E

137. no. 2. Anger is a normal stage in the death and dying process. Although it may be directed at nurses, it is usually displaced anger. The nurse should respond in a way that indicates acceptance and empathy while encouraging her to express feelings. Option no. 1 indicates that the nurse has interpreted the client's anger as personal. Option no. 3 is a defensive remark that avoids the client's feelings and may increase her guilt. Option no. 4 is a withdrawal reaction and may be helpful to the nurse, but it leaves the client with unresolved feelings. P/L, IM, PC

138. no. 3. Frequently, nurses have been directly or indirectly affected by problems associated with alcohol and are not able to assist the client in a helping manner until they discern their own attitudes. After the nurse is able to explore his or her own feelings about alcoholism, options no. 1, no. 2, and no. 4 would be appropriate. A/NM, IM, PC

139. no. 4. Dying at home is a reasonable request that should be supported. The nurse can assist the client in making arrangements. Option no. 1 is not helpful because they need further information about the possibilities of a home death. Discharge planning falls within the purview of nursing, and it is appropriate for the nurse to discuss this with the family. No data suggest denial of seriousness at this time. P/L, IM, PC

140. no. 1. Elevation is critical to decrease edema and resulting circulatory compromise. Feeding difficulties have no relationship to the foot problem. Infants having casts with plaster foot molds should be turned with legs supported on pillows or blankets to avoid pressure on the toes. Option no. 3 is used for a fractured femur. C/M, PL, PS

141. no. 3. All the other options are appropriate for Mr. Arnold, but immediately using relaxation techniques would be most beneficial as a short-term goal. A/NM, PL, PC

142. no. 2. Information about the complications of ulcer may be the least helpful. The client has not experienced any complications, so the client can use denial and choose not to comply. A/NM, IM, PC

143. no. 3. This is the only option leading to a measurable outcome. The only true measurement of successful teaching is if the parents can apply the brace. C/M, EV, H

144. no. 1. This suggests resolution of the most comprehensive and realistic goals for the client. Anger is not the end stage of the grief process; the expectation is to move beyond this phase. Option no. 3 is not realistic. Independence is an important achievement, but dealing with the emotional impact of impending death is more important. P/L, EV, PC

145. no. 2. Hypovolemic shock can occur quickly after a perforation, so IV access for fluid replacement must be done first and quickly. Options no. 1, no. 3, and no. 4 are all appropriate once the client is stable. The client initially should be maintained in semi-Fowler's position to localize the gastric contents to one area of the peritoneum. Preoperatively only deep breathing or incentive spirometer is taught to minimize movement of bowel contents. After surgical repair, turning, coughing, and deep breathing would be appropriate to implement. A/NM, IM, PS

146. no. 1. Indomethacin (Indocin) is irritating to the stomach and duodenum and can cause or aggravate ulcers.

Magnesium and aluminum hydroxide (Maalox) is an antacid that will help, not aggravate, the ulcer. Acetaminophen (Tylenol) is a nonnarcotic, nonsalicylate analgesic that will not aggravate ulcers. Atropine is an anticholinergic drug that decreases gastric secretions. A/NM, AN, PS

147. no. 3. Mr. Seele needs decreased, not increased, sensory stimuli at this time. With sleep deprivation, the client may have impaired judgment, so protecting this client from self-injury would be important. Although this client is in the manic episode, he may be able to care for his personal hygiene with assistance. P/E, PL, E

148. no. 3. The priority is to determine whether cervical changes have occurred so that an appropriate plan of care can be designed. A contraction stress test would be contraindicated for a client experiencing the possibility of premature labor. An internal monitor cannot be applied unless membranes are ruptured. There is no evidence that delivery is imminent. CBF/I, AS, E

149. no. 4. Wearing a bib at mealtimes is essential to prevent aspiration of spilled foods or fluids into the stoma, but a plastic bib is contraindicated. A fabric bib should be worn to protect from aspiration. Plastic would prevent exchange of oxygen and carbon dioxide. C/O, EV, H

150. no. 2. An irregular pulse is characteristic of a disturbance of electrical stimulation or conduction in the heart. This is more commonly found in clients with heart disease, severe acid-base imbalance, or electrolyte imbalance. Jaundice occurs when bilirubin accumulates in the skin, sclerae, and other tissues in the body. These findings relate to the obstruction of the bile ducts and liver cells. Edema, the ascites, occurs from decreasing plasma protein levels and increasing portal pressure. In addition, sodium is retained as a result of increased aldosterone levels from the lack of aldosterone breakdown from the failed liver. Ecchymosis occurs with vitamin K deficiency from fat malabsorption and defective synthesis of factors II, VII, IX, and X by a failed liver. A/NM, AS, PS

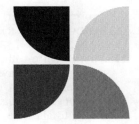

Answers and Rationales: Practice Test 3

151. no. 1. Clients with liver disease have an increased tendency to bleed. This is caused either by a failure to absorb vitamin K or because the liver is unable to use vitamin K to form prothrombin. If the client's bile duct is obstructed, absorption of vitamin K is reduced. Even if vitamin K is absorbed, damaged liver cells usually cannot synthesize adequate amounts of clotting factors. With a decrease in platelets the finding is usually petechiae on the anterior chest wall, not bruising easily. A/NM, AN, PS

152. no. 3. Advancing the suction catheter further than 0.5 cm beyond the end of the tracheostomy tube can cause trauma to the trachea. To prevent prolonged obstruction of the airway, suctioning should require no more than 3 to 4 seconds. To prevent hypoxia, it is often advisable to hyperoxygenate before and after suctioning. C/O, IM, PS

153. no. 4. A complication of this procedure is accidental penetration of a blood vessel, causing hemorrhage, or penetration of a biliary vessel, causing chemical peritonitis from the leakage of bile into the abdominal cavity. These complications would be manifested as abdominal pain and unstable vital signs. Pressure to the biopsy site can be applied by positioning the client in the right lateral recumbent position after the procedure. Bed rest is prescribed for the client for 24 hours after the procedure. During the procedure the client is positioned supine with the right arm under the head. A/NM, PL, E

154. no. 1. Regular uterine contractions can be painless and still produce cervical changes resulting in irreversible labor and delivery. A pregnant woman should report contractions >4 per hour whether they are painful or painless. Other options decrease risk of preterm birth through adequate hydration and perfusion of uterine muscle, avoidance of urinary tract infections, early detection of contractions, and avoidance of oxytocin production through orgasm and nipple stimulation. CBF/A, EV, H

155. no. 1. Cellular function in the liver depends on tissue-building materials supplied by amino acids derived from proteins. Clients with liver disease *with no evidence of encephalopathy* need high-protein, high-calorie, low-sodium diets. A/NM, PL, PS

156. no. 4. It is important to decrease environmental (sensory) stimulation for these clients and, at the same time, provide close observation. Taking him to the recreation room may be too stimulating. He may not be able to sleep at this time because of being in a new environment. Developing social skills while in a manic episode is impossible. P/E, IM, PC

157. no. 3. Clients with ascites experience dyspnea, resulting from pressure exerted upward against the diaphragm. High Fowler's position reduces this pressure. The client needs rest to reduce metabolic demands on the liver and should keep activities to a minimum with quiet rest in bed for most of the day. A/NM, IM, PS

158. no. 3. With her history of hypertension, cerebral hemorrhage is the most probable cause of the CVA. Transient ischemic attacks produce sudden neurologic deficits; these usually disappear within minutes or 24 hours. A cerebral aneurysm and meningitis do not result in these types of findings. A/SP, AN, PS

159. no. 1. This determines a child's ability to handle information. Options no. 2, no. 3, and no. 4 are factors for consideration but are not as important as no. 1. C/I, AS, H

160. no. 1. A positive Babinski's reflex is extension or dorsiflexion of the great toe and the fanning of the other toes when a hard object is applied to the lateral surface of the sole, starting at the heel and going over the ball of the foot, ending beneath the great toe. The normal response to plantar stimulation in adults is to plantar-flex the foot and flex all toes (called a negative Babinski's reflex). A/SP, AS, PS

161. no. 3. Offering the bedpan q2h is the first step in the initiation of bladder training, which is part of rehabilitation. The 2-hour interval is gradually lengthened as control is gained. Catheters can introduce bladder infections and should be avoided when possible. Wearing a diaper may cause embarrassment and skin breakdown. Restricting fluids to control incontinence would be inappropriate. A/SP, PL, PS

162. no. 4. Polycythemia is characterized by an increased number of red blood cells, which results in increased blood viscosity. Increasing fluids prevents dehydration and reduces hemoconcentration. C/O, EV, PS

163. no. 4. There is no such thing as hysterical aphasia. In expressive aphasia, the client has difficulty in selecting, organizing, and initiating motor speech. Expressive aphasia is also termed motor, Broca's, or nonfluent aphasia. In contrast, the client with receptive (sensory, Wernicke's, or fluent) aphasia generally has impaired auditory comprehension and auditory feedback. A/SP, AN, PS

164. no. 1. Initial care of the client with bipolar disorder, manic phase would focus on physical problems such as poor nutrition, hygiene, and sleep and rest problems. Promoting increased physical activity would promote exhaustion. Increased sensory stimuli would overload the client. Working on low self-esteem is not appropriate during this period because the client is easily distracted. P/E, IM, PC

165. no. 4. The normal heart rate for a 4-year-old is approximately 100 beats per minute; a heart rate of 90 beats per minute would indicate that the child is resting comfortably. C/I, EV, PS

166. no. 2. The occipital lobe holds the visual center; the medulla deals with essential functions (e.g., temperature); the parietal lobe deals mainly with sensory function. A/SP, AN, PS

167. no. 1. Tocolytic drugs stimulate type II beta-receptors, resulting in vasodilation and hypotension. To compensate, the maternal heart rate increases even to the point of cardiac failure. For this reason, tocolytic drugs are usually discontinued if the pulse rate exceeds 140 beats per minute. CBF/I, IM, PS

168. no. 4. Encourage the client to speak at any possible opportunity. Although time consuming, it is more therapeutic for the client. Options no. 1, no. 2, and no. 3 discourage the rehabilitation of verbal communication. A/SP, IM, E

169. no. 2. Infusion of blood too rapidly may lead to hypervolemia, which in turn may lead to heart failure. C/O, AN, PS

170. no. 2. Magnesium sulfate is being given to this client to stop the contractions of preterm labor. There is no indication that this client has increased blood pressure or potential convulsions. These findings would be more consistent with a medical diagnosis of pregnancy-induced hypertension. There is no indication of fetal distress. CBF/I, EV, PS

171. no. 1. Have the family continue to encourage the client's efforts. If the aphasia is expressive, she may be able to choose another word to communicate her needs. A/SP, IM, H

172. no. 1. Lithium has a narrow therapeutic index. Therefore clients must be closely observed for signs of lithium toxicity. Lithium is not addicting, nor does it produce severe sedation. It is often given with antipsychotic agents during the acute phase of manic episode. P/E, AN, PS

173. no. 3. Keeping him in semi-Fowler's position is important to prevent aspiration, a frequent complication after a CVA. Although the other options may be appropriate, client safety comes first. A/SP, PL, E

174. no. 2. The child is experiencing an allergic reaction. The transfusion should be stopped immediately, but the patency of the IV line is maintained as a route for emergency drugs, if they become necessary. C/O, IM, PS

175. no. 1. Initial damage to any tissue creates edema and impairs functioning. As the cerebral edema decreases, muscle function begins to return and can improve for a period of up to 6 months. The most dramatic changes in functional gains generally occur within the first 3 months after the onset of the stroke. Option no. 4 is

correct; however, it is too general a statement to best answer this specific question about paralysis. A/SP, AN, PS

176. no. 3. Once a therapeutic serum level is attained, it takes 7 to 10 days for a clinical response to lithium. Therefore antipsychotic drugs that have a therapeutic response time that can be measured in minutes are used to alleviate the acute symptoms of mania until lithium begins to take effect. Clients with bipolar disorder, manic episode do not have schizophrenia, but both have psychotic features. Antipsychotic drugs do not reduce lithium toxicity or increase the beneficial effects. P/E, AN, PS

177. no. 3. There is no research data that suggest lithium therapy causes irreversible side effects with long-term use. Lithium therapy does produce side effects such as nausea, vomiting, dizziness, headache, impaired vision, and diarrhea, among other symptoms. Clients with bipolar disorder, manic episode often report liking the euphoric feeling, and once the lithium takes effect, clients fear having to face their underlying depression. P/E, AN, PS

178. no. 2. The presence of fetal hemoglobin prevents sickling; it begins to decrease around 4 to 6 months of age, and the child eventually develops symptoms of the disease. C/O, IM, PS

179. no. 4. These signs are all indicative of a gestational age of less than 40 weeks. Lanugo and vernix are shed in utero as the fetus matures. Palmar and plantar creases increase with age. Development in the ears, breast tissue, and scrotum occurs with age. Testes begin descent at approximately 36 weeks of gestation. Dark-red skin in the premature infant is reflective of lack of subcutaneous fat. Parchmentlike skin is typical of the postterm infant. CBF/N, AN, PS

180. no. 4. The preterm infant is at greater risk for heat loss than the full-term infant. The nurse must keep this in mind while carrying out routine delivery-room procedures. Drying the infant is important to prevent heat loss by evaporation. Metabolism is dysfunctional because of impaired enzyme systems. Thus maintaining body temperature is more difficult for the preterm baby. Vernix and lanugo are more abundant in the preterm infant. Hypoglycemia is more likely in preterm infants because of perinatal stress and decreased glycogen stores. CBF/N, AN, PS

181. no. 1. Children with sickle cell disease have an increased susceptibility to infections. The exact cause is unknown, but supporting data suggest that many organisms thrive in a state of diminished oxygen and that phagocytosis is reduced in a hypoxic state. C/O, AN, PS

182. no. 3. Rehabilitation attempts to reduce the impairments and disability in stroke and to restore and develop physical and psychologic functioning. A/SP, PL, PS

183. no. 1. Hydration promotes hemodilution, which in turn decreases blood viscosity and prevents further sickling; hydration also interferes with the cycle of stasis, thrombosis, and ischemia. C/O, PL, PS

184. no. 3. With the help of significant others or family,

rehabilitation efforts are continued over the long term, resulting in a more optimal recovery. A/SP, AN, H

185. no. 3. Daily skin checks are done to note any bleeding. Pink urine may be from hematuria and must be reported immediately. Foods high in vitamin K will enhance the clotting mechanism and counteract the effects of the drug. Prothrombin levels, not activated partial thromboplastin times, are measured in clients receiving warfarin (Coumadin). A/SP, IM, PS

186. no. 4. Prerenal azotemia refers to a decreased blood flow to the kidneys. Poisons cause renal azotemia. A/E, AN, PC

187. no. 2. Clients with bipolar disorder, manic episode experience sensory-perceptual disturbance and inability to cope. Calling the physician for discharge orders would not be appropriate when the client is agitated and shows bizarre grooming. Assessing the client's abilities realistically would be done at some point, but when the client is demanding, and disorganized, this is not the time. Distraction only works temporarily and may increase irritation when the real issue is not addressed. P/E, IM, PC

188. no. 2. Hyperkalemia is an immediate and life-threatening problem associated with renal failure. Clients on hemodialysis have diet and fluid restrictions. Hemodialysis sustains a client until renal transplant is scheduled. A/E, PL, PS

189. no. 3.

$$\frac{5 \text{ mg}}{1 \text{ ml}} = \frac{2 \text{ mg}}{x \text{ ml}}$$

$$5x = 2 = \frac{2}{5} = 0.4 \text{ ml}$$

C/I, IM, PS

190. no. 1. Competitive games, group debates, and physical movement serve to escalate aggression and irritability and should be avoided. P/E, IM, PC

191. no. 4. Nasal flaring is the only indication of respiratory distress listed. The nares flare to take in more oxygen to compensate for hypoxia. CBF/N, A/N, PS

192. no. 3. Sickle cell disease is an autosomal recessive disease. Both parents are carriers; therefore with each pregnancy Mrs. Henderson has a 25% chance of having a child with the disease, a 50% chance of having a child with the trait, and a 25% chance of having a child without the disease or the trait. C/O, IM, H

193. no. 3. The hemodialysis machine works on the simple physical principles of filtration, osmosis, and diffusion. It cannot duplicate the complex endocrine functions of the kidneys (e.g., the production of erythropoietin). The other options reflect the purposes of hemodialysis. A/E, PL, PS

194. no. 4. Postoperative renal shutdown is usually reversible. A/E, IM, PC

195. no. 4. This option describes manic behavior and does not meet discharge criteria. Option no. 1 indicates the client is in good control of his feelings. Option no. 2 indicates the client has an awareness of underlying feelings of depression. Option no. 3 indicates the client will not use hostility to threaten others into doing what he wants. P/E, EV, PC

196. no. 1. Emphasis is on heart rate, which is usually counted for 1 full minute in order to detect any dysrhythmias or bradycardia. Pulses should also be routinely checked, especially distal to the puncture site, after the procedure. C/O, AS, PS

197. no. 4. Conversion reaction is the loss or alteration of physical function that is not explained by any physical disorder or underlying medical condition. It is postulated that the behavior is reinforced by the gain it represents to the client by repressing some unacceptable feeling or desire. P/A, AN, PC

198. no. 2. Lethargy is a symptom of a high BUN. Disequilibrium syndrome is caused by the rapid decline of electrolytes or wastes. A/E, AS, PS

199. no. 1. Lee can shower the next day, but baths should be avoided for several days. The pressure dressing should be removed the next day and the area inspected for redness, drainage, or swelling. An adhesive bandage is then placed over the site. He should wait several days before any strenuous activity. Aspirin can increase the potential for bleeding. C/O, EV, H

200. no. 3. This is the result of a backup of blood in the right ventricle, which enlarges to accommodate the extra volume. C/O, AN, PS

201. no. 4. The shift of too much blood into the dialyzer may produce symptoms of hypovolemic shock. Accidental disconnection of the tubing may also result in rapid exsanguination and hypovolemic shock. A/E, PL, PS

202. no. 2. It is most important to determine his understanding and allow him to express his feelings. Option no. 4 is contraindicated; option no. 3 is too severe a measure. C/O, PL, E

203. no. 2. Repression of feeling controls anxiety and internal conflicts. The tension generated is converted into the presenting symptom, which is symbolic. A fixation at the oral stage of development produces defense mechanisms of sublimation and displacement, not conversion. Suppression of feelings is a conscious effort to eliminate feelings of discomfort. Conversion is an unconscious, intrapsychic conflict. Sublimation is the process of altering and expressing an unacceptable feeling into a socially acceptable one. P/A, AN, PC

204. no. 2. Regional heparinization prevents clotting in the hemodialyzer without subjecting the client to the risks of systemic anticoagulation. Protamine sulfate is used to counteract the heparin when the blood is returned to the client. A/E, PL, PS

205. no. 2. Blood flow must be maintained in the cannula to prevent clotting. A tight dressing constricts flow. A/E, IM, PS

206. no. 4. Focusing on physical symptoms and expressing thoughts tend to reinforce symptoms of a conversion disorder. The other options do not focus on physical symptoms. P/A, IM, PC

207. no. 2. Checking for excess bleeding is the next priority because hemorrhage is the more common complication in the immediate postoperative period. Palpation of the bladder is usually done instead of percussion. A/E, IM, PS

208. no. 4. Because her defect was mild, repair should be complete. She should not be encouraged to develop a chronically ill, dependent personality. C/O, PL, H

209. no. 1. Postoperative clients should void within 8 to 12 hours after surgery. At this time, it is most appropriate to assess the client's status by asking if the client feels the need to urinate. Catheterization is done as a last resort when other measures (e.g., no. 3 and no. 4) are ineffective. Further assessment of the client's need to void comes before interventions such as options no. 3 and no. 4. A/E, IM, PS

210. no. 4. The client's temperature should be taken orally, not rectally. Avoid the supine position, sitting for prolonged periods, and sitting on highly inflated rubber rings, all of which increase venous stagnation in the rectal area. A/E, IM, PS

211. no. 4. All the statements represent possible secondary gains, which reinforce the conversion reaction. P/A, AN, PC

212. no. 2. Use an open-ended comment to encourage the child's own expressions. The other options are judgmental or discourage sharing of comments by the child. C/I, IM, PC

213. no. 2. This option gives the client the opportunity to voice his concerns. The other options assume the cause of the client's worry. A/E, IM, PS

214. no. 1. To avoid postoperative infection, the client should do perineal care after each stool and have sitz baths as needed to clean the incision or to provide for comfort. A/E, IM, H

215. no. 3. This skill comes at age 6. The child should be able to do the other skills listed. C/O, AS, H

216. no. 2. Increased pain with bowel movements is a symptom of anal stricture, and the client should notify the physician. The client should drink 2500 to 3000 ml of fluid daily and eat a low-residue, soft diet for the first postoperative week. The client will usually have had a first bowel movement before the client is discharged. A/E, IM, H

217. no. 4. Sitting upright, leaning forward with mouth open, drooling, and dysphagia are classic signs of epiglottitis. C/O, AN, PS

218. no. 3. It is critical to minimize the physical complaints and stress the positive aspects of the client's behavior to avoid reinforcement of the sick role. Confrontation often increases defensiveness and meets resistance because of the client's need for denial. Supportive measures may provide secondary gain and increase dependency. The client is not psychotic; therefore such medication is inappropriate. P/A, IM, PC

219. no. 2. Research and observations of infants who have not been touched have shown that there are differences in the behavior of these babies when they are compared with babies who have received normal mothering. CBF/N, AN, E

220. no. 4. The majority of side effects of external radiation are dependent on the specific site being radiated. Because the client's cancer site is the lung, radiation will result in irritation of the lung mucosa, resulting in dyspnea. A/CA, AS, PS

221. no. 4. Skin markings must not be removed in any way. If they are inadvertently washed off, markings are redrawn only by the radiation technician. A/CA, PL, PS

222. no. 2. It is important to understand the difference between external and internal radiation so that the nurse can be accurate when correcting the client's misconceptions. He is not radioactive and does not need to limit contact with others. Options no. 1, no. 3, and no. 4 are incorrect. A/CA, IM, PC

223. no. 1. An adequate airway is the primary objective in treating any child with a respiratory problem. C/O, PL, PS

224. no. 4. Encourage the client to participate in self-care as much as possible, but provide periods of uninterrupted rest in a quiet environment between periods of activity. A/CA, PL, PS

225. no. 4. The two chief symptoms of cancer of the cervix are metrorrhagia (vaginal bleeding or spotting at irregular intervals and between periods) and a watery vaginal discharge. Options no. 1 and no. 3 are findings of advanced lesions of the cervix. A/CA, AS, PS

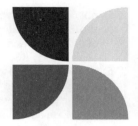

Answers and Rationales: Practice Test 4

226. no. 1. Because of exposure to carbon monoxide an altered mental and neurological status may occur. The other options are appropriate during some aspect of treatment, but initial attention must be diverted to her physical and mental status. P/E, IM, E

227. no. 3. A change in heart rate (i.e., increasing heart rate) is an early sign of hypoxia. Options no. 2 and no. 4 are signs of lower airway involvement; no. 1 is characteristic of spasmodic croup. C/O, AS, PS

228. no. 1. Determine Joe's hypersensitivity to the medication. Penicillin products are at high risk for causing allergic reactions. C/O, IM, E

229. no. 3. It is desirable for parents to take an active role as care providers for their infants. This will promote attachment and help develop their comfort and confidence in caring for the infant at home. CBF/N, PL, PC

230. no. 2. This response encourages the client to express feelings of hopelessness. Though anger may be present, the affect in no. 2 suggests hopelessness. The probability of her discussing or even recognizing anger at this time is minimal. Option no. 1 is a form of reassurance, which is rarely therapeutic. The nurse cannot presume to know what the client will be experiencing later. Option no. 4 would reinforce the client's persistence to attempt suicide and reinforce feelings of hopelessness rather than instill a sense of hopefulness that something could be different. It also conveys a lack of empathy from the nurse. P/E, IM, PC

231. no. 4. The Croupette concentrates the cool mist. This facilitates the heavy, cool water droplets reaching deeper into the respiratory tract to reduce edema and soothe irritated mucous membranes. Although the Croupette will also accomplish options no. 1, no. 2, and no. 3 to some extent, they are not the primary goals. C/O, PL, PS

232. no. 4. The most common form of tracheoesophageal fistula is one in which the proximal esophageal segment terminates in a blind pouch. When the child swallows saliva, water, or milk, it accumulates in the blind pouch, resulting in excessive salivation or aspiration. Other options are not symptoms of tracheoesophageal fistula. CBF/N, AN, PS

233. no. 4. Cancer of the endometrium tends to be slow spreading. Once it has spread to the cervix, invaded the myometrium, or spread outside the uterus, the prognosis is poor. A/CA, AN, PS

234. no. 3. Loosely tucking the tent edges will allow mist and oxygen to escape; edges should be firmly tucked around the mattress. All other options are necessary because of the child's age and problem. C/O, IM, E

235. no. 2. Menstruation will cease after a hysterectomy, but as long as the ovaries are left in place, they will continue to function, and surgical menopause will not occur. A hysterectomy is removal of the uterus and usually the cervix. A/CA, IM, PS

236. no. 4. Menstrual irregularities occur with menopause, but these do not include dysmenorrhea (menstrual cramps) and mittelschmerz. A/CA, AN, PS

237. no. 1. Though all options provide useful information to assess suicide potential, the presence of a viable suicide plan greatly increases the risk. Although determining recent major stressors is necessary, it is not particularly helpful in deciding suicide potential. P/E, IM, E

238. no. 2. A specific gravity of 1.005 indicates adequate hydration status. The other options are values that are not measures of hydration. C/O, AS, PS

239. no. 3. A serious complication of a hysterectomy is the accidental ligation of the ureter during surgery. These symptoms would be found if that had occurred. A/CA, AS, PS

240. no. 4. Close observation is imperative in suicide prevention. Although observation may be easier on a closed unit, an open unit is satisfactory as long as the client can be watched closely. A locked psychiatric unit does not imply that the client is being closely watched. A double room would assist the client only during client-client interactions. However, other clients are not responsible for supervision. P/E, IM, E

241. no. 1. Vaginal packing is not used after an abdominal hysterectomy. Crying spells may be related to her change in body image. A/CA, IM, H

242. no. 2. The inflamed mucosa of the bladder is the most likely cause of the spasms that lead to symptoms of urgency. The other options are incorrect. The client probably has cystitis. A/E, AN, PS

243. no. 2. Imaginary friends are normal for this age group. Because this is normal behavior, the other options are not warranted. C/H, IM, PC

244. no. 4. Paroxetine takes 2 to 3 weeks to produce therapeutic effects (reduce depressive symptoms). It is too early to determine if the medication is ineffective. Suicidal ideations are not a side effect of this medication. It is too early for the medication to be changed. P/E, AS, PS

245. no. 2. Tying shoelaces, jumping rope, and walking backward are activities performed by a typical 5- to 6-year-old. C/H, AS, H

246. no. 3. Vitamin C is the only choice given that will best acidify urine. Commercial juices may be too dilute to affect urine acidity. Large quantities of juice help by flushing out the urinary tract. A/E, IM, PS

247. no. 2. Preschoolers fear body mutilation, especially genital-rectal procedures and intrusions, because of their level of psychosexual development. Their understanding of body integrity is still developing. C/I, PL, IM, PC

248. no. 2. Vigorous nasotracheal suctioning may easily disrupt the integrity of the suture line, so it is contraindicated. Gentle oropharyngeal suctioning would be indicated if the infant cannot handle oral secretions. Intravenous fluids will be necessary until the infant can be fed through a gastrostomy tube. Elevation of the head of the bed at 30 degrees promotes pooling of secretions at the catheter tip if an indwelling nasal catheter is in use. Skin care will prevent skin breakdown and infection. CBF/N, IM, PS

249. no. 3. Manipulation is a dominant characteristic of antisocial personality disorder. These clients often lack sensetivity and have difficulty relating to others because of inner feelings of abandonment. Although it is possible that this particular nurse has superior abilities, it is likely that a number of other staff also have superior abilities. Clients such as Miss Epstein are rarely motivated to change. Any adaptive behavioral changes happen very slowly. P/SM, AN, PC

250. no. 1. Sulfisoxazole (Gantrisin) is excreted by the kidneys and not absorbed and is therefore more active in the urine than other antibiotics. The others listed are absorbed systemically. A/E, AN, PS

251. no. 4. Adolescents need privacy and an opportunity to express their feelings about illness and treatment options. Their thoughts and feelings should be listened to attentively and respectfully. C/MO, IM, H

252. no. 3. Amniotic fluid is continually produced by the mother. A normal fetus swallows and excretes the amniotic fluid while in utero. If there is a gastrointestinal obstruction or neurologic problem that interferes with swallowing in the fetus, the amniotic fluid accumulates and results in hydramnios. CBF/N, AN, PS

253. no. 3. Lack of opportunity to identify with healthy role models, such as parents, results in a poorly developed and unsocialized superego. These clients often have developmental histories suggesting that early needs were not met adequately. They also have histories of conduct disorder, truancys, stealing, and lying. There are no data suggesting below-average intelligence. P/SM, AS, PC

254. no. 1. *E. coli* is the most common cause of urinary tract infections and is sensitive to sulfisoxazole (Gantrisin). *Pseudomonas* and *Klebsiella* infections are more commonly found in the respiratory system, and *Salmonella* infection is more commonly found in the gastrointestinal tract. A/E, AN, PS

255. no. 3. The other options are characteristic of osteoarthritis. Rheumatoid arthritis has familial tendencies and commonly occurs between the ages of 25 and 55 years. A/M, AS, PS

256. no. 3. An interdisciplinary treatment approach is necessary to achieve consistency in setting limits on behavior. Clients with antisocial personality disorders need firm and consistant limit-setting. The client is not likely to do well in a group setting because there is no internalized impulse control. The client needs a matter-of-fact attitude and firm limits. The client will mistake sympathy for weakness and try to manipulate staff more. P/SM, IM, E

257. no. 3. These findings are consistent with a diagnosis of a hydatidiform mole. Because pregnancy-induced hypertension is usually a disease of late pregnancy, if hypertension occurs in early pregnancy a hydatidiform mole should be suspected. Anemia occurs as a result of blood loss. Signs and symptoms in options no. 1 and no. 4 are not consistent with a diagnosis of hydatidiform mole. CBF/A, AS, PS

258. no. 3. Extensive blood loss during surgery and subsequent decreased renal perfusion necessitate close monitoring of urine output. Decreased or absent urine output could signal acute renal failure. Paralytic ileus is common after surgery and not unexpected 6 hours postop. Postoperative pain is usually considerable. C/MO, AS, EV, PS

259. no. 1. The sedimentation rate is elevated and is the most consistent lab finding in rheumatoid arthritis. The serum white blood cell count is usually slightly elevated, the client is usually anemic, and protein antibodies or rheumatoid factor is present in 80% of clients. Synovial fluid is not tested in either type of arthritis. A/M, AS, PS

260. no. 2. Older children are more prone to develop a headache after lumbar puncture than younger children. Because the headache is related to postural changes, lying flat in bed reduces the development of headache. C/SPP, EV, PS

261. no. 2. Stiffness is more pronounced in the early morning; it diminishes with use of the joint in rheumatoid arthritis. A/M, AS, PS

262. no. 2. Safety and precision make ultrasound the diagnostic technique of choice for women with suspected molar pregnancy; no fetal skeleton is revealed. Other options will not provide necessary diagnostic data. CBF/A, AN, PS

263. no. 4. Clients with antisocial personality disorders have no lasting attachments or sense of loyalty. They attempt to achieve pleasurable ends at the expense of others. P/SM, AN, E

264. no. 4. Increasing calories and weight would place extra stress on joints. Added calcium would cause serum calcium to be high with increased risk of frozen joints. The client needs rest with spacing of activities to facilitate treatments for this systemic disease. Putting the head of the bed in high position prevents stress and strain on the joints when the client gets out of bed. A/M, PL, E

265. no. 4. Options no. 1, no. 2, and no. 3 are definite signs

of respiratory distress. Irregular respirations may occur for many other reasons and are frequently normal in young children. C/O, AS, PS

266. no. 1. The current methods of removing a molar pregnancy are dilation and curettage and hysterotomy. Betamethasone therapy is done to accelerate fetal lung maturation in preterm labor. Vacuum extraction is a technique used instead of forceps to deliver a fetus. Laser therapy is not a treatment for a molar pregnancy. CBF/A, IM, PS

267. no. 3. Ambivalence is exemplified by these opposing behaviors. Ambivalence is demonstrated in behaviors described in the question. Further information is necessary to determine whether guilt is present. Option no. 1 is questionable. P/SM, AN, PC

268. no. 1. Pillows under major joints contribute to the complication of flexion contractures. Options no. 2. and no. 4 prevent contractures. Option no. 3 maintains skin integrity. A/M, IM, E

269. no. 3. After realizing how inappropriate past behavior was, the client often feels depressed. Depression occurs as a consequence of dealing with difficulties in therapy and an emerging awareness of how his behavior affects others. Dysthymic disorder refers to a chronic, milder depression. A major depressive episode more severe psychologic and physiologic disturbances. The client may begin to think his prognosis is not good, but such thoughts would not be as likely to occur at this time as option no. 3. P/SM, EV, PC

270. no. 3. Epinephrine is a beta-adrenergic agent that strengthens myocardial contractions and increases blood pressure, heart rate, and cardiac output. The vasoconstrictive effects predispose the child to tachycardia as well as elevated blood pressure, pallor, weakness, tremors, and nausea. C/O, AS, PS

271. no. 4. Massage tends to further traumatize swollen, inflamed, and painful joints. Cold packs produce an anesthetic effect. Heat or cold can both be used effectively in the treatment of arthritis to decrease muscle spasms. A/M, IM, PS

272. no. 3. Intake and output and specific gravity are good indicators of hydration. Hydration helps liquefy secretions and enables the child to expel the mucus. Option no. 1 is contraindicated. Position of choice is high Fowler's position. Option no. 4 is unnecessary. C/O, PL, E

273. no. 2. Choriocarcinoma, a neoplastic process that often follows a hydatidiform mole, has a tendency to undergo rapid, widespread metastasis. The client's human chorionic gonadotropin levels will be monitored for at least 1 year. Molar pregnancies do not place the client at higher risk for the remaining options. CBF/W, AN, H

274. no. 3. More appropriate interactions with others demonstrates a decrease in antisocial behavior. Motivation for impressing the staff is difficult to discern. His feelings for the other client are not known. The behavior described does not indicate apathy. P/SM, EV, PC

275. no. 4. Inflamed joints should not be exercised. All joints need not be exercised at all times. An appropri-

ate exercise regimen must be flexible and adjustable. The other options are correct. A/M, EV, H

276. no. 3. Aspirin in high doses increases the risk of bleeding; thus stools and urine should be examined. A/M, IM, PS

277. no. 4. Tachycardia is the only manifestation of aminophylline toxicity listed. Other manifestations include headache, hypotension, vomiting, and nervousness. C/O, EV, PS

278. no. 2. This option both acknowledges the client's concern and allows him to discuss it. Options no. 1 and no. 4 establish a behavioral limit with the client; however, these responses also minimize the chance of the client sharing any feelings with this nurse. Option no. 3 completely dismisses and avoids the feelings behind (or underlying) this client's request. P/E, IM, PC

279. no. 4. Adustment disorder, depressed mood is related to precipitating stress and personal loss. In Larry's case, loss of freedom of movement and the possibility of the loss of his arm have caused adjustment disorder, depressed mood. A common response is angry and demanding behavior. Withdrawal from alcohol probably would have occurred within 24 to 72 hours after hospitalization. Boredom usually manifests as complaining and restlessness, not yelling and demanding. The current behavioral presentation is not consistent with psychosis. However, one would want to continue monitoring him for a possible delirium syndrome. P/E, AN, PC

280. no. 1. Epinephrine relieves bronchospasm. It does not liquefy secretions (a subemetic dose of syrup of ipecac does this), nor does it increase antibody formation. The drug increases (not reduces) airway diameter. C/O, AN, PS

281. no. 1. Several months of therapy are required before effectiveness can be determined. The drug is commonly given deep intramuscularly. Adverse effects most commonly occur late, often after treatment has been discontinued. A/M, AN, PS

282. no. 1. A change in environment affects concentration, but confusion is usually minimal unless the client is fatigued. The unfamiliar is overwhelming to a person with brain damage. The client's level of fatigue must be considered to obtain accurate assessment data. A/SP, AS, E

283. no. 2. Expiratory wheezing is the result of air attempting to pass through narrowed bronchial lumens. Option no. 1 characterizes croup and laryngotracheobronchitis; no. 4 relates to croup; expirations in asthma are prolonged. C/O, AS, PS

284. no. 3. Because of the concern about choriocarcinoma, it is generally recommended that pregnancy be avoided for 1 year after a molar pregnancy. CBF/W, IM, H

285. no. 2. Involve clients in their care with mutual goal setting and by promoting self-responsibility. These actions can enhance client compliance. Use arm sling and leg cast only during transport; these restrict range of motion if used continuously. Food trays and equipment should be positioned on the client's unaffected

side, which would have normal strength and feeling. A/SP, PL, E

286. no. 2. Active listening allows the gathering of more information and provides an opportunity for psychosocial intervention. Options no. 3 and no. 4 may be appropriate after further assessment. Option no. 1 is not an independent nursing action. P/A, IM, PC

287. no. 3. This is the optimal way to facilitate eating. Feeding clients increases dependency. Chewing and swallowing may never be completely restored. Liquids are generally more difficult to handle than solids. A/SP, IM, PS

288. no. 2. Subcutaneous is the preferred route. On occasion, it may be given IM, but the gluteal sites should be avoided. There is no epinephrine preparation suitable for sublingual use. The IV route may be used only if the drug is adequately diluted. C/O, IM, PS

289. no. 3. The fact that the client asked the nurse for a date, to go bowling in particular, is the clue to her concern. Options no. 1 and no. 4 are possibilities; however, the specific activity for the date is bowling, which would require a healthy arm. She is taking a risk with this request, which could embarrass her, not the nurse. P/E, AN, PC

290. no. 3. Fluid and dietary iron may need to be increased if anemia is present. Avoiding tampons is unnecessary. Prophyllactic antibiotics. Once normal nonpregnant levels of serum chorionic gonadotropin are reached, follow-up protocol includes testing every month for 6 months, then every 2 months for the next 6 months. This allows early detection of malignancy. CBF/W, EV, H

291. no. 4. A cerebrovascular accident is an upper motor neuron lesion; therefore spastic, not flaccid, paralysis is present. Clients should participate in exercises but cannot be expected to initiate and remember their own exercise program. A/SP, PL, E

292. no. 3. Reflection. It encourages the client to express her feelings about the loss of her foot. Option no. 1 does not address her fears or concerns and will only provide the nurse with a factual option, not an exploration of feelings. Option no. 2 is a threat which, with an adolescent, will probably precipitate a power struggle. Option no. 4 will be seen as punishment and humiliation in front of a peer wh could be beneficial in helping the client to verbalize her fears. P/E, IM, PC

293. no. 3. Pulmonary function tests are used for diagnosis of asthma by revealing obstruction, air trapping, and decreased expiratory airflow. They are also used as guidelines for management of asthma. Young children can perform the measurements at home via a peak flow meter. C/O, PL, H

294. no. 2. Pregnancy tests are based on the presence of human chorionic gonadotropin in the blood or urine of the woman. CBF/A, AS, PS

295. no. 2. These behaviors are characteristic of left-brain lesions near the motor cortex. In contrast, right-brain lesions result in perceptual and spatial disabilities. A/SP, AS, PS

296. no. 2. These behaviors are signs of anxiety. Confusion is usually manifested by disorientation and memory disturbances. Yelling, threats, and demands would indicate anger or agitation. A suspicious client may exhibit agitation but the main symptom is distrust or paranoia. P/A, AN, PC

297. no. 3. Most pressure is on the ischial tuberosities when sitting. Any redness that does not resolve 20 minutes after the pressure is relieved indicates risk for tissue breakdown. A/SP, AS, PS

298. no. 3. Once the lesions have dried, chickenpox is no longer communicable, and the child can return to school. A fever may be gone by the time the rash appears. Option no. 4 indicates that the child is still contagious. C/SPP, IM, H

299. no. 3. Home pregnancy tests have a high degree of accuracy (about 97%) if instructions are followed exactly. Both false-positives and false-negatives can occur if the woman is taking certain drugs, has certain diseases, or does not follow test directions. Home pregnancy tests are immunologic tests that have been refined by pharmaceutical companies to detect human chorionic gonadatrophin in a first-voided morning urine sample within 2 to 3 minutes. CBF/A, AN, PS

300. no. 3. Anger is implied in her getting back at her friend. Option no. 1 is not an acceptance of the "getting back" theme but an inference of what the client may be feeling or thinking. A reflective statement uses part of what the client has already stated, i.e., "You are going to get back at your friend." Option no. 4 would be the outcome of using any one of the previously stated communication techniques. P/E, IM, PC

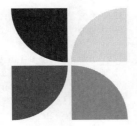

Answers and Rationales: Practice Test 5

301. no. 1. Although teratogenic effects may be specific depending on the causative agent, the greatest danger exists during the formation of the organ systems, or organogenesis, which typically is completed by the end of the eighth week of pregnancy. CBF/A, IM, H

302. no. 4. Firm and consistant limit setting will make the client feel more secure and help reduce fear. Limiting the number of nurses who care for the client facilitates the implementation of a consistent approach. Ignoring or meeting the inappropriate demands only serves to escalate unacceptable behavior. P/E, IM, PC

303. no. 3. Painting with watercolors allows the child to use imagination for expression of feelings and ideas; it also promotes development of fine motor skills, which is important at this age. C/SPP, IM, H

304. no. 4. Stress the importance of taking medications daily. In the partial or total removal of the endocrine gland, the hormones supplied by that gland commonly need to be replaced. If on steroid therapy it is important for the patient to inform a physician about the medication when ill or having surgery so that the dosage can be temporarily increased. A/NM, IM, H

305. no. 2. Decreased steroid production after an adrenalectomy can result in loss of sodium and water in copious amounts. In the absence of aldosterone, sodium is lost. Hypovolemic shock can occur quickly if the crisis is untreated. Also, potassium rises to dangerous levels, causing life-threatening dysrhythmias. A/NM, AN, PS

306. no. 3. Harsh limitations promote rebellion. Limit setting is needed but should be balanced with privileges. Negotiating, family conferences, contracting, and withholding privileges are appropriate for adolescents. C/H, EV, PC

307. no. 2. The ductus arteriosus and foramen ovale allow most of the fetal blood to bypass the fetal lungs. Circulation to the lungs of the fetus is needed only for nutrition of the lungs because oxygen exchange occurs across the placental barrier. The ductus venosus allows fetal blood to bypass the fetal liver. CBF/A, IM, H

308. no. 1. Manifestations of a situational crisis are a precipitating event, the spouse moving out and probable separation and divorce, and signs and symptoms of profound emotional pain and agitation. Any depressive symptoms would be related to the current situation and loss. Options no. 3 and no. 4 are diagnoses

that are not consistent with the clinical symptoms. P/T, AN, PC

309. no. 4. After the stress of surgery, addisonian crisis is a possibility if there has not been adequate steroid replacement. Change in blood pressure, typically a drop in pressure, is a first indication of this problem and must be reported immediately. A/NM, AS, PS

310. no. 2. Keeping the child's fingernails short and clean decreases the chance of the child acquiring a secondary infection of the pruritic lesions of chickenpox. C/SPP, IM, PS

311. no. 2. Having the client verbalize the meaning of the body changes is essential before a comprehensive plan of care can be implemented. A/NM, IM, E

312. no. 1. Cortisone, the glucocorticoid of choice, will be taken on a daily basis for the remainder of life. When there is an increase in stress, the dosage may need to be temporarily increased. With total removal of a gland, replacement therapy is indicated. With partial removal, follow-up of serum hormone levels without hormone replacement may be possible. A/NM, IM, E

313. no. 1. Varicella is an airborne virus, and respiratory isolation procedures should be used to prevent its spread. C/SPP, IM, H

314. no. 4. Crisis intervention deals with here-and-now problems and help the client and family to find coping mechanisms effective in dealing with stress in the environment. Adaptive coping skills can be explored without knowing the cause of the problem. Insight and increased self-knowledge are valuable but may not always produce behavioral change. Crises provide opportunities for clients to form healthier coping behaviors. The discomfort of the high anxiety provides leverage for the nurse to assist the client in learning how to problem solve and develop more effective coping. Giving advice reinforces the person's sense of powerlessness. P/T, AN, PC

315. no. 1. Crisis intervention involves assessment of the client's support systems, current and previous coping patterns, and the precipitating event. Options no. 2, no. 3, and no. 4 can be behavioral manifestations of someone experiencing a crisis state; however, they are more indicative of chronic maladaptive behavior. The crisis intervention focuses on the here-and-now and not chronic problems. P/T, AS, PC

316. no. 1. This selection is best for high protein, low calories and sodium, and high potassium. Complex carbohydrates should also be included. A/NM, IM, PS

317. no. 3. Cushing's syndrome results in increased gluconeogenesis; hyperglycemia occurs, resulting in a diabetic state, and polyphagia is common. A/NM, AN, PS

318. no. 4. A paroxysmal cough that worsens at night is characteristic of pertussis. The other three options are characteristic of chickenpox. C/SPP, AS, PS

319. no. 2. The placenta provides a semipermeable membrane across which exchange occurs by osmosis. In addition, diffusion, facilitated diffusion, active transport, and pinocytosis occur. Oxytocin is produced by the maternal posterior pituitary gland. Viruses readily pass through the placenta. Maternal and fetal blood do not mix unless there is a break in the placental barrier. CBF/A, IM, H

320. no. 2. Initially, it is necessary to determine immediate problems and how they are viewed by the client. Reassurance at this time seldom lowers anxiety and tends to make the client feel misunderstood. Advice given before the problem is identified and feelings are explored is usually not taken because the client's anxiety is too high to make use of the suggestion. It is preferable to encourage the client come up with his own solutions after the distorted perceptions have been corrected and his anxiety lowered. Rather than contacting the wife, explore with the client who his support system is, and encourage him to contact someone with whom he can share feelings. P/T, IM, E

321. no. 4. Birthing centers are designed for low-risk gravidas. Most freestanding birthing centers are staffed with nurse-midwives; complications are handled by obstetricians in a hospital setting. A wide variety of medications are available according to client preference and safety considerations. Generally the family unit is kept together throughout the birthing process. CBF/I, EV, E

322. no. 4. When a client cries, reflect the feeling and ask for more information. Some clients will want privacy, but this should be clarified with the client before the nurse automatically leaves a client alone to cry. Premature reassurance impedes communication. Although antianxiety medications are commonly used to reduce tension and gain control over themselves, crying is a healthy emotional outlet and should be supported rather than suppressed with medication. P/T, IM, E

323. no. 2. Corticosteroids' antiinflammatory action relieves airway obstruction by reducing edema. They can be inhaled or given IV when the usual drugs (e.g., epinephrine) are not effective. Steroids do not reduce anxiety, mobilize secretions, or relieve bronchospasms. The other asthma drugs achieve these actions. C/O, AN, PS

324. no. 4. Normally, cortisol levels are highest between 6 AM and 8 AM and decrease during the evening hours, with a nadir around midnight. A client with Cushing's disease will have elevated levels regardless of wake pattern, sleep pattern, or time. A/NM, AS, PS

325. no. 3. Increased amounts of mineral corticoids will cause increased sodium and water retention with loss of potassium in the urine. A/NM, AN, PS

326. no. 2. Adrenocortical steroids interrupt normal linear growth in children when used over a prolonged time. C/O, AN, PS

327. no. 4. The usual cause of asthma is an allergy or hypersensitivity to a foreign protein. A fish would be the most logical choice of pet for an asthmatic child. C/O, IM, H

328. no. 2. The nurse can refer clients such as this one to health maintenance organization (HMO) for crisis intervention and for continued therapy or necessary referrals. Inpatient psychiatric treatment or day care is not indicated at this time. Professional evaluation would be indicated first before any referral to a self-help group. P/T, IM, PC

329. no. 2. The nurse is paraphrasing what the client said to encourage feedback. Option no. 1 is a direct question that limits clarification of feelings. Option no. 3 does not respond to the expressed concern, and no. 4 is a meaningless statement when the client has not had an opportunity to fully express his feelings. C/CA, IM, PC

330. no. 1. Because of increased cortisol levels, clients with Cushing's disease have a low tolerance for stress; in addition, the accuracy of diagnostic tests performed is dependent on minimizing stress. Fluids may be given but usually not in liberal amounts. Explaining tests and procedures as well as providing diversional activities would be done; however, neither are the first nursing concern. A/NM, PL, PS

331. no. 4. Crises are time limited and are usually resolved within 6 weeks. Once a week appointment is usually sufficient and allows time for the client to implement new coping behaviors and be supported during the crisis. P/T, PL, PC

332. no. 3. The information given suggests she has experienced personal growth. The goal of crisis intervention is to mobilize emotional support and develop adaptive coping skills. This has been achieved. Even though the client has been traumatized and is the same person she was 8 weeks ago, her coping has become adaptive and enhances her life, so she is functioning at a higher level. P/T, EV, PC

333. no. 3. This provides sound control for the other clients' benefit and allows Roberto to have his request. Music with earphones is also helpful for pain control and relaxation. C/CA, IM, E

334. no. 4. Adrenal atrophy results in hypocorticism (Addison's disease). A pituitary tumor might produce an increased ACTH that would stimulate the adrenal cortex to produce more cortisol and cortisone. An adrenal tumor might overproduce steroids. A/NM, AN, PS

335. no. 1. Increased cortisone leads to sodium retention and higher levels of free cortisol. A/NM, AS, PS

336. no. 3. Hydroxyzine causes sedation and does not stimulate the central nervous system. The others are all actions of hydroxyzine. C/CA, AN, PS

337. no. 4. Do not avoid Tommy and his parents; they may be unable to ask for the help that they need (a common problem for persons in crisis). Provide both privacy and emotional support. C/CA, PL, PC

338. no. 3. Amphetamine and other central nervous system stimulants, such as cocaine, produce these symptoms.

These symptoms are not chief manifestations of heroin intoxication, alcohol intoxication, or cocaine withdrawal. P/SU, AN, PS

339. no. 1. Allow the client to select another individual to take on the supporting role. If no one is available, it is helpful to assign one nurse. CBF/I, IM, PC

340. no. 1. Touching an irritable and suspicious client is inappropriate because the client's agitation may escalate and increase the risk of aggression. The other options are appropriate measures and should be initiated as soon as possible. P/SU, AN, PS

341. no. 3. This indicates that the presenting part of the fetus is at the perineum; delivery will be very soon. Other options can occur before or during labor and are not indicative of imminent birth. CBF/I, AS, PS

342. no. 3. The toothbrush and peroxide solution might further damage an ulcerated and infected mouth. Doing nothing is not an appropriate measure because discomfort will be increased. C/CA, IM, PS

343. no. 4. Cushing's syndrome is characterized by excessive amounts of cortisone. This delays wound healing (antiinflammatory) and interferes with calcium metabolism, leading to osteoporosis. Other findings include easy bruising, thin, transparent skin, sodium and water retention, potassium loss, hyperglycemia, and truncal obesity. A/NM, AS, PS

344. no. 1. Fingernails should be kept short to prevent scratching and injury to skin with pruritus. The other answers are inappropriate for a terminally ill client. C/CA, IM, PS

345. no. 2. It is essential to provide guidelines for normal versus abnormal recovery and teach related assessment skills for self-monitoring. The other options are important but can be addressed during follow-up visits. CBF/P, IM, H

346. no. 3. Exploring the content of the delusion or arguing with the client only reinforces the delusion. The nurse should acknowledge to Ms. Ortez that it must be upsetting to feel as she does. This will promote trust by providing empathy. Thus the nurse begins to build the relationship with the client. If the nurse focuses on the content and details of the delusion or acknowledges the delusion as reality, the delusion is given credibility, which reinforces it. P/S, IM, PC

347. no. 4. Although other goals are appropriate over a longer period, promoting attachment is the best short-term goal. CBF/P, PL, H

348. no. 1. According to Kübler-Ross, Mrs. Ackers is denying the consequences of the terminal phase of Paul's illness. C/CA, AN, PC

349. no. 3. Bladder fullness is a priority assessment if the client has spinal cord injuries. There is loss of bladder reflex to empty during spinal shock that occurs within 30 minutes of injury. A/SP, AS, PS

350. no. 3. Mannitol is an osmotic diuretic. When it is discontinued, there is a temporary increase in fluid retention. A/SP, AN, PS

351. no. 3. Presenting reality is the best response. Tell the client who you are. Communication should avoid reinforcing the client's delusion. In option no. 1, the nurse does not understand how the client feels and the

response could serve as a reinforcement of her delusional system. Ignoring her comment can cause her anxiety to rise, or she may interpret the nurse's silence as agreement. Rational explanations tend to make the client hold more firmly to the delusion. P/S, IM, PC

352. no. 2. This is a period of peak blood volume (increase of 30% to 50% during pregnancy) and maximum cardiac output. As a result, cardiac decompensation may occur. Risk of premature delivery is not the priority. HELLP syndrome is a complication of PIH; DIC is a complication of hemorrhage. CBF/A, AN, PS

353. no. 3. This is indicative of decreased total blood volume because hematocrit is a measure of packed red blood cells per deciliter of blood volume. C/SPP, AS, H

354. no. 1. The speech center is located in the left posterolateral side of the frontal lobe (Broca's center). A/SP, AS, PS

355. no. 3. These symptoms are indicative of fluid overload resulting in congestive heart failure. C/SPP, AS, PS

356. no. 4. These are the early symptoms of congestive cardiac failure and must be promptly recognized and treated. Other options are not true statements. CBF/A, EV, H

357. no. 4. The nurse cannot talk the client out of her suspicions. Serving foods in sealed containers may diminish the client's anxiety. It is also possible that the action may not, but it allows her some control about whether to eat. Option no. 2 may lead the client to conclude that the nurse believes there may be some reality to her delusion *or* is refuting her belief. Tasting the food is a rational explanation that serves to reinforce the delusion. P/S, IM, PC

358. no. 2. Combining an antipsychotic agent with an antianxiety agent lowers the dose of the former to produce therapeutic effects. Side effects of antianxiety agents are not related to this combination. Neither drug induces agranulocytosis. Medication compliance and improved self-care deficits are not directly correlated with these medications. P/P, AS, PS

359. no. 2. Restriction of visitors is unnecessary if they are healthy and are instructed in proper isolation technique. C/SPP, PL, E

360. no. 2. Heparin is the drug of choice when an anticoagulant is required because its large molecular weight prevents it from crossing the placenta. Penicillin is used prophylactically to prevent subacute bacterial endocarditis. Digitalis is commonly used to treat arrhythmias in pregnancy. Although it does cross the placenta, there is no evidence that it causes adverse fetal effects. Diuretics may be used to treat edema associated with congestive heart failure. CBF/A, AN, PS

361. no. 3. These measures will decrease cerebral edema, which will reduce the intracranial pressure. The other measures may be employed later. A/SP, AN, PS

362. no. 2. Myasthenia gravis is exacerbated by infection, emotional stress, menses, pregnancy, surgery, or accidental administration of curare, quinine, or quinidine. The other options would not be discussed by the nurse but by the physician. A/SP, IM, PS

363. no. 2. Forceps application reduces the stress and exertion of pushing. Vaginal delivery is the preferred method of delivery for cardiac clients. Risk of infection is secondary to reduced cardiac strain during second stage labor. CBF/I, IM, PS

364. no. 1. Withdrawal can occur if the client cuts back the amount of alcohol consumed, as well as if drinking is stopped altogether. Ambulatory care nurses must always evaluate cardiovascular status; however, Mr. Fincher's history and presenting clinical picture are more consistent with withdrawal. Increased anxiety is only one symptom of alcohol withdrawal. Peripheral neuropathy usually indicates chronic alcoholism, and a depressive reaction may be alcohol induced or underlay alcoholism. Physical and mental status must be assessed continuously. P/SU, AS, PS

365. no. 1. A urinary output of 10 ml/hr is abnormally low. However, the first measure is always to see if the catheter is patent. If it is, the next step would be to notify the physician. C/SPP, IM, PS

366. no. 3. Muscle rigidity and tremors at rest are symptoms of Parkinson's disease. A/SP, AS, PS

367. no. 4. Proteins and carbohydrates are needed for wound healing and tissue replacement. The other options do not achieve these goals primarily. C/SPP, PL, PS

368. no. 4. Myasthenia gravis frequently causes weakness in muscles innervated by cranial nerves IX and X, which is associated with difficult swallowing, regurgitation, and aspiration. A/SP, AS, E

369. no. 3. Korsakoff's syndrome is also known as alcohol amnestic disorder due to thiamine deficiency. Korsakoff's syndrome produces severe memory impairment, manifested by memory lapses and confabulation. Persons with chronic alcoholism often suffer from chronic gastritis, paresthesias, and a fatty liver; however, Korsakoff's syndrome is a dementia associated with an underlying general medical condition. P/SU, AS, PS

370. no. 4. Pyridostigmine (Mestinon) is absorbed too quickly on an empty stomach. However, if the client is having symptoms, she may need to take the medication, or part of it, before a meal to aid chewing and swallowing. A/SP, IM, H

371. no. 3. Weakness becomes worse on exertion and at the end of the day (as opposed to morning). Rest typically increases muscle strength. A/SP, IM, H

372. no. 3. Fantasy, play therapy that allows expression of emotions, is best for preschoolers. C/I, IM, E

373. no. 4. The semirecumbent, or semi-Fowler's, position allows for maximum functioning of her heart and respiratory system. A left side-lying position may also be used to correct hypertension or for delivery. CBF/I, IM, PS

374. no. 1. Helping the client to find new adaptive coping skills without alcohol is a long-term goal of treatment. Short-term goals would include learning to handle specific situations. Clients with chronic alcoholism need support from friends and family and increased emotional support to assist them through difficult times. Reality therapy has not been found to be effective in treating alcoholism. P/SU, IM, PC

375. no. 1. Breast-feeding is permissible if there are no cardiac problems during labor and delivery and immediately postpartum. Rooming-in is possible only with assistance and as the mother desires. A gradual increase in activity during the postpartum period is recommended. CBF/P, PL, PS

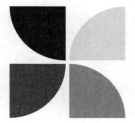

Answers and Rationales: Practice Test 6

376. no. 1. Hypospadias is located anywhere along the ventral surface of the penile shaft. In mild cases, the opening is just off center of the glans; in the most severe cases, it is on the perineum. C/E, AS, PS

377. no. 3. Although disulfiram (Antabuse) does cause tachycardia, it also causes a drop, not an increase, in blood pressure and respiratory depression. A pulsating headache (from dilation of peripheral blood vessels) and vomiting do occur; however, a generalized flushing becomes apparent rather than pallor. Although blurred vision does occur, dry skin does not because the person experiences profuse sweating. P/SU, IM, PS

378. no. 2. Myasthenia gravis can be aggravated by pregnancy. Medication will need careful management during pregnancy but may not be able to prevent problems. A/SP, IM, PS

379. no. 2. Myasthenia gravis is caused by an autoimmune process that impairs receptor function at the myoneural junction. A/SP, AN, PS

380. no. 3. Family therapy looks on the presenting problem as a family problem. Family therapy does not focus on any one individual; instead, it aims at getting a better understanding of the relationship between the client with alcoholism and family members. Its goal is to help the family members communicate more effectively in order to find adaptive ways to meet their needs. The family therapy sessions would not be centered on getting a client to stop drinking, but on having the members express themselves clearly on important matters, including the drinking issue, and on helping the members to develop effective communications skills. P/SU, PL, PC

381. no. 2. Swelling in the upper part of the body is significant; dependent edema of the lower extremities is not. The blood pressure rise in option no. 1 is not significant enough to indicate a problem. A weight gain of 1 pound per week is expected in the last two trimesters of pregnancy. Protein in the urine, not glucose, would be a significant finding. CBF/A, AN, PS

382. no. 3. Nausea and vomiting are unrelated to hypospadias. Urinary retention is due to obstruction of flow and is not the case with hypospadias. Ambiguous genitalia may be seen in conjunction with hypospadias in severe cases, but it is not the norm. The abnormal stream direction is often the first indication. C/E, AS, PS

383. no. 3. Recurrent nightmares, hypervigilance and difficulty in concentration are all symptoms commonly found in posttraumatic stress disorder. Hallucinations that involve insects are generally a part of delirium such as alcohol withdrawal. P/A, AS, PC

384. no. 4. The primary problem is a generalized vasospasm leading to uterine insufficiency. There is a decrease in plasma proteins as a result of protein loss into the urine through damaged kidneys, and there is a decrease in glomerular filtration as a result of vasoconstriction. Sodium and water retention is augmented by an increase in aldosterone. Cardiac output falls as the result of hypovolemia. CBF/A, AN, PS

385. no. 1. The client experiencing posttraumatic stress disorder has a sense of isolation and believes that no one understands his pain. In establishing a relationship, the nurse must create an accepting and empathetic environment. It is important to identify past coping behaviors and to teach the client relaxation techniques; however, this will prove easier after a therapeutic relationship has been established. Arranging a couples' session meeting is not needed to establish the nurse-client relationship. P/A, IM, H

386. no. 1. Family history is important because certain genitourinary anomalies are familial. Childhood illness, immunizations, and toilet training do not have significance for embryonic development (and detection) of these anomalies. C/E, AS, PS

387. no. 4. Diversion of urinary flow is usually accomplished with a urethral-bladder catheter. A nephrostomy tube is uncommon because the kidneys are not usually involved. Explanations to the child and parents are important along with an explanation of the expected outcome so that there are no surprises. C/E, PL, PS

388. no. 3. Ampicillin is in the penicillin family and should not be given to someone who is allergic to penicillin. A/O, IM, PS

389. no. 3. Although encouraged ventilation of feelings might include crying or an angry outburst, the continued expression of anger and rage can lead to loss of control or increase tension and rage rather than reducing it. Encourage the client to describe thoughts rather than feelings and think through how posttraumatic experiences affect current relationships in society. Assist the client by discussing ways to control anger and gain a perspective on current experiences. As the nurse

Key to abbreviations may be found on p. 255.

communicates confidence that he or she will help him find solutions, gain a sense of the "normalcy" of reactions and that problems can be resolved. P/A, IM, PS

390. no. 4. The 5-year-old has not developmentally defined his sexuality completely. Fear of mutilation is common to this age group. Fear of punishment for misdeeds is common in the preschool child. C/E, AN, PC

391. no. 4. There is no cure for pregnancy-induced hypertension except delivery of the child. The aim of all treatment is to prevent progression of the disease to eclampsia. CBF/A, PL, PS

392. no. 3. The right and left mainstem bronchi are not symmetric; the right bronchus is shorter and wider and continues from the trachea in a vertical course. This anatomic difference facilitates aspiration into the right lung. A/O, AN, PS

393. no. 2. The client will need continued support after she leaves the hospital. Self-help groups are an effective way to increase social interactions and support, and explore new coping methods and problem solving. Unless both the client and her husband have had an opportunity to explore the reason for their separation, moving back with her husband might cause increased stress. Lorazepam might be useful as adjunctive therapy for reduction of anxiety, but it is not the best long-term solution for the client. Because the client's job is probably not what has caused the increase in her anxiety, a job-training program might not be necessary after the client's emotional state is stabilized. P/A, EV, E

394. no. 4. Fluid intake of at least 3 L per day facilitates the expectoration of bronchial secretions. A/O, PL, PS

395. no. 3. Wiping from front to back when cleansing is important to prevent contamination of the urethral meatus with *Escherichia coli* from the anal area. C/E, EV, H

396. no. 3. A decreased respiratory rate indicates central nervous system depression from the magnesium sulfate. The urinary output listed is within normal limits. The drug produces hypoactive reflexes and indirectly lowers blood pressure. CBF/A, AS, PS

397. no. 3. Of the options provided, no. 3 is most critical. In high-stress situations, it is important for the nurse to provide emotional support as an integral aspect of the care. Notifying the police is important and will also be done. The client may or may not need a referral to a psychiatric clinical specialist. Most often, rape crisis advocates are called. Crisis intervention includes emotional support and is part of the emergency room nurse's or clinical specialist's role. Pregnancy concerns can be dealt with later. P/SM, IM, PC

398. no. 2. Sedatives can have this effect. Antineoplastic drugs usually suppress bone marrow. Antibiotics may increase the risk of superinfections. Penicillin-type drugs more commonly cause hypersensitivity reactions. A/O, AN, PS

399. no. 3. Normalizing the client's feelings conveys understanding and acceptance. Furthermore, it helps the client's understanding of her responses to the rape. Of-

fering a telephone number she may call for help if she wishes is another way to provide support. Numerous questions are inappropriate and tire a client. It is not important that the client discuss the rape at this time unless she wishes to do so. Not all rape survivors want to discuss the rape. How a client copes does not depend on what her initial reaction is like. P/SM, IM, PC

400. no. 1. Notifying the physician is most appropriate. Medications are ordered by the physician and then given by the physician or nurse. Option no. 3 may help decrease fluid loss but should be a secondary action. Parents can be called after the physician is notified. C/E, EV, PS

401. no. 4. Findings on physical examination of the chest may include dullness to percussion, diminished breath sounds, crackles, and a pleural friction rub. Audible wheezing is a symptom of narrowed bronchioles in hyperinflated lungs such as those found in clients with asthma. A/O, AS, PS

402. no. 1. Magnesium sulfate is used to depress the central nervous system. It also reduces blood pressure and produces diuresis, but this is not its main action. CBF/A, AN, PS

403. no. 3. Staff will often negate or deny the seriousness of a traumatic event to decrease their own anxiety arising from unresolved issues, such as a rape. Sometimes staff will look for ways in which the client was responsible for the rape. However, it is much healthier for a nurse to accept that people are vulnerable and to be aware of the emotional pain that awareness can cause. This self-awareness can increase the nurse's effectiveness in providing emotional support. Option no. 1 is not likely; people rarely lie about being raped. Responses to rape vary and include both high-anxiety behavior and a seemingly calm external demeanor. P/SM, AN, PC

404. no. 2. A follow-up urine culture is done 1 to 2 weeks after completing the antibiotic to make certain the causative organism is eradicated. C/E, EV, H

405. no. 2. Most toddlers are able to point to their body parts by 15 to 18 months of age. All other options are too advanced for a toddler. C/H, AS, H

406. no. 4. The goal of crisis-intervention therapy is to return clients to a precrisis level of functioning or higher. Crisis intervention can be effective whether or not the client develops insightful understanding about her feelings. It deals with the immediate event and does not aim at understanding earlier conflicts. Developing effective coping skills reduces the deleterious impact of rape. Crisis intervention is brief; the focus is on the here and now; treatment is short term and time limited. P/SM, PL, PC

407. no. 4. The early phase of a crisis is a time when here-and-now issues are dealt with by the client. Options no. 1, no. 2, and no. 3 are all important and necessary components of the assessment. Successful resolution of a crisis parellels the client's ability to mobilize effective coping skills and support systems. P/SM, AS, PC

408. no. 2. Exogenous steroids cause adrenal gland hypofunction. The body may not be able to respond in times of stress. A/SP, AN, PS

409. no. 4. Toddlers will resist invasive procedures, so it is best to proceed confidently. Obtain assistance to restrain the child and be matter-of-fact so the child does not feel that what is happening is a punishment or the result of being "bad." The child is too young to benefit from options no. 1 and no. 3. Deferring the exam is not appropriate. C/H, IM, PC

410. no. 3. When the client seems to be losing control, the first action should be to help the client cope with the contractions through breathing and relaxation. Analgesia should not be used in early labor. There is no need to call the physician at this time. Increasing the IV with the oxytocin will increase the contractions. CBF/I, IM, PC

411. no. 1. Clients may find the crisis situation overwhelming and misdirect their anger at staff, family, or friends. There are no data to suggest that the staff hurt her. Survivors of rape often feel powerless. These statements may also be a way of increasing control. P/SM, AN, PC

412. no. 2. This option allows the client to focus on her feelings without judging her or pushing her to discuss issues she is not comfortable talking about. Option no. 3 avoids dealing with the client's anger and is not therapeutic. Option no. 4 tries to talk the client out of her anger rather than encouraging her to express angry feelings. P/SM, IM, PC

413. no. 1. A saddle block is an intradural anesthetic that affects the sensory and motor pathways. The client therefore does not have the involuntary urge to push during the second stage of labor. This is desirable if forceps are indicated. That ability is not lost with the other types of anesthetic listed. CBF/I, AN, PS

414. no. 1. Playing with a toy will divert the child's attention from the task of learning independent toileting skills. C/H, IM, H

415. no. 1. Stopping steroids suddenly would mimic addisonian crisis, the major complication of which is cardiovascular collapse. A/SP, AN, PS

416. no. 3. The toddler often has physiologic anorexia and is more likely to accept small portions of a variety of foods. This approach also allows the toddler to exert autonomy by making choices. C/H, IM, H

417. no. 2. Pain patterns of angina vary from individual to individual but usually are the same in one individual. A change may indicate new ischemic areas. Anginal pain frequently occurs with stress or after eating a heavy meal. The client needs to purchase a fresh supply of nitroglycerin if the current medication does not cause a tingling sensation under the tongue. Nitroglycerine prescriptions are usually written for prn use and refilled as needed. A/O, IM, H

418. no. 4. Rape is a crisis situation, but many times the survivor has adequate coping mechanisms and social supports to handle the trauma. Option no. 1 describes conditions that lessen the potential for crisis. Coping mechanisms and social supports are terms used in crisis theory. If the client stayed with a friend and was

able to manage the stress, a crisis may not occur. P/SM, AN, PC

419. no. 2. Propranolol (Inderal) is a beta-adrenergic blocking agent. As such, it blocks the bronchodilator effect of sympathetic (adrenergic) stimulation and is contraindicated for all chronic obstructive lung conditions. It is also contraindicated in cardiac failure, cardiogenic shock, and second- or third-degree AV heart block. It is not contraindicated for MI, CVA, or thrombophlebitis. A/O, AN, PS

420. no. 3. Hemorrhage is the most common complication after tonsillectomy. Bleeding and clotting times are necessary to determine whether the child is at risk for hemorrhage and to serve as a baseline value postoperatively. C/SPP, AS, E

421. no. 2. Contractions should not last more than 90 seconds. The blood pressure increase is not significant. Fetal heart rate accelerations during the stimulation of a contraction are considered normal. A resting period of at least 30 seconds should occur between contractions. CBF/I, AS, PS

422. no. 3. During the school-age period, most children lose their primary teeth and develop their permanent teeth. By adolescence, all deciduous teeth should be gone. Options no. 1 and no. 2 are periods when deciduous teeth are erupting. C/SPP, AN, PC

423. no. 1. Secondary prevention refers to early treatment to prevent long-term illness. Crisis-intervention helps the client mobilize emotional support and resources. Tertiary prevention refers to treatment of chronic, long-term problems. Crisis intervention does not aim for insight, although insights may occur. P/SM, AN, PC

424. no. 2. There is no indication that propranolol causes GI or urinary bleeding, so there is no need to check stools and urine for occult blood during propranolol therapy. Propranolol does cause bradycardia and hypotension, so the blood pressure should be closely monitored, and the client should be instructed to change positions slowly. Propranolol can cause bronchospasms, so the client should be assessed for dyspnea and respiratory difficulties. A/O, IM, PS

425. no. 2. Cheese is high in fat and sodium content, which makes it unsuitable for a cardiac client. Eating smaller meals is important because of the increased incidence of angina after eating a heavy meal. In addition, exercise should be avoided after eating because it increases the workload of the heart. Fat consumption should be reduced. Fish and chicken are appropriate low-fat, high-protein foods. Caffeine should be limited because it may increase the heart rate. A/O, PL, H

426. no. 2. Preventing a rape would be primary prevention. Emergency care after the rape is an example of secondary prevention. Hospitalization may be indicated for life-threatening situations, such as a sucide attempt after the rape. Option no. 4 is a legal action and not a type of prevention. P/SM, AN, H

427. no. 1. There is no attending underlying medical condition or actual loss of function. Clients with hypochondriasis are preoccupied with a fear of having a grave illness. There is no medical basis for their concerns. Hypochondriasis is not a psychotic disorder. P/A, AS, PC

428. no. 4. Color, along with heart rate, reflex irritability, muscle tone, and respirations, is evaluated as part of the Apgar score. CBF/N, AS, PS

429. no. 4. The use of play to prepare a child for surgery is an effective teaching strategy and helps to decrease anxiety. Although there is some truth to option no. 3, option no. 4 describes a wider application of play. C/I, PL, PC

430. no. 1. Minimizing the risk of a respiratory infection carried by others would be important preoperatively. C/I, IM, PS

431. no. 2. Clients are responsible for their own health care and have a right to choose their own habits. The nurse has a right to insist on a model of health behavior in class. A/O, PL, H

432. no. 2. A low-fiber diet has been associated with an increased risk of colorectal cancer, possibly by promoting a slow stool transit time and fecal stasis, which gives potential carcinogens more contact time with the intestinal lining. X-ray exposure is associated with leukemia. A high intake of smoked foods is associated with gastric cancer. Alcohol abuse has been linked to laryngeal cancer. A/E, AS, H

433. no. 4. Anxieties are displaced onto the body in an effort to cope. Although hypochondriasis is a replacement of behavior, it does not produce adaptation. It is not a voluntary exclusion of anxiety from the conscious level as in repression. Clients with hypochondriasis do not attempt to justify their behavior, nor do they have a conscious understanding about their behavior. P/A, AN, PC

434. no. 2. A cardiac angiography or catheterization is done to confirm heart disease, determine the extent of heart disease, obtain cardiac pressures, measure oxygenation in the blood, and measure the contractility of the heart as measured by the ejection fraction, >50% being normal. A cardiac catheterization does not dilate coronary blood vessels, force oxygen to the myocardium, or bypass the blocked coronary artery. A/O, AN, PS

435. no. 3. The lower GI series (barium enema) requires a specific dietary and bowel-cleansing protocol before the exam. The day before the exam the client is restricted to clear liquids for lunch and supper. The client is then NPO after midnight. The bowel is cleansed with magnesium citrate and bisacodyl (Dulcolax) the evening before the exam and suppositories or tap water enemas until clear the day of the exam. The rationale is that the bowel must be free of fecal debris for the barium to outline the intestinal surfaces. Any solid food the day of the exam is contraindicated. Options no. 1, no. 2, and no. 4 are appropriate preprocedural interventions. A/E, IM, PS

436. no. 3. Frequent swallowing is often an early sign of bleeding from the operative site after a tonsillectomy. The other options are normal after a tonsillectomy. C/SPP, AS, PS

437. no. 1. An experienced nurse should be available to

mothers who are beginning breast-feeding to provide assistance with proper technique during the first period of reactivity for the infant. Using the situation is a more effective teaching strategy than verbal or written information. CBF/P, IM, H

438. no. 4. Symptoms occur as an attempt to cope with stress and the ability to gain insight may decrease the need for secondary gain. Allowing her to talk about her physical symptoms provides secondary gain and reinforces preoccupation with illness. Physical symptoms must be assessed and treated, not minimized or avoided. P/A, IM, PC

439. no. 3. Sodium polystyrene sulfonate (Kayexalate) enemas reduce serum potassium levels. Cleansing enemas reduce bacteria, old blood, and fecal matter in the bowel; antibiotics reduce gastrointestinal flora. The client is restricted to clear liquids for 2 or 3 days before the surgery to control fecal accumulation. Gastrointestinal decompression may be required during the preoperative period if the client has a total or partial bowel obstruction from the tumor. A/E, PL, PS

440. no. 4. Clubbing, or a thickening and flattening of the finger and toe tips, is believed to occur because of chronic tissue hypoxemia and polycythemia. Chronic conditions that affect the oxygen-carrying capabilities of the blood may also be responsible. Acute conditions do not cause clubbing. C/O, AN, EV, PS

441. no. 3. Colostrum, secreted for 2 to 3 days after birth, has a high protein level, which facilitates binding of bilirubin and helps minimize neonatal jaundice through elimination in stool. All other statements are true. CBF/P, IM, PS

442. no. 4. An exaggeration of premorbid personality traits determines the behaviors exhibited in dementia. There is no correlation between the amount of brain impairment and amount of alcohol ingested to the severity of psychologic symptoms. The degree of orientation the client exhibits on admission may vary over time. P/C, AS, PC

443. no. 2. A single-barreled colostomy is always permanent. When the sigmoid colon has been preserved, regulation of bowel evacuation is possible, because stools are more formed here. Some such ostomates will be able to go without a colostomy bag. Others may find varying need for one, depending on their diet and success with irrigation. Sanguineous drainage from the stoma is abnormal and should be reported to the physician. A/E, AN, PS

444. no. 1. This statement is a myth. Because of incomplete myelinization of the spinal cord, there is a delayed reaction between the time of pain and body reaction, but the infant will still feel pain. C/I, AN, PS

445. no. 1. The bluish color is a sign of decreased vascularity of the tissue. The physician should be notified of this finding. The stoma should appear slightly pale immediately after surgery, then reddish-pink and moist in the postoperative phase. A/E, AN, PS

446. no. 3. Behavioral manifestations are most frequently noted in children experiencing pain. This is especially true of young children, who may not have the vocabulary to communicate pain, and in children who fear injections for pain relief. C/I, EV, PS

447. no. 2. The passage of flatus signals the return of gastrointestinal motility. Flatus may also appear as air in the colostomy bag. Rectal temperatures are contraindicated; the rectum was removed and the anal area was sutured or packed with a dressing after an abdominoperineal resection. Oral intake is not usually begun for several days. If the client is a diabetic or is receiving hyperalimentation, serum glucose levels, such as Accuchecks (peripheral stick glucose checks), are done. A/E, PL, PS

448. no. 4. The thick, puttylike mucilaginious meconium blocks the lumen of the small intestine, usually at or near the ileocecal valve, causing intestinal abstruction. Manifestations include abdominal distention, vomiting, constipation, and increased dehydration. C/NM, IM, PS

449. no. 3. Memory impairment that affects knowledge of time occurs first, then confusion of place, and finally confusion of person. P/C, AS, PC

450. no. 4. Consistancy of routine and staff structure and a sense of security. In coordinating the client's schedule, it is important to avoid excessive stimulation and variations, which might only serve to confuse the client further. Making numerous introductions may be futile because of client's loss of memory for recent events is impaired. P/C, IM, PC

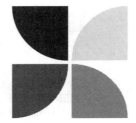
451. no. 4. The irrigation catheter with a cone may be inserted until snug or up to 4 inches. Use 1000 ml of water or less to irrigate; more may produce abdominal cramping. To prevent further electrolyte imbalance do not irrigate if diarrhea is present. The catheter tip should be lubricated with a water-soluble lubricant such as K-Y jelly. Antibiotic preparations are not necessary. A/E, IM, E

452. no. 3. Ostomates sometimes find that odor is reduced by taking charcoal or bismuth subcarbonate, with the physician's approval. Clear liquids such as tea and water are advised during diarrhea, and the physician should be notified in order to monitor electrolyte imbalances. Stool softeners such as docusate sodium (Colace) can help prevent hard stools. Laxatives are not advised. Carbonated beverages can exacerbate cramping. A/E, IM, H

453. no. 2. An elevated sweat chloride level is the definitive diagnostic test for cystic fibrosis. Trypsin from duodenal secretions is sometimes measured if the sweat chloride results are questionable. C/NM, AS, PS

454. no. 2. Confabulation is a process whereby experiences are imagined to fill in memory blanks. It is a form of protection against anxiety. Amnesia is loss or lack of memory. Dissociation is defined as segments of the personality or mental processes separating from the conscious mind. Free association is a process whereby the client is encouraged to describe thoughts or feelings as they occur. P/C, IM, PC

455. no. 3. Respiratory synacytial virus (RSV) bronchiolitis is a lower airway condition and is usually associated with thick secretions. Option no. 1 is indicative of upper airway conditions. Conjunctivitis is not usually present, and most infants are febrile. C/I, O, AS, PS

456. no. 1. These are the only foods listed that are not known gas producers. Legumes, onions, peas, cabbage, carbonated beverages, nuts, and chewing gum often cause gas. Milk can cause gas in clients with a lactose intolerance. Foods that caused gas before the surgery will continue to cause a problem with gas production after surgery. A/E, EV, H

457. no. 4. This motion is the only one listed that uses the quadriceps muscles. It increases their strength. A/M, IM, PS

458. no. 1. An immediate short-term goal would be that the client is able to confidently initiate the process of

breast-feeding. Breast-feeding is generally done on demand with an expectation of 8 to 12 feedings each 24 hours for the first 3 to 4 weeks. Supplements can interfere with adequate milk production and are unnecessary. Infant nutrition and hydration needs are met completely with breast milk. CBF/P, PL, H

459. no. 3. This response conveys empathy and emotional support. Continued contact is important for both father and family. The client with dementia will be aware of a caring person even though he may not always display recognition. Although it is true that Mr. Ochato is probably disoriented by his new surroundings, chances are that he will still not know his daughter or any other family members tomorrow because of the nature of Alzheimer's disease. P/C, IM, H

460. no. 2. Hemorrhage is a risk because the large vessels have been severed. The first postoperative day is too early for the client to accept the loss and look at the stump. Heat to the surgical area is inappropriate. The pain after amputation is commonly mild. Phantom pain should always be taken seriously and medicated for as requested by the client. A/M, IM, PS

461. no. 3. Poor memory of recent events is common in this condition. Aphasia is not necessarily associated with this dementia, but may be found in clients with vascular dementia. Refusal to cooperate and social withdrawal are also not limited to dementia. P/C, AN, PC

462. no. 2.

$$\frac{250 \text{ mg}}{1.2 \text{ ml}} = \frac{100 \text{ mg}}{x \text{ ml}} \quad \frac{100(1.2)}{250} = 0.48 \text{ ml}$$

C/NM, IM, PS

463. no. 4. Incontinence may occur frequently in a client with this syndrome. The nurse needs to convey empathy and understanding as well as institute nursing measures that will decrease its occurrence. Options no. 1, no. 2, and no. 3 convey a lack of understanding of dementia plus an unnecessary annoyance with the client that is nontherapeutic. He will probably be unable to work with the nurse to discover how to prevent his incontinence or change his clothes and clean up. P/C, IM, PC

464. no. 3. This position prevents hip contracture. Lotion is contraindicated for the stump; it keeps the skin soft, which increases the risk of skin breakdown. Elevating the stump after the first 24 hours results in flexion contractures, and a pillow between the thighs promotes abduction fixation. Both of these result in difficulty walking with the prosthesis. A/M, IM, PS

465. no. 2. Encouraging the client to reminisce about her life as a surgeon is valuable in maintaining her sense of value and integrity. It also helps decrease feelings of isolation and promotes a sense of continuity. Options no. 1, no. 3, and no. 4 reflect the client's disorientation; the nurse should not reinforce the client's confusion and disorientation. P/C, IM, PC

466. no. 3. The weight of the client should be carried on the wrists and palms. The weight should not be carried on the axilla area because this pressure can damage the radial nerve and cause paralysis of the elbow and wrist extensor muscles. The axillary bar should be 1 to 2 inches below the axilla. Crutches should be 16 inches shorter than the client for best fit. The elbow should be fully extended when a step is taken. In the three-point gait (the most common crutch-walking gait), both crutches are moved forward with the involved leg. The unaffected leg is then moved forward. A/M, IM, PS

467. no. 3. Even the most withdrawn client with schizophrenia is sensitive to other's feelings, even though they themselves communicate little verbally and may be unaware of their feelings. Clients diagnosed with paranoid schizophrenia generally demonstrate social isolation related to impaired ability to trust and are unreceptive to receiving attention from others. Response to treatment is generally slow. Electroconvulsive therapy is most successfully used with depressed clients and is not the first line of treatment for schizophrenia. P/W, AS, PC

468. no. 2. Virazole works by inhibiting the replication of RSV, which is simply messenger RNA. Because RSV is not bacterial, antibiotics are not necessary, and Virazole is administered only in a hospital setting. C/I, O, AN, PS

469. no. 4. Keeping the bladder empty will prevent urinary stasis, a common cause of cystitis. Although a nutritious diet is important, it only prevents infection indirectly by preventing anemia. Sixty-four ounces of clear, noncaffeinated liquid per day should be encouraged. CBF/P, IM, PS

470. no. 2. Applesauce helps disguise the taste of the enzymes; also, the cellulose in the applesauce retards the otherwise instant action of the enzymes. C/NM, EV, PS

471. no. 3. Pancreatitis is an inflammation of the pancreas, which leads to pancreatic tissue change, edema, swelling, ductal obstruction, necrosis, and hemorrhage. Autodigestion of the pancreas by the pancreatic enzymes has been suggested as a possible cause of the disease. The two major causes are high alcohol consumption and gallstones. There appears to be no relationship between race and incidence of pancreatitis. A/NM, AN, PS

472. no. 3. Hallucinations are the most common. Hallucinations temporarily decrease anxiety by delaying interaction with someone real. Delusion is a fixed, false belief that may be persecutory, grandiose, or somatic in nature and cannot be corrected with reasoning. Il-

lusion is a misinterpretation of a real sensory experience. Projection refers to attributing one's negative ideas and feelings to other people. P/P, AN, PC

473. no. 4. The exocrine portion of the pancreas secretes more than 500 ml of pancreatic juice daily that contains water, bicarbonate, electrolytes, and enzymes. The primary enzymes are amylase, lipase, chymotrypsinogen (converts to chymotrypsin), and trypsinogen (converts to trypsin). The enzyme pepsin is secreted by the stomach. Sucrase, lactase, dipeptidase, and maltase are enzymes secreted by the intestine. A/NM, AN, PS

474. no. 2. Psychosis related to an underlying medical condition such as an adverse drug reaction must be assessed, particularly if there is evidence of change in physical status. The other conditions also manifest symptoms of psychosis, but before a psychiatric diagnosis is made a differential diagnosis is crucial to treating clients appropriately. P/P, AN, PS

475. no. 1. Chronic pancreatitis causes degeneration of the islet cells, thereby decreasing production and secretion of insulin, which elevates the blood glucose level. Severe, steady, boring abdominal pain is a hallmark of pancreatitis. Serum amylase and lipase will be elevated. The abdomen will be distended related to intestinal hypomotility and chemical peritonitis. A/NM, AS, PS

476. no. 1. Fats are incompletely metabolized, and calcium ions are bound to fats; thus calcium ions are not absorbed in normal amounts. A/NM, AN, PS

477. no. 4. The retreat from reality of the client with schizophrenia is derived from internal ideas and desires not shared by others—autism. Aloofness refers to social distance and withdrawal. Ambivalence is having simultaneous conflicting feelings or attitudes toward a person or object. Apathy is a lack of interest and concern. P/W, AN, PC

478. no. 1. Clients with pancreatitis are given anticholinergic drugs to decrease secretions and relax spasms. The client will be kept NPO initially to rest the GI tract and then will be started on clear liquids once the acute phase has passed. IV fluids will be given to maintain fluid and electrolyte balance. Once the clear liquids are tolerated, the client will be given a bland, low-fat diet with no alcohol or caffeine to minimize stimulation of the pancreas. A/NM, PL, PS

479. no. 1. Agranulocytosis is the most serious side effect of clozapine. Other symptoms are not common side effects of clozapine. P/W, AN, PC

480. no. 3. Meperidine is preferred for the treatment of the pain of pancreatitis because it produces less spasm of the sphincter of Oddi. A/NM, AN, PS

481. no. 1. Nausea and vomiting and vomiting are not common side effects of phenothiazine neuroleptics. The other options are all noted side effects of phenothiazines; however, the most common side effects are extrapyramidal side effects such as akathesia, dystonias, and tremors. Prolixin is a high-potency antipsychotic agent, and use can also lead to development of tardive dyskinesia, an irreversible movement disorder. P/W, AS, PS

482. no. 1. Levels of pain will vary in the foot and leg. However, as the gangrenous area develops, pain decreases because of the nerve destruction that occurs. Despite the occurrence of gangrene, infection, or inflammation, pain may be totally absent in the client with advanced neuropathy or gangrene. A/NM, AS, PS

483. no. 2. Because clozapine increases the risk of agranulocytosis this drug is absolutely contraindicated in these clients. Other symptoms do not contraindicate taking this medication. P/P, AN, PS

484. no. 4. Pulmonary involvement is the leading cause of illness and death in children with cystic fibrosis. The major goal is to decrease the incidence of pulmonary infections to promote adequate oxygenation and increase life expectancy. C/NM, EV, H

485. no. 1. When the bladder is not emptied, it may push the uterus upward and to the side of the abdomen. On percussion, a full bladder emits a dull sound. Catheterization is not appropriate. Perineal pressure would not be related to bladder distention or urge to void. Intake and output alone would not indicate urinary retention. CBF/P, AS, PS

486. no. 4. A slow breathing pattern is desirable in early labor to ensure adequate oxygenation to the fetus. Modified paced breathing or accelerated breathing are useful in active labor. Panting is carried out if the client has the desire to push when it is not indicated. CBF/I, IM, H

487. no. 1. Benztropine mesylate (Cogentin) is effective in relieving the symptoms of parkinsonism caused by antipsychotic medications. This is an appropriate dosage and can be given parenterally if indicated. Trihexyphenidyl (Artane) is another good antiparkinson drug; however, the dose is 5 mg bid, not 15 mg. The use of anxiolytic agents (Buspar, Ativan) are not appropriate because these drugs do not have a direct effect on the extrapyramidal system. P/W, AN, PS

488. no. 4. Haloperidol is used parenterally every 7 to 21 days for outpatients. The other statements are false. Haloperidol has a mild anticholinergic sedating effect and extrapyramidal effect. Tolerance and addiction to antipsychotics are not substantiated in the literature, although mild withdrawal symptoms (e.g., headaches, irritability, and nausea) can occur after rapid discontinuation. P/W, AN, PS

489. no. 4. An immediate priority for the nurse is to determine the client's psychologic response to the physiologic happening: in this case, the death of a part of his body. The three ways of assessing a psychologic response are included in this option. A/NM, AS, PS

490. no. 1. Milieu therapy creates an environment that improve the physical and emotional condition of the client by providing positive living and learning experiences. The other options are an integral part of milieu therapy but not the overall goal. P/W, PL, E

491. no. 2. A footboard is not used; footdrop is not a concern because the client will not be on bed rest for long. The nursing actions are directed at promoting circulation by the prevention of pressure areas from developing in dependent areas. A/NM, PL, E

492. no. 3. When bed rest is prescribed for a client, fluids are increased, not decreased, to prevent urinary stasis. A/NM, PL, E

493. no. 2. Effective communication is a critical aspect of family therapy. Other options are not limited to family therapy, and no form of therapy can reduce the genetic link of bipolar disorder. P/E, PL, PS

494. no. 4. Refer families with children who have inherited disorders such as cystic fibrosis for genetic counseling. New screening tests are being developed for the prenatal detection of cystic fibrosis. C/NM, IM, H

495. no. 2. Keeping the area dry prevents moisture from promoting the growth of infection and macerating the skin. The other options would interfere with this. A/NM, PL, PS

496. no. 3. The client's symptoms represent severe anxiety. Mild anxiety does not produce the discomfort that this client is experiencing; it motivates growth and creativity. Moderate anxiety, which narrows the perceptual field, can be redirected with help, and clients can feel challenged to cope. The severely anxious person might have a greatly reduced perceptual field or develop a denial of existing feelings with selective inattention. Although problem solving is difficult, it is not impossible. P/A, AN, PC

497. no. 3. Decelerations can be detected early if fetal heart tones are evaluated during and soon after contractions, because they occur at this time. CBF/I, AS, PS

498. no. 2. The correct actions are stated in this option. Dakin's solution is used to debride the area, and petroleum jelly is a precautionary and preventive measure to protect the healthy tissue. A/NM, AN, PS

499. no. 4. The immediate goal is to reduce the client's anxiety. The focus is not immediately on the relationship, although trust in relationships with the nurse will occur. An immediate goal of gaining insight is impossible because a severe level of anxiety blocks cognitive functioning. P/A, PL, E

500. no. 4. Lice nits attach firmly to the hair shaft; dandruff flakes off easily. Lice do not cause areas of alopecia (ringworm does). Itching can occur with lice or dandruff. C/SPP, AS, PS

501. no. 3. Infection will increase the blood glucose level; thus the need for insulin increases. Infection results in a stress response in the body. Thus serum glucose levels will increase. Note that typically everything in life increases the need for insulin except exercise, which decreases the need for insulin. A/NM, AN, PS

502. no. 1. Persons in a panic state need to feel that someone understands their terror and that they will not be left alone. Reassurance minimizes the experience and distress of the present. Clients in panic must not be left alone because panic is experienced as dread and terror. Acting out or verbal expression of true feelings of anger and helplessness would be blocked. P/A, IM, PC

503. no. 4. The fetus is in a posterior presentation, resulting in fetal pressure on the mother's back. Squatting and hands and knees positions allow rotation of the fetal head to an anterior position, relieving the cause of back pain. Other options will not relieve or treat the pain. CBF/I, IM, PS

504. no. 1. A priority is to determine the client's perception of the condition before any teaching takes place. Remember, assessment occurs before planning or implementing nursing care, especially client education. A/NM, IM, PC

505. no. 2. Enlarged lymph nodes often accompany head lice. Honey-colored vesicles are characteristic of impetigo. Alopecia and ringlike lesions are characteristic of ringworm (tinea). C/SPP, AS, PS

506. no. 2. The fetal heart rate should be checked every 5 minutes for 15 minutes after rupture of the membranes because of the possibility of cord prolapse, an emergency situation that can be detected by a changed fetal heart rate pattern. CBF/I, IM, PS

507. no. 2. Clients may not want medication but may come to recognize their need for it and therefore ready themselves. Respond to the anxiety, not to the client's remark. The first remark is authoritarian and defensive. It makes an assumption that the client cannot refuse ordered medication. Options no. 3, and no. 4 are patronizing and discount the client's fear of addiction. P/A, IM, PC

508. no. 3. Gout is a disease of faulty purine metabolism and is characterized by increased amounts of uric acid, which forms into renal stones. The other options are all associated with calcium stones and are not indicated by the client's history. A/E, AN, PS

509. no. 4. These signs are indicative of delivery of the placenta, which signals the end of the third stage. Other signs of placental separation include a firmly contracted uterus, a change in uterine shape from discoid to globular, and a lengthening of the umbilical cord. Option no. 1 is indicative of delivery of the baby (end of second stage). Option no. 2 is the end of the first stage. Option no. 3 is not related to stage of labor. CBF/I, AN, PS

510. no. 1. Kwell shampoo can cause neurotoxicity if used more often than prescribed. The shampoo directions explicitly state not to shampoo more frequently than once a week. Laundering, but not disinfecting, clothing is helpful as a secondary activity. C/SPP, IM, E

511. no. 3. Use the assessment process to identify the factors that precipitated the client's present stage of anxiety. Be specific. Anxious clients need great assistance to stay focused. Option no. 1 is generalized and assumes a high level of awareness on the part of the client. Option no. 2 assumes a connection between client's job situation and the anxiety with little input from client. Clients with severe anxiety do not know how to help themselves. P/A, AS, PC

512. no. 2. The ability to communicate with the client is essential to the quality of care. A/NM, AS, E

513. no. 3. Lice are most often spread by sharing personal articles (e.g., comb or hat). C/SPP, AN, PS

514. no. 2. About the sixth week of pregnancy, the lower uterine segment becomes much softer than the cervix (Hegar's sign). Palpation of the fetal outline is possible at approximately 26 weeks. Quickening occurs between 16 and 20 weeks of gestation. Fetal heart rate can be detected at about 12 weeks by doppler device. CBF/A, AS, PS

515. no. 3. Drowsiness and dizziness are the most common side effects of lorazepan. The client's high level of anxiety (panic) does not manifest itself in drowziness and dizziness. The most common withdrawal symptoms include restlessness, agitation, seizures, and arise from abrupt cessation or reduction of medication. There is no indication that the client has not eaten today. P/A, AN, PS

516. no. 2. Respiratory status is always the primary concern. Blood pressure, heart rate, and mental status would be the next priority. A/NM, AS, PS

517. no. 2. A single shampoo with Kwell kills the ova in nearly all cases. If observable nits are no longer present, the nurse and parent can safely assume that the child's condition is no longer communicable. C/SPP, IM, H

518. no. 1. Uncomplicated bereavement is characterized by a loss, sleeping and appetite disturbances, or decreased energy. She may be experiencing anxiety about being alone, but the symptoms indicate feelings of depression. Psychosis would include more severe symptoms such as disorganized and incoherent thinking. There is no indication of bipolar disorder, depressed episode. P/E, AN, PC

519. no. 4. The major and potentially most serious effect of chronic lead poisoning is neurologic damage. Therefore frequent assessment of neurologic status is imperative. C/SPP, AS, PS

520. no. 2. During the admission process, a family member fluent in both languages is the best person to help gather the essential data. In the Spanish culture, the family plays an important role in the care of the client and the success of treatment. A/NM, IM, E

521. no. 2. An indication of adaptive responses is resumption of activities of daily living. There is no evidence in the situation to suggest that the client is suspicious or paranoid. When clients self-care abilities improve, this indicates that the immobility imposed by depressed feelings is lifting. Options no. 1 and no. 3 reflect a person with a psychosis, and no. 4 reflects a goal for a person with anxiety. P/E, PL, E

522. no. 4. Allowing the siblings to room together will promote security for each of them because they are familiar with each other. C/SPP, IM, PC

523. no. 1. Mrs. Keyser's symptoms are manifestations of abnormal grief. She is not psychotic, there is not enough information about her father to link him with her present state, and she has effective communication skills. P/L, AN, PS

524. no. 3. This response is client centered and reflects the nurse's empathy. Option no. 1 gives false reassurance and minimizes the client's feelings and situation. Option no. 2 may help the nurse feel better by getting out of the situation, but it may not meet the client's need. The nurse can offer to help the client express feelings but should not pressure the client to talk. P/E, IM, PC

525. no. 4. This is not specifically a goal for the care of this client, although it is a behavior that could be expected at a later date, when the client is more comfortable and adjusted to her condition. A/NM, PL, E

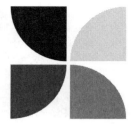

Answers and Rationales: Practice Test 8

526. no. 3. CaNa$_2$ EDTA is potentially toxic to the kidneys and can cause damage that can result in oliguria. The drug is administered IV, unless the child has encephalopathy. C/SPP, AS, PS

527. no. 1. The five-digit obstetric history notation includes number of *pregnancies* (gravida), number of *term* births, number of *preterm* births, number of *abortions,* and number of living *children.* This client has been pregnant four times including this current pregnancy. She has had 1 term delivery, 1 preterm delivery, 1 miscarriage (abortion), and has 3 living children. Gravida, term, and preterm count number of *pregnancies,* not number of fetuses. Multiple births are only included in the living children category. CBF/A, AS, PS

528. no. 1. Clients who are depressed and abruptly improve may have made the decision to commit suicide or may now be feeling better and have the energy to act on suicidal thoughts. Discharging the client or giving him a pass as soon as he improves is premature. P/E, AN, PC

529. no. 2. The practice of abdominal splinting facilitates postoperative performance of coughing and deep breathing. This is a priority because of the fact that a client performing these exercises will have less likelihood of respiratory complications. Respiratory stability is always a priority. A/S, PL, PS

530. no. 3. In the toddler, medication should be administered intramuscularly in the anterolateral thigh (vastus lateralis muscle). C/SPP, IM, PS

531. no. 3. When a depressed client becomes critical with others, it signals that the anger is moving from being inwardly directed to being directed out. This is a sign that the depression is lifting. An indication of regression would be returning to an earlier developmental level. The client is neither threatening the staff nor exhibiting suicidal behavior. P/E, EV, PC

532. no. 4. Improved mental well-being of a client is evidenced by an increased ability to carry out activities of daily living or self-care activities. When the depression is less incapacitating, the client has more energy to act. Option no. 1 reflects improvement from an anxiety disorder, no. 2 reflects improvement from psychosis, and no. 3 reflects improvement from paranoia. P/E, EV, PC

533. no. 3. Separating food and fluids can help control nausea and vomiting. The mother should be counseled to avoid food with high fat content, strong odor, or intense spiciness, but not foods high in fiber. Dry carbohydrates before arising and 5 or 6 small meals per day are recommended. CBF/A, IM, PS

534. no. 3. After the client has received preoperative sedation, he is no longer considered competent to sign the operative permit. The other options are true but unrelated to preoperative medication. A/S, IM, E

535. no. 2. This tells Raymond what is expected of him but also gives him an outlet for his fears. The other options either increase fear or belittle him. C/SPP, IM, PC

536. no. 4. In the second half of pregnancy, palpation of the uterus using Leopold's maneuver determines the position of the fetus. CBF/A, AS, PS

537. no. 2. Alcohol withdrawal involves four stages. Signs and symptoms occurring in stage I (8 hours or more after cessation of drinking) include mild tremors and nervousness. In stage II, symptoms include hyperactivity and disorientation. Mr. McKay was admitted on the previous day, and sufficient time had elapsed without alcohol ingestion, resulting in several signs of alcohol withdrawal. Major signs of cocaine withdrawal are primarily psychologic and behavioral and include severe depression and suicidal ideations. LSD does not produce major physical withdrawal symptoms. Opioid withdrawal consists of abdominal cramps, diaphoresis, and rhinorrhea, but no alterations in mental status. P/SU, AN, PS

538. no. 4. The circulating nurse is responsible for ensuring the safety of the client and preventing any harm from positioning. A/S, PL, E

539. no. 1. This menu is highest in vitamin D, calcium, and phosphorus, which are needed to aid in excreting lead from the bones. C/SPP, IM, H

540. no. 3. Contractions that occur at irregular intervals and are relieved by walking are Braxton Hicks' contractions. CBF/A, AN, PS

541. no. 4. Whenever a client talks with the nurse about another staff member, especially in a demeaning manner, the nurse should consider the possibility that the client is trying, consciously or unconsciously, to manipulate her to gain a sympathetic response. The nurse's role is to focus on the problem the client is having rather than give the desired response. Mrs. Myers is describing her reaction to the nurse, not this nurse's weaknesses. There are no data to suggest a thought disorder. P/SM, EV, PC

Key to abbreviations may be found on p. 255.

542. no. 4. The conscious interpretation of pain takes place in the cerebral cortex. A/S, AN, PS

543. no. 4. Lead does not interfere with platelet production or bleeding and clotting mechanisms. The other tests are used to monitor effects of lead poisoning. C/SPP, AN, PS

544. no. 3. Achievement of age-appropriate developmental milestones indicates there has been no permanent neurologic damage. C/SPP, EV, H

545. no. 3. The client with borderline personality disorder tends to have a pervasive lack of concern and empathy for others. The client with a personality disorder has minimal insight and poor impulse control, which results in acting-out behavior. Compliance and passivity are seen in clients with low self-esteem who depend on others for validation. Option no. 4 is also incorrect because these clients lack insight into their problems. P/SM, AS, PC

546. no. 3. This rate is too slow to be a fetal heart rate. The nurse is most likely hearing a uterine souffle as blood rushes through the placenta. This rate is the same as the mother's pulse. If the mother's pulse rate is not 96, further assessment would be required. CBF/A, AN, PS

547. no. 1. Movement of the client from the operating room table to the postanesthesia room may cause a transient drop in blood pressure. This may be a normal response to the anesthetic agents. The nurse must monitor the client for a further drop in blood pressure. The nurse must also evaluate what is normal for this client. A/S, IM, PS

548. no. 2. Standing a male client who is experiencing postoperative urinary retention at the bedside may facilitate voiding. Waiting is not appropriate, and explanations will not solve the problem. Catheterization may eventually be necessary but is not the first step. A/S, IM, PS

549. no. 2. Because this may be an arterial bleed, it is most important to control the amount of blood loss. Pressure should be placed above the puncture site where the vessel was entered. Amy should also be placed flat on the floor. Walking her back to bed will increase the rate of bleeding. C/O, IM, PS

550. no. 1. Clients with personality disorders consistently engender uncomfortable feelings of anger, frustration, helplessness, and defensiveness in staff. The deliberate, manipulative behaviors are blatant enough that there is no confusion about what is happening. Staff reactions toward the client with a personality disorder are usually negative rather than positive. An absence of feelings is sometimes seen in response to clients with schizophrenia, and boredom can be experienced with withdrawn, depressed clients. P/SM, AS, PC

551. no. 4. The contraction stress test uses medication to assess fetal response to maternal contractions. The nonstress test neither uses medication nor is used to diagnose PIH. Ultrasound is used to determine gestational age. CBF/A, AN, PS

552. no. 3. When secretions are retained, they block the small alveoli and cause them to collapse. The resul-

tant inflammation often leads to pneumonia. A/S, AN, PS

553. no. 2. Both mother and neonate are at risk because of prolonged rupture of membranes before delivery. Once membranes rupture, microorganisms can ascend into the uterus, causing chorioamnionitis. Mother and infant are both assessed for developing infection. CBF/P, AN, PS

554. no. 4. Turning the head to locate sounds should be present before 4 months of age. All other options are age appropriate. C/H, AS, H

555. no. 1. Because staff feel so frustrated and upset with clients with personality disorders, these clients are rarely sought out. Reinforcing positive behavior is an effort to reward the client with attention. Options no. 2 through no. 4 tend to foster the client's chronic manipulative behavior. P/SM, IM, PC

556. no. 2. Regression and increased demands for attention are common occurrences in older siblings, and parents need to be alerted to expect this behavior. The 2-year-old requires the security and confidence that her mother as well as her father loves her in spite of the new baby. Option no. 1 is not developmentally appropriate for a 2-year-old. C/H, IM, E

557. no. 3. Immunizations should be postponed if the child has a febrile illness. This is a nursing decision. The child's symptoms do not warrant referral to a physician at this time. C/H, IM, PS

558. no. 1. Observe the interaction between Lucida and her father. Abusers frequently do not offer appropriate comfort or support to the distressed child. The abused child frequently appears wary of the caregivers or does not seek them out for comfort and affection. Options no. 2, no. 3, and no. 4 may prove useful, but no. 1 will provide the most important information to assess child abuse. P/SM, AS, PC

559. no. 2. During any seizure, restraining the client can create more trauma than the seizure itself. Other options listed are appropriate to protect client safety. A/SP, IM, E

560. no. 2. All other assessments are normal in the postpartal period. A temperature elevated above 100.4°F (38°C) indicates sepsis. Leukocytosis normally occurs after delivery and may be related to the stress of labor and delivery. A process of diuresis begins after delivery and may be pronounced at night. The client eliminates excess fluid through the skin and urinary tract in an attempt to return to normal water metabolism. Hematocrit should be slightly elevated or returning to prepregnant levels by 2 days postpartum. CBF/P, AN, PS

561. no. 1. All the choices listed are important, but instituting seizure precautions is the priority. A/SP, IM, PS

562. no. 3. Dexamethasone (Decadron) is the only corticosteroid that crosses the blood-brain barrier. It is the most commonly used steroid in clients with neurologic damage because of its antiinflammatory action. A/SP, AN, PS

563. no. 2. Taking hold, or maternal independence, usually occurs 2 to 10 days postpartum and is characterized by anxiety, readiness to learn, and mood swings. Taking in occurs 1 or 2 days postpartum and is characterized by dependence, focus on self, and reviewing the birth. Letting go, or bursting out, occurs 10 days to 6 weeks postpartum and is characterized by interdependence, realistic role transition, and new norms. CBF/P, AN, PC

564. no. 3. All suspected cases of child abuse must be reported to the child protective services agency. Personnel cannot be prosecuted for defamation of character if their suspicions prove to be incorrect. Option no. 1 is not helpful at this time and would create further problems. The law requires the use of protective services rather than directly involving the police. Doing nothing jeopardizes the child's life. P/SM, IM, E

565. no. 3. The extrusion reflex is present until approximately 4 months of age. Although the infant may be hungry, she cannot bring solids to the back of her mouth yet. The child will outgrow this with practice. Altering eating patterns or foods because of this may establish poor feeding habits. C/H, IM, H

566. no. 4. A spontaneous bowel movement may be delayed until several days after delivery. Within 24 hours following delivery, the fundus should have begun involution and be located below the umbilicus. The breasts should be soft at this time because breast milk does not come in until 2 to 3 days after delivery. Lochia rubra is typical at this time. CBF/P, AN, PS

567. no. 2. Although identification of support systems is important, the ability to deal with any negative feelings is imperative in establishing a working relationship. The family's present and past coping patterns do have value, but it has a lower priority and is more likely to be obtained after a relationship is established. Option no. 4 has a lower priority and does not necessarily facilitate an effective working relationship. P/SM, IM, PC

568. no. 2. Hydronephrosis is caused when the ureter is obstructed and urine backs up and distends the kidney. Nephrosis, also called nephrotic syndrome, is an abnormal condition of the kidney from glomerular disease, thrombosis of a renal vein, or as a complication of many systemic diseases. Classic findings are marked proteinuria, hypoalbuminemia, and edema. A/E, AN, PS

569. no. 2. The shorter, wider, straighter eustachian tube in the young child predisposes the child to develop otitis media. Mechanical or functional obstruction of the eustachian tube results in accumulation of secretions and negative pressure in the middle ear. C/SPP, AN, PS

570. no. 2. The perineum should be wiped from front to back to prevent contamination of the vagina or urinary meatus. Clean tap water may be used for perineal care: sterile water is not necessary. The perineum should be washed with mild soap and water at least once a day. CBF/P, IM, E

571. no. 1. Attendance at a parent-support group indicates that the client might be willing to invest time and that there is some motivation to change. Bringing gifts and calling the hospital do not necessarily indicate a commitment to furthering parenting skills. Attendance at the parents' group (which deals with feelings and needs of parents and children) demonstrates interest, motivation, and commitment. P/SM, EV, H

572. no. 2. Unless the pain is controlled, there is little chance the stone will be safely passed. All of the other choices would be actions to take after pain is controlled. Also, based on Maslow's hierarchy of needs, the physiologic need of pain relief takes priority. A/E, IM, PS

573. no. 1. Hearing loss and subsequent delayed speech development may be a result of recurrent otitis media, especially when it occurs in infancy. C/SPP, EV, H

574. no. 2. To prevent nipple cracking, air-drying after each nursing period is suggested. Alcohol causes drying of the nipples with an increase in the chance of skin breakdown. Feeding positions should be rotated to change the site of maximum suck stress on the nipple. The infant should get the nipple and areola into his mouth when sucking to prevent nipple trauma and breakdown. CBF/P, EV, H

575. no. 1. A lack of empathy for others, poor impulse control, and difficulty managing stress are major symptoms of borderline personality disorder. Such clients make unrealistic appraisals of others and usually do not demonstrate ritualistic or fearful behaviors. Ritualistic behavior is seen in compulsive personalities. Intense fear of rejection, disapproval, and inability to make simple decisions are major symptoms of dependent personality disorder. P/SM, AS, PC

576. no. 1. Inorganic calcium stones occur in alkaline urine and often follow a urinary tract infection. A/E, AN, PS

577. no. 1. The mother is dependent in the taking-in phase. She needs to integrate the birth experience and be mothered so that she can mother her infant. Options no. 2 and no. 3 indicate the taking-hold phase. Option no. 4 is consistent with the letting-go phase. CBF/P, AN, PC

578. no. 2. This game teaches a sense of object permanence, which gradually develops from 4 to 8 months. Options 1 and 4 relate to older children, while option 3 lists an activity seen with younger children. C/H, PL, H

579. no. 2. Appetite, sleep, and concentration disturbances along with a sad mood and irritability are symptoms of a major depressive episode when underlying medical conditions are ruled out. Administering an antidepressant is the most appropriate consideration at this time. Antipsychotic and antimanic agents are useful in the treatment of psychosis and bipolar disorder, respectively. Electroconvulsive therapy is not generally used as the first line of treatment for depression unless there are major physical contradictions. P/E, AN, PS

580. no. 2. Dark-red, "currant jelly" stools indicate the onset of bowel necrosis from gangrene. C/E, AS, PS

581. no. 3. It is safe to resume sexual intercourse by the third or fourth week if bleeding has stopped and the episiotomy has healed. Most couples resume intercourse before the 6-week checkup. CBF/P, IM, H

582. no. 2. Vitamin C, when given in large (1 g) daily doses, is excreted through the urine to acidify it. A/E, AN, PS

583. no. 4. All options may occur, but the specific reason is to prevent loss of bladder tone. A/E, AN, PS

584. no. 3. Manipulation is characteristic behavior of clients like Mrs. Lord. These clients seldom ruminate, lose contact with reality, or have ritualistic behavior. Increased feelings of suspiciousness are generally associated with psychotic disorders. Hallucinations occur in psychotic individuals and clients using street drugs (e.g., cocaine or PCP). Although depersonalization and splitting occur and are serious distortions of reality, actual psychosis is the exception rather than the rule. Depersonalization is not a characteristic symptom of borderline personality disorder. P/SM, AS, PC

585. no. 2. Metrorrhagia is bleeding between periods. It may be the first sign of cervical cancer. CBF/W, AN, PS

586. no. 2. Bethanechol (Urecholine) is a cholinergic drug, which mainly increases bladder tone and promotes urination. Reglan, also a cholinergic, mainly stimulates peristalsis and increases esophageal sphincter tone. A/E, AN, PS

587. no. 4. Nursing notes should include clear, measurable, and specific descriptions. A/O, AS, PS

588. no. 4. The average 9-month-old infant may be able to say "mama" or "dada" but has not learned to articulate other words yet. C/H, AS, H

589. no. 3. This is another sign of endometritis. Lochia would have a red-brown color and may be either foul smelling or odorless. An increase in thirst is most likely a result of dehydration. Diastasis recti is separation of the abdominal muscle as a result of weakened muscles and is unrelated to infection. CBF/P, AN, PS

590. no. 4. Because clients with borderline personality disorder have a tendency to manipulate and use others, they should not be asked to assist staff with other clients. Clients with borderline personality disorder require firm limits on their behavior because they have little inner control. A firm, consistent, and positive attitude will help strengthen the client's ego, which will help the client manage stress more effectively. By expecting the client to act in a realistic, mature way, less regression should occur. P/SM, IM, PC

591. no. 4. Consistent limit setting is necessary in order to teach the client with borderline personality disorder to relate to others in socially acceptable ways. The client has little internal control and needs to learn control of impulsivity and acting-out behavior. Clients with borderline personality disorder distort social problem areas and blame others for their problems. This client will antagonize others with critical and hostile complaints and verbal abuse. P/SM, IM, PC

592. no. 2. Ophthalmia neonatorum is an eye disease of infants that causes blindness. It is passed from mother to infant through a birth canal infected with gonorrhea or other pathogens such as chlamydia. Antibiotic eye ointments, such as erythromycin or tetracycline, or penicillin drops prevent this. Retinopathy of prematurity is caused by prolonged exposure to high oxygen levels. *Treponema pallidum* is the organism that causes syphilis. Chemical conjunctivitis is a side effect of antibiotic eye medication. CBF/N, AN, PS

593. no. 4. Clients with borderline personality disorder manipulate to avoid facing and working on their own problems. Genuine social skill development occurs gradually. Impulse control is demonstrated when client shows restraint, not when focusing on other clients' problems. There is no evidence that the client is learning problem-solving skills. P/SM, EV, PC

594. no. 2. A gunshot wound is grossly contaminated, and an abdominal wound would bleed profusely; clean towels would be appropriate. A/O, AN, PS

595. no. 3. Acrocyanosis (blue hands and feet) is due to poor peripheral circulation. CBF/N, AN, PS

596. no. 3. Although all these goals are important, the child is especially at risk for dehydration and electrolyte imbalance because of vomiting associated with intussusception. C/E, PL, E

597. no. 4. This approach is demonstrating consistent limit setting in a matter-of-fact way. A firm and consistent approach is necessary, so it is important not to ignore the incident. The nurse is responsible and accountable for meeting with the client. Threatening to call her physician reflects a negative reaction to the client. P/SM, IM, PC

598. no. 4. The nasogastric tube may be obstructed, causing the abdominal distention. Inserting a rectal tube is contraindicated because the infant has had lower intestinal tract surgery. C/E, IM, E

599. no. 2. Removing or disturbing the knife in a chest wound can cause severe damage or massive hemorrhage. The knife acts as a tamponade to the affected sites. Cleaning or covering the knife may cause it to move, which may result in further damage and bleeding. A/O, IM, PS

600. no. 2. Internal thoracic injury leads to an air leak within the tissues and thereby causes subcutaneous emphysema. A/O, AN, PS

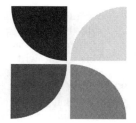

Answers and Rationales: Practice Test 9

601. no. 4. If Keith lives in an endemic area, it is most important that Mrs. Kohlberg check him after playing. Option no. 3 is not realistic. Keith should wear light-colored clothes, preferably a T-shirt and long pants with socks. Insect repellents will probably be useless unless they contain the chemical DEET. C/SPP, AN, H

602. no. 3. A ruptured bladder causes the sensation of needing to void. The urine is actually collecting in the peritoneal cavity. A urethral tear typically results in blood seepage around the catheter. A/O, AN, PS

603. no. 2. Grasping the tick with tweezers just behind its neck and then turning clockwise will loosen the tick's grip and make removal easier. Vaseline around the tick will make removal more difficult. A tick should not be pried loose, and the heat will only irritate the tick and cause it to feed and regurgitate its contents more quickly. C/SPP, IM, H

604. no. 1. This procedure is essential to prevent the administration of incompatible blood, which could result in the client's death. It is essential to check the client's blood band on the client's arm. Just checking the chart does not ensure that the client receives the correct blood. Options no. 3 and no. 4 are important but do not require two nurses. A/O, IM, E

605. no. 2. Separation anxiety begins at about 8 months of age and can cause extreme distress for the infant in this age group. C/E, AN, H

606. no. 3. A history of hepatitis disqualifies a potential blood donor for life. The other options do not disqualify a person from blood donation. A/O, AS, PS

607. no. 3. When breast-fed, an infant's stool is light yellow and mushy. Stools go through a transitional process from black meconium in the first 24 hours to a greenish-yellow (transitional) color to a breast-fed or bottle-fed stool on the fifth day of life. CBF/N, AN, PS

608. no. 1. An activity box will promote continued development of fine motor skills and hand-eye coordination and allow the infant some activity within the confines of his hospital crib. C/E, IM, H

609. no. 4. Daily staff conferences must be held to discuss client behaviors and plan a consistent approach for all three shifts; clients with borderline personality disorder have an amazing ability to split the staff. Although clinical and administrative aspects of the matter must be explored by nursing management, better methods than that described in option no. 3 can be taken if staff behavior becomes problematic. P/SM, IM, PC

610. no. 2. Normal saline is used because it is an isotonic solution. A/O, AN, PS

611. no. 3. Bleeding under the skin at the IV site indicates infiltration or leaking around the site. All the other options given are findings of a transfusion reaction. A/O, AS, PS

612. no. 1. Infants should not be switched to whole milk (or 2% low-fat milk) until 1 year of age. Other options are appropriate for a 10-month-old. C/E, IM, H

613. no. 4. Phenylalanine is an amino acid found in milk. If testing occurs before 48 hours of age, the mother's breast milk is not sufficiently established to give an accurate result. Therefore it may be necessary to re-test the infant later. CBF/N, AN, PS

614. no. 2. The client with borderline personality disorder needs limits and does not have the ability to adaptively set personal limits and rules. Analyzing requests, holding daily staff conferences, and using written care plans are effective in decreasing manipulation and consequently staff anger as well as splitting of staff. P/SM, IM, PC

615. no. 3. It is imperative that the blood be stopped, the tubing be disconnected at the IV site, and the IV needle be left in place and kept patent with a new IV tubing and normal saline to administer other fluids and medications to counteract the reaction. Option no. 2 is a second action, and no. 1 is a third action. A/O, IM, E

616. no. 2. Perfect matches of all four HLAs are found in monozygotic twins and 25% of natural siblings (born of the same pair of parents). The degree of compatibility of remaining siblings varies. A/E, IM, PS

617. no. 1. Removing the nipple frequently while feeding breaks the suction, causing the child to swallow more air. This also frustrates the child, and crying further aggravates the problem. Breast-feeding is permitted, but it is more difficult. C/NM, IM, E

618. no. 2. The amount of lanugo decreases while plantar creases increase with increasing gestational age. These are elements of the modified Dubowitz scale. Determining gestational age by physical examination most often involves the Dubowitz assessment, which provides the correct gestational age within 2 weeks (in 95% of infants). CBF/N, AS, PS

Key to abbreviations may be found on p. 255.

619. no. 2. Clients are often prevented from beginning resolution of their grief when they are unable to attend funerals of loved ones. Options no. 1, no. 3, and no. 4 are all possible explanations for why he is thin and socially withdrawn, but he is having a delayed grief response because his physical condition prevented him from going through the normal funeral ritual. P/E, AN, PC

620. no. 1. Azathioprine (Imuran) is a potent drug that produces immunosupression by inhibiting purine synthesis in cells. It is used in renal transplants to prevent organ rejection. The client should avoid crowds and infectious individuals, because infection is a serious consequence in a client who is immunocompromised. The client is instructed to report chills, fever, sore throat, and fatigue immediately. Azathioprine does not stimulate kidney output or increase the number of circulating antibodies. In fact, leukopenia occurs during therapy. Azathioprine does not significantly alter blood pressure, so frequent monitoring is not required. A/E, IM, PS

621. no. 1. This child will swallow a lot of air because of the abnormal openings. The other answers are contraindicated. C/NM, PL, PS

622. no. 4. Rejection is the body's reaction to foreign tissue. Symptoms of kidney rejection include a swollen and tender kidney, weight gain, fever, elevated blood pressure, decreased urine output, elevated serum creatinine levels, anorexia, malaise, and drowsiness. The white blood cell count does not rise. A/E, AS, PS

623. no. 2. An Isolette should be maintained at a temperature of 92° to 94°F (33.3° to 34.4°C). An infection in the neonate, not the mother, may be accompanied by an elevated or subnormal temperature. CBF/N, AN, PS

624. no. 1. Opening up and irrigating a closed sterile urinary drainage system increases the risk of infection in the immunosuppressed client. Reverse isolation will be maintained to protect the client from infection. Frequent turning and repositioning is required to prevent pneumonia. The stools must be routinely checked for blood because of the high risk of gastrointestinal bleeding with immunosuppressant drug therapy and the stress response to the overall therapy. A/E, PL, E

625. no. 3. Independence is encouraged by allowing him to select foods that appeal to him. Option no. 1 imposes another person on him and places a burden on the other client. Option no. 2 causes isolation and self-absorption. Option no. 4 is a good second choice if he will not select his own foods. P/E, IM, PS

626. no. 3. A witnessed, cosigned donor card is appropriate for the client who is a minor. A/E, IM, H

627. no. 1. Most surgeons prefer to repair the palate before the child develops faulty speech patterns. By 12 to 18 months of age, palatal growth has progressed enough to allow surgery. Although some surgeons prefer to wait until 4 or 5 years of age to allow complete palatal development, by that age the child's speech will have been permanently affected by the deformity. C/NM, AN, PS

628. no. 2. Prednisone is prescribed for its immunosuppres-

sive effects. Withdrawal of the drug makes it more likely that the body will reject the transplanted tissue. Increased risk of infection and psychosis are two side effects of prednisone. Anemia will not occur if prednisone is stopped. A/E, AN, PS

629. no. 3. Newborns lose up to 10% of their birth weight in the first few days after birth. Because this is expected weight loss, support the mother in her efforts to breast-feed. The normal neonate will void 6 to 10 times a day by the end of the first week of life. This is indicative of adequate hydration. Supplementary or replacement fluids can interfere with the supply and demand balance of breast milk production. CBF/N, IM, PS

630. no. 1. To correctly evaluate chest pain, it is essential to obtain an accurate description. Also, this question can elicit the client's knowledge about heart attacks. This will provide a basis for the discharge teaching plan. Option no. 4 is closed-ended, only giving a partial description and closing off other descriptions of the pain. Option no. 2 is important, but it is not the most relevant choice. It is also too general a question. A better question is, "Are you taking any medication to prevent or to stop the chest pain?" Option no. 3 assumes that the client smokes cigarettes. A/O, IM, PS

631. no. 4. These are appropriate nursing measures to promote sleep. Options no. 1, no. 2, and no. 3 are all stimulating actions that would increase arousal. P/E, IM, PS

632. no. 1. An electrocardiogram (ECG) reflects the electrochemical activity of the heart (i.e., the transmission of the cardiac impulse through the heart muscle). Information about heart perfusion, contraction, and integrity, which is evaluated by a cardiac catheterization, is inferred from ECG information but not measured directly. A/O, AN, PS

633. no. 2. Voiding is monitored to determine if edema from surgical trauma has closed off the urethra. Feeding the baby who has just been circumcised is comforting and essential because it is recommended that feedings be withheld for several hours before the procedure. The penis is checked hourly for bleeding; infection would not appear until much later. A sterile petrolatum-jelly dressing rather than dry gauze should be used on the newly circumcised penis to prevent it from sticking to the diaper. CBF/N, IM, PS

634. no. 4. When an organ such as the heart is damaged, it releases specific enzymes into the bloodstream. Options no. 1, no. 2, and no. 3 are incorrect. A culture and sensitivity is used to detect causative organisms of an infection. Arterial blood gas studies determine how well the blood is oxygenated and the acid-base balance of the body. A/O, AN, PS

635. no. 1. Clients with dysthemic disorder usually feel best in the morning and worse as the day progresses. P/E, PL, E

636. no. 2. Options no. 1, no. 3, and no. 4 do not relate to chest pain in any way. A/O, AN, PS

637. no. 3. The coronary arteries fill, and the aortic and pulmonary valves close during ventricular diastole. This is why diastolic pressures greater than 90 might result in angina. A/O, AN, PS

638. no. 4. Speech and hearing problems are common after this repair because of the necessary change in the palate arch and concomitant change in eustachian tubes. Contractures of the mandible are unrelated to this repair. C/NM, AN, H

639. no. 1. Eczema is most often seen in infancy. The most frequent cause is cow's milk and egg albumin allergy. The infant is at highest risk for developing an allergic response because the immune system is still not fully mature. C/SPP, AS, PS

640. no. 4. With traditional phototherapy, the unclothed infant is placed under a bank of lights to modify the bilirubin and make it excretable in urine and feces. Temperature fluctuations are possible; therefore infants must be monitored. Sufficient intake is required to eliminate the bilirubin through the gastrointestinal tract and prevent dehydration. Watery stools are common. Fluid loss is replaced by increasing the fluid volume offered to the neonate by 25%. Blood pressure is not relevant. CBF/N, PC, PS

641. no. 3. 1/150 grain = 0.4 mg. A/O, AN, PS

642. no. 2. Resolution of grief is exhibited by the ability to reminisce about both the positive and negative aspects of a relationship in a realistic manner. Crying is a normal response but will occur less often and for shorter periods. Detachment is a sign of abnormal grieving. Being able to talk about concerns shows an ability to deal with the reality of the loss but does not show resolution; it shows the beginning of the working phase in dealing with the grief. P/E, EV, PC

643. no. 2. Before treatment can be effective, the allergen that is causing the problem must be identified. C/SPP, PL, PS

644. no. 2. Active phase (stage one) generally spans from 4 to 7 cm dilation and is accompanied by moderate discomfort in most women. Latent phase spans 0 to 3 cm and is accompanied by less frequent contractions and mild discomfort. Transition phase is from 8 to 10 cm with intense contractions and pain. Second stage is from complete dilation until the birth of the infant. CBF/I, AN, PS

645. no. 3. Sublingual nitroglycerin appears in the bloodstream in about 2 minutes and peaks in 4 minutes; the effect begins to disappear in 10 minutes. The sublingual form should be taken at the onset of chest pain and every 5 minutes until the pain is relieved for a maximum of three doses. The client should be taken to the nearest emergency room if the pain is not relieved after three doses. A/O, IM, PS

646. no. 1. Because of its venous dilating effect, nitroglycerin may cause headache, hypotension, and dizziness. Other side effects of nitroglycerin include flushing, increased heart rate, a rebound effect from the decreased preload, and nausea. Shock, convulsions, hypertension, and loss of consciousness are not side effects of nitroglycerin. A/O, AS, PS

647. no. 3. Fresh nitroglycerin tablets cause a burning, tingling sensation. Sublingual nitroglycerin should be taken at the onset of chest pain. The client should not wait until the pain is severe. Sublingual nitroglycerin is not taken with meals. Headache and flushing are normal side effects so the physician does not need to be notified. A/O, IM, H

648. no. 3. Soaps are drying agents and are not used. Lipid lotions or agents are not good cleansing agents. Warm water increases itching; cool water promotes chilling and loss of body heat. Tepid baths soothe irritated skin and decrease itching. C/SPP, PL, PS

649. no. 1. Demerol should be given late enough in the labor that it does not slow the labor (active phase), yet not so late that it causes the newborn to be "sleepy" when delivered (transition). The situation given describes the optimum time to administer the pain medication. CBF/I, IM, PS

650. no. 1. The diagnosis of "psychologic factors affecting medical condition" is used when there is a clear relationship between the environment and the initiation or exacerbation of a physical condition. The client is not always aware of the relationship. Personality and hereditary factors may have contributed to the clients' physical problem, but the condition has been exacerbated by a stressful working environment. P/A, AN, PS

651. no. 2. Normal tidal volume is about 500 cc. A/O, AN, PS

652. no. 3.

$$\frac{100 \text{ mg}}{1 \text{ ml}} \times \frac{75 \text{ mg}}{x \text{ ml}} = 100 \, x = 0.75 \text{ ml}$$

OR

75/100 ml × 1 ml = 75/100 = 0.75 ml

CBF/I, IM, PS

653. no. 2. The amount of dead space in the respiratory tract increases with chronic obstructive pulmonary disease. Usual dead space is 100 to 150 ml. A/O, AS, PS

654. no. 3. Fowler's position with a slight forward lean best increases the expansibility of the lungs with minimal energy expenditure. A/O, IM, PS

655. no. 2. This is an age-appropriate activity that would provide a distraction for the child without giving her anything to scratch with. Working with clay requires more coordination than the average 2-year-old has; additionally, the clay may prove irritating to her skin condition. Although building columns with blocks is age appropriate for her, she may use the blocks to scratch or irritate her eczema. Until her eczema clears, she should play with safe objects with rounded edges. Although the average 2-year-old is able to hold a crayon and make circular and linear lines, they do not typically associate these markings with specific objects. C/SPP, IM, H

656. no. 2. The high P_{CO_2} is balanced by an increased bicarbonate, resulting in a pH of 7.40. The pH is within normal range (7.35 to 7.45); thus the client has physiologically compensated. If the pH is abnormal, the client is said to be in a decompensated state. A/O, AN, PS

657. no. 2. Wool is not used because it can irritate the skin. Synthetic materials are substituted for wool in coats, hats, gloves, etc. C/SPP, IM, H

658. no. 4. An emphysema client with an illness has the greatest risk of metabolic acidosis. A respiratory rate of 48 reflects a potential uncompensated state. The normal state of a client with chronic obstructive pulmonary disease may be compensated respiratory acidosis. A/O, AN, PS

659. no. 3. A client with chronic obstructive pulmonary disease adjusts to an increased Pco_2 and a decreased Po_2. This is why $Po_2 < 80$ is maintained for the stimulation of respirations. A/O, AN, PS

660. no. 3. The effects of selected medications on the fetus are generally heightened by increasing the dosage, giving the drug intravenously, and administering the agent close to delivery. CBF/I, AN, PS

661. no. 4. Terminally ill clients are least likely to experience a sense of control. They do, however, experience a sense of loss, disturbance in self-concept and anxiety. P/L, AS, PS

662. no. 4. Close-fitting clothes cause irritation and perspiration and increased itching. These should be avoided. Loose-fitting, one-piece clothing prevents access for itching. C/SPP, EV, H

663. no. 4. This client's electrolyte levels will not be affected by suctioning him. A/O, AN, PS

664. no. 3. Serum sodium of less than 130 mEq/L is indicative of hyponatremia. The posterior fontanelle is closed either at birth or within 2 months of age; normal specific gravity is between 1.010 and 1.020, and the heart rate, although slightly elevated, is not significant at this time. C/NM, EV, PS

665. no. 1. For clients with chronic obstructive pulmonary disease, the breathing stimulus is based on a low Po_2 (from 60 to 80 mm Hg). Administration of more than 2 to 3 L of oxygen impairs the respiratory drive. A/O, IM, PS

666. no. 4. Oral poliovirus vaccine is contraindicated in children who are immunosuppressed and in children who have household members who are immunosuppressed. The oral polio vaccine is composed of live, attenuated polioviruses. C/SPP, AN, H

667. no. 1. The client is slightly hypoxemic, but not cyanotic. This means his Po_2 is around 50 mm Hg. The normal range of Po_2 for COPD clients is usually 60 to 80 mm Hg. A/O, AS, PS

668. no. 2. Emphysema produces bronchiolar and alveolar changes that cannot be reversed. Treatment is aimed at relieving symptoms and liquefying and loosening secretions. A/O, AN, PS

669. no. 1. Acquired immunodeficiency syndrome is characterized by destruction of the immune system, including white blood cell production. A differential of white blood cells will give an indication of cell maturity and lymphocyte dysfunction. C/SPP, EV, PS

670. no. 2. Many drugs can cause suppression of the bone marrow and result in aplastic anemia. Vitamin B_{12} malabsorption is from a lack of intrinsic factor in the stomach; this is pernicious anemia. Genetic factors contribute to thalassemia, found in Mediterranean populations. A/O, AN, PS

671. no. 2. Expressing concerns and feelings can help the client understand the relationship between feelings and physical illness so that management of the environment can become more effective. Leisure activities may help reduce the client's stress, but psychosomatic illnesses will recur if the client does not learn effective stress-reducing activities. Continued repression of emotional tension in a stressful environment will increase the risk of a recurrence of illness. Option no. 4 is a good first step, but the client needs to learn how to express emotions. P/A, EV, H

672. no. 4. Skin color is affected by many things other than oxygenation, including cardiac output, hot or cold environment, anemia, and trauma. A/O, AS, PS

673. no. 2. The immense metabolic needs of the proliferating leukemic cells cause bone marrow depression and reduce red blood cell production. C/CA, AN, PS

674. no. 1. A bone marrow sample will allow evaluation of the marrow condition and number of erythrocytes, leukocytes, and thrombocytes. Schilling's test is to identify pernicious anemia. A differential blood cell count is commonly used to differentiate between a viral and bacterial infection. A/O, AN, PS

675. no. 3. Platelets are involved in clotting and coagulation and are decreased in number because of leukocytosis. C/CA, AS, PS

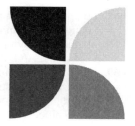

Answers and Rationales: Practice Test 10

676. no. 3. Antacids may neutralize the highly acidic gastric juice and thereby prevent a fatal chemical pneumonitis if vomiting and aspiration occur during anesthesia. CBF/I, AN, PS

677. no. 1. Chest pains, shortness of breath, hyperventilation, tingling sensation in the fingers, and worrying all the time are symptoms of a generalized anxiety disorder. The other disorders are also anxiety disorders with worrying all the time being characteristic of generalized anxiety disorders. P/A, AS, P, S.

678. no. 2. When providing nursing care to a client who has a low hemoglobin, conserve the client's energy. With low hemoglobin, less oxygen will be carried and available to the cells. Maintenance of fluid and electrolyte balance is important for any client but is not specific to someone with a diagnosis of aplastic anemia. A/O, PL, E

679. no. 1. Intramuscular injections can precipitate bleeding and are to be avoided. C/CA, PL, PS

680. no. 2. The thyroid, the regulator for the metabolic rate, produces and releases more thyroid hormones in hyperthyroidism. The increased hormones increase the metabolic rate. The increased metabolic rate leads to elevated vital signs, nervousness, and weight loss. This results in increased activity in and demands on all body systems. A/NM, AS, PS

681. no. 2. Occiput refers to vertex presentation; the words right and posterior refer to those portions of the maternal pelvis. Option no. 1 is correct but does not answer the client specifically; no. 3 and no. 4 are incorrect. CBF/I, IM, H

682. no. 3. Tachycardia is usual in hyperthyroidism, and a further increase in cardiac rate indicates thyroid crisis, a more toxic state. Cold intolerance, sensitivity to narcotics, and lethargy are symptoms of hypothyroidism. A/NM, AS, PS

683. no. 2. This indicates that Samuel is aware that myelosuppression occurs and is temporary. C/CA, EV, E

684. no. 3. Assigning the client to a private room may promote rest by decreasing stimulation. A/NM, PL, E

685. no. 3. The nurse's response encourages the client to express her feelings and redirects her from blaming the nurse to discussing what is bothering her. This response does not blame or judge. To back down because of an angry outburst will encourage further use of that behavior in difficult situations. Option no.

2 creates a power struggle between the client and the nurse. Option no. 4 is demeaning and leaves the client feeling more frustrated. P/A, IM, PC

686. no. 1. This is the most realistic nursing plan because it is supportive to the family without overburdening them. Options no. 2, no. 3, and no. 4 place too much responsibility on the family and do not allow them a respite. C/CA, PL, H

687. no. 1. A major consequence of malpresentation is the lengthening of labor through decreased efficiency of contractions, longer time for the presenting part to descend, and weaker forces working on the cervix, all of which slow dilation. Breech births are associated with trauma and higher neonatal morbidity. External cephalic version may be attempted. Usually a cesarean delivery occurs. CBF/I, AN, PS

688. no. 3. In a euthyroid state, a controlled thyroid situation, the client requires a regular diet. The client in a hyperthyroid state would have increased hunger as a result of the increased metabolic rate and would require a high-protein, high-calorie intake. A/NM, PL, PS

689. no. 3. The infant's temperature normally drops immediately after birth if the infant is not dried and well wrapped. The large body surface area and the difference in external temperature from the mother's internal temperature predispose the infant to chilling. The infant must be warmed immediately. One way to do this is placement under a radiant warmer. Bathing should be postponed until the temperature is 97.6° F for 2 hours. Neither administration of oxygen nor notification of the pediatrician is warranted. CBF/NR, IM, PS

690. no. 1. These symptoms are characteristic of hypothyroidism. The client will need an increase in the exogenous hormone. Lifelong daily replacement of thyroid hormones will be given to this client as indicated from the results of routine thyroid study results. A/NM, AN, H

691. no. 3. Leukocytosis (an elevated white blood cell count of greater than 10,000) is present with a bacterial infection. All other options are indicative of acute pyelonephritis. A/E, AS, PS

692. no. 1. Cold increases an infant's metabolic rate because of inability to shiver. This increases both oxygen and calorie consumption, necessitating the administration of more oxygen and calories. If they are unavailable, the infant develops metabolic acidosis,

Key to abbreviations may be found on p. 255.

which is manifested by lowered blood pH. CBF/N, AN, PS

693. no. 2. The most common sources of salmonella infection are poultry and eggs. Other sources include dogs, cats, hamsters, and pet turtles. C/NM, AN, PS

694. no. 4. Grunting is an abnormal breathing pattern, usually indicative of respiratory distress. Cephalohematoma, a collection of blood between the bone and periosteum, is the result of pressure sustained at birth, usually requiring no treatment. Milia, resulting from blocked sebaceous glands, is a normal newborn characteristic. Acrocyanosis, bluish coloration of the extremities caused by inadequate peripheral circulation, is a normal finding. CBF/N, AN, PS

695. no. 3. Collaboration with the nurse is an effective way for a client to receive help in decision making. Taking an excessively assertive stand with clients is an ineffective way to teach them how to make decisions. Giving more responsibility to the client's wife will not help. A client is less likely to follow orders when he has not actively participated in their development. P/A, PL, E

696. no. 3. Synthesis of vitamin K by *E. coli* bacteria occurs in the intestinal tract. Newborns have a sterile intestinal tract and lack the vitamin, which is essential in the formation of prothrombin and for normal blood clotting. CBF/N, AN, PS

697. no. 3. Phenazopyridine hydrochloride (Pyridium) is a local analgesic to the urinary tract and stops burning on urination. A/E, AN, PS

698. no. 3. Acrocyanosis can be present in a normal neonate because of immature peripheral circulation. Average pulse rate is 100 to 160 and respirations are 30 to 60 and irregular. CBF/N, AN, PS

699. no. 2. Increased fluids will help treat the symptoms of infection (i.e., elevated temperature, dysuria). A/E, PL, PS

700. no. 3. The female urethra is short, and its proximity to the vagina predisposes the client to infection. Bacterial contamination can result from sexual intercourse, and emptying the bladder before and after intercourse reduces this risk. Voiding every 2 hours is recommended to prevent urinary infections. A/E, IM, H

701. no. 4. Uncoordinated eye movements are a normal finding in full-term neonates because they have poor control of eye muscles. The normal heart rate is 100 to 160. Jaundice in the first 24 hours is considered pathologic. Nasal flaring is a sign of respiratory distress. CBF/N, AN, PS

702. no. 4. During the first few days after birth, the infant may lose 5% to 10% of her birth weight because of loss of excess fluid and minimal intake of nutrients. An 8-ounce weight loss is 7%. Supplementing is not necessary and may interfere with milk production. A 1-pound weight loss would be in excess of 10%. CBF/NR, IM, PS

703. no. 2. The posterior fontanel is closed by 2 months, and the anterior closes at 12 to 18 months. Although the anterior fontanel can be an indicator of dehydration at 6 months, the weight of the infant is a more

reliable sign of fluid loss and dehydration. C/NM, AS, PS

704. no. 3. The azo dye in phenazopyridine hydrochloride (Pyridium) stains the urine reddish-orange. It is important to inform the client when the initial dose is given, so that the client does not think something is wrong when the client voids. A/E, IM, PS

705. no. 2. Approximately 50% of full-term newborns develop jaundice around the third day of life in the absence of disease or a specific cause. This is called physiologic jaundice because of the rapid breakdown of fetal cells, resulting in an increase in bilirubin. This subsides approximately 5 to 7 days after birth without treatment. The level of jaundice described is not excessive and therefore not associated with pathology (liver dysfunction or infection). There is no blood type discrepancy, which would predispose to erythroblastosis fetalis. CBF/N, AN, PS

706. no. 4. A medical history would be important to assess for conditions affecting the course of pregnancy. Because this is the first prenatal visit, it would not be possible to determine a pattern of weight gain yet. Cervical dilation determination would not be appropriate at this time. Plans for childbirth would be appropriate in the third trimester. CBF/A, AS, PS

707. no. 1. The infant with a potassium deficit has muscle weakness and hyporeflexia, is anorexic, and develops cardiac dysrhythmias, rather than apnea. C/NM, AS, PS

708. no. 3. The "DS" product denotes double strength. A/E, AN, PS

709. no. 2. Chorionic villus sampling, removal of tissue from the fetal portion of the placenta, is done between 8 and 14 weeks for genetic testing and gives rapid results. Urine estriol determines placental function. Liver enzymes, platelets, and glucose determine maternal status. CBF/A, IM, PS

710. no. 3. Apple juice, which has a high osmolality, will tend to increase the number of stools and potentiate a dehydrated state. The other components are all parts of the BRATTS diet: bananas, rice, applesauce, tea, toast, saltines. C/NM, PL, PS

711. no. 4. Methenamine decomposes to formaldehyde and ammonia. The urine should be maintained at a pH of 5.5 or less for the most effective treatment. A/E, AN, PS

712. no. 4. Options no. 1, no. 2, and no. 3 will help prevent vascular pooling without greatly increasing oxygen demand. Coughing may increase intracranial pressure. A/SP, IM, E

713. no. 3. The myelomeningocele sac must be protected because the sac is prone to tears and subsequent infection, such as meningitis. C/SPP, PL, PS

714. no. 4. There is not enough information to make a judgment about the child's growth. Information concerning his previous growth pattern, his dietary habits and exercise patterns, and hereditary influences (growth of family members) is needed before conclusions can be drawn. C/H, AN, PS

715. no. 2. Natural rewarming is the least invasive and safest method of regaining the normal body temperature after induced hypothermia. A/SP, PL, PS

716. no. 4. Fetal limb abnormalities are not associated with smoking. Smoking increases the risk of all other complications listed. Nicotine and carbon monoxide are ingredients of tobacco linked with adverse effects. They result in vasoconstriction and inactivation of hemoglobin. CBF/A, AN, PS

717. no. 4. Cardiac irregularity is the most common complication of rewarming. A/SP, AS, PS

718. no. 2. Maintenance of proper positioning for a lumbar puncture is important. A lumbar puncture produces no risk to the respiratory system. An incision is not made. A/SP, IM, E

719. no. 3. Maternal isoimmunization in the Rh-negative expectant mother may occur if the baby inherits the father's Rh factor; therefore it should be determined if the father of the baby is Rh-positive. All other data would require no action. CBF/A, AN, PS

720. no. 2. During the acute phase, bed rest and passive range of motion will help conserve energy while maintaining good joint mobility. A/SP, PL, PS

721. no. 1. Unequal pupils indicate a possibility of increased intracranial pressure (ICP). With increased ICP a lumbar puncture is dangerous because of the risk of brain stem herniation from a sudden decrease in pressure when spinal fluid escapes. A/SP, AS, PS

722. no. 4. These are danger signs that indicate activity intolerance for mother or fetus. Swimming is allowed throughout pregnancy as long as membranes are intact. Exposure to very high temperatures such as are found in saunas and hot tubs should be avoided because they can increase the mother's own body temperature and subsequently harm the fetus. The Kegel exercise helps strengthen the pubococcygeal muscle, not relieve leg cramps. CBF/A, IM, H

723. no. 3. Results of visual-acuity testing are abnormal for the child's age, and he should be referred for a more comprehensive evaluation at once. Option no. 4 is wrong; options no. 1 and no. 2 are inappropriate. C/H, PL, PS

724. no. 1. Because Felicia has had the full recommended series, she will not need any additional immunizations until she is 11 to 12 years old; then she will need measles, mumps, rubella vaccines. C/H, PL, PS

725. no. 4. Poor reality testing is a problem for clients with a psychotic disorder; it is not a symptom of a physical disorder with psychologic factors. Dependency issues, indecision, and excessive controlling behavior are all characteristic of clients with psychologic factors affecting medical condition. P/A, AS, PC

726. no. 4. Meningitis is often accompanied by photophobia, a visual intolerance to light; therefore the client will be more comfortable in a dark room. With photophobia, lights cause discomfort in the eyes and are unlikely to cause a seizure. A/SP, AN, PS

727. no. 1. Myelomeningocele location along the spinal cord can reveal information about the child's future ability to ambulate. C/SPP, EV, PS

728. no. 1. Excessive milk intake limits ingestion of iron-rich foods. C/O, AS, PS

729. no. 1. The baby will contract herpes through the birth canal if delivered vaginally. This virus has a devastating effect on newborns, and many of those infected die. CBF/A, IM, PS

730. no. 3. An increase in alphafetoprotein is indicative of neural tube defects in the fetus. Lung maturity is assessed in late pregnancy by determining the L/S ratio; a ratio of 2:1 indicates fetal lung maturity. Gestational age and fetal growth are more appropriately evaluated using serial ultrasonography. Placental functioning is not assessed by amniocentesis. CBF/A, AN, PS

731. no. 3. This is the only remedy known to eliminate the cramp quickly. The other methods listed do not work. CBF/A, IM, PS

732. no. 2. Iron-deficiency anemia can cause symptoms including pallor, fatigue, irritability, decreased exercise tolerance, decreased growth rate, and poor muscle tone. C/O, AS, PS

733. no. 4. Stools, after administration of an oral iron preparation, will become a tarry-green color. Other options are expected. C/O, EV, H

734. no. 2. The body will attempt to compensate for hypothermia therapy, and the vital signs will initially become elevated; later, they will decrease. A/SP, AS, PS

735. no. 1. A hemoglobin of 11 to 15.5 g/dl is within normal limits and is a valid measure of improvement in anemia. A hematocrit of 28% is abnormally low. Neither the platelets nor the white blood cell count is affected by nutritional anemia. C/O, EV, PS

736. no. 3. Swelling and discomfort from varicosities caused by impeded venous return can be decreased by lying down or sitting with the legs elevated. Relief measures are aimed at promoting venous return. Thus increased periods of sitting (causing popliteal pressure) and constricting garments should be avoided. CBF/A, EV, PS

737. no. 4. Pregnancy-induced hypertension is the development of hypertension (increase of 30/15 from baseline) with proteinuria, edema, or both after the twentieth week of gestation. Normal fluid retention is reflected in lower extremity edema in late pregnancy. Data do not support a diagnosis of cardiac decompensation or pyelonephritis. CBF/A, AN, PS

738. no. 1. Weight loss is typical of diabetes in children. Because glucose is unable to enter the cells, the body quickly is in a state of starvation. C/NM, AS, PS

739. no. 3. During hypothermic therapy the client's skin must be protected from frostbite, which is most commonly caused by skin contact with the hypothermic blanket. A/SP, AS, PS

740. no. 2. Regular insulin is the only type given intravenously because it can act quickly to reduce the blood-glucose level. C/NM, AN, PS

741. no. 3. The let-down reflex causes milk to be pushed through the lacteal ducts. Oxytocin is released from the posterior pituitary for action on the myoepithelial cells of the mammary glands. As these cells contract, milk moves from the duct system to the lactiferous sinuses for ultimate delivery to the infant. The other

options listed relate to milk secretion or production and not to the let-down reflex. CBF/P, EV, PS

742. no. 1. Circulation slows at low temperatures, which predisposes the client to the formation of emboli. A/SP, AN, PS

743. no. 2. Shortness of breath, diaphoresis, palpitations, and an apprehension of closed spaces are symptoms of a phobic disorder (i.e., claustrophobia). P/A, AS, PS

744. no. 2. He can exchange food items within each list (e.g., one vegetable for another vegetable from the same list), but he cannot exchange a vegetable for another food (e.g., meat or fruit). C/NM, PL, E

745. no. 3. Tremors or a shaky feeling indicates hypoglycemia and impending insulin shock. Other options indicate hyperglycemia. C/NM, AS, E

746. no. 2. Recommended daily allowance for lactation includes 2700 calories (nonpregnant 2200), 65 g of protein (nonpregnant 50), 1200 μg of calcium (nonpreg-

nant 800), and 280 μg folic acid (nonpregnant 180). Iron is unchanged at 15 μg. CBF/P, IM, PS

747. no. 4. The gag and corneal reflexes are not lost until the client is completely comatose; an earlier sign of deteriation is a fading of the senses. A/SP, EV, PS

748. no. 4. Nuchal rigidity, (the neck becomes rigid when flexion is attempted), results from meningeal irritation or cerebral hemorrhage. This does not usually occur with concussions. A/SP, AN, PS

749. no. 1. In addition to the intercostal muscles, the medulla and the cranial nerves may also be affected with this pattern of paralysis. Respiratory findings generally are not the result of increased intracranial pressure or the effect of bacteria. Ascending paralysis is typically associated with a postviral infection. A/M, AN, PS

750. no. 3. The motor division of cranial nerve VII is specific, and controls the musculature of the face. A/M, AS, PS

Index

A

ABCs approach, 8
Abdomen
  bleeding from, 240-241
  trauma to, 242
Abdominal hysterectomy, 209-210, 269
Abdominoperineal resection, 80
Abortion
  inevitable, 148
  missed, 132-133, 148
  threatened spontaneous, 132, 147, 148
Above-the-knee amputation, 92
Abruptio placentae, 133-134, 139, 149
Absence seizures, 120
Absolutes as clue, 8
Abstinence, alcohol, 222
Abuse
  alcohol, 29, 32-33, 52, 55, 201, 221, 222, 263
  child, 28, 51, 238, 239, 287, 288
  crack cocaine, 52
  heroin, during pregnancy, 141, 154
  spouse, 28-29, 51
  substance, 34, 56, 218-219, 237
    during pregnancy, 141, 154
Acetaminophen, 124, 161
Acetazolamide, 121
Acetylcholine, 120
Acid-base imbalances, 61, 64
  in child, 168
Acidosis
  metabolic, 10, 104, 246, 293
  respiratory, 65, 106
Acquired immunodeficiency syndrome, 97, 127, 247, 293
  pregnancy and, 152
Acrocyanosis, 241, 289, 295
Acromegaly, 72, 111
Acrophobia, 42
ACTH; see Adrenocorticotropic hormone
Acting-out behavior of adolescents, 29, 51-52
Activated partial thromboplastin time, 106
Activities, age-appropriate, 216
Activity intolerance for mother or fetus, 296
Addison's disease, 74, 104, 112, 274
Addisonian crisis, 61, 74, 112, 216, 273, 279
Adenocarcinoma of rectum, 94
Adenoidectomy, tonsillectomy and, 159, 160, 179
Adjustment, postpartal, 239
Adjustment disorder, depressed mood, 213, 271
Admission assessment, 234
Adolescent(s)
  acting-out behavior of, 29, 51-52
  demanding, 216
  development, 216
Adoption, 136, 150
Adrenalectomy, 216, 217, 273
Adrenalin, 61, 104
Adrenergic agents, 60, 104
Adrenocortical insufficiency, 112
Adrenocorticotropic hormone, 225
Adult, nursing care of, 59-127
Adult respiratory distress syndrome, 106
Aerosolized drugs for child with asthma, 165
Affective strategies to promote success on
    NCLEX-RN, 6-7
Afterpains, 140-141, 153
Age
  as cue, 4
  gestational, determination of, 243
Age-appropriate activities, 216
Age group of patient as clue, 8
Aggression, 27, 29, 50
Agitated depression, 24, 47
Agoraphobia, 17, 41-42
AIDS; see Acquired immunodeficiency syndrome
Airway, establishing, 104

Airway obstruction in child, 164
Alanine aminotransferase, 109
Al-Anon, 33, 55
Albumin-globulin ratio, 262
Albuterol, 182
Alcohol
  abstinence from, 222
  abuse of; see Alcoholism
  hallucinations from, 110
  MAO inhibitors and, 47
  withdrawal from, 33-34, 55, 275, 276, 286
Alcoholic, recovering, 33, 55-56
Alcoholics Anonymous, 33, 55, 56
Alcoholism, 29, 32-34, 52, 55, 56, 72, 111, 201, 221, 222, 263
Aldactone; see Spironolactone
Aldosterone, 262
Alkaline phosphatase, 262
Alkalosis
  metabolic, in child, 185
  respiratory, 64
Allopurinol, 93, 124, 125, 173, 187
Alphafetoprotein, 296
ALT; see Alanine aminotransferase
Aluminum hydroxide antacids, 114
Aluminum hydroxide gel, 68, 108
Alzheimer's disease, 20, 44, 229
Ambivalence, 271
Amebiasis, 115
Aminophylline, 213, 271
Amitriptyline, 45
Ammonia, 110, 111
Amnesia, 282
Amnestic disorders, 46
Amniocentesis, 252
Amniotic fluid, meconium-stained, 134, 149, 150
Amniotic fluid embolus, 152
Amoebae, stool specimen for, 78, 115
Amoxicillin-clavulanic acid, 164
Amphetamine, 274
Amphogel; see Aluminum hydroxide gel
Amphotericin B, 107
Ampicillin, 164, 168, 169, 182, 184-185, 209, 223, 230, 277
Amputation
  above-the-knee, 92
  adaptation to, 92
  arm, 92
  below-the-knee, 229-230
  care after, 123, 282
Amylase, 109
Anal stricture, 268
Analgesics, maternal, effect on fetus of, 246
Analysis, 2
  gastric, 196-197, 260
Anaphylaxis, 113
Anemia, 248, 296
  aplastic, 247, 293
  hemolytic, 182
  iron-deficiency, 296
    in child, 252, 253
    during pregnancy, 135, 150
  pernicious, 293
  secondary to postpartum hemorrhage, 141, 153
Anesthesia
  epidural, 138, 151
  general, 237
    for cesarean section, 138, 152
  regional, for cesarean section, 138, 152
  spinal, low, 140
Anesthetic(s), 45
  maternal, effect on fetus of, 246
Anesthetic spray, topical, 5
Anger, 14, 40, 225, 263, 271
  depression and, 23, 47

Angina, 62, 225, 226, 244, 245, 279
  pain of, 106, 279
Angiography, cardiac, 226
Anorexia nervosa, 18-19, 43
Antabuse; see Disulfiram
Antacids, 294
Antepartal care, 135, 150
Anterior chamber of eye, 87, 120
Antianxiety agents, 220
Antibiotics, 154, 278
Anticholinergics, MAO inhibitors and, 47
Anticipatory grieving, 62, 105
Anticoagulants, 106
Antidepressants, 191, 256
  selective serotonin reuptake inhibitor (SSRI), 45
  tricyclic, 24
    side effects of, 48
Antidiabetic agents, MAO inhibitors and, 47
Antidiuretic hormone, 116
  inappropriate secretion of, 116
Antigen, carcinoembryonic, 115
Antineoplastic chemotherapy after mastectomy, 96
Antineoplastic drugs, 278
Antiparkinsonian drugs, 85
Antipsychotic medications, restlessness from, 44
Antiretroviral therapy, 161
Antisocial personality disorder, 211, 212, 270
Anxiety, 14, 15, 16-17, 19, 39, 41, 43, 232, 233, 234, 253, 284, 285, 290
  controlling, 6-7
  mild versus moderate, 41
  normal, 16, 41
  psychosis and, 54
  separation; see Separation anxiety
Anxiety disorder, 16, 41, 46
  generalized, 214, 248
Aorta, coarctation of, 167
Apgar score, 226, 280
Aphasia, 83, 117
  expressive, 204, 265, 266
  types of, 265
Aplastic anemia, 247, 293
Apnea in newborn, 143, 155
Appendectomy, 69, 159, 171, 186
Appendicitis, 68, 115, 236
Appendix, ruptured, 171, 186
  repair of, 9
Aqua k-pad, 165
Aquamephyton; see Vitamin K
Arm, amputation of, 92
Arrhythmia, sinus, in child, 166, 183
Artane; see Trihexyphenidyl
Arterial blood gases, 67, 108, 246
Arterial insufficiency of lower extremities, 73-74
Arteriovenous shunt, 207
Arthritis, 93
  gouty, 93
  rheumatoid, 123, 211, 212, 213, 270
Ascending paralysis, 254, 297
Ascites, 105, 111, 199, 203, 262, 265
  esophageal varices with, 70
ASO titer, 184
Aspartate aminotransferase, 109
Aspiration, 278
Aspiration pneumonia, 223
Aspirin, 93, 105, 106, 124, 148, 213, 271
Assay, Western blot, 127
Assessment, 2; see also specific assessment
AST; see Aspartate aminotransferase
Asterixis, 200, 263
Asthma, 213, 214, 217, 218, 246-247, 249, 271, 274
  bronchial, 214
  in child, 165, 168, 182, 212
  pneumonia and, 247
  psychologic factors affecting, 252
Astraphobia, 42

Atelectasis, 65, 107
Ativan; *see* Lorazepam
Atonic bladder, 118
Atrial septal defect, 167
Atrophy, optic nerve, 89
Atropine sulfate, 45, 121, 221
Attachment
  parent-infant, 136, 150
  with preterm infant, 209, 269
Augmentin; *see* Amoxicillin-clavulanic acid
Aura, 181
Autism, 231
Autografts, 85
Autonomic dysreflexia, 118, 260
Avascular necrosis of femoral head, 92
Aventyl; *see* Nortriptyline
Axillary lymph node dissection, 96
Azathioprine, 243, 290
Azotemia, 104
  prerenal, 205-206, 267

B

Babinski's reflex
  bilateral, in adult, 203-204, 265
  in child, 155
Bacteria in urine, 211, 270
Bacterial infection, 294
Bacterial meningitis, 251, 252, 253
Bacterial pharyngitis, 160, 180
Bacterial pneumonia, 223, 224
Bactrim DS; *see* Sulfamethoxazole-trimethoprim
BAL; *see* Dimercaprol
Balloon, esophageal, 110
"Bandage, shrinker," 123
Barbiturate-addicted infants, 154
Barbiturates, 56
  MAO inhibitors and, 47
  withdrawal syndrome from, 52
Bargaining, 40
Barium enema, 226, 280
Battered woman, 28-29, 51
Bed rest, 284
Bed rest, joint complications with, 251
Bed-wetting by child, 158-159, 160, 178-179
Behavior
  age-appropriate, 241
  demanding, 41
  "good client," 40
  incongruent, 14, 39
  manic, 26, 27, 28, 49, 50
  reinforcement of, 41
  ritualistic, 18, 42, 43
  withdrawn, 40
Behavior-modification program, 41, 56
Below-the-knee amputation, 229-230
Bence Jones protein, 256
Benztropine mesylate, 231, 284
Bereavement, uncomplicated, 234-235, 236, 285
Bethanechol, 240, 289
Bilateral myringotomy, 160, 179
Billroth I procedure, 108
Billroth II procedure, 108
Biopsy
  breast, 96
  liver, 203, 265
Biot's respirations, 116
Bipolar disorder, manic episode, 26-27, 28, 48, 49, 50,
    201, 203, 204, 205, 206, 232, 263, 264,
    265-266, 267
Birth, preterm, 203, 205, 265
Birthing center, 217, 219, 274
Bisacodyl, 280
Bite, tick, 242
Bivalving of cast, 123
Bladder
  atonic, 118
  cancer of, 192, 199
  carcinoma of, 75, 113
  decompression drainage of, 240
  distention of, after vaginal delivery, 198
  emptying, by postpartum woman, 231
  paralysis of, 118
  rupture of, 290

Bladder training, 265
Bleeding
  from abdomen, 240-241
  adrenergic agents for, 60
  assessment of, 122
  during delivery, excessive, 138
  esophageal, 71, 110
  gastrointestinal, severe, 8
  internal, 125
  postpartal, 140, 141, 153
  during pregnancy, 131, 132, 133, 148, 149
Blindness, 120
  partial, 117
Blood
  components of, infusion of, 204, 266
  donation of, 242, 290
  loss of, 60
Blood buffers, 104
Blood gases, arterial, 67, 108, 246
Blood pressure, measuring, 10
Blood tests
  for child, 159
  pregnancy, 251
Blood transfusion, 242
  flushing IV tubing after, 172-173, 187
  reaction to; *see* Transfusion reaction
Blood urea nitrogen, 267
Bone, demineralization of, 118
Bone marrow depression, 95
Borborygmi, 108
Borderline personality disorder, 237, 240, 241, 242,
    288, 289, 290
Bowel
  obstruction of, 79, 115
  perforated, 81
Bowel sounds, 115
Brace, Milwaukee, 172, 211
Bradycardia, sinus, 198, 261
Brain damage, 214
Brain injury, 220
BRATTS diet, 184
Breast
  biopsy of, 96
  cancer of, 15, 95, 96, 124, 125, 126, 127
  fibrocystic disease of, 124
  self-examination of, 5, 95, 96
Breast-feeding, 139, 140, 152, 153, 226, 227, 229,
    239-240, 242, 253, 280, 282, 288, 297
  after cesarean section, 138, 152
  contraceptives and, 140, 153
  diabetes mellitus and, 135, 150
  mastitis and, 142, 154
  nutrition during, 253
Breathing
  CPR to restore, 60
  mouth, 117
  pursed-lip, 65, 106
Breech presentation, 249
Broca's aphasia, 265
Bronchi, 278
Bronchial asthma, 214
Bronchiolitis, RSV, 164, 181, 229, 230, 282
Bronchogenic carcinoma, 66, 94, 107
Bronchoscopy, 66
Brudzinski's sign, 82, 117
Bryant's traction for child, 172
Buck's extension, 91
Buck's traction, 123
Buffers, blood, 104
Bulging fontanel, 155
Bupropion hydrochloride, 22, 46, 191, 257
Burns, 85, 118, 220, 221
  airway management with, 118
  in child, 162, 180
    fluid loss from, 162, 180
    nutrition and, 162, 180-181
  contractures caused by, 118-119
  fluid balance and, 118
Buspar; *see* Buspirone
Buspirone, 232
Bypass graft, femoral-popliteal, 74

C

C4 spinal cord injury, 84
C7, fracture of, 84
Calcitonin, 111
Calcium
  loss of, fracture and, 259
  low level of, 76, 113, 114
Calcium disodium EDTA, 161, 180, 236, 286
Calcium gluconate, 111, 149
Calculi, renal; *see* Kidney stones
Calendar method of contraception, 153
Calories, diet low in, 217
CaNa$_2$ EDTA; *see* Calcium disodium EDTA
Cancer
  bladder, 192, 199
  breast, 15, 95, 96, 124, 125, 126, 127
  cervical, 95, 124, 125-126, 208, 209-210, 268, 269
  child with, 173, 187
  colon, 80, 94, 115, 227
  colorectal, 226, 227
  endometrial, 209, 269
  of esophagus, 67, 108
  laryngeal, 90, 94
  liver, 201
  lung, 94, 124-125
    radiation for, 208
  mouth care for client with, 219
  ovarian, 94, 124
  predisposing factors to, 122
  prevention of, 226
  rectal, 80
  terminal, 199-200, 201, 262
  testicular, 94
  uterine, 15
  warning signs of, 93, 124
Cancer cells, 126
Cancer-related checkups, 93, 124
Cararact, extraction of, 88
Carbonic anhydrase inhibitors, 89, 121
Carcinoembryonic antigen, 115
Carcinoma
  bladder, 75, 113
  bronchogenic, 66, 94, 107
Cardene; *see* Nicardipine
Cardiac angiography, 226, 280
Cardiac arrest, 62, 280
Cardiac catheterization, 206-207
  in child, 166, 183, 238-239
Cardiac dysfunction, 226
Cardiac-enzyme studies, 62, 105
Cardiac enzymes, 244
Cardiac output, decreased, 63
Cardiac tamponade, 103
Cardiogenic shock, 62, 105
Cardiopulmonary resuscitation, 60
Cardiovascular disease, smoking and, 226
Cardiovascular status, 191
Care environment, safe effective, 3
Care plan, formulation of, 40
Carotid dressage, 183
Carotid studies, Doppler, 117
Cast
  application of, for clubfoot, 200, 263
  bivalving of, 123
  care of, 91, 122
  dry, 90-91
  fiberglass, 122
  plaster, 122
CAT; *see* Computer Adaptive Testing
Cataract, 88
  congenital, 154
Cataract lenses, 121
Catatonic type of schizophrenia, 32
Catheter
  Foley, 80, 114
  urinary, 78, 114
Catheterization, cardiac, 206-207
  in child, 166, 183, 238-239
Ceftriaxone, 169
Cells, cancer, 126
Central cyanosis, 106
Central venous pressure, 103-104
Cephal hematoma, 295

Cerebral edema, 219
Cerebral embolism, 123
Cerebral hemorrhage, 265
Cerebral palsy in child, 162
Cerebrospinal fluid, 117
Cerebrovascular accident, 83, 203, 204, 205, 213, 265, 266, 271
Cervical dilation and effacement, 137, 151
Cervical implant for cancer, 95, 126
Cervical spine, injury to, 84, 85
Cervix
    cancer of, 95, 124, 125-126, 208, 209-210, 268
    incompetent, 132-133, 148
Cesarean section, 138-139, 152, 248
    breast-feeding after, 138, 152
    care after, 138, 139, 152
Checkups, cancer-related, 124
Chelation therapy, 161
Chemical conjunctivitis, 151
Chemical dependence; see Abuse
Chemotherapy, 94-95, 96, 125
    in child, 173, 187
    nausea and vomiting from, 94
Chest
    circumference of, in newborn, 142, 154
    injuries to, 60, 103
    pain in, 104, 244, 291
    percussion of, 65
Chest physical therapy with postural drainage, 164, 181, 182
Cheyne-Stokes respirations, 81, 105, 116
Chickenpox, 160-161, 180, 215, 271, 274
Child
    death of, 19-20, 44
    dying, 218
    expression of emotions by, 40
    hospitalized, nursing care plan for, 165
    injection for, 236
    laboratory tests for, 159
    nursing care of, 157-187
    nutrition for, 158, 159, 178, 179
    pain in, 227, 280
    poisonous ingestions by, 161, 180
    preoperative preparation of, 226
    reaction of, to hospitalization, 169, 170, 184, 185, 234
    seizures in, 163, 181
    surgery for, 159-160, 179
    views of death by, 15, 40
    vision testing in, 251-252
    weight of, 251
Child abuse, 28, 51, 238, 239, 287, 288
Childbearing family, nursing care of, 129-155
Childbirth; see also Delivery
    discharge after, 139, 140
    menstruation following, 141, 153
Childbirth education programs, 131, 148
Chills, postpartum, 140, 153
Chlamydia infection in neonate, 151
Chloasma, 147
Chlordiazepoxide, 55
Chlorothiazide, 74
Chlorpromazine, 30, 53, 55
Cholecystectomy, 69-70, 109
Cholecystitis, 69, 109, 115
Cholecystogram, 69, 109
Cholesterol, diet low in, 63, 193, 258
Cholinergic crisis, 87
Cholinergic drugs, 120
Chorea, Sydenham's, 192, 257, 258
Choriocarcinoma, 271
Chorionic gonadotropin, human, in urine, 147
Chorionic villus sampling, 295
Chronic obstructive pulmonary disease, 246, 247
Chronic obstructive pulmonary edema, 64-65, 106, 293
Chvostek's sign, 111
Cimetidine, 118, 201
Circulatory structures, fetal, 143, 155, 216
Circumcision, 244, 291
Cirrhosis, 70, 71, 72, 110, 199, 200, 202, 203, 264, 265
Citrucel; see Methylcellulose
Claudication, intermittent, 112

Claustrophobia, 42
Cleft lip, 162, 169, 185, 243, 245
Cleft palate, 169, 185, 243, 244, 245, 291
Clomid; see Clomiphene
Clomiphene, 200
Cloth extremity restraints, 198, 261
Clozapine, 231, 283, 284
Clubbing of fingers and toes, 227, 280
Clubfoot, 200, 201, 263
Coagulation, disseminated intravascular, 104, 149
Coagulation factors, 183
Coarctation of aorta, 167
Cocaine, 274
Cocaine-addicted infants, 154
Cocaine intoxication, 52
Cocaine withdrawal, 275
Codeine, 104
Coffee and gastric acidity, 108
Cogentin; see Benztropine mesylate
Cognitive strategies to promote success on NCLEX-RN, 4-6
Cold stress, 6
Colectomy and ileostomy, 79
Colitis, 115
    ulcerative, 79, 115
Collecting appliance, 192
Colon
    cancer of, 80, 94, 115, 227
    polyps in, 115
    resection of, 172
    sigmoid, removal of, 80
    tumors of, 115, 125
Colorectal cancer, 226, 227
Colostomy, 80, 94, 115, 229
    care of, 79-80, 115
    double-barrel, 172
    irrigation of, 79, 80, 115, 229, 282
    sigmoid, single-barreled, 227, 280
    transverse, 79
Colostomy stoma, 227
Colostrum, 227, 280
Coma, 87, 117, 120
    diabetic, in child, 169-170
    nonketotic, hyperglycemic hyperosmolar, 73
Comminuted fracture, compound, 194
Common sense in test taking, 11
Communication
    with non-English-speaking client, 234, 285
    therapeutic, 5-6
Communication test items, 5-6
Compartment syndrome, 91, 123, 262
Compensation, 42
Complete blood count in child, 187
Compound comminuted fracture, 194
Compromised perfusion of vital organs, 60, 103
Compromised pulmonary function, 223-224
Computer Adaptive Testing, 2; see also NCLEX-RN
Concussion, 81, 116, 122
Condom, 153
Conduct disorder, 25, 29, 215
Confabulation, 282
Confidence in test taking, 8-11
Confusion, 228
    postoperative, 121
Congenital anomalies, testing for, 250
Congenital cataracts, 154
Congenital heart defects, 166, 183
Congenital heart disease, 220
Congenital hip dysplasia, 163, 181
Congestion, lung, fluid intake and, 223
Congestive heart failure, 63, 105, 275
    during pregnancy, 150
Conjunctivitis, chemical, 151
Consciousness, level of, 82
    assessment of, 116
Consolidation, lung, 106
Constipation, 10, 123
    during pregnancy, 130, 147
    from immobilization, 91
Contamination, salmonella, 249
Content in test taking, 11
    knowledge of, 10
Continuous portable suction device, 96

Contraception
    breast-feeding and, 140, 153
    douching for, 148
Contraction(s), 279
    Braxton Hicks', 237, 286
    premature ventricular, 62
    uterine, after delivery, 153
Contraction stress test, 190, 256, 264, 287
Contractures
    burns causing, 85, 118-119
    flexion, 117, 271
Control in test taking, 11
Conversation, monopolizing, 40
Conversion, 267
Conversion disorder, 206, 207, 208, 267
Conversion reaction, 267
Convulsions from pregnancy-induced hypertension, 149; see also Seizure(s)
COPD; see Chronic obstructive pulmonary disease
Coping, ineffective, 22
Coping mechanisms as cue, 4
Cor pulmonale, 106
Corticosteroids, 119, 122, 182, 274
    long-term, 224, 225
    previous use of, 61
Corticotropin-releasing factor, 225
Cortisol, 274
Cortisol test, plasma, 217
Cortisone, 74, 273, 274
Coughing after gastric surgery, 68
Coumadin; see Warfarin sodium
Countertraction, 194-194, 259
Cozaril; see Clozapine
Crack cocaine intoxication, 52
Cramps, leg, during pregnancy, 252
Cranial nerves, 89, 121
Craniotomy, 81-82
    transfrontal, 111
Creatine kinase-MB isoenzyme, 105
Crisis intervention, 30, 44, 52, 217, 218, 273, 274, 278-279
Crisis intervention approach, 225, 278
Cromolyn sodium, 164, 182
Croupette, child in, 209, 269
Crutch-walking, 230, 283
Crying client, 217, 274
Cues in test items, 4
Cuffed tracheostomy tube, 82
Cushing's disease, 111, 274
Cushing's syndrome, 217, 218, 219, 273, 275
Cyanosis, 122
    central, 106
Cyanotic heart defects in child, 183, 184
Cystectomy, 75
    and urinary diversion, 192, 258
Cystic fibrosis, 170-171, 186, 227, 229, 230, 231, 232, 282, 284
Cystitis, 210, 270, 282
    postpartum, 230
Cystoscopy, 74, 77, 113
Cytology testing, 94

D

Dakin's solution; see Sodium hypochlorite and boric acid
Dandruff, 233
Death
    child's, 19-20, 44
    child's view of, 159, 173, 179, 187
    grief reaction to, 14-15, 16
    home, 263
    of newborn, 139
Decadron; see Dexamethasone
Decelerations in fetal heart rate, 137, 151, 191, 257
Decerebrate posturing, 81, 116
Decision-making skills in depressed patient, 24
Decompression drainage of bladder, 240
Decorticate posturing, 116
Decubitus ulcers, 40, 83, 117, 215, 271
Dehydration, 10, 112
    in child, 168-169, 184, 185, 246, 250
Delayed wound healing, 109
Delirium tremens, 52, 70, 110

Delivery; *see also* Childbirth
 bleeding after, 140, 141, 153
 care after, 140-141, 195, 238, 239, 259
 cesarean; *see* Cesarean section
 excessive bleeding during, 138
 expected date of, 130, 147
 forceps, 225
 genital herpes during, 252, 296
 hemorrhage after, 139, 140, 141, 153
 mitral valve prolapse and, 220-221
 precipitous, 152
 sexual activity after, 240, 288
 transfusions after, 139
 vaginal, 137, 151
  bladder distention after, 198
Delusional disorder, 220
Delusional system, persecutory, 52
Delusions, 35, 57, 196, 259, 260, 283
Demanding client, 16, 41
Dementia, 227, 229, 230, 282
 vascular, 214-215
Demerol; *see* Meperidine
Demineralization, bone, 118
Denial, 40, 53, 104, 126, 261, 262
 of grief, 40
Depressant-withdrawal syndrome, 52
Depression, 14, 15, 20-21, 22, 23, 24, 25, 40, 41, 44,
  45, 190, 196, 197, 209, 210, 236, 243, 244, 245,
  260, 261, 271, 286, 288
 agitated, 24, 47
 anger and, 23, 47
 assessment for, 22
 bone marrow, 95
 classification of, 46
 group therapy for, 21, 45-46
 guilt and, 196, 260
 after mastectomy, 96
 with psychomotor retardation, 20, 47, 49
 psychotic, 25, 48
 reactive (situational), 40, 126, 260
 self-esteem and, 23, 47
 suicide and, 21, 22, 23, 45, 46, 48, 286
Depressive episode, major, 23-24, 47
Desensitization, gradual, 42
Desquamation of neonatal skin, 154
Detachment, retinal, 88
Development
 fetal, 216, 217
  teratogen exposure during, 216
 hospitalization affecting, 242
Developmental milestones, 158, 161, 164, 166,
  167-168, 178, 180, 183, 184, 208, 210, 224,
  238, 268, 270, 287
Dexamethasone, 84, 118, 125, 219, 239, 287
Diabetes, gestational, 134, 143, 155
Diabetes insipidus, 82, 111, 116
Diabetes mellitus, 9, 73, 74, 112, 198, 234, 235, 237
 breast-feeding and, 135, 150
 in child, 169-170, 185, 253, 296
 infection in client with, 233, 284
 newborn of woman with, 143, 150, 155
 pregnancy and, 134-135, 149-150
Diabetic coma in child, 169-170
Diabetic mothers, infants of, 143, 150, 155
Diagnex Blue Test, 260
Dialysis
 peritoneal, 77, 114
 regional heparinization during, 207, 267
Diamox; *see* Acetazolamide
Diaphragm
 contraceptive, 153
 paralysis of, 118
Diarrhea
 in child, 246, 249, 251
 watery, 168, 184
Diastasis recti, 289
Diazepam, 57, 219, 263, 285
 withdrawal syndrome from, 52
Dibenzepine, MAO inhibitors and, 47
Dicumarol, 106
Diet
 high-protein, high-potassium, low-sodium,
  low-calorie, 217

Diet—cont'd
 low-cholesterol, 63
 low-fat, low-sodium, low-cholesterol, 193, 258
 sodium-restricted, 106
 sugar-restricted, 198
Diffusion, 105
Digitalis, 63, 64, 105, 220, 275
Digitalis toxicity, 105
Digoxin, 105, 261
 for child, 166-167, 183
Digoxin toxicity, 183
Dilantin; *see* Phenytoin
Dilation
 and curettage, 271
 and effacement, 137, 151
Dilaudid, 104
Diltiazem, 105
Dimenhydrinate, 88, 111, 120
Dimercaprol, 236
Diplopia, 120
Discharge after childbirth, 139, 140
Discharge evaluation, 50
Discharge planning, 22, 46
Discharge teaching, 9
Disequilibrium syndrome, 114, 206, 267
Disorientation, 228
Displacement, 42, 53
Dissection, axillary lymph node, 96
Disseminated intravascular coagulation, 104, 149
Disseminated intravascular coagulation syndrome, 149
Dissociation, 282
Distractors as clue, 8
Disulfiram, 33, 55, 222, 277
Diuresis, 287
Diuresis, uncontrolled, 116-117
Diuretics, 275
Diuril; *see* Chlorothiazide
Diversion, urinary, 192-193, 257
Diverticula, 116
Diverticulitis, 81, 115, 116
Diverticulosis, 81
Dopamine, 119
 for shock, 60, 103
Doppler carotid studies, 117
Double-barrel colostomy, 172
Douching for contraception, 132, 148
Down syndrome, 162, 181
Drainage
 of bladder, decompression, 240
 postural, chest physical therapy with, 164, 181, 182
 wound, 191, 256
Dramamine; *see* Dimenhydrinate
Dressage, carotid, 183
Drug withdrawal, 33-34, 56
 in newborn, 141-142, 154
Dry cast, 90-91
Dubowitz scale, 290
Dubowitz assessment, 290
Ductus arteriosus, 155, 273
 patent, 167, 184
Ductus venosus, 155
Dulcolax *see* Bisacodyl
Dumping syndrome, 68, 108
Duodenal ulcer, 67, 108, 197
 perforation of, 201, 263
Dying, stages of, 40
Dying child, 218
Dying client, 15, 200, 262-263
Dysphagia from stroke, 204
Dysplasia, hip, congenital, 163, 181
Dyspnea, 63, 105
Dysreflexia, autonomic, 118, 260
Dysthymic disorder, 244, 271, 291

E

Ear infections, 239
Ears of neonate, assessment of, 142, 154
Ecotrin, 124
Ectopic pregnancy, 133, 148-149
Eczema, 245, 246, 292
Edema
 cardiac failure causing, 63, 105
 cerebral, 219

Edema—cont'd
 pulmonary, 10, 63, 123
  chronic obstructive, 64-65, 106
  from IV fluids, 152
Edrophonium, 120, 221
Effacement, cervical dilation and, 137, 151
Effexor; *see* Venlafaxine
Ego-defense mechanisms, 17
Egophony, 106
Ejaculation, 118
Elbow, fracture of, 198, 199, 262
Elderly nursing home residents, introduction to, 14
Electrocardiogram, 244, 291
Electroconvulsive therapy, 21-22, 24-25, 45, 46, 48
Electrode, scalp, internal, for fetal monitoring, 137,
  151, 152
Electrode patches to monitor cardiac activity, 197, 261
Electroencephalogram, 119
ELISA, 127
Embolism, cerebral, 123
Embolus(i)
 amniotic fluid, 152
 fat, 122, 123
  after fracture, 91
 pulmonary, 106
Emergency room assessment, 219
Emmetropia, 120
Emotional lability, 117
Emotions, child's expression of, 40
Emphysema, 241, 289, 293
Encephalopathy, 263
 hepatic, 71, 110
Endocarditis, 4-5
Endocrine gland, removal of, 216
Endometrial cancer, 209, 269
Endometritis, postpartal, 241, 289
Endoscopy, 199, 262
 gastric, 67
Endotracheal tube for child, 164, 182
Enema, barium, 226, 280
Environment, safe effective, 3
Enzymes
 cardiac, 244
 pancreatic, 170, 186, 230, 283
Epidural anesthesia, 138, 151
Epiglottitis, 208, 209, 268
Epilepsy, 119, 120
Epinephrine, 61, 104, 122, 182, 271
Epinephrine toxicity, 212, 270-271
Episiotomy, 140, 153
Epistaxis, 90
Epstein's pearls, 143, 155
Equipment, hypothermia, 104
Erection, 118
Ergonovine, 153
Erythema, 107
Erythema toxicum in newborn, 154
Erythrocyte sedimentation rate, 109, 184
Erythrocytosis, 125
Erythromycin, 258
Erythromycin ophthalmic ointment, 241, 289
Escherichia coli, 270
Esophageal balloon, 110
Esophageal bleeding, 71, 110
Esophageal varices, 111, 199
 with ascites, 70
Esophagitis, 67
Esophagus, cancer of, 67, 108
Essence, words of, as clue, 8
Estrogen deficiency, 123
Estrogen excess, 111
Estrogen therapy, 210
Evaluation, 2
Excretory function of liver, 199, 262
Exercise(s)
 for diabetic client, 112
 during pregnancy, 251, 296
 quadriceps-setting, 229
Exhibitionism, 52
Exophthalmos, 110
Expected date of delivery, 130, 147
Expressive aphasia, 204, 265, 266
Extension, Buck's, 91

External radiation treatments, 94, 125
External rotation in lower extremities, 123
External shunt, 77, 114
Extraction, cataract, 88
Extremities, lower
  arterial insufficiency of, 73-74
  external rotation in, 123
Extrusion reflex, 288
Eye(s)
  anterior chamber of, 87, 120
  care of, for newborn, 137, 151
  foreign object in, 87-88, 120
  lens of, 87
  of neonate, assessment of, 142, 154
  surgery on, 88, 121
Eye drops, mydriatic, 88, 89

F

Facial nerve, 254
Failure-to-thrive syndrome, 167, 168, 184
Fainting spell, 234
  in child, 166
Fall, 197
Fallot, tetralogy of, 167, 184
Family
  of dying client, 15, 40
  involvement of, in treatment process, 31, 54
Family therapy, 56, 277, 284
Fantasy, 276
Farsightedness, 87
Fat, diet low in, 193, 258
Fat emboli, 122, 123
  after fracture, 91
Febrile seizures, 163, 181
Fecal incontinence, 230
Fecalith, 109
Feedings, gastrostomy tube, for child, 168, 184
Femoral-popliteal bypass graft, 74
Femur
  fracture of, 90
  head of, avascular necrosis of, 92
Ferrous gluconate, 153
Ferrous sulfate, 153
Fertility, male, 118
Fetal distress, 150, 151
Fetal heart monitor, 191
Fetal jeopardy, 151
Fetal presentation, 248, 249
Fetus
  circulatory structures of, 143, 155, 216
  development of, 216, 217, 296
  teratogen exposure during, 216
  effects of maternal analgesic and anesthetics on, 246, 293
  heart rate of, 237, 284, 285
  monitoring of, 137, 151
  heart sounds of, 232
  hypoxia of, 149
  left occiput posterior position for, 233
  monitoring of, 137, 151
  position of, 284, 294
Fever
  in neonate, 243-244
  postoperative, 224
  rheumatic, 167, 184
  in child, 192, 193, 257, 258
  before surgery, 160, 179
Fiber in diet, 280
Fiberglass cast, 122
Fibrin, dissolving, 11
Fibrocystic breast disease, 124
Fibrosis, cystic, 170-171, 186, 227, 229, 230, 231, 232
Fingers, clubbing of, 227, 280
Fistula, tracheoesophageal, 210, 211, 270
  in infant, 209, 269
Fixation, 267
Flaccid paralysis, 118
Flatus, 281, 282
Flexion contractures, 117, 271
Florinef; see Fludrocortisone acetate
Fludrocortisone acetate, 74
Fluent aphasia, 265
Fluid balance, burn care and, 118
Fluid intake, lung congestion and, 223

Fluid loss from burns in child, 162, 180
Fluid replacement with shock, 60
Fluid retention during pregnancy, 253
Fluid therapy for dehydration, 168-169
Fluids, IV, 5
  for child, 163, 181
  rapid infusion of, 138, 152
5-Fluorouracil, 81, 94, 125
Fluoxetine, 190, 256
Fluphenazine decanoate, 231-232
Foley catheter, 80, 114
Follicle-stimulating hormone, 263
Fontanel(s), 295
  bulging, 179-180
  palpation of, 144, 155
Foot, gangrene of, 233
Foot drop, 257
Foramen ovale, 273
Forceps delivery, 225
Foreign object in eye, 87-88, 120
Fowler's position, 66, 107, 292
  for congestive heart failure, 105
Fracture(s), 122
  C7, 84
  calcium loss with, 259
  compound comminuted, 194
  elbow, 198, 199, 262
  fat embolus after, 91
  femur, 90
  hip, 91
  leg, 194
  ulnar, 91
Free association, 282
Fremitus, tactile, increased, 106
Friction rub, pleural 106
5-FU; see 5-Fluorouracil
Fundus
  after delivery, 153
  massage of, 151, 152
Furosemide, 63, 64, 105
Fusion, spinal, 84
  laminectomy and, 93

G

Gait, parkinsonian, 85, 119
Galactorrhea, 72, 111
Gangrene, 231, 232, 233, 283-284, 288
Gantrisin; see Sulfisoxazole
Garamycin; see Gentamicin
Gas(es)
  arterial blood, 67, 108, 246
  intestinal, 229, 281, 282
Gastrectomy, subtotal, 68, 108
Gastric analysis, 196-197, 260
Gastric endoscopy, 67
Gastric regurgitation, 67, 108
Gastric suction tube, 80, 115
Gastric ulcers, 67, 68, 108
Gastroduodenostomy, 108
Gastroesophageal reflux, 67, 108
  in child, 196, 260
Gastrointestinal bleed, severe, 8
Gastrojejunostomy, 108
Gastrostomy tube feedings for child, 168, 184
General anesthesia, 237
  for cesarean section, 138, 152
Generalized anxiety disorder, 214, 248
Genital herpes, 193, 194, 195, 258, 259
  delivery of woman with, 252
Gentamicin, 65, 107
Gestational age, determination of, 243
Gestational diabetes, 134, 143, 155
Gland
  endocrine, removal of, 216
  prostate; see Prostate gland
Glasgow Coma Scale, 116
Glaucoma, 88-89, 120, 121
Glomerulonephritis in child, 171, 186
Glucagon, 170, 185
Glucocorticoid, 74
  deficiency of, 104
Glucose tolerance tests, 185
Glutamic-oxaloacetic transaminase, serum, 109
Glycosylated hemoglobin, 185

Gonadal-stimulating hormone, 111
Gonadotropin(s), 263
  human chorionic, in urine, 147
Gonorrhea, 195, 259
Gonorrheal ophthalmia neonatorum, 151
"Good client" behavior, 40
Gout, 93, 124, 285
Gouty arthritis, 93
Gradual desensitization, 42
Graft, femoral-popliteal bypass, 74
Grand mal seizure, 87, 119
  in child, 163, 181
Granulocytic leukemia, acute, 94
Grasp reflex in newborn, 143, 155
Grief, 126, 218, 285
  denial of, 40
Grief group for senior citizens, 14
Grief reaction, 14-15, 16, 40-41, 234
Grief resolution, 245, 290-291
Grieving, anticipatory, 62, 105
Grooming, 194, 258
Group therapy, 14, 241, 248-249
  for depression, 21, 45-46
Grunting, 295
Guaiac testing, 108
Guillain-Barré syndrome, 90, 122, 254
Guilt
  depression and, 196, 260
  expression of, 49
Gunshot wound, 241, 289
Gynecomastia, 111

H

Haldol; see Haloperidol
Hallucinations, 31, 32, 35, 52, 54, 56, 194, 230, 231, 258, 283, 289
  during alcohol withdrawal, 33
  alcoholic, 110
Hallucinogens, 56
Haloperidol, 31, 45, 54, 57, 220, 232, 284
Hand-washing, obsessive-compulsive, 17-18, 42
Head and neck surgery, 90
Head circumference of newborn, 142, 154
Head injury, 82, 117
Head lice, 233, 234, 284, 285
Headache(s), 19
  after lumbar puncture and myelogram, 118, 211
  migraine, 248-249
    psychologic factors affecting, 252
  spinal, 118
  postpartal, 139, 152
Healing, wound, delayed, 109
Health promotion/maintenance, 3
Heart, dysfunction of, 117
Heart defects, congenital, 166, 183, 184
Heart disease
  congenital, 220
    diet and, 279-280
  labor and, 221
  mother with, 221
  pregnancy and, 135, 150, 220, 221, 276
Heart failure
  chronic, 63-64
  congestive, 63, 105
    during pregnancy, 150
  left-sided, 63, 105
  right-sided, 105, 106
Heart problems, monitoring for, 197
Heart rate
  for child, 266
  fetal, 237, 284, 285
    monitoring of, 137, 151
Heart sounds, fetal, 232
Hegar's sign, 285
Hemarthrosis, 183
Hematoma, 259
Hematuria, 113
Hemianopia, 117
Hemiplegia, 214
Hemodialysis, 77, 205, 206, 207, 267
Hemoglobin,
  glycosylated, 185
  low, 294
Hemolytic anemia, 182

Hemophilia, 165-166, 182-183
Hemoptysis, 106
Hemorrhage
  cerebral, 265
  postpartal, 138, 139, 140, 141, 153
  subconjunctival, in newborn, 154
  after tonsillectomy, 160, 179
Hemorrhoidectomy, 207-208
Heparin overdose, 64, 106
Heparin sodium, 64, 104, 106, 114, 220, 275
Heparinization, regional, during dialysis, 207, 267
Hepatic encephalopathy, 71, 110
Hepatitis
  infectious, 70
  serum, 154
  viral, 70
Hepatitis B secondary to substance abuse, 141, 154
Heroin abuse during pregnancy, 141
Heroin withdrawal in newborn, 141-142, 154
Herpes, genital, 193, 194, 195, 258, 259
  delivery of woman with, 252, 296
Hip, fracture of, 91
Hip dysplasia, congenital, 163, 181
Hip nailing, 92, 123
Hip prosthesis, 92, 123
  displacement of, 191, 257
Hip replacement, total, 123, 190, 191, 192, 257
Hirschsprung's disease, 171-172, 186
Histoplasmosis, 66, 107
History, obstetric, 236, 286
HIV; see Human immunodeficiency virus
HIV-positive child, 161, 180
HIV-positive woman
  in labor, 139, 152
  pregnancy and, 139, 152
HIV status of child, 161, 180
Hodgkin's disease, 96-97, 127
Homans' sign, 106
Home death, 263
Hormone(s)
  adrenocorticotropic, 225
  antidiuretic, 116
    inappropriate secretion of, 116
  follicle-stimulating, 263
  gonadal-stimulating, 111
  luteinizing, 263
  melanocyte-stimulating, 225
Hospitalization
  child's reaction to, 159, 169, 170, 179, 184, 185,
    210, 234, 270
  development affected by, 242
Hospitalized child, nursing care plan for, 165
Human chorionic gonadotropin in urine, 147
Human immunodeficiency virus, 127, 213, 247
  transmission of, 97, 161, 180
Human needs, categories of, 2-3
  test item focus suggested by, 3
Humidification oxygen therapy, 168, 184
Humulin-R; see Regular human insulin
Hydatidiform mole, 211-212, 213, 270
Hydramnios, 270
Hydration status, 271
  of child, 210, 269, 246
Hydrocephalus, 163
Hydrochlorothiazide, 125
Hydrocortisone, 217
Hydronephrosis, 288
Hydroxyzine, 218, 274
Hygiene, personal, 194, 258
Hyperadrenal function, 218
Hyperbilirubinemia in neonate, 143, 155, 245
Hypercoagulation, 61, 104
Hyperglycemia, 112, 185
Hyperglycemic hyperosmolar nonketotic coma, 73
Hyperkalemia, 76-77, 105, 106, 113, 114, 267
  in child, 180
Hyperosmolar nonketotic coma, hyperglycemic, 73
Hyperpituitarism, 111
Hyperresonance, 106
Hypersensitivity reaction, 124
Hypertension, 75, 113, 193, 258
  portal, 71, 110, 262
  pregnancy-induced, 134, 149, 222, 223, 224, 270,
    278, 296

Hyperthyroidism, 110, 111, 248, 249, 294
Hypertrophy, prostate, 77, 78, 114
Hyperventilation during labor, 136-137, 151
Hypocalcemia, 72, 76, 111, 113, 114, 231
Hypochondriasis, 19, 43, 226-227, 280
Hypocorticism, 274
Hypoglycemia, 73, 112, 170, 185, 297
  in neonate, 143, 155
Hypoglycemic reaction, 112
Hypokalemia, 250, 295
Hyponatremia, 76, 293
Hypoparathyroidism, 11, 294
Hypophysectomy, 72, 111
Hypopituitarism, 111
Hypospadias, 222, 223, 277
Hypotension
  adrenergic agents for, 60
  from antipsychotic or neuroleptic drugs, 54
  postural, 106
Hypothermia, 61, 251, 295-296
  in open-heart surgery, 167, 183
  therapy for, 253
Hypothermia equipment, 104
Hypotonicity, Down syndrome and, 181
Hypovolemic shock, 267, 273
  after burn, 85
Hypoxemia, 106
Hypoxia, 64, 106
  fetal, 149
Hysterectomy, 95, 209-210, 269
Hysterical aphasia, 265
Hysterostomy, 271

I

Idealization, 256
Identification, 256
Ileal conduit stoma, 192
Ileostomy, 115
  colectomy and, 79
Ileostomy bag, 192
Ileus
  meconium, 227
  paralytic, 113, 120-121
Illness
  psychiatric, 219-220, 292
  psychologic factors affecting, 247, 252
  terminal, 201, 218, 219, 246, 249, 293
    skin care for, 219
Illusion, 52, 283
Imaginary playmate, 210, 269
Imipramine, 24, 48, 57
Immobility for child, 199, 200, 262
Immobilization
  constipation from, 91
  of spinal cord, 117
Immunizations, 159, 179, 164, 182, 238, 252, 287, 296
  for HIV-positive child, 247
Immunodeficiency syndrome, acquired; see Acquired
    immunodeficiency syndrome
Immunodeficiency virus, human; see Human
    immunodeficiency virus
Impetigo in newborn, 154, 285
Implant, cervical, for cancer, 95, 126
Implementation, 2
Impulses, visual, transmission of, 89
Imuran; see Azathioprine
Incompetent cervix, 132-133, 148
Incongruent behavior, 14, 39
Incontinence
  fecal, 230
  after prostatectomy, 114
  stress, 257
Independence in depressed client, 23, 47
Inderal; see Propranolol
Indocin; see Indomethacin
Indomethacin, 263-264
Induction of labor, 224, 225
Inevitable abortion, 148
Infant(s); see also Child
  of diabetic mothers, 150
  nutrition and, 164, 181-182, 239, 243
  postmature, 192, 258
  preterm; see Preterm infant

Infant(s)—cont'd
  term, 155
    preterm infant compared to, 205, 266
    weight gain for, 164, 181
Infant-parent attachment process, 136, 150
Infant-parent interaction, 142, 143, 144, 154
Infarction, myocardial, 8, 9, 61-63, 104-105
Infection
  bacterial, 294
  in casted leg, 91
  chlamydia, in neonate, 151
  diabetic client with, 233, 284
  ear, 239
  kidney, 250
  in neonate, 143, 155
  at operative site, 190
  postpartal, 238
  potential, 122
  urinary tract, 75, 113, 223, 224, 251, 295
Infectious hepatitis, 70
Information giving, 5
Infusion
  of blood components, 204, 266
  of IV fluids, rapid, 138, 152
Infusion rate for child, 163, 181
Ingestions, poisonous, by child, 161, 180
INH; see Isoniazid
Injection
  for child, 236
  intramuscular, for infant, 159, 179
  insulin, 73
  for toddler, 236
Insomnia, 17, 22, 46
Insulin, 253
  deficiency of, 112
  needs for, during pregnancy, 134, 150
  regular human, 73
Insulin injections, 73, 296
Insulin shock, 116, 253
Intal; see Cromolyn sodium
Integrated nursing examination, 2
Intellectualization, 256
Interaction
  parent-infant, 142, 154
  present, 39
Intermittent claudication, 112
Internal bleeding, 125
Internal scalp electrode for fetal monitoring, 137, 151,
  152
Interview, 5
Intestinal gas, 229
Intracranial pressure
  changes in, 81
  increased, 220, 238
    in child, 163, 179-180, 181
  positioning and, 116
Intramuscular injection for infant, 159, 179
Intraocular pressure, 121
  measurement of, 88-89
Intrauterine device, 153
Intravascular coagulation, disseminated, 104, 149
Intravenous pyelogram, 75, 77, 114
Introjection, 42, 45
Intussusception, 240, 241
  in child, 185, 289
  reduction of, 172, 187
Iontophoresis, pilocarpine, 186
Ipecac, syrup of, 180
Iris, prolapse of, 121
Iron-deficiency anemia
  in child, 252, 253, 296
  during pregnancy, 135, 150
Iron intake during pregnancy, 130, 135, 147
Irrigation of colostomy, 79, 80, 115, 229, 282
Irritation, meningeal, 117
Ischemic attack, transient, 82
Isocarboxazid, 45, 57, 190-191, 256
Isoenzymes, cardiac, 105
Isoimmunization, maternal, 296
Isolation
  reverse, child in, 221, 291
  social, 14
Isolette, newborn in, 143, 144, 155, 243-244, 291
Isoniazid, 66, 107

Isordil; *see* Isosorbide dinitrate
Isosorbide dinitrate, 193, 258
IV fluids, 5
    for child, 163, 168, 181, 184
    rapid infusion of, 138, 152
IV tubing, flushing, after blood transfusion, 172-173, 187

J

Jaundice, 72, 107
    neonatal, 154, 250, 295
Joint complications of bed rest, 251
Joint surgery, 190

K

Kaposi's sarcoma, 127
Kayexalate; *see* Sodium polystyrene sulfonate
KCl; *see* Potassium chloride
Kernig's sign, 117
Ketoacidosis, 73, 116, 253
Key words, 4
    as clue, 8
Kidney failure, 76, 104, 113, 267, 270
    chronic, 76, 113
Kidney infection, 250
Kidney stones, 75, 113, 233, 239, 240, 288
Kidney transplant, 243, 244
Klebsiella, 270
Knife wound, 241
Korsakoff's syndrome, 33, 55, 221, 276
Kussmaul's respirations, 76, 116
Kwell shampoo, 233, 285

L

Lability, emotional, 117
Labor, 191, 201, 219, 231, 245, 248, 256, 264, 284, 292
    active stage of, 137
    HIV-positive woman in, 139, 152
    hyperventilation during, 136-137, 151
    induction of, 137, 139, 190, 224, 225, 256
    patient teaching during, 136, 150
    preterm, 147, 204, 205, 266
    second stage of, 151
    signs of, 131, 148
    third stage of, 233
    transitional phase of, 131-132, 136, 148
    true, 148
    woman with heart disease in, 221
Laboratory tests for child, 159
Lactic dehydrogenase isoenzyme, 105
Lactose intolerance, temporary, 184
Lactulose, 110
Lamaze classes, 131
Lamaze techniques, 148
Laminectomy and spinal fusion, 93
Large bowel obstruction, 79, 115
Larynx, cancer of, 90, 94
Lasix; *see* Furosemide
Lead poisoning, 234, 237, 285, 287
Left-sided heart failure, 63, 105
Leg
    casted, infection in, 91
    fracture of, 194
Leg cramps during pregnancy, 252
Lens(es)
    cataract, 121
    of eye, 87
    opacity of, 121
Leopold's maneuvers, 237, 286
Let-down reflex, 253, 296, 297
Letting go, 288
Leukemia, 248, 249
    in child, 173, 187
    granulocytic, acute, 94
    lymphoblastic, acute, 247, 248
    lymphocytic, in child, 172, 173, 187
Leukocytosis, 125, 287, 293, 294
Levodopa, 85-86, 119
Levopa; *see* Levodopa
Levothyroxine, 249
Librium; *see* Chlordiazepoxide
Lice, head, 233, 234, 284, 285
Lidocaine, 62, 105, 122

Ligation, tubal, 132, 148
Light reflexes, pupillary, 81, 116
Lip, cleft, 162, 169, 185, 243, 245
Lipase, 109
Lithium carbonate, 26, 27, 45, 49, 50, 204, 205, 266
Lithium toxicity, 26, 49, 50
Liver
    biopsy of, 203, 265
    cancer, 201
    dysfunction of, 70, 71
    excretory function of, 199, 262
Liver failure, 71, 200, 263
Liver flap, 263
Liver tremor, 263
Lobectomy, upper, 67
Locations as clue, 8
Lochia rubra, 153
Log rolling, 124
Loose teeth, 160, 225
Lopressor; *see* Metoprolol
Lorazepam, 19, 43-44, 55, 220, 223, 232, 233, 234, 278
Loss, feelings of, 40
Lower extremities
    arterial insufficiency of, 73-74
    external rotation in, 123
Lower gastrointestinal tract study, 226, 280
LSD; *see* Lysergic acid diethylamide
Lumbar myelogram, 97
Lumbar puncture, 83, 251, 296
    headache after, 118, 211, 270
Luminal; *see* Phenobarbital
Lumpectomy, 96
Lung
    aspiration into, 278
    cancer of, 94, 124-125
        radiation for, 208, 268
    chronic obstructive disease of, 246, 247, 293
    compromised function of, 223-224
    congestion in, fluid intake and, 223
    consolidation in, 106
    secretions in, postoperative, 238
Lung volumes, 246, 292
Luteinizing hormone, 263
Lying by child, 158, 178
Lymph nodes, axillary, dissection of, 96
Lymphangiography, 97, 127
Lymphedema after axillary lymph node dissection, 96
Lymphoblastic leukemia, acute, 247, 248
Lymphocytic leukemia in child, 172, 173, 187
Lymphoma, 218
Lysergic acid diethylamide, 34-35, 56

M

Maalox; *see* Magnesium and aluminum hydroxide
Mafenide acetate, 85, 118
Magnesium and aluminum hydroxide, 263, 264
Magnesium citrate, 280
Magnesium hydroxide, 109
Magnesium sulfate, 134, 149, 204, 266, 278
Mammogram, 124
Mandelamine; *see* Methenamine mandelate
Manic behavior, 26, 27, 28, 49, 50
Manic episode, bipolar disorder, 26-27, 28, 48, 49, 50, 201, 203, 204, 205, 206, 263, 264, 265-266, 267
Manipulation, 237, 270, 286, 289
Mannitol, 219, 275
MAO inhibitors, 256-257
Marplan; *see* Isocarboxazid
Marrow, bone, depression of, 95
Mask
    of pregnancy, 147
    Venturi, 65, 107
Massage
    fundal, 151, 152
    uterine, 153
Mastectomy, 95-96, 126-127
Mastitis, breast-feeding and, 142, 154
Masturbation by child, 159, 179
Mathematical calculations, 5
McDonald's procedure, 132-133, 148
Measles, 148
Meconium ileus, 227

Meconium staining, 134, 149, 150
Medication, preoperative, 236; *see also* specific medication
Melanocyte-stimulating hormone, 225
Melena, 106
Mellaril; *see* Thioridazine
Membranes, rupture of, 136, 150-151, 233, 287
    artificial, 139
Meniére's syndrome, 88, 120
Meningeal irritation, 117
Meningitis, 83, 296
    bacterial, 251, 252, 253
    in child, 160, 180
Menopause, 210, 269
Menstruation following childbirth, 141, 153
Mental health problems, psychosocial problems and, 13-57
Mental retardation in child, 162, 181
Mental stressors, 11
Meperidine, 55, 69, 104, 109, 204, 218, 231, 245, 246, 283, 292
Mestinon; *see* Pyridostigmine
Metabolic acidosis, 10, 104, 246, 293
Metabolic alkalosis in child, 185
Metamucil; *see* Psyllium hydrophilic mucilloid
Methenamine mandelate, 240, 251, 295
Methotrexate, 94, 173, 187
Methylcellulose, 125
Methylergonovine, 193, 258
Methergine; *see* Methylergonovine
Methylxanthines, 182
Metoclopramide, 125, 289
Metoprolol, 63, 194, 258
Metrorrhagia, 240, 289
Microclotting, diffuse, 61
Microthrombi, 104
Migraine headaches, 248-249
    psychologic factors affecting, 252
Milia, 155, 295
Milieu therapy, 232, 284
Milk ejection reflex, 253
Milk production, 140, 153
Miller-Abbott tube, 79, 115
Milwaukee brace, 172, 211
Mineralocorticoids, deficiency of, 104
Minimal change nephrotic syndrome, 186
Miotics, 89, 121
Missed abortion, 132-133, 148
Missed questions, patterns of, 10
Mitral stenosis, 220
Mitral valve prolapse, 220-221
Mittelschmerz, 148, 262
Modified radical mastectomy, 95-96
Molar pregnancy, 211, 271
Mole, hydatidiform, 211-212, 213, 270
Mongolian spots, 152, 154
Monitor, fetal heart, 191
Monitoring, fetal, 137, 151, 152
Monoamine oxidase inhibitors, 23-24, 45, 47
Monopolizing conversation, 40
Mood swings, 27-28
Moro reflex, 143, 155
Morphine sulfate, 69, 104, 109, 113, 206
Mothers
    diabetic, infants of, 150
    teenage, 28, 51
Motor aphasia, 265
Motor function, assessment of, 85
Motor vehicle accidents, 213, 214
Mottling of neonatal skin, 154
Mouth breathing, 117
Mouth care, 219
    for unconscious patient, 83
Mouth sores from chemotherapy, 94
Mouth-to-nose resuscitation, 60
Mouth ulcers, 219
MTX; *see* Methotrexate
Mucus, suctioning, 65, 107, 246
Multiple-choice tests, acing, 8-11
Multiple sclerosis, 86, 119
Muscle spasms, 118
    with multiple sclerosis, 86, 119
    after spinal cord injury, 84

Myasthenia gravis, 87, 120, 220, 221, 222, 276, 277
  pregnancy and, 222
Myasthenic crisis, 87, 120
Mycobacterium tuberculosis, 107
Mycomyst, 247
Mydriatic eye drops, 88, 89
Mydriatics, 121
Myelogram, lumbar, 84-85
  headache after, 118
Myelomeningocele, 162-163, 181, 251, 252, 295, 296
Myocardial infarction, 8, 9, 61-63, 104-105
Myocardial pump failure, 63
Myopia, 120
Myringotomy, 88
  bilateral, 160, 179

N

Nägele's rule, 147
Nailing, hip, 92, 123
Narcotics, 151
  for burned child, 162
  MAO inhibitors and, 47
Narcotics Anonymous, 56
Nardil; *see* Phenelzine sulfate
Nasal packing, 90
Nasogastric tube, 68, 75, 90, 109, 113, 122, 289
Nasotracheal suctioning, 270
National Council of State Boards of Nursing, 2, 3
Nausea
  nasogastric tube and, 113, 289
  of pregnancy, 236, 286
  and vomiting, 72
    from chemotherapy, 94
NCLEX-RN
  categories of human needs portion of, 2-3
  format for, 2-3
  nursing process portion of, 2
  preparation and review of, 4
  preparing for, 1-11
  scoring of, 3-4
  success on, keys to, 4-7
  test items on, 2, 3, 5-6
Neck and head surgery, 90
Necrosis
  avascular, of femoral head, 92
  vascular, 123
Negativism of toddler, 158, 178
Neomycin, 71, 110, 111, 115, 263
Neonate
  apnea in, 143, 155
  assessment of, 142, 154, 249, 250
  care of, 138
  chest and head circumferences of, 142, 154
  death of, 139
  of diabetic mother, 143, 155
  drug withdrawal in, 141-142, 154
  eye care for, 137, 151
  fever in, 243-244
  hyperbilirubinemia in, 143, 155
  hypoglycemia in, 143, 155
  infection in, 143, 155
  jaundice in, 154, 295
  reflexes of, 143, 155
  refusal to care for, 143, 155
  siblings of, 139, 152
  "spitting up" by, 143, 155
  stroking of, 155
  temperature of, 249, 294
  vitamin K for, 250
  weight of, 244, 250, 291, 295
Neostigmine, 121
Neo-Synephrine; *see* Phenylephrine
Nephritis in child, 191
Nephrosis in child, 171, 186, 190, 191, 256, 257, 288
Nephrotic syndrome, minimal change, 186, 288
Nerve(s)
  cranial, 89, 121
  facial, 254
  olfactory, 121
  optic, 89, 121
    atrophy of, 89
  peroneal, palsy of, 91
Nerve palsy, peroneal, 122

Neural tube defects, 296
Neurobiologic model of psychiatric illness, 25-26, 49
Neurogenic spinal shock, 118
Newborn; *see* Neonate
Nicardipine, 63
Nicotine and gastric acidity, 108
Night-light for child, 158, 178
Nipples, cracked, from breast-feeding, 239-240, 288
Nitroglycerin, 104, 245, 279, 292
Nodes, lymph, axillary, dissection of, 96
Nonfluent aphasia, 265
Nonketotic coma, hyperglycemic hyperosmolar, 73
Nonstress test, 238
Nortriptyline, 20, 44
Nose drops, vasoconstrictive, 90, 122
Nuchal rigidity, 253-254, 297
Nursing assistant, tasks for, 6
Nursing examination, integrated, 2
Nursing home residents, elderly, introduction to, 14
Nursing process, 2
  as clue, 8
  test item focus suggested by, 2
Nutrition
  breast-feeding and, 253, 297
  for burned child, 162, 180-181
  child's, 158, 159, 178, 179
  infant and, 164, 181-182, 239, 243
  during pregnancy, 130, 135, 147
  toddler and, 225
Nutritional intake, 20, 44
Nystagmus in newborn, 154

O

Obesity, 196, 260
Obsessive-compulsive disorder, 17-18, 42, 43
Obstetric history, 236, 286
Obstruction
  airway, in child, 164
  bowel, 79, 115
    large-bowel, 79, 115
    small-bowel, 79, 115
Obstructive pulmonary disease, chronic, 246, 247, 293
Obstructive pulmonary edema, chronic, 64-65, 106
Occupational therapy for client with overactive
    behavior, 28, 51
Odor, infection and, 122
Olfactory nerve, 121
One-to-one relationships, 40
Opacity, lens, 121
Open-heart surgery, hypothermia in, 167, 183
Operating room table, positioning on, 237
Operative site, infection at, 190
Ophthalmia neonatorum, 151, 241, 289
Opiates, 56
  withdrawal syndrome from, 52
Optic nerve, 89, 121
  atrophy of, 89
Oral contraceptive, breast-feeding and, 140
Organ transplant, 243
Organic brain syndrome, 280
Organs, vital, compromised perfusion of, 60, 103
Orgasms, 118
Osmosis, 105
Osteoarthritis, 93, 123-124, 270
Osteogenic sarcoma, 172
Osteoporosis, 123
Ostomy, 229
Otitis, chronic, 88
Otitis media, 239, 288
Ovarian cancer, 94, 124
Over-the-counter pregnancy tests, 130
Overhydration, 220
Ovulation, signs of, 132, 148, 199, 262, 263
Ovum, release of, 130, 147
Oxygen for myocardial infarction, 62
Oxygen therapy, humidification, 168, 184
Oxygenation, 117
Oxytocin, 137, 139-140, 151, 152, 153, 190, 224, 225,
    256, 296

P

Pacemaker, permanent, 198, 261-262
Packing, nasal, 90

Pain
  anginal, 106, 244, 245
  assessment for, 82
  chest, 104, 244, 291
  child and, 227, 280
  management of, in child, 184, 204
  perineal, postpartal, 140, 153, 195, 259
  reaction to, 109
    assessment of, 116
Palate, cleft, 169, 185, 243, 244, 245, 291
Palsy
  cerebral, in child, 162
  peroneal nerve, 91, 122
Pancreas, 231, 283
  exocrine function of, 70, 109
Pancreatic enzymes, 170, 186, 230, 283
Pancreatin, 109
Pancreatitis, 70, 109, 116, 230, 231, 283
Panic attack, 17, 41, 233, 284
Pap smear, 93-94, 124
Paralysis
  ascending, 254, 297
  of bladder, 118
  of diaphragm, 118
  flaccid, 118
Paralytic ileus, 113, 120-121
Paranoia; *see* Schizophrenia, paranoid-type
Paranoid personality disorder, 30, 53
Paranoid schizophrenia, 31, 47, 283
Paraphrasing, 274
Parathyroidectomy, 73
Parent-infant attachment process, 136, 150
Parent-infant interaction, 142, 143, 144, 154
Parents, hospitalized child and, 173, 187
Parents Without Partners, 44
Paresthesias, peripheral, 112
Parkinson's disease, 85-86, 119, 276
Parkinsonian gait, 119
Parkinsonian side effects, 55
Parnate; *see* Tranylcypromine
Paroxetine, 45, 190-191, 256, 269-270
Partial blindness, 117
Partial thromboplastin time, activated, 106
Patches, electrode, to monitor cardiac activity, 197,
    261
Patent ductus arteriosus, 167, 184
Patient teaching during labor, 136, 150
Paxil; *see* Paroxetine
Pearson attachment, 194-195, 259
Pedophilia, 52
Penicillin, 130, 151, 160, 180, 182, 194, 220, 258,
    275, 277, 278
  prophylactic, 4, 289
Peptic ulcer, 118, 196, 260
Peptic ulcer disease, 68
Percussion, chest, 65
Perforated bowel, 81
Perforation of duodenal ulcer, 201, 263
Perfusion of vital organs, compromised, 60, 103
Perineal care, 239
Perineal pain, postpartal, 140, 153, 195, 259
Perineal prostatectomy, 78, 114
Peripheral paresthesias, 112
Peritoneal dialysis, 77, 114
Peritonitis, 68-69
Pernicious anemia, 293
Peroneal nerve palsy, 91, 122
Persecutory delusional system, 52
Personal hygiene and grooming, 194, 258
Personality disorder, 46, 238, 287, 289
  antisocial, 211, 212, 270
  borderline, 237, 240, 241, 288, 290
Pertussis, 274
Petit mal seizure, 87, 120
Petroleum jelly, 232
Pharyngitis, bacterial, 160, 180
Phenazopyridine hydrochloride, 250, 295
Phenelzine sulfate, 45, 191, 256
Phenobarbital, 220
Phenothiazines, side effects of, 55
Phentolamine mesylate, 125
Phenylephrine, 122
Phenylalanine, 290

Phenylketonuria, 151, 243
  tests for, 151
Phenytoin, 55, 86, 119, 163, 181, 220
Phlebitis, 106
Phobia, 52
Phobic disorders, 17, 42, 253, 297
Phosphorus, elevated, 113, 114
Photophobia, 296
Phototherapy for neonate, 143, 155, 245, 292
Physical restraints, 29, 52
Physical stressors, 11
Physical therapy, chest, with postural drainage, 164,
  181, 182
Physiologic integrity, 3
Physiologic jaundice, 154, 295
Pica, 147
Pilocarpine, 121
Pilocarpine iontophoresis, 186
Pin, Steinman, 194, 195, 259
Pin care for child in traction, 199, 262
Pinworms, 161, 180
Pitocin; *see* Oxytocin
Pituitary tumor, 72, 111
Placenta
  delivery of, 285
  function of, 217, 274
Placenta previa, 133-134, 149
Planning, 2
Plasma cortisol test, 217
Plaster cast, 122
Pleural friction rub, 106
Pneumocystis carinii pneumonia, 127
Pneumonectomy, partial, 66
Pneumonia, 65, 106
  aspiration, 223
  asthma and, 247
  bacterial, 223, 224
  in child, 171, 208
  Pneumocystis carinii, 127
Poison prevention, 161
Poisoning, lead, 234, 237, 285, 287
Poisonous ingestions by child, 161, 180
Polioviris vaccine, 293
Polycythemia, 125, 204, 265
Polydipsia with diabetes, 185
Polyphagia with diabetes, 185
Polyps, colon, 115
Polyuria with diabetes, 73, 185
Portacaval shunt, 200, 262
Portal hypertension, 71, 110, 262
Position; *see also* specific position
  intracranial pressure and, 116
  on operating room table, 237
Postmature infant, 192, 258
Postoperative fever, 224
Postoperative vital signs, 238
Postpartal adjustment, 239
Postpartal care, 238, 239
Postpartal hemorrhage, 138, 153
Postpartal infection, 238
Postpartal teaching, 219
Postpartum chills, 140, 153
Posttraumatic stress disorder, 19, 20, 44, 52, 222, 223,
  277
Postural drainage, chest physical therapy with, 164,
  181, 182
Postural hypotension, 106
Posturing
  decerebrate, 81, 116
  decorticate, 116
Potassium
  diet high in, 217
  normal level of, 113
Potassium chloride, 168, 184, 197, 261
Potassium iodine, saturated solution of, 111
Practice questions, reviewing, 10-11
Precipitous delivery, 152
Prednisone, 86, 125, 191, 219, 244, 256, 291
Preeclampsia, 147
Pregnancy, 130-140, 234
  AIDS virus and, 152
  bleeding during, 132, 133, 148, 149
  blood tests in, 251

Pregnancy—cont'd
  couple's needs during, 130, 147
  danger signs of, 130, 131
  diabetes mellitus and, 134-135, 149-150
  ectopic, 133, 148-149
  exercise during, 251, 296
  first trimester of, 130, 131, 250
  fluid retention during, 253
  heart disease and, 135, 150
  heroin abuse during, 141
  high-risk, 135, 150
  HIV-positive woman and, 139, 152
  leg cramps during, 252
  mask of, 147
  maternal heart disease during, 220
  molar, 211, 271
  nausea of, 236, 286
  nutrition during, 130, 135, 147
  signs of, 130, 147
  smoking during, 143, 251, 296
  teenage, 135-136, 150
  in widowed client, 16
Pregnancy-induced hypertension, 134, 149, 222, 223,
  224, 270, 278, 296
Pregnancy test, 214, 215, 271
  over-the-counter, 130
Premature ventricular contractions, 62
Prematurity, retinopathy of, 289
Prenatal teaching, 251
Preoperative medication, 236
Preoperative preparation of child, 226
Prerenal azotemia, 205-206, 267
Presbyopia, 120
Preschooler, nursing care of, 190
Present interaction, 39
Presentation, fetal, 138, 248, 249
Pressure
  blood, measuring, 10
  central venous, 103-104
  intracranial; *see* Intracranial pressure
  intraocular, 121
Preterm birth, 203, 205, 265
Preterm infant, 208, 268
  mother and, 209, 269
  respiratory distress in, 206, 267
  term infant compared to, 205, 266
Preterm labor, 147, 204, 205, 266
Preventil; *see* Albuterol
Priority action, 5
Pro-Banthine; *see* Propantheline bromide
Procainamide, 105
Proctoscopic examination, 78, 115
Proctosigmoidoscopy, 78, 115
Projection, 42, 45, 53, 256, 283
Prolactin, 111, 153
Prolapse
  of iris, 121
  mitral valve, 220-221
Prolixin; *see* Fluphenazine
Propantheline bromide, 68, 109
Propranolol, 225, 226, 279
Prostate gland
  examination of, 77, 114
  hypertrophy of, 77, 78, 114
  transurethral resection of, 77-78, 114
Prostatectomy, 77, 78, 114
Prosthesis
  fitting, after above-the-knee amputation, 92
  hip, 92, 123
  displacement of, 191, 257
Protamine sulfate, 106
Protein
  Bence Jones, 256
  diet high in, 217
  intake of, during pregnancy, 131, 148
Prothrombin times, 106, 262
  in cirrhosis, 110
Prozac; *see* Fluoxetine
Pruritus, 111
  skin care for, 219
Pseudomonas, 270
Psychiatric illness, 219-220
  neurobiologic model of, 25-26, 49

Psychoanalysis, 56
Psychologic factors affecting illness, 247, 252, 292
Psychomotor retardation, depression with, 20, 47, 49
Psychosis, 53, 54, 283
  anxiety and, 54
Psychosocial integrity, 3
Psychosocial and mental health problems, 13-57
Psychosocial stressors, 11
Psychotic depression, 25, 48
Psychotic disorder, 231
Psychotic episodes, 34, 35
Psychotic symptoms from LSD, 34
Psychotropic drugs, indications for, 30, 53
Psyllium hydrophilic mucilloid, 116
Pulmonary edema, 10, 123
  acute, 63
  chronic obstructive, 64-65, 106
  from IV fluids, 152
Pulmonary embolus, 106
Pulmonary stenosis, 203, 207
Puncture, lumbar, 83, 251, 296
  headache after, 118, 211, 270
Pupillary light reflexes, 81, 116
Pupillary responses, 116
Purified protein derivative skin test for tuberculosis,
  65-66, 107, 183
Purine, restriction of, 124
Purpura, 107
Pursed-lip breathing, 65, 106
Pyelogram, intravenous, 75, 77, 114
Pyelonephritis, 249, 250
Pyloric stenosis, 169, 185
  in child, 197, 198, 260-261
Pyloroplasty, vagotomy and, 197, 261
Pylorotomy, 169
Pyridium; *see* Phenazopyridine hydrochloride
Pyridostigmine, 87, 120, 220, 221, 276
Pyridoxine, 107, 119

Q

Quadriceps-setting exercises, 229, 282
Quantitative sweat chloride test, 186
Questions
  misreading, 10-11
  missed, patterns of, 10
  practice, reviewing, 10-11
Quickening, 285

R

Radiation for lung cancer, 208, 268
Radiation syndrome, 208
Radiation treatments, external, 94, 125
Radical mastectomy, modified, 95-96
Radium implant, cervical, 95
Rancho Los Amigos Scale, 116
Ranitidine, 197, 231, 261
Rape, 29-30, 52, 223, 224-225, 226, 278, 279, 280
Rationalization, 42, 45, 261
Reaction
  conversion, 267
  hypersensitivity, 124
  transfusion, 204-205, 290
Reactive depression, 40, 126, 260
Receptive aphasia, 265
Recovering alcoholic, 33, 55-56
Rectum
  adenocarcinoma of, 94
  cancer of, 80
Reflection, 41, 271
Reflex(es)
  Babinski's, bilateral, in adult, 203-204, 265
  extrusion, 288
  let-down, 253, 296-297
  milk ejection, 253
  pupillary light, 81, 116
  gastroesophageal, 67, 108
    in child, 196, 260
Regional anesthesia for cesarean section, 138, 152
Regional heparinization during dialysis, 207, 267
Regitine; *see* Phentolamine mesylate
Reglan; *see* Metoclopramide
Regression, 31, 53, 184, 287
Regular human insulin, 73, 112

Regurgitation
gastric, 67, 108
by neonate, 155
Rehabilitation after stroke, 117
Rehydration process, 251
Reinforcement of behavior, 41
Rejection, 291
Renal calculi; see Kidney stones
Renal failure; see Kidney failure
Replacement, total hip, 123, 190, 191, 192, 257
Repression, 53
Resection
abdominoperineal, 80
colon, 172
transurethral, of prostate, 77-78, 114
Reserpine, MAO inhibitors and, 47
Resolution, 40
Resonance, 106
Respiration
Biot's, 116
Cheyne-Stokes, 81, 105, 116
in congestive heart failure, 105
Kussmaul's, 76, 116
Respiratory acidosis, 65, 106
Respiratory alkalosis, 64
Respiratory distress, 61, 114, 209, 212
in preterm infant, 206, 267
Respiratory distress syndrome, adult, 106
Respiratory syncytial virus bronchiolitis, 164, 181,
229, 230, 282
Response(s)
misreading, 10-11
pain, assessment of, 116
pupillary, 116
selecting, 10-11
Responsiveness, sympathetic, 11
Restatement, 41
Restlessness from antipsychotic medications, 44
Restraints, 29, 52, 261
alternatives to, 29, 52
cloth extremity, 198, 261
Resuscitated client, 60
Resuscitation
cardiopulmonary, 60
mouth-to-nose, 60
successful, 62
Retardation
mental, in child, 162, 181
psychomotor, depression with, 20, 47, 49
Retention, urinary, 77, 257
Retinal detachment, 88, 120
Retinopathy of prematurity, 289
Reverse isolation, child in, 221, 291
Rewarming process, 251
Reye's syndrome, 148
Rh-negative mother, 141, 153
Rheumatic fever, 167, 184
in child, 192, 193, 257, 258
Rheumatoid arthritis, 123, 211, 212, 213, 270
Rhinoplasty, 89-90, 121-122
Rh₀(D) immune globulin, 141, 153-154
RhoGAM; see Rh₀(D) immune globulin
Ribavirin, 283
Rifampin, 66, 107
Right-sided heart failure, 105, 106
Rigidity, nuchal, 253-254, 297
Rimactane; see Rifampin
Ringworm, 285
Risk factors as cue, 4
Risperdal; see Risperidone
Risperidone, 195, 259
Ritodrine, 153
Ritualistic behavior, 18, 42, 43
Rivalry, sibling, 148, 238
Rivaviran, 181, 230
Rocephin; see Ceftriaxone
Rooming-in, 152
ROP, 248
Rotation, external, in lower extremities, 123
RSV; see Respiratory syncytial virus
Rubella
exposure to, 6
pregnancy and, 132, 148
Rubeola, 148

Rule of nines, 85, 118
Rumination, 23, 46-47
Rupture of membranes, 136, 150-151, 233, 287
artificial, 139
Ruptured appendix, 171, 186
repair of, 9
Ruptured bladder, 290

S

Saddle block, 279
Salicylates, 124
Salmonella, 270, 295
contamination with, 249
Samples, sputum, 124
collection of, 94
Sampling Chorionic villus, 295
Sarcoma
Kaposi's, 127
osteogenic, 172
Saturated solution of potassium iodine, 111
Scalp electrode, internal, for fetal monitoring, 137,
151, 152
Schilling test, 127, 293
Schizophrenia, 31-32, 54, 195
catatonic type, 32
chronic undifferentiated, 194, 258
paranoid type, 31, 47, 192, 193, 194, 230, 257, 258,
259
School-age child, nutrition and, 159, 179
Sclerosis, multiple, 86, 119
Scoliosis, 172, 187, 211
Scopolamine, 121
Scoring of NCLEX-RN, 3-4
Seclusion, 50
indications for, 34, 56
Secretion(s)
of antidiuretic hormone, inappropriate, 116
lung, postoperative, 238
Sedatives, 278
Seizure(s), 8-9, 86-87, 119, 120, 238, 287
absence, 120
in child, 163, 181
febrile, 163, 181
grand mal, 87, 119
petit mal, 87, 120
tonic-clonic, 119-120
Selective serotonin reuptake inhibitor (SSRI)
antidepressant, 45, 256
Self, therapeutic use of, 5
Self-esteem, increasing, 23, 47
Self-exploration by child, 159, 179
Self-help groups, 278
Semi-Fowler's position, 110, 124
for congestive heart failure, 105
Sengstaken-Blakemore tube, 71, 110, 199, 262
Sensory aphasia, 265
Separation anxiety in child, 169, 179, 183, 185, 190,
192, 257, 290
Septal defect
atrial, 167
ventricular, 166, 183, 206, 207
Sepsis, 287
Septic shock, 74-75, 113
Sertraline, 22, 24, 46, 47, 191
Serum glutamic-oxaloacetic transaminase, 109
Sexual activity
after delivery, 240, 288
douche after, 132, 148
after myocardial infarction, 62
after spinal cord injury, 84
Sexually transmitted diseases, 194, 258
Shirodkar procedure, 148
Shock, 60, 122
cardiogenic, 62, 105
dopamine for, 60, 103
fluid replacement with, 60
hypovolemic, 267, 273
after burn, 85
insulin, 116, 253
septic, 74-75, 84, 113, 117-118
"Shrinker" bandage, 123
Shunt
arteriovenous, 207
external, 77, 114

Shunt—cont'd
portacaval, 200, 262
ventriculoperitoneal, 163, 181
Sibling of newborn, 139, 152
Sibling rivalry, 148, 238
Sibling visitation program, 132
Sickle cell crisis, 165, 167, 182, 205, 206, 266
Sickle cell disease, 205, 266, 267
child with, 165, 182
inheritance of, 139, 152
Sickledex, 182
SIDS; see Sudden infant death syndrome
Sigmoid colostomy, 80
single-barreled, 227, 280
Silvadene; see Silver sulfadiazine
Silver nitrate, 118, 151
Silver sulfadiazine, 162, 180
Sinus arrhythmia in child, 166, 183
Sinus bradycardia, 198, 261
Situational crisis, 216
Situational depression, 126
Skeletal traction, 194, 195, 259
child in, 199, 200, 262
Skin of newborn, assessment of, 142, 154
Skin care for cancer and pruritus, 219
Skin test, purified protein derivative, for tuberculosis,
65-66, 107
Sleep, promoting, 244
Sleeping, child's, 158
Small-bowel obstruction, 79, 115
Smear, Pap, 93-94, 124
Smoking
cardiovascular disease and, 226
during pregnancy, 143, 251, 296
Social isolation, 14
Sodium
diet low in, 106, 193, 217, 258
low level of, 76
Sodium bicarbonate, 68, 240
Sodium citrate, 248
Sodium hypochlorite and boric acid, 232
Sodium phosphate, 240
Sodium polystyrene sulfonate, 280
Sodium-restricted diet, 106, 193, 217, 258
Solu-Cortef; see Hydrocortisone
Souffle, uterine, 287
Sounds
bowel, 115
heart, fetal, 232
tympanic, 106
Spanish-speaking client, 234, 235, 285
Spasms, muscle, 118
with multiple sclerosis, 86, 119
after spinal cord injury, 84
Specimen, stool, for amoebae, 78, 115
Speech center of brain, 204, 266
Spinal anesthesia, low, 140
Spinal cord
immobilization of, 117
injury to, 84, 118, 196, 266
Spinal fusion, 84
laminectomy and, 93
Spinal headache, 118
postpartal, 139, 152
Spinal shock, 84, 117-118
Spine, cervical, injury to, 84, 85
Spinnbarkheit, 262
Spironolactone, 262
"Spitting up" by neonates, 143, 155
Splint, Thomas, 194-195, 259
Splinting, 65, 107, 286
Spouse
abuse of, 28-29, 51
death of, 14-15, 16
Sputum samples, 124
collection of, 94
Staining, meconium, 134, 149
Stapedectomy, 88
Status epilepticus, 119, 181
Steatorrhea, 186
Steinman pin, 194, 195, 259
Stem, systematic reading of, 9-10
Stenosis
mitral, 220

Stenosis—cont'd
    pulmonary, 203, 207
    pyloric, 169, 185
        in child, 197, 198, 260-261
Steroids, 279
    in children, 218
Stimulants, 56
Stoma
    colostomy, 227
    ileal conduit, 192
    urinary, 75, 113
Stomach, surgery on, 60
Stomatitis from chemotherapy, 94
Stool
    of breast-fed infant, 242, 290
    incontinence of, 230
Stool guaiac slide test, 124
Stool specimen for amoebae, 78, 115
Stork bites in newborn, 154
Strabismus in newborn, 154
Stress, 245-246, 248
    Addison's disease and, 112
    reduction of, 6-7
    ulcers and, 201, 263
Stress disorder, posttraumatic, 19, 20, 44, 52, 222,
        223, 277
Stress incontinence, 257
Stress test, contraction, 190, 256
Stressors, 11
Stricture, anal, 268
Stridor, 105
Stroke, 82-84, 117, 203, 204, 205, 213-214, 215, 265,
        266
    rehabilitation after, 117
Stroking of newborn, 155
Stump care, 92
Subconjunctival hemorrhage in newborn, 154
Subcutaneous emphysema, 241, 289
Sublimation, 42, 45, 261, 267
Substance abuse, 34, 56, 218-219, 237
    during pregnancy, 141, 154
Substitution, 42
Subtotal gastrectomy, 68, 108
Subtotal thyroidectomy, 72-73, 111, 249
Sucking reflex, 155
Suction device, continuous portable, 96
Suction tube, gastric, 80, 115
Suctioning
    of endotracheal tube in child, 164, 182
    of mucus, 65, 107, 246
    nasotracheal, 270
    of tracheostomy tube, 203, 265
Sudden infant death syndrome, 163-164, 181
Sugar-restricted diet, 198
Suicidal gestures, 47
Suicidal ideations, 240
Suicide, 23, 45, 47, 192, 257, 209, 210, 269
    depression and, 21, 22, 23, 45, 46, 48, 286
Sulfamethoxazole-trimethoprim, 250
Sulfamylon; see Mafenide acetate
Sulfisoxazole, 270
Sulfobromophthalein test, 262
Sulfonamides, 211
Suppression, 42, 261
Surgery
    for child, 159-160, 179
    eye, 88, 121
    fever before, 160, 179
    gastric, 60
    head and neck, 90
    joint, 190
    open-heart, hypothermia in, 167, 183
    preparation of child for, 226
    vital signs after, 238
    voiding after, 238
Suspiciousness, 30, 31, 53
Sweat chloride test, 186, 282
Sydenham's chorea, 192, 257, 258
Sympathetic responsiveness, 11
Sympathomimetics, MAO inhibitors and, 47
Synthroid; see Levothyroxine
Syphilis, 195, 259
    neonatal, 151
    during pregnancy, 130, 147

T

T-tube, 69, 109
Tachycardia, 117, 261
Tactile fremitus, increased, 106
Tagamet; see Cimetidine
Taking-hold phase, 239, 287
Taking-in phase, 239, 240, 287-288
Talipes equinovarus, 200, 263
Tamponade, cardiac, 103
Teaching
    discharge, 9
    patient, during labor, 136, 150
    postpartal, 219
    prenatal, 251
Teaching/learning, 5
Teasing, 51
Teenager, pregnancy in, 28, 51, 135-136, 150
Teeth, loose, 160, 225
Telangiectasia in newborn, 154
Temper tantrums in child, 167, 184
Temperature
    of neonate, 249, 294
    taking, in child, 169, 185
Tensilon; see Edrophonium
Tension, reducing, 6-7
Teratogen exposure during fetal development, 216
Term infant, 155
    preterm infant compared to, 205, 266
Terminal cancer, 199-200, 201, 262
Terminal illness, 201, 218, 219, 246, 249, 262, 293
    skin care for, 219
Test(s)
    blood, pregnancy, 251
    Computer Adaptive, 2; see also NCLEX-RN
    for congenital anomalies, 250
    contraction stress, 190, 256, 264, 287
    cytology, 94
    glucose tolerance, 185
    guaiac, 108
    laboratory, for child, 159
    multiple-choice, acing, 8-11
    nonstress, 238
    personal responses to, 6
    phenylketonuria, 151
    plasma cortisol, 217
    pregnancy, 214, 215, 271
        over-the-counter, 130
    purified protein derivative skin, 65-66, 107, 183
    quantitative sweat chloride, 186
    Schilling, 127, 293
    stool guaiac slide, 124
    sulfobromophthalein, 262
    sweat chloride, 186, 282
    tuberculin, 65-66, 107, 166, 182, 183
    vision, for child, 251-252
Test items, practice, reviewing, 10-11
Testicular cancer, 94
Testicular self-examinations, 125
Testing; see Test(s)
Tetracycline, 289
Tetralogy of Fallot, 167, 184
Therapeutic communication, 5-6
Therapeutic use of self, 5
Thioridazine, 32
Thomas splint, 194-195, 259
Thoracotomy, 66
Thoracotomy tube in child, 167, 183
Thorazine; see Chlorpromazine
Threatened abortion, 132, 147, 148
Thrombocytopenia, 125
Thrombophlebitis, 64, 106, 113
    preventing, 114
    venous, 112
Thromboplastin time, activated partial, 106
Thrush, 155
Thumb sucking, 167
Thyroidectomy
    subtotal, 72-73, 111, 249
    total, 111
Tick, removal of, 242, 290
Tick bite, 242
Time parameters as clue, 8
Timolol, 121

Tinea, 285
Tissue typing, 243
Tocolytic drugs, 266
Toddler, 158, 178, 279; see also Child
    injection for, 236
    negativism of, 158, 178
    nutrition for, 225
Toes
    clubbing of, 227, 280
    gangrene of, 231, 232
Tofranil; see Imipramine
Toilet training, 158, 178, 225
Tonic-clonic seizures, 119, 120
Tonic neck reflex, 155
Tonometer, 88-89, 121
Tonsillectomy, 225, 226, 279, 280
    and adenoidectomy, 159, 160, 179
    care after, 160, 179
Topical anesthetic spray, 5
Total hip replacement, 123, 190, 191, 192, 257
Total thyroidectomy, 111
Toxoplasmosis during pregnancy, 131, 148
Toys, age-appropriate, 168, 184, 240, 242
Tracheoesophageal fistula, 210, 211, 270
    in infant, 209, 269
Tracheostomy, 164, 182
    in child, 201-202, 264
Tracheostomy tube
    cuffed, 82
    suctioning of, 203, 265
Traction, 123
    Bryant's, for child, 172
    Buck's, 91, 123
    skeletal, 194, 195, 259
        child in, 199, 200, 262
Training, bladder, 265
Transfrontal craniotomy, 111
Transfusion, blood, 242
    after delivery, 139
    flushing IV tubing after, 172-173, 187
Transfusion reaction, 173, 187, 204-205, 242-243, 2●
Transient ischemic attack, 82, 117
Transitional phase of labor, 131-132, 136, 148
Transplant
    kidney, 243, 244
    organ, 243
Transurethral resection of prostate, 77-78, 114
Transverse colostomy, 79
Tranylcypromine, 256
Trauma, 239
    abdominal, 242
Tremor, liver, 263
Tricyclic antidepressants, 24
    MAO inhibitors and, 47
    side effects of, 48
Trihexyphenidyl, 231, 284
Trousseau's sign, 76, 111, 113
True labor, 148
Trunk of neonate, assessment of, 142, 154
Trypsin, 109
Tubal ligation, 132, 148
Tube(s)
    endotracheal, for child, 164, 182
    gastric suction, 80, 115
    Miller-Abbott, 79, 115
    nasogastric, 68, 75, 90, 109, 113, 122, 289
    Sengstaken-Blakemore, 71, 110, 199, 262
    thoracotomy, in child, 167, 183
    tracheostomy
        cuffed, 82
        suctioning of, 203, 265
    tympanostomy, placement of, 179
Tube feedings, gastrostomy, for child, 168, 184
Tuberculin test, 65-66, 166, 182, 183
Tuberculosis, 65-66, 107
    in child, 166, 183
Tumor(s)
    colon, 115, 125
    pituitary, 72, 111
    Wilms', in child, 173, 187
TURP; see Transurethral resection of prostate
Tympanic sounds, 106
Tympanostomy tube, placement of, 179

U

Ulcer(s)
 decubitus, 40, 83, 117, 215, 271
 duodenal, 67, 108, 197
  perforation of, 201, 263
 gastric, 67, 68, 108
 mouth, 219
 peptic, 68, 118, 196, 260
 psychologic factors affecting, 252
 stress and, 201, 263
Ulcerative colitis, 79, 115
Ulna, fracture of, 91
Unconscious client, 81, 82
Unequal pupillary light reflexes, 81
Uniform Anatomical Gift Act, 244
Upper gastrointestinal series, 196, 260
Upper lobectomy, 67
Urea-splitting organisms, 240
Urecholine; see Bethanechol
Urgency, 210, 269
Uric acid, 125
 levels of, 95
Urinary catheter, 78, 114
Urinary diversion, 192-193, 257
Urinary retention, 77, 257
Urinary stoma, 75, 113
Urinary tract infection, 75, 113, 223, 224, 251, 295
Urine
 bacteria in, 211, 270
 human chorionic gonadotropin in, 147
 output of, for child, 184
 pH of, 240
Uterine souffle, 287
Uteroplacental insufficiency, 151
Uterus
 cancer of, 15
 contraction of, after delivery, 153
 massage of, 153

V

Vaccine, poliovirus, 293
Vaginal bleeding during pregnancy, 131
Vaginal delivery, 137, 151
 bladder distention after, 198
Vagotomy, 68, 108
 and pyloroplasty, 197, 261

Valium; see Diazepam
Valsalva's maneuver, 62, 105
Variable decelerations for fetus, 137, 151
Varicella, 160-161, 180, 215, 216, 217, 271, 273
Varices, esophageal, 111, 199
 with ascites, 70
Varicose veins, 253, 296
Vascular dementia, 214-215
Vascular necrosis, 123
Vasoconstrictive nose drops, 90, 122
Vasopressin, 110
Vegetarians, pregnancy and, 131
Veins, varicose, 253, 296
Venlafaxine, 191
Venous thrombophlebitis, 112
Ventilation, 40, 247
Ventilator, "fighting," 82
Ventolin; see Albuterol
Ventricular contractions, premature, 62
Ventricular septal defect, 166, 183, 206, 207
Ventriculoperitoneal shunt, 163, 181
Venturi mask, 65, 107
Vertex presentation, 138
Vertical reading, 10
Villus sampling, chorionic, 295
Vincristine, 173, 187
Viral hepatitis, 70
Virazole; see Ribaviran
Virus, human immunodeficiency; see Human
   immunodeficiency virus
Vision, child's, assessment of, 251-252
Visitation program, sibling, 132
Vistaril; see Hydroxyzine
Visual acuity, 87
Visual acuity examination, 120, 296
Visual capacity of newborn, 142, 154-155
Visual impulses, transmission of, 89
Visual loss, 87
Vital organs, compromised perfusion of, 60, 103
Vital signs, postoperative, 238
Vitamin B_1, 109
Vitamin B_6, 107, 119
Vitamin B_{12} malabsorption, 293
Vitamin C, 109, 240, 270, 289
Vitamin D, 109
Vitamin E, 109

Vitamin K, 106, 115, 250, 265, 267
Voiding, postoperative, 207, 238, 268, 287
Vomiting
 in child, 251
 nausea and, 72
  from chemotherapy, 94

W

Walker, 92, 123
Warfarin sodium, 64, 106, 205, 267
Water-seal chest drainage system, 66, 67, 107-108
Watery diarrhea, 168, 184
Weight
 child's, 251
 infant's gain in, 164, 181
 neonate's, 244, 250, 291, 295
Weight loss, 244
 with diabetes, 185
Wellbutrin; see Bupropion hydrochloride
Wernicke's aphasia, 265
Western blot assay, 127
Wheezing, 278
Wide-angle glaucoma, 89
Wilms' tumor, in child, 173, 187
Withdrawal
 alcohol, 33-34, 55, 275, 276, 286
 depressant, 52
 drug, 33-34, 56
  in newborn, 141-142, 154
Withdrawn behavior, 31, 32, 40
Woman, battered, 28-29, 51
Words of essence as clue, 8
Wound
 gunshot, 241, 289
 knife, 241
Wound drainage, 191, 256
Wound healing, delayed, 109

X

Xylocaine; see Lidocaine

Z

Zantac; see Ranitidine
Zoloft; see Sertraline
Zyloprim; see Allopurinol

Simulate the NCLEX Test on either the MAC disk or DOS disk

Instructions for Disk Start-Up

DOS Version

System Requirements

A computer with at least 324 of RAM (Random Access Memory) available is needed for this program. This computer must be IBM PC or 100% compatible. This program operates on a high density (HD) disk only.

For these examples we assume that your A drive is your floppy drive, and your C drive is your hard drive. Please substitute the letter of your floppy drive for A if your floppy drive letter is different. Substitute the letter of your hard drive for C if your hard drive letter is different.

Start-up (floppy drive):

1. Turn your computer on
2. At the prompt, insert the disk into your A drive
3. Type A: and press <Enter>
4. Type MOSBY and press <Enter>
5. Follow the instructions on the screen

Start-up (hard disk):

1. Turn your computer on
2. At the prompt, insert the disk into your A drive
3. Type C: and press <Enter>
4. Type MD/MOSBY and press <Enter>
5. Type CD/MOSBY and press <Enter>
6. Type COPY A:*.* and press <Enter>

The software is now installed on your hard drive. Once the software is installed, start the software by following these directions:
1. Type CD/MOSBY and press <Enter>
2. Type MOSBY and press <Enter>
3. Follow the directions on the screen

MAC Version

System Requirements

Mac 68XXX or Power Mac with a total of at least 1 MB of RAM is needed for this program.

Start-up:

1. Insert the disk into your diskette drive, then open it.
2. Select the installer and follow the instructions for installation.

The software is now installed on your hard drive. Once the software is installed, start the software by following these directions:
1. Open the MOSBY folder.
2. Select the MOSBY program.
3. Follow the directions on the screen

WRITE DOWN THE PASSWORD THAT YOU HAVE SELECTED.
YOUR DISK WILL BE BRANDED WITH THIS INITIAL ENTRY.